Metabolic Syndrome: Diagnosis and Treatment

Metabolic Syndrome: Diagnosis and Treatment

Editor: Damian Wayne

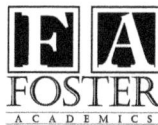

FA
FOSTER
ACADEMICS

www.fosteracademics.com

www.fosteracademics.com

FA FOSTER
A C A D E M I C S

Cataloging-in-Publication Data

Metabolic syndrome : diagnosis and treatment / edited by Damian Wayne.
    p. cm.
Includes bibliographical references and index.
ISBN 978-1-63242-848-6
1. Metabolic syndrome. 2. Metabolism--Disorders--Diagnosis. 3. Metabolism--Disorders--Treatment.
4. Syndromes. I. Wayne, Damian.
RC662.4 .M48 2019
616.399--dc23

Foster Academics,
118-35 Queens Blvd., Suite 400,
Forest Hills, NY 11375, USA

ISBN 978-1-63242-848-6 (Hardback)

Contents

Preface

This book aims to highlight the current researches and provides a platform to further the scope of innovations in this area. This book is a product of the combined efforts of many researchers and scientists, after going through thorough studies and analysis from different parts of the world. The objective of this book is to provide the readers with the latest information of the field.

Metabolic syndrome is a cluster of any three conditions, among central obesity, high blood sugar levels, high blood pressure, low serum high-density lipoprotein and high triglycerides levels. There exists a strong association between metabolic syndrome and the risk of development of Type 2 diabetes and cardiovascular disease. Accumulation of fat around the stomach and abdomen is the primary symptom of metabolic syndrome. Its common causes include stress, physical inactivity, aging, diabetes, coronary artery disease and lipodystrophic disorders. Physical exercise and healthy diet are useful in preventing it. This book brings forth some of the most innovative concepts and elucidates the unexplored aspects of metabolic syndrome. It includes some of the vital pieces of work being conducted across the world, on various topics related to the treatment of metabolic syndrome. The book is appropriate for students seeking detailed information in this area as well as for experts.

I would like to express my sincere thanks to the authors for their dedicated efforts in the completion of this book. I acknowledge the efforts of the publisher for providing constant support. Lastly, I would like to thank my family for their support in all academic endeavors.

Editor

A Combined Treatment with Myo-Inositol and Monacolin K Improve the Androgen and Lipid Profiles of Insulin-Resistant PCOS Patients

Vincenzo De Leo*, Maria Concetta Musacchio, Valentina Cappelli, Alessandra Di Sabatino, Claudia Tosti and Paola Piomboni

Molecular Medicine and Development Department, Obstetrics and Gynecology Clinic, University of Siena, Italy

Abstract

Objective: We sought to assess and compare the effects of myo-inositol combined with monacolin k (Group A) versus inositol only (Group B) and metformin (Group C), on the clinical, hormonal, metabolic and lipid profiles of insulin-resistant PCOS patients.

Study design: 60 insulin resistant PCOS patients were randomly assigned into three groups. All groups were treated for 6 months with either myo-inositol and monacolin k, inositol only or metformin. Patients clinical, hormonal and metabolic profiles were compared between all groups, and within each group, prior and following the aforementioned treatment.

Results: All treatment arms improved patients' clinical, hormonal and metabolic profiles, with a tendency toward better results in patients using the combination of myo-inositol and monacolin k.

Conclusion: The combined treatment with the natural products: monacolin K and myo-inositol represents a valid and well tolerated alternative to the common medical therapy, improving the PCOS related symptoms, with minimal side effects.

Keywords: Cholesterol; Inositol; Insulin resistance; Monacolin k; PCOS

Introduction

Polycystic Ovary Syndrome (PCOS) is a multifactorial endocrinopathy, affecting 5-10% of reproductive age women. The clinical presentation varies from eumenorrhea and a sonographic picture of polycystic ovaries but with subtle phenotypic abnormalities or signs of hyperandrogenism, to advanced Stein and Leventhal syndrome [1,2] and its associated long- term sequelae. Moreover, most women with PCOS also exhibit metabolic syndrome features, including insulin resistance, obesity and dyslipidaemia [3-5]. For a long time, treatments for PCOS were focused on androgen suppression and induction of ovulation. More recently it has been clearly demonstrated that the effective reduction of insulin resistance obtained with metformin restores regular menstrual cycles, ovulation and therefore fertility [6,7]. This substance has an insulin-sensitizing activity and it is currently used to reduce blood sugar levels in patients with diabetes mellitus since it improves the peripheral utilization of glucose, acting on the liver by increasing insulin sensitivity and inhibiting glucose production, whereas it improves glucose storage and utilization in skeletal muscle cells [8,9]. Interestingly it is been clearly demonstrated that metformin improves insulin action at least in part, by increasing insulin mediated release of D-Chiro-Inositol Phosphoglycan (DCI-IPG) in PCOS women [10].

The Inositol Phosphoglycans (IPGs) are putative mediators in non-classical insulin signaling cascade for glucose uptake and use, they play an important role in cell development and morphogenesis. Insulin-resistant PCOS women display decreased insulin-stimulated release of D-Chiro-Inositol (DCI)-Containing IPGs (DCI-IPGs) during an oral glucose tolerance test, as compared to control women [11], which was related to impaired coupling between insulin action and the release of the DCI-IPG [12,13].

Oral nutritional supplementation with inositol, part of the vitamin B complex (B8) and an intracellular second messenger, was demonstrated to enhance insulin sensitivity and improves the clinical and hormonal characteristics of PCOS patients [14-18]. Moreover, inositol supplementation was shown to restore spontaneous ovulation with the consequent increase in conception, either alone [19-21] or when combined with gonadotropins [22].

Systemic inflammation associated with endothelial vascular dysfunction and metabolic dysfunction are commonly present in women with PCOS, with the consequent exaggerated risk for Cardiovascular Disease (CVD), compared with those without PCOS [23-25]. Moreover, Triglyceride (TG), Low-Density Lipoprotein (LDL) and non-high-density lipoprotein (HDL) cholesterol levels are also higher in PCOS as compared with non-PCOS women. Red yeast rice, a Chinese dietary supplement, has gained popularity due to its properties as a natural statin. It contains varying amounts of natural monacolin K (mevinolin) - a metabolite of Monascus rubber, which specifically inhibit 3-hydroxy-3-methylglutaryl (HMG)-CoA reductase, the rate-limiting enzyme in cholesterol synthetic pathway [18].

Monacolin K was suggested to have a similar effect on lipid metabolism, as shown for the mechanism of action of pharmacological statins [26], and it was demonstrated to effectively reduce the levels of cholesterol in patients with hypercholesterolemia [27]. Moreover, its ability to inhibit steroid synthesis was claimed to be responsible for the observed decrease in hyperandrogenism, which may further restore ovulation in those PCOS patients, as was already demonstrated following the use of simvastatin alone or in combination with metformin [28]. Furthermore, the antioxidative properties of statins and monacolin K, may further control cellular proliferation and improve ovulatory function [29].

---

*Corresponding author: Prof. Vincenzo De Leo, Molecular Medicine and Development Department University of Siena, Italy,
E-mail: vincenzo.deleo@unisi.it

Prompted by these findings, we sought to assess and compare the effects of myo- inositol combined with monacolin k versus inositol alone and versus metformin treatment, on the clinical, hormonal, metabolic and lipid profiles of insulin-resistant PCOS patients.

Patients and Methods

The study population consisted of 60 PCOS patients, aged between 24 and 32 years, with insulin resistance (as evaluated by homeostasis model assessment of insulin resistance-HOMA index). Informed consent was obtained from all patients before participation in the study, and the study was approved by the Clinical Research Committee. All patients met the PCOS criterion of the recent ESHRE/ASRM consensus [1], with the exclusion of other endocrinopathies. HOMA index was calculated as the product of fasting plasma insulin (mU/L) and glucose (mmol/L) concentrations divided by 22.5 [23,30].

Upon enrollment, all patients underwent a basic workup, including the completion of a referral status form that covered demographic

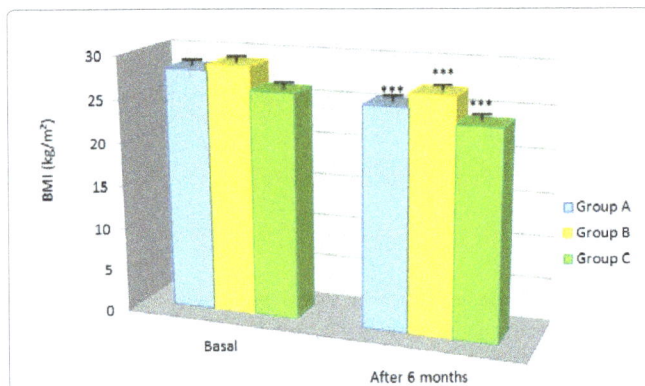

Figure 1: Evaluation of basal BMI and after 6 months of treatment in women treated with monacolin k + myo-inositol (group A), inositol only (group B), or metformin (Group C). Values are presented as median and IC 95%. *=p<0.05, **=p<0.005, ***=p<0.001.

characteristics, basic medical and gynecological history and comprehensive physical examination, including Body Mass Index (BMI) and Ferriman-Gallwey score [28] evaluations. We considered hirsute women with Ferriman-Gallwey score >8 [31,32]. Moreover, blood was drawn from all patients for hormonal [FSH, LH, Total Testosterone (TT), free Testosterone (fT), SHBG and Androstenedione (A)], metabolic (glucose, insulin) and lipid (total cholesterol, LDL, HDL, triglycerides) profiles.

Eligible women were randomly assigned into three groups. Group A (n=20) achieved myo-inositol 1,5 g and monacolin k 3 g (AZELIP-ProgineFarmaceutici), twice a day, for 6 months; and Group B (n=20) was treated with a galenic preparation containing inositol 1,5 g twice a day for 6 months and Group C (n=20) was treated with metformin 850 mg twice a day, for 6 months.

After 6 months of therapy, all patients had repeated the aforementioned evaluations.

Statistical analysis

Statistical analysis was performed by SPSS statistical software version 17 (SPSS I Chicago, IL, USA), with Mann-Whitney test, as appropriate. Results are presented as medians ± confidence interval (IC) 95%; p< 0.05 was considered significant.

Results

The baseline clinical, hormonal, metabolic and lipid profiles were comparable between the three study groups (Table 1). Following 6 months of treatment, the duration of the menstrual cycles was significantly shortened in all study groups (Table 1). Moreover, while all the BMI (Table 1 and Figure 1) and the Ferriman-Gallwey (Table 1) were significantly improved after 6 months of treatments in the three study groups, the reductions were pronounced in group A (myo-inositol+monacolin k) compare to group B (inositol only).

While, we observed no differences in FSH levels following the 6-months, LH levels were significantly reduced in all three patient

	GROUP A			GROUP B			GROUP C		
	BASAL	AFTER 6 MONTHS	P	BASAL	AFTER 6 MONTHS	P	BASAL	AFTER 6 MONTHS	P
BMI (kg/m²)	28.2 ± 1.3	25.7 ± 1.1	0.001	28.8 ± 0.7	27.1 ± 1	0.001	26.2 ± 0.5	24 ± 0.6	0.001
Menstrual cycles(days)	45-60	30-35	0.001	45-60	33-38	0.001	45-60	30-38	0.001
F.Gallwey (score)	11.7 ± 2.7	7 ± 3.9	0.001	11 ± 1	9 ± 4	0.035	11 ± 2	9 ± 1	0.035
LH (mU/ml)	10.3 ± 1.3	7.3 ± 0.4	0.001	11.1 ± 0.7	8.6 ± 0.4	0.001	11.5 ± 1.1	7.9 ± 0.7	0.001
FSH (mU/ml)	4.5 ± 0.3	5.8 ± 0.6	0.040	5.5 ± 0.2	6.1 ± 0.3	0.040	4.9 ± 052	5.8 ± 0.3	0.040
T (pg/ml)	0.8 ± 0.1	0.5 ± 0.1	0.040	1 ± 0.1	0.8 ± 0.1	0.040	0.8 ± 0.1	0.6 ± 0.1	0.040
fT (pg/ml)	1.2 ± 0.2	0.6 ± 0.1	0.001	1.3 ± 0.4	1.1 ± 0.3	0.032	1.3 ± 0.2	0.8 ± 0.1	0.040
A (ng/ml)	2.0 ± 0.1	0.9 ± 0.1	0.001	2 ± 0.2	1.7 ± 0.1	0.048	2.6 ± 0.2	1.8 ± 0.2	0.001
SHBG (nMol/L)	42.5 ± 3.2	96 ± 10.8	0.001	38 ± 3.2	50 ± 2.7	0.367	39 ± 3.7	85 ± 5.6	0.001
Glucose(mg/dl)	99.5 ± 2.1	91 ± 1.7	0.001	100 ± 1.4	95 ± 2.1	0.001	100.5 ± 3.1	92.5 ± 4.2	0.001
Insulin (mU/ml)	14.1 ± 2.8	10.2 ± 1.1	0.001	14.5 ± 0.8	11 ± 0.6	0.001	15 ± 0.7	10.9 ± 0.6	0.001
HOMA	3.8 ± 0.42	2.5 ± 0.4	0.001	3.8 ± 0.3	2.7 ± 0.3	0.001	3.2 ± 0.4	2.4 ± 0.3	0.001
Total Cholesterol (mg/dl)	220 ± 12.4	194 ± 8.15	0.001	220.7 ± 5.7	211.2 ± 5.3	0.040	236 ± 5.2	206 ± 3.8	0.040
HDL (mg/dl)	59.5 ± 3.4	68.5 ± 3.2	0.001	62.1 ± 4.3	63.1 ± 4.1	0.359	58 ± 4.2	70 ± 6.4	0.040
TG (mg/dl)	164 ± 9.4	134.2 ± 9.4	0.001	155.5 ± 9.1	137.4 ± 15.1	0.008	165.5 ± 4.1	144.5 ± 12	0.036
LDL (mg/dl)	127.5 ± 13.1	96.5 ± 7.3	0.001	198.8 ± 7.9	174.4 ± 7.1	0.036	198.5 ± 4.7	167.5 ± 5.8	0.036

Clinical, hormonal, metabolic and lipidic profiles of the two study group, before and following 6 months of treatment. (Group A: inositol plus monacolin; Group B: inositol only; Group C metformin). Data are presented as median ± confidence interval (IC) 95%. P values are significative if p<0.05

Table 1: Clinical, hormonal, metabolic and lipidic profiles of the three study groups.

groups with a consequent improvement and normalization of the LH/FSH ratio to a level below 2 (Table 1).

Androgens levels (TT, fT and A) were significantly reduced in all three groups following treatment (Table 1), but to a lesser degree in group B and C, as compared to A. This probably results from the significant increase in SHBG levels observed following treatment with myo-inositol + monacolin k (group A, p<0.001), but not with inositol only (group B, p=0.367).

Considering the glycemic profile, glucose and insulin levels, as well as the HOMA-index were significantly reduced following treatment in both study groups (Table 1). These reductions were more pronounced following treatment in group A, compared to B (Figure 2).

Regarding the lipid profile (Table 1 and Figure 3), total cholesterol level was reduced in all three group but significantly only in group A treated with myo-inositol monacolin k. The same pattern was observed

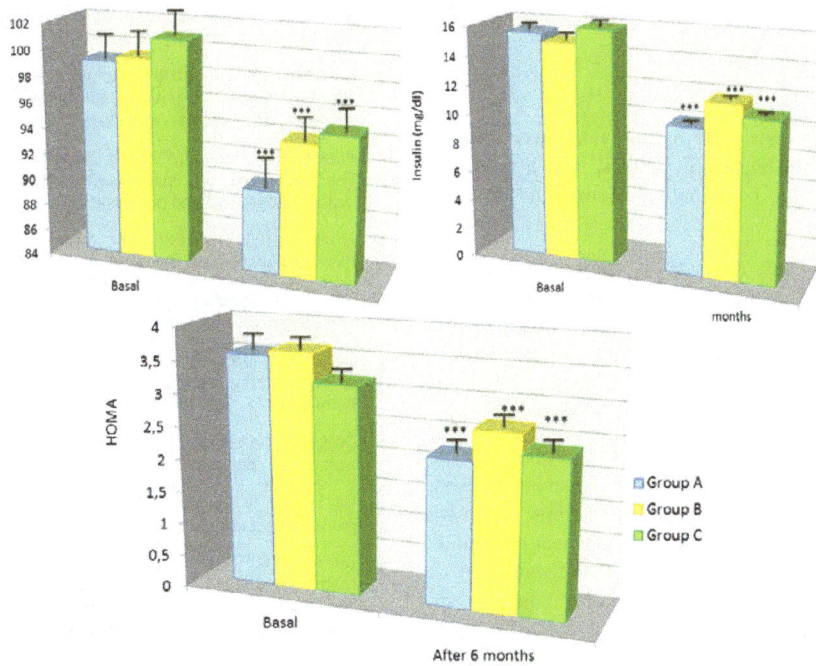

Figure 2: Representation of HOMA, insulin and glucose at basal time and after 6 months of treatment with monacolin k + myo-inositol (group A), only inositol (group B) or metformin (Group C). Values are presented median and IC 95%.. *=p<0.05, **=p<0.005, ***=p<0.001.

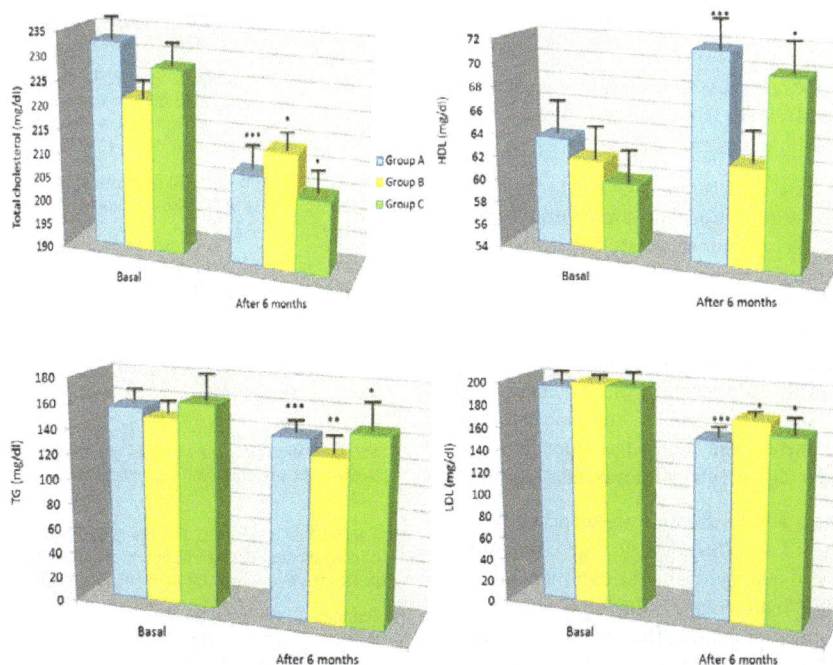

Figure 3: Cholesterol (Chol.), triglicerides (TG), HDL and LDL values at basal time and after 6 months treatment with monacolin k + myo-inositol (group A), inositol only (group B), or metformin (Group C). Values are presented as median and IC 95%. *=p<0.05, **=p<0.005, ***=p<0.001.

for TG and LDL-cholesterol with significantly reduction in group A, (Figure 3). Furthermore treatment with myo-inositol and monacolin K (group A) resulted in a significant increase in HDL cholesterol level, no change in inositol only instead (Group B) and metformin treatment (Group C) (Table 1 and Figure 3).

Almost all women in each group have endured well the two treatments: only two women in group A and one in group B reported moderate diarrhea carefully controlled with lactic ferments intake, while the women treated with metformin (Group C) reported severe side effects like nausea and diarrhea and two women interrupted the treatment.

Discussion

In the present study, we demonstrated that all treatments improved patients' clinical, hormonal and metabolic profiles, with a tendency toward better results using the combination of myo-inositol and monacolin k.

Our data confirm previous observations demonstrating the beneficial effect of inositol on overweight, hyperinsulinemic and hirsute PCOS patients with menstrual irregularities [17,20]. Moreover our study confirms that metformin can improve metabolic aspects in PCOS patient, even if the literature is discrepant about metformin effects on lipid, menstrual and ovulation characteristics [8,9,33,34].

Actually, after 6 months of therapy all study groups have demonstrated shorter menstrual cycles, lower Ferriman-Gallwey scores and decreased BMI and LH/FSH ratio. Observations, which are probably the consequence of weight loss and improvement in insulin-resistance, associated with inositol intake. In fact, the reduction in BMI was more pronounced in group A (myo-inositol + monacolin k), compare to group B (inositol only).

Ferriman-Gallwey score, as well as androgen levels were significantly reduced in all study groups, with a tendency toward a better improvement following the combined treatment with myo-inositol and monacolin k. This probably results from the significant increase in SHBG levels observed following treatment with myo-inositol+monacolin k [34,35].

While glucose, insulin and HOMA index were significantly decreased in all groups, the HOMA index in patients treated with myo-inositol and monacolin k were within the normal range.

Regarding the lipid profile, total cholesterol, triglycerides and LDL levels were significantly reduced in all groups, with a more pronounced reduction in LDL following the combined treatment with myo-inositol and monacolin k. Moreover, while HDL cholesterol was not significantly modified in inositol therapy, the combined treatment with myo-inositol and monacolin k significantly rised in HDL levels. The reduction of plasma lipids has a significative role, since PCOS patients show an increased risk of cardiovascular disease [9], the aforementioned observations emphasize the important role of myo-inositol and monacolin k intake on lipid metabolism, and more specifically in improving lipid profile and reducing patients' cardiovascular risk.

Since metformin and statins administrations are associated with several side effects such as nausea, vomiting, gastric pain causing the end of therapy [36], the combined treatment with the natural products: monacolin k and myo-inositol represents a valid alternative, well tolerated and with a similar mode of action. This new combination of myo-inositol and monacolin k may oppose the etiopathologies responsible for the onset and deterioration of PCOS related symptoms, and may represents a reasonable alternative to other treatments

modalities, such as combined oral contraceptive or antiandrogenic drugs, which are associated with a variety of side effects, especially in adolescents. Moreover this natural choice is much more accepted by patients and clinicians who consider metformin only an antidiabetic drug and then other uses are "off label" [37].

References

1. Rotterdam ESHRE/ASRM- Sponsored PCOS Consensus Workshop Group (2004) Revised 2003 consensus on diagnostic criteria and long-term health risks related to polycystic ovary syndrome. Fertil Steril 81: 19-25.

2. Stein IF, Leventhal ML (1935) Amenorrhea associated with bilateral polycystic ovaries. Am J Obstet Gynecol 29: 181-191.

3. Dunaif A, Graf M, Mandeli J, Laumas V, Dobrjansky A (1987) Characterization of groups of hyperandrogenic women with acanthosis nigricans, impaired glucose tolerance, and/or hyperinsulinemia. J Clin Endocrinol Metab 65: 499-507.

4. Robinson S, Kiddy D, Gelding SV, Willis D, Niththyananthan R, et al. (1993) The relationship of insulin insensitivity to menstrual pattern in women with hyperandrogenism and polycystic ovaries. Clin Endocrinol (Oxf) 39: 351-355.

5. Franks S (2006) Genetic and environmental origins of obesity relevant to reproduction. Reprod Biomed Online 12: 526-531.

6. Glueck CJ, Streicher P, Wang P (2002) Treatment of polycystic ovary syndrome with insulin-lowering agents. Expert Opin Pharmacother 3: 1177-1189.

7. De Leo V, la Marca A, Ditto A, Morgante G, Cianci A (1999) Effects of metformin on gonadotropin-induced ovulation in women with polycystic ovary syndrome. Fertil Steril 72: 282-285.

8. De Leo V, La Marca A (2002) Metformin and FSH for induction of ovulation in women with polycystic ovarian syndrome. Hum Reprod 17: 2481-2482.

9. De Leo V, la Marca A, Petraglia F (2003) Insulin-lowering agents in the management of polycystic ovary syndrome. Endocr Rev 24: 633-667.

10. Baillargeon JP, Iuorno MJ, Jakubowicz DJ, Apridonidze T, He N, et al. (2004) Metformin therapy increases insulin-stimulated release of d-chiro-inositol-containing inositolphosphoglycan mediator in women with polycystic ovary syndrome. Clin Endocrinol Metab 89: 242-249.

11. Baillargeon JP, Nestler JE, Ostlund RE, Apridonidze T, Diamanti-Kandarakis E (2008) Greek hyperinsulinemic women, with or without polycystic ovary syndrome, display altered inositols metabolism. Hum Reprod 23: 1439-1446.

12. Baillargeon JP, Iuorno MJ, Apridonidze T, Nestler JE (2010) Uncoupling Between Insulin and Release of a D-Chiro-Inositol–Containing Inositolphosphoglycan Mediator of Insulin Action in Obese Women With Polycystic Ovary Syndrome. Metab Syndr Relat Disord 8: 127-136.

13. Cheang KJ, Baillargeon JP, Essah PA, Ostlund RE Jr, Apridonize T, et al. (2008) Insulin-stimulated release of D-chiro-inositol-containing inositolphosphoglycan mediator correlates with insulin sensitivity in women with polycystic ovary syndrome. Metabolism 57: 1390-1397.

14. Nestler JE, Jakubowicz DJ, Reamer P, Gunn RD, Allan G (1999) Ovulatory and metabolic effects of D-chiro-inositol in the polycystic ovary syndrome. N Engl J Med 340: 1314-1320.

15. Iuorno MJ, Jakubowicz DJ, Baillargeon JP, Dillon P, Gunn RD, et al. (2002) Effects of d-chiro-inositol in lean women with the polycystic ovary syndrome. Endocr Pract 8: 417-423.

16. Gerli S, Mignosa M, Di Renzo GC (2003) Effects of inositol on ovarian function and metabolic factors in women with PCOS: a randomized double blind placebo-controlled trial. Eur Rev Med Pharmacol Sci 7: 151-159.

17. Genazzani AD, Lanzoni C, Ricchieri F, Jasonni VM (2008) Myo-inositol administration positively affects hyperinsulinemia and hormonal parameters in overweight patients with polycystic ovary syndrome. Gynecol Endocrinol 24: 139-144.

18. Zacchè MM, Caputo L, Filippis S, Zacchè G, Dindelli M, et al. (2009) Efficacy of myo-inositol in the treatment of cutaneous disorders in young women with polycystic ovary syndrome. Gynecol Endocrinol 25: 508-513.

19. Papaleo E, Unfer V, Baillargeon JP, De Santis L, Fusi F, et al. (2007) Myo-inositol in patients with polycystic ovary syndrome: a novel method for ovulation induction. Gynecol Endocrinol 23: 700-703.

20. Papaleo E, Unfer V, Baillargeon JP, Chiu TT (2009) Contribution of myo-inositol to reproduction. Eur J Obstet Gynecol Reprod Biol 147: 120-123.

21. Gerli S, Papaleo E, Ferrari A, Di Renzo GC (2007) Randomized, double blind placebo-controlled trial: effects of myo-inositol on ovarian function and metabolic factors in women with PCOS. Eur Rev Med Pharmacol Sci 11: 347-354.

22. Raffone E, Rizzo P, Benedetto V (2010) Insulin sensitiser agents alone and in co-treatment with r-FSH for ovulation induction in PCOS women. Gynecol Endocrinol 26: 275-280.

23. Amsterdam ESHRE/ASRM-Sponsored 3rd PCOS Consensus Workshop Group (2012) Consensus on women's health aspects of polycystic ovary syndrome (PCOS). Hum Reprod 27: 14-24.

24. Legro RS (2003) Polycystic ovary syndrome and cardiovascular disease: a premature association? Endocr Rev 24: 302-312.

25. Diamanti-Kandarakis E, Kandaraki E, Christakou C, Panidis D (2009) The effect of pharmaceutical intervention on lipid profile in polycystic ovary syndrome. Obes Rev 10: 431-441.

26. Sokalska A, Piotrowski PC, Rzepczynska IJ, Cress A, Duleba AJ (2010) Statins inhibit growth of human theca-interstitial cells in PCOS and non-PCOS tissues independently of cholesterol availability. J Clin Endocrinol Metab 95: 5390-5394.

27. Feuerstein JS, Bjerke WS (2012) Powdered red yeast rice and plant stanols and sterols to lower cholesterol. J Diet Suppl 9: 110-115.

28. Kazerooni T, Shojaei-Baghini A, Dehbashi S, Asadi N, Ghaffarpasand F, et al. (2010) Effects of metformin plus simvastatin on polycystic ovary syndrome: a prospective, randomized, double-blind, placebo-controlled study. Fertil Steril 94: 2208-2213.

29. De Leo V, Musacchio MC, Palermo V, Di Sabatino A, Morgante G, et al. (2009) Polycystic ovary syndrome and metabolic comorbidities: therapeutic options. Drugs Today (Barc) 45: 763-775.

30. Hosker JP, Matthews DR, Rudenski AS, Burnett MA, Darling P, et al. (1985) Continuous infusion of glucose with model assessment: measurement of insulin resistance and beta-cell function in man. Diabetologia 28: 401-411.

31. FERRIMAN D, GALLWEY JD (1961) Clinical assessment of body hair growth in women. J Clin Endocrinol Metab 21: 1440-1447.

32. Goodman N, Bledsoe M, Cobin R, Futterweit W, Goldzieher J, et al. (2001) American Association of Clinical Endocrinologists Hyperandrogenism Guidelines. Endocrine Practice 7: 120-134.

33. Tang T, Lord JM, Norman RJ, Yasmin E, Balen AH (2010) Insulin-sensitising drugs (metformin, rosiglitazone, pioglitazone, D-chiro-inositol) for women with polycystic ovary syndrome, oligo amenorrhoea and subfertility. Cochrane Database Syst Rev.

34. De Leo V, Di Sabatino A, Musacchio MC, Morgante G, Scolaro V, et al. (2010) Effect of oral contraceptives on markers of hyperandrogenism and SHBG in women with polycystic ovary syndrome. Contraception 82: 276-280.

35. Lee CL, Pan TM (2012) Development of Monascus fermentation technology for high hypolipidemic effect. Appl Microbiol Biotechnol 94: 1449-1459.

36. Practice Committee of American Society for Reproductive Medicine (2008) Use of insulin-sensitizing agents in the treatment of polycystic ovary syndrome. Fertil Steril 90: S69-73.

37. Hsia Y, Dawoud D, Sutcliffe AG, Viner RM, Kinra S, et al. (2012) Unlicensed use of metformin in children and adolescents in the UK. Br J Clin Pharmacol 73: 135-139.

Development and Validation of Metabolic Syndrome Prediction and Classification-Pathways using Decision Trees

Brian Miller[1]* and Mark Fridline[2]

[1]School of Sport Science & Wellness Education, The University of Akron, Akron, OH; Doctoral Student, Health Education and Promotion, School of Health Sciences, Kent State University, Kent, OH, USA
[2]Department of Statistics, The University of Akron, Akron, OH, USA

Abstract

Purpose: The purpose of the current investigation was to create, compare, and validate sex-specific decision tree models to classify metabolic syndrome.

Methods: Sex-specific Chi-Squared Automatic Interaction Detection, Exhaustive Chi-Squared Automatic Interaction Detection, and Classification and Regression Tree algorithms were run in duplicate using metabolic syndrome classification criteria, subject characteristics, and cardiovascular predictor variable from the National Health and Nutrition Examination Survey cohort data. Data from 1999-2012 were used (n=10,639; 1999-2010 cohorts for model creation and 2011-2012 cohort for model validation). Metabolic Syndrome was classified as the presence of 3 of 5 American Heart Association National Heart Lung and Blood Institute Metabolic Syndrome classification criteria. The first run was made with all predictor variables and the second run was made excluding metabolic syndrome classification predictor variables. Given that the included decision tree algorithms are non-parametric procedures, all decision tree models were compared to a logistic regression based model to provide a parametric comparison.

Results: The Classification and Regression Tree algorithm outperformed all other decision tree models and logistic regression with a specificity of 0.908 and 0.952, sensitivity of 0.896 and 0.848, and misclassification error of 0.096 and 0.080 for males and females, respectively. Only one predictor variable outside of the metabolic syndrome classification reached significance in the female model (age). All metabolic syndrome classification predictor variables reached significance in the male model. Waist circumference did not reach significance in the female model. Within each model, 5 female and 3 male pathways built off of <3 American Heart Association National Heart Lung and Blood Institute Metabolic Syndrome classification criteria resulted in an increased likelihood of presenting Metabolic Syndrome.

Conclusion: The proposed pathways show promise over other current metabolic syndrome classification models in identifying Metabolic Syndrome with <3 predictor variables, before current classification criteria.

Keywords: Cardiovascular disease; Metabolic syndrome; Decision trees; Diabetes; NHANES

Introduction

Metabolic syndrome (MetS) is a constellation of cardiometabolic predictor variables that when presented in tandem increases the risk of cardiovascular disease (CVD) and insulin resistance [1,2]. The prevalence of this classification affects approximately 1 in 3 adults in the United States [3]. Due to the high prevalence of this syndrome, proper identification of persons with MetS is imperative in order to prevent and/or modify the multiple predictor variables associated with CVD related morbidity and mortality as well as its high healthcare costs [1,2,4,5]. Furthermore, utilization of pathways for MetS classification could guide health education professional interventions before the onset of related morbidity and mortality. Using Decision Trees (DT) as a preliminary pre-metabolic syndrome classification criterion could improve outcomes associated with the development of MetS or could halt the progression of MetS and its relative consequences [6].

Classification of metabolic syndrome

Although there have been numerous attempts to harmonize classification models for MetS, there remains a lack of consensus amongst the leading organizations with particular disagreement based on predictor variable cut-off points as well as which predictor variables should be considered in making the MetS classification [1,7-9]. More recently, there has been support for MetS to be considered as a pre-morbid condition intended to inform health educators and clinicians

on relative risk of developing CVD rather than a clinical diagnosis [6,10]. In lieu of a clinical diagnosis, MetS can provide a research framework for establishing a unified cardiometabolic pathophysiology, quantifying chronic disease risk, guiding clinical management decisions, and providing a concise methodology to inform public health and health education professionals of the relationship of clustering predictor variables [10].

Classification criteria based on the leading models from the national cholesterol

Education Adult Treatment Panel III (ATPIII), the International Diabetes Federation (IDF), the World Health Organization (WHO), and the American Heart Association National Heart Lung and Blood Heart Institute (AHA/NHLBI) risk models are limited in their usefulness because they classify MetS based on predictors with binary thresholds [1,2]. There currently exists limited evidence-based research that considers the severity of these MetS cardiometabolic predictor variables, their interactions with one another, and their relationship

*Corresponding author: Brian Miller, School of Sport Science & Wellness Education, InfoCision Stadium 317, The University of Akron, Akron, OH, 44325-5103, USA, E-mail: bm25@zips.uakron.edu

to CVD. A major limitation within these models is the dichotomous nature of predictor variable identification [6,10]. However much like obesity, there are varied clinical implications based on the severity of predictor variables used to define MetS where the dichotomized cut-off points for each predictor variable might be clinically ambiguous. Furthermore, current MetS classification models lack consideration for established CVD predictor variables such as patient demographics (i.e. race/ethnicity and socioeconomic status), smoking [3] and previous cardiovascular events [11]. The creation of clinically feasible pathways for MetS classification that both stratifies each predictor variable based on its severity and then considers the interaction effect as predictor variable clusters could be invaluable for reducing risk of cardiovascular morbidity and mortality [5].

Decision trees

DT methodologies have been shown to be effective tools for the classification and prediction of cardiometabolic chronic disease such as MetS and insulin resistance [6,12-14]. However, with the exception of Miller, Fridline, Liu & Marino and Stern et al. other models have been based on international samples. To the best of our knowledge, no published pathways for MetS classification derived from DT methodologies have been built, validated, and implemented in clinical practice [6,14].

DTs are powerful classification and prediction techniques that analyze how both categorical and continuous predictor variables best combine to create pathways explaining the outcome of a given binary response variable according to statistical tests in tandem with "if-then" logic [6,14,15]. In DT algorithms, the data set is partitioned into two or more mutually exclusive subsets in each split with the goal of producing subsets of the data which are as homogeneous as possible with respect to the response variable. This nonparametric modeling technique shows promise over traditional regression techniques in that DT's make no assumptions about the underlying data including mutlicollinearity, are able to handle missing variables, are easily interpreted by non-statisticians, and consider the effects of variable clusters in relation to sample subsets unlike regression which considers the effect of each variable within the entire sample.

Chi-squared automatic interaction detection

The Chi-Squared Automatic Interaction Detection (CHAID) algorithm proposed by Kass operates using a series of merging, splitting, and stopping steps based on user-specified criteria as follows [16]. The merging step operates using each predictor variable where CHAID merges non-significant categories using the following algorithm: (1) Perform cross-tabulation of the predictor variable with the binary target variable. (2) If the predictor variable has only 2 categories, go to step 6. (3) $\chi 2$ -test for independence is performed for each pair of categories of the predictor variable in relation to the binary target variable using the $\chi 2$ distribution ($df=1$) with significance (α_{merge}) set at 0.05. For nonsignificant outcomes, those paired categories are merged. (4) For nonsignificant tests identified by $\alpha_{merge} > 0.05$, those paired categories are merged into a single category. For tests reaching significance identified by $\alpha_{merge} \leq 0.05$, the pairs are not merged. (5) If any category has less than the user-specified minimum subset size, that pair is merged with the most similar other category. (6) The p-values for the merged categories are adjusted using a Bonferroni correction to control for Type I error rate.

The splitting step occurs following the determination of all the possible merges for each predictor variable. This step selects which predictor is to be used to "best" split the node using the following

algorithm: (1) $\chi 2$-test for independence using an adjusted p-value for each predictor. (2)The predictor with the smallest adjusted p-value (i.e., most statistically significant) is split if the p-value less than the user-specified significance split level (α_{split}) is set at 0.05; otherwise the node is not split and is then considered a terminal node.

The stopping step utilizes the following user-specified stopping rules to check if the tree growing process should stop: (1) If the current tree reached the maximum tree depth level, the tree process stops. (2) If the size of a node is less than the user-specified minimum node size, the node will not be split. (3) If the split of a node results in a child node whose node size is less than the user-specified minimum child node size value, the node will not be split. The parent node is the level where the data set divides into child nodes that can themselves become either parent nodes or end in a terminal or decision node. (4) The CHAID algorithm will continue until all the stopping rules are met.

Exhaustive CHAID (E-CHAID) proposed by Biggs, DeVille, and Suen uses the basic CHAID algorithm with more computationally intensive merging and testing of response variables [17]. In the E-CHAID algorithm, there is no reference to any α_{merge} value. Rather category merging continues until only two categories remain. Therefore, careful considerations should be made for over-fitting when the E-CHAID algorithm is used for large data sets with large amounts of continuous predictor variables.

Classification and regression trees

Unlike CHAID based algorithms, the Classification and Regression Tree (CART) algorithm proposed by Breiman, Freidman, Stone, and Olshen builds purely binary trees [18]. Therefore, CART pathways are easier to understand as parent nodes are always split into 2 child nodes that partition data to maximize homogeneity of each subset. In the CART procedure, the maximum tree is produced followed by tree pruning to avoid over-fitting.

The first step in the tree growing process is to find each predictor variables best split. In the CART algorithm, the splitting step employs a statistical calculation known as the Gini Impurity Function. This function is a measure of how often a randomly selected case would be incorrectly predicted; therefore it is used to determine the optimal binary split of the parent node into the child nodes. In the next step when the stopping rules are satisfied, the best possible split is chosen for the predictor variable when the impurity decreases the most from the parent node to the child nodes. This impurity decrease is quantified by the Gini Improvement Measure, which measures the decrease in impurity from the parent node to the child node. The parent node will be split when the change in impurity is maximized.

Logistic regression

Logistic Regression (LR) is a widely utilized statistical technique in binary response prediction [19]. However, LR output can be tedious to interpret and requires considerations for mutlicollinearity and missing values. These models are used when the response variable (y) is binary with the response variable taking the value of 1 with probability of success π or the value of 0 with probability of failure $1 - \pi$, and the predictor variables (xi) are either categorical or continuous values represented by the following equation:

$$ln\left[\frac{\pi(x_i)}{1-\pi(x_i)}\right] = ln\left[\frac{P(y_i = 1/x_i)}{P(y_i = 0/x_i)}\right] = \beta + \sum_{i=1}^{p}\beta_i x_i$$

Where $\beta 0$ is a constant and βi are the coefficients of the predictor variables in the model. The LR equation, called the likelihood function, is used for estimating the regression model coefficients. The maximum likelihood estimation method uses an iterative procedure to find the model coefficients that best match the pattern of observations in the sample data. Interpretation of the model comes from transforming the LR coefficients for each predictor variable by taking the exponential of the coefficients ($e\beta i$) to determine the influences of each predictor variable on the response variable in terms of the odds ratio. To determine if each model coefficient is statistically significant, the Wald statistic is used.

Purpose

The central hypothesis states that the decision tree pathways derived from DT algorithms using data from National Health and Nutrition Examination Survey (NHANES) cohorts would detect the presence of MetS in adults with <3 AHA/NHLBI MetS predictor variables. The current investigation had two aims. The first aim was to develop and validate sex-specific pathways for MetS classification using multiple DT derived methodologies. The second aim was to compare each DT model with and without MetS classification criteria.

Materials and Methods

Data management

The study sample was derived from National Health and Nutrition Examination Survey (NHANES) data made publically available by the Centers for Disease Control and Prevention (CDC). This included 7 cohorts from 1999-2012 collected in 2-year intervals. The data was arranged in a column-wise format with each subject given a sequence identifier. Data management was performed with dataset merging and data subset functions using SPSS version 22 (SPSS Inc., Chicago, IL). The final sample size for inclusion in model development was $n=10,639$ (male: $n=5,474$; female: $n=5,165$). The current investigation was approved by the Institutional Review Board.

The inclusion criteria were based on the following parameters: Age range of 18-59 years, 12 hour fasting protocol for laboratory values, abstinence from alcohol and/or tobacco use prior to laboratories, and a negative exam for pregnancy for females. The age criteria was chosen based on Ford, Li, and Zhao [3] where the highest prevalence of MetS was exhibited after 59 years of age. This decision was made in order to create pathways to detect MetS before onset of MetS with traditional classification criteria based on the high prevalence of MetS beyond age 59. Participants with missing data based on the MetS classification criteria were excluded due to the inability/uncertainty in making a complete MetS classification. The 1999-2010 cohorts were reserved for model creation (training) and the 2011-2012 cohort was reserved for model validation. Both of the training and validation sets were separated by sex. The distributions of all parameters were the same between training and validation sets. Blood pressure readings were the average of 4 blood pressure collections per subject. An indicator of cardiovascular events was built off of the presence of 1 of 5 cardiovascular events including congestive heart failure, coronary heart disease, angina, heart attack, and/or stroke.

Metabolic syndrome classification

The MetS classification was defined as the presence of 3 of 5 predictor variables based on the clinical classification model proposed by the AHA/NHLBI, see Table 1 [1].

Statistical analysis

The DT models were developed using CHAID, E-CHAID, and CART algorithm analysis using SPSS version 22 (SPSS Inc., Chicago,

IL). Each DT analysis was run in duplicate with parent nodes defined at 250 subjects, child node defined at 100 subjects, and significance for all statistical tests within each DT set at ≤ 0.05. Maximum tree depth was user specified at 5 levels. The NHANES cohort data was divided by sex to create sex-specific models for MetS classification with the 2011-2012 cohort reserved for model validation. Each DT algorithm was run twice with the first model including all possible predictor variables and the second without any AHA/NHLBI MetS classification criteria. Predictor variables included the AHA/NHLBI MetS classification criteria in addition to binary smoking status, American Heart Association Blood Pressure Classification, anthropometrics [height (cm), weight (kg), Body Mass Index (BMI) (kg/m^2), and weight classification)], marital status, socioeconomic status measured via Family Poverty to Income ratio (PIR) (a measure of adjusted family income to relative poverty threshold), and race/ethnicity. Each DT was assessed using classification specificity, sensitivity, and classification error expressed as proportions. Sensitivity quantifies the proportion of correctly classified MetS and specificity gives the proportion of correctly classified non-MetS.

Within the CART algorithm, DT predictor variables were ranked by level of importance related to MetS. The best DT model was chosen and described for each node using the total proportion of MetS and no-MetS classification and a MetS Index describing the estimated probability of MetS compared to the overall prevalence of MetS in the NHANES cohort. For both the training and validation sets, MetS classification threshold was set at the current MetS prevalence within the NHANES cohort in accordance with Stern et al. who used DT models to explain insulin resistance. In this study the classification threshold of the response variable was set at the response variable's prevalence within the study cohort [14]. Instead of maintaining the 50% classification threshold for the response variable, the optimal classification cut-off point was set to maximize the sum of theoretical sensitivity and specificity, as determined from the cohort data. This decision was made to increase the number or correctly classified cases of MetS.

Stepwise Forward Logistic Regression (LR) was performed on the predictor variables used to define MetS as a parametric classification comparison. This procedure was used to approximate the predictive power of the DT techniques. The classification threshold was set at the current prevalence of MetS within the NHANES cohort as mentioned previously. The final LR model was corrected for multicollinearity problems between the predictor variables by removing highly correlated predictor variables. Within LR, severe multicollinearity can cause instability in the model coefficients when highly correlated variables are included in the model. Variables with large amounts of missing data were excluded.

Measure	Defining Cut-off Points
Elevated Waist Circumference[1]	
Male	>94 cm
Female	>80 cm
Elevated Triglycerides[2]	≥ 150 mg/dl
HDL Cholesterol[2]	
Male	<40 mg/dl
Female	<50 mg/dl
Blood Pressure[2]	≥130 mmHg Systolic and/or ≥ 80 mmHg Diastolic
Fasting Plasma Glucose[2]	≥100 mg/dl

[1]Values based on lowered AHA/NHLBI Guidelines [1]
[2]Drug therapy for dyslipidemia, hypertension, and/or hyperglycemia were alternate indicators meeting the criteria for MetS for that risk factor

Table 1: National Health Lung & Blood Institute Metabolic Syndrome Classification Criteria.

Results

Model performance

The average prevalence of MetS within the NHANES cohort was 33.1%. Subject characteristics are displayed in Table 2. The best performing models based on specificity and sensitivity for both males and females (Table 3) were the CART models considering all study parameters as contenders for inclusion. The classification error of each of the best performing models were also the lowest of the DT and LR models at 0.096 and 0.080 for the male and female model, respectively.

Best performing female model

The first split within the DT was based on Triglycerides (TG) which corroborates with the ranked order of importance in Figure 1. The second level was on splits based on either High Density Lipoprotein Cholesterol (HDL-C) or Fasting Plasma Glucose (FPG). All MetS classification risk-factors were present in the model with the exception of Waist Circumference (WC). The only non-MetS predictor variable

that the algorithm identified as statistically significant was age for the female cohort (Table 4 and Figure 2) with age greater than 46 years were 6.3 times more likely to be classified with MetS. However, this predictor variable was present in the lowest level within the model. Within the female cohort, all the terminal nodes with significant risk of Mets (MetS Index>1) were based on <3 MetS classification criteria. Within the female model the terminal node with the highest likelihood of presenting with MetS using <3 AHA/NHLBI MetS classification criteria is interpreted as a female patient presenting with TG<150 mg/dl, FPG100 mg/dl, and HDL<50 mg/dl. The probability of MetS for this pathway is 0.969 which results in being 2.910 times more likely to than the average likelihood of presenting with MetS (Table 4, Terminal Node 9).

Best performing male model

The first split within the DT was based on TG which corroborates with the ranked order of importance in Figure 3. All second level splits were based on WC. Considering the risk-factors ranked by importance,

	Male			Female		
Parameter	Total	MetS	No Mets	Total	MetS	No Mets
Age at Screening (year)	36 ± 13	42 ± 11	33 ± 12	37 ± 12	43 ± 11	34 ± 12
Family PIR	2.60 ± 1.65	2.69 ± 1.67	2.55 ± 1.63	2.48 ± 1.67	2.35 ± 1.64	2.53 ± 1.68
Weight (kg)	86.0 ± 19.9	97.2 ± 19.9	79.8 ± 17.0	75.3 ± 20.3	86.9 ± 21.7	70.1 ± 17.3
Standing Height (cm)	175.7 ± 7.7	175.8 ± 7.7	175.6 ± 7.8	162.2 ± 7.0	161.7 ± 7.0	162.4 ± 7.0
Body Mass Index (kg/m²)	27.8 ± 5.8	31.4 ± 5.6	25.8 ± 4.8	28.6 ± 7.3	33.1 ± 7.6	26.5 ± 6.2
Waist Circumference (cm)	96.8 ± 15.8	107.9 ± 13.8	90.8 ± 13.3	93.4 ± 16.6	104.9 ± 15.4	88.2 ± 14.3
Total cholesterol (mg/dl)	193 ± 42	205 ± 45	186 ± 39	192 ± 41	204 ± 45	186 ± 38
LDL-cholesterol (mg/dl)	117 ± 35	124 ± 36	114 ± 35	113 ± 34	122 ± 37	109 ± 32
HDL-cholesterol (mg/dl)	48 ± 13	41 ± 11	52 ± 13	56 ± 15	48 ± 13	60 ± 15
Triglyceride (mg/dl)	147 ± 149	225 ± 212	105 ± 68	115 ± 97	179 ± 144	87 ± 41
Systolic Blood Pres (mmHg)	121 ± 14	127 ± 15	118 ± 12	115 ± 15	123 ± 18	111 ± 12
Diastolic Blood Pres (mmHg)	72 ± 12	77 ± 12	69 ± 11	69 ± 11	74 ± 11	67 ± 10
Fasting Glucose (mg/dl)	104 ± 34	118 ± 48	97 ± 18	99 ± 29	115 ± 44	92 ± 14

Based on Collective Sum of 1999-2012 NHANES Cohorts

Table 2: Sample Characteristics.

		Training			Validation		
Sex	Model	Specificity[1]	Sensitivity[2]	Risk[3]	Specificity[1]	Sensitivity[2]	Risk[3]
Male	CHAID	0.815	0.866	0.167	0.850	0.870	0.172
	E-CHAID	0.814	0.834	0.179	0.796	0.835	0.191
	CART	**0.908**	**0.896**	**0.096**	**0.900**	**0.856**	**0.115**
	LR	0.843	0.878	0.144	0.827	0.853	0.164
	CHAID-MetS	0.654	0.865	0.271	0.597	0.839	0.319
	E-CHAID-MetS	0.718	0.807	0.250	0.686	0.785	0.289
	CART-MetS	0.608	0.898	0.289	0.558	0.881	0.330
	LR-MetS	0.746	0.776	0.244	0.738	0.811	0.239
Female	CHAID	0.889	0.822	0.132	0.870	0.756	0.160
	ECHAID	0.838	0.837	0.162	0.838	0.782	0.179
	CART	**0.952**	**0.848**	**0.080**	**0.939**	**0.811**	**0.100**
	LR	0.881	0.854	0.127	0.878	0.835	0.134
	CHAID-MetS	0.722	0.754	0.268	0.689	0.786	0.282
	ECHAID-MetS	0.718	0.755	0.271	0.698	0.777	0.284
	CART-MetS	0.767	0.732	0.244	0.753	0.731	0.254
	LR-MetS	0.770	0.706	0.249	0.733	0.724	0.270

CHAID = X^2 Automatic Interaction Detection, E-CHAID = Exhaustive X^2 Automatic Interaction Detection, CART = Classification and Regression Tree, LR = Logistic Regression
Bold values indicate best performing models
[1]Specificity = Proportion of correctly classified non-MetS cases
[2]Sensitivity = Proportion of correctly classified MetS cases
[3]Risk = MetS misclassification defined as total proportion of MetS misclassification

Table 3: Model Performance.

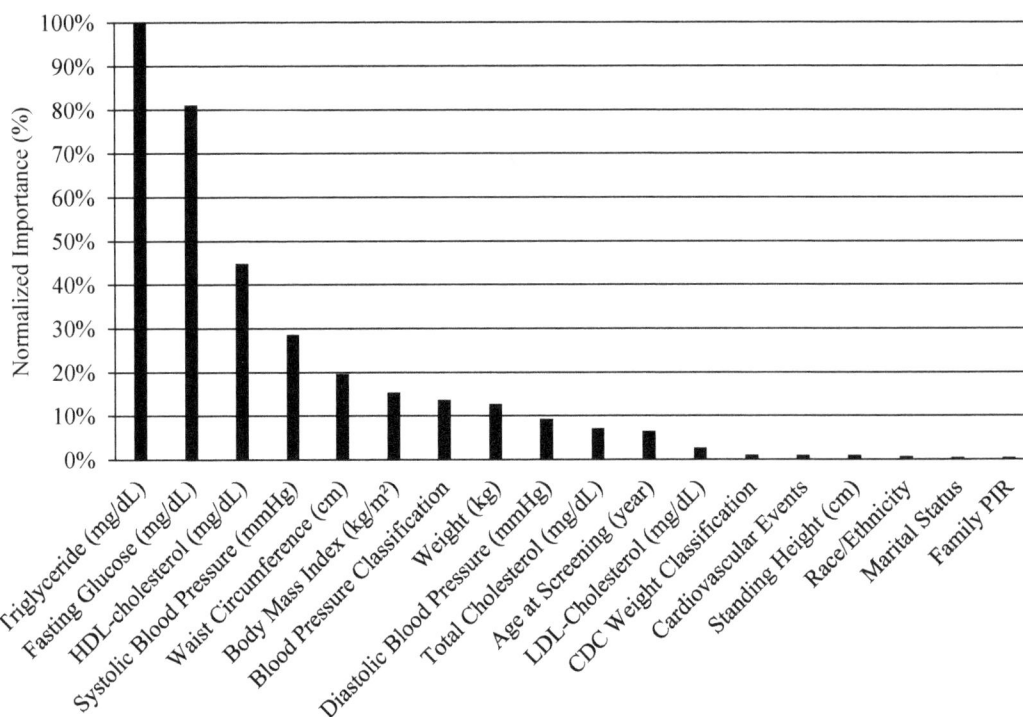

Figure 1: Female CART Decision Tree Ranked Order of Normalized Importance.

Terminal Node	Level 1	Level 2	Level 3	Level 4	Level 5	MetS[1]	MetS Index[2]
9	TG<150	**FPG ≥ 100**	**HDL-C<50**	*	*	0.969	2.910
5	**TG ≥ 150**	**HDL-C<50**	*	*	*	0.962	2.889
12	**TG ≥ 150**	HDL-C ≥ 50	**FPG ≥ 100**	*	*	0.956	2.871
14	TG<150	**FPG ≥ 100**	HDL-C ≥ 50	**SBP ≥ 130**	*	0.897	2.694
16	TG<150	**FPG ≥ 100**	HDL-C ≥ 50	SBP<130	Age ≥ 46	0.391	1.174
11	**TG ≥ 150**	HDL-C ≥ 50	FPG<100	*	*	0.330	0.991
8	TG<150	FPG<100	**SBP ≥ 131**	*	*	0.304	0.913
15	TG<150	**FPG ≥ 100**	HDL-C ≥ 50	SBP<130	Age<46	0.062	0.186
7	TG<150	FPG<100	SBP<131	*	*	0.024	0.072

TG = Triglycerides (mg/dl), WC = Waist Circumference (cm), FPG = Fasting Plasma Glucose (mg/dl), SBP = Systolic Blood Pressure (mmHg), HDL-C = High Density Lipoprotein Cholesterol (mg/dl), Age (years)
Bold values indicate that the predictor reached the MetS threshold within the AHA/NHLBI MetS Classification Criteria
* Indicates no further node splits within level
[1] Probability of MetS Classification
[2] MetS Index = Estimated probability of MetS compared to the overall prevalence of MetS in the NHANES cohort (33.1%)

Table 4: Female CART Decision Tree Model Performance.

BMI was in the top predictor variables. However this predictor variable did not appear in the model. Within the male DT, there were 3 pathways that resulted in a significant increase in likelihood of MetS (MetS Index>1) was based on <3 MetS criteria (Table 5 and Figure 4). Within the male model the terminal node with the highest likelihood of presenting with MetS using <3 AHA/NHLBI MetS classification criteria is interpreted as a male patient presenting with TG ≥ 150 mg/dl, WC<94 cm, and a FPG>100 mg/dl. The probability of MetS for this pathway is 0.655 which results in being 1.967 times more likely to than the average likelihood of presenting with MetS (Table 5, Terminal Node 10).

Discussion

The purpose of the current investigation was to create, compare, and validate sex-specific DT models to classify MetS. DT models were derived using CHAID, E-CHAID, and CART algorithms based on the presence of MetS as the response variable and the MetS classification criteria, predictor variables from cardiovascular risk model and subject characteristics as the predictor variables whose values were obtained from 1999-2012 NHANES data [3,6,10,11,13]. MetS is classified by the presence of 3 of 5 criteria defined by AHA/NHLBI classification guidelines [1].

This study has multiple novelties. First, these models are based on large amounts of data that is representative of adults in the United States. Second, the pathways derived from this model show promise in accurately classifying sex-specific MetS using fewer measurements than traditional classification criteria. Third, unlike traditional MetS classification models, the pathways of the current investigation do not provide universal cutoffs for each predictor variable. Rather, these pathways consider the clustering and multilevel interactions among predictor variables to identify stepwise pathways to classify MetS. Finally, each pathway describes the likelihood of developing MetS.

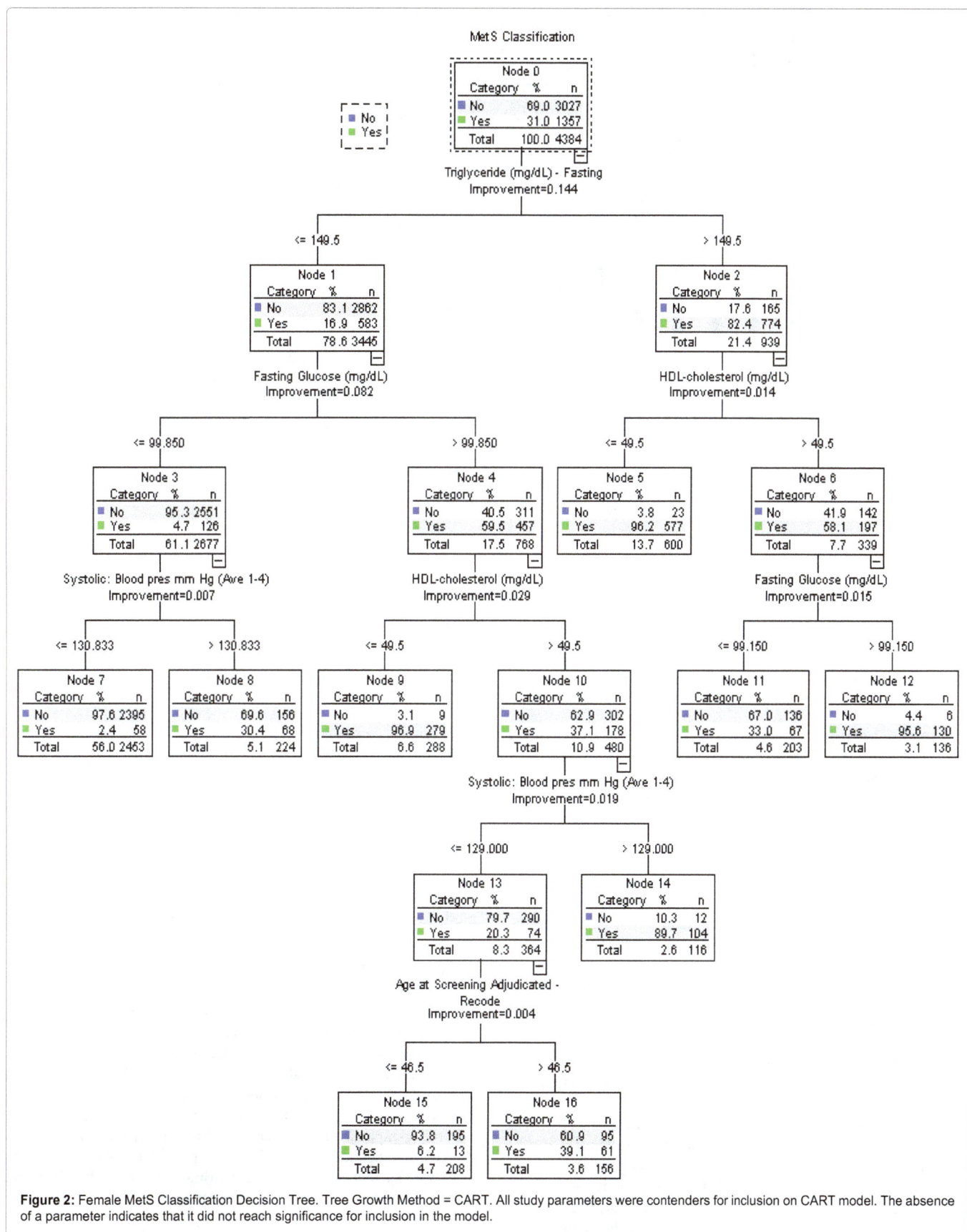

Figure 2: Female MetS Classification Decision Tree. Tree Growth Method = CART. All study parameters were contenders for inclusion on CART model. The absence of a parameter indicates that it did not reach significance for inclusion in the model.

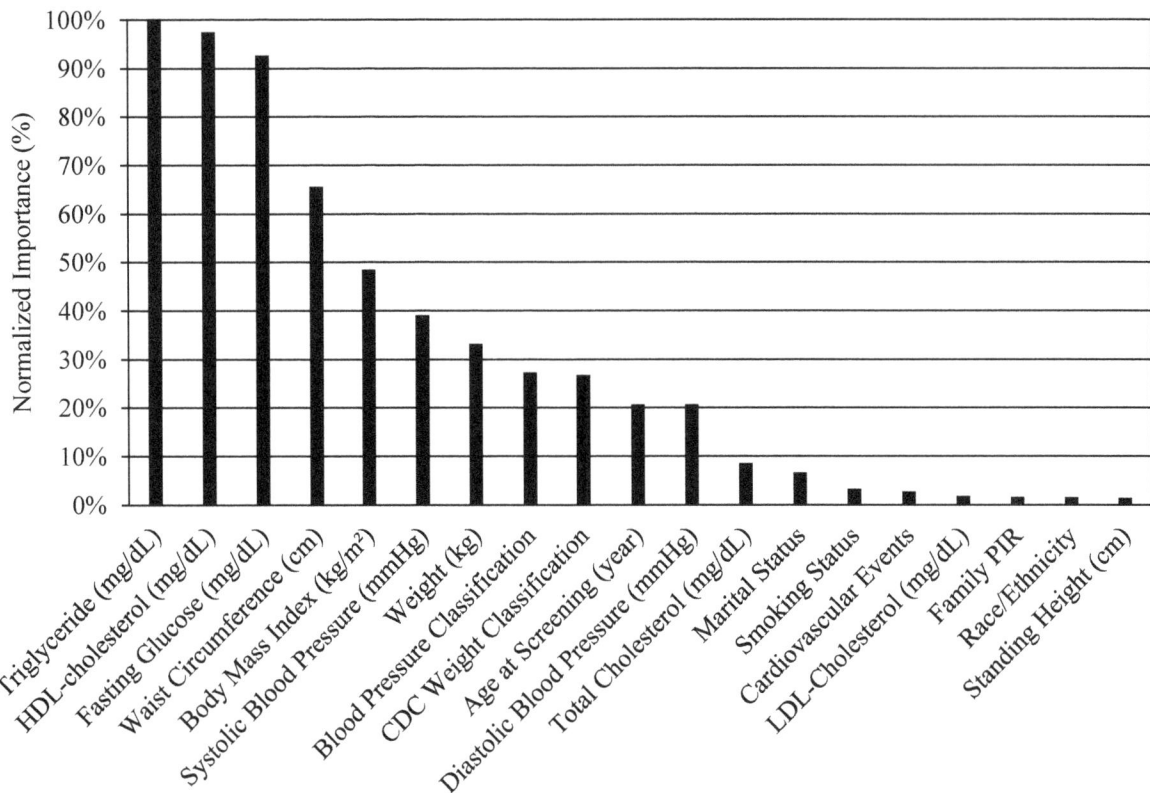

Figure 3: Male CART Decision Tree Ranked Order of Normalized Importance.

In this study the prevalence of MetS within the NHANES cohort, a representative sample of the United States adult population, was 33.1% which approximates Ford, Li, & Zhao's study that found the prevalence of MetS within the NHANES cohort to be 34.3% [3].

The first level split indicates the risk-factor with the highest association with MetS. The first level split was based on TG which corroborates with Worachartcheewan et al. who used CART to classify MetS in a sample of Thai men and women [13]. The results of this study also corroborate with Miller, Fridline, Liu, & Marino who used the CHAID algorithm to classify MetS in a sample of young adults using NHANES data. The best performing model in this study was built as a user-specified first level split on WC [6]. When the algorithm was not user-specified, the CHAID algorithm identified TG as the first level split. Interestingly in this study, the proposed CHAID model with the user-specified first split on WC outperformed the CHAID algorithm without first-level split specification and the logistic regression model in both overall sensitivity and classification accuracy for MetS.

There were notable differences between the male and female models. The first was that WC was present in the male model but not the female model. This phenomenon might be based on the body fat distribution of women prior to menopause that occurs in women at or near the age split identified by the DT model [20]. This suggests that a moderate increase in adiposity would not result in a significant increase in central adiposity. Therefore the WC measurement might not be warranted in women. Conversely for men, the body fat distribution would contribute to increases in central adiposity as body fat increases. This finding corroborates with Hari et al. who compared sex-specific differences between multiple MetS classification models and found that measures of central adiposity, specifically WC, were more profound

for males than females [21]. Future investigation regarding this phenomenon is warranted considering that physicians and health professionals recommend WC measurements for both sexes.

Also notable was the close relationship between WC and BMI based on the normalized order of importance in Figures 1 and 4. Both WC and BMI have been shown to be a strong proxy of visceral adiposity [22]. However, BMI only considers the relationship of weight to height and does not consider actual body composition and girth measurements. Central adiposity has been identified as a strong predictor of MetS and a strong contributor to BMI and Despres et al. demonstrated a strong correlation between BMI and WC which suggests the interchangeability of measures [22]. Given that WC was more significantly associated with MetS than BMI, the inclusion of WC most likely diminished the effect of BMI in the DT models. Therefore WC seems to be a more sensitive predictor of MetS than BMI.

Also interesting in the female model was the inclusion of a non-MetS classification criterion parameter, age. Although this factor was not present in a high-risk MetS pathway (MetS Index>1), age $\geq$ 46 years were 6.3 times likely to present with MetS than females within this pathway with an age<46 years. One suggestion for the split based on age was at 46 years relates to the cardiometabolic changes related to menopause. However, a review by Barret-Conner of menopause in relation to CVD risk in women delineated the direct relationship between menopause and CVD risk [23]. The methodology of the current investigation was unable to explain the inclusion of this predictor. Further investigation exploring the relationship between central adiposity and likelihood of presenting with MetS for women by age and pre, peri, and post-menopause is warranted.

A successful improvement in current methodologies using the

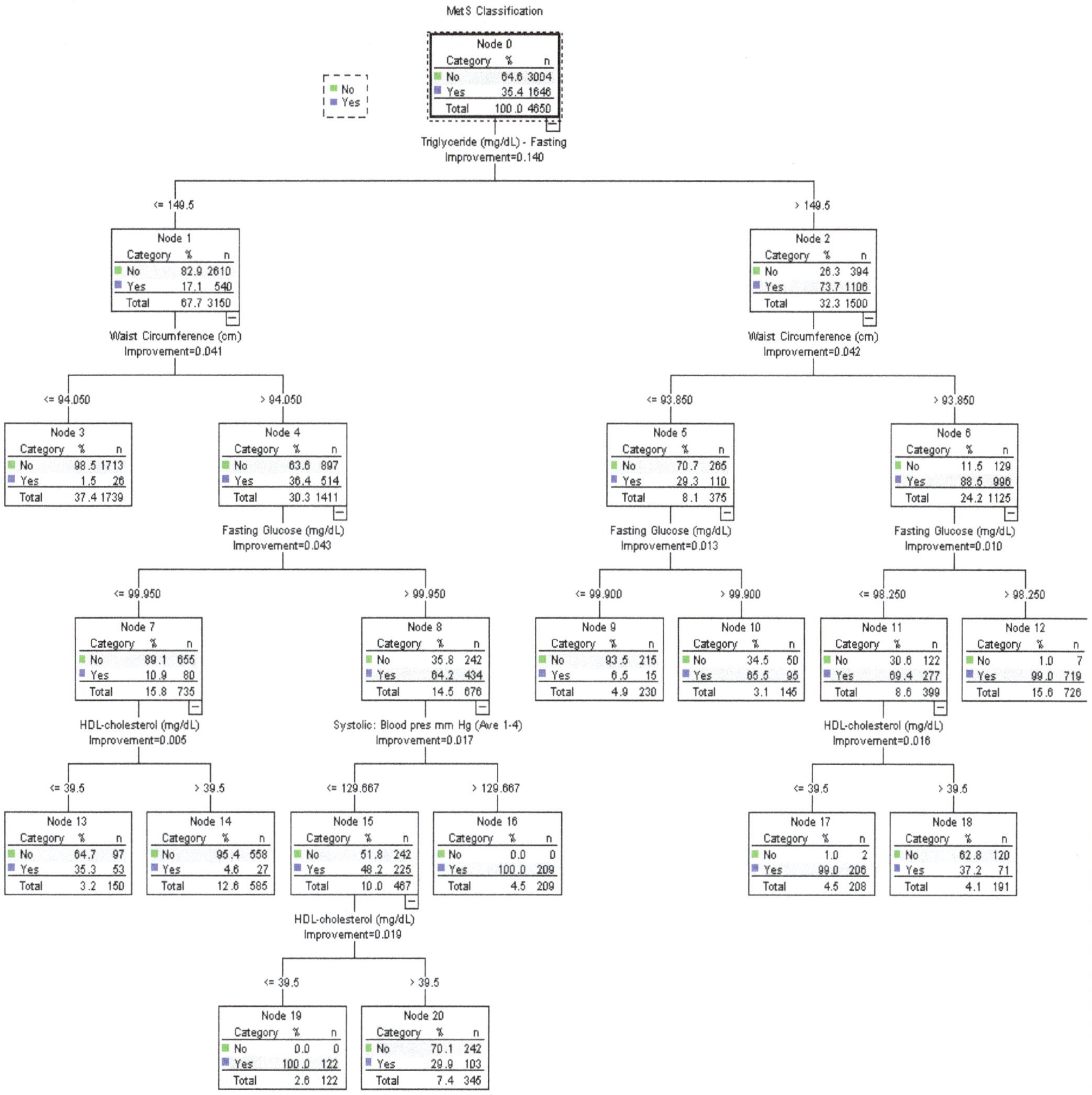

Figure 4: Male MetS Classification Decision Tree. Tree Growth Method = CART. All study parameters were contenders for inclusion on CART model. The absence of a parameter indicates that it did not reach significance for inclusion in the model.

models developed in the current investigation in relation to other classification models would be the classification of MetS with less than 3 risk-factors and/or identify the MetS risk of multiple clustering combinations of predictor variables. In the female model all of the pathways leading to increased risk of MetS were based on less than 3 predictor variables. However, in the male model only one pathway required less than 3 predictor variables for MetS classification. Clinical application of these pathways can inform health educators and/or clinicians identifying high risk pathways and focusing on interventions that could shift a patient to a lower risk pathway.

Conclusions

In summary, the current investigations findings suggest that DT-based pathways to classify MetS and likelihood of presenting with MetS could detect MetS before other classification models. Within the female model, waist circumference measures did not reach significance as a predictor variable. However, age did reach significance for inclusion in the female model. Five of the pathways with increased likelihood of MetS in the female model were built using ≤ 2 MetS AHA/NHBLI classification criteria. Three of the pathways with increased likelihood of MetS in the male model were built using ≤ 2 MetS AHA/NHLI

Terminal Node	Level 1	Level 2	Level 3	Level 4	Level 5	MetS[1]	MetS Index[2]
16	TG<150	**WC > 94**	**FPG ≥ 100**	**SBP > 130**	*	1.000	3.003
19	TG<150	**WC > 94**	**FPG ≥ 100**	SBP<130	**HDL-C<40**	1.000	3.003
12	**TG ≥ 150**	**WC ≥ 94**	FPG > 98	*	*	0.990	2.973
17	**TG ≥ 150**	**WC ≥ 94**	FPG ≤ 98	**HDL-C<40**	*	0.990	2.973
10	**TG ≥ 150**	WC<94	**FPG ≥ 100**	*	*	0.655	1.967
9	**TG ≥ 150**	WC<94	FPG<100	*	*	0.650	1.952
18	**TG ≥ 150**	**WC ≥ 94**	FPG ≤ 98	HDL-C ≥ 40	*	0.372	1.117
13	TG<150	WC ≤ 94	FPG<100	**HDL-C<40**	*	0.353	1.060
20	TG<150	**WC>94**	**FPG ≥ 100**	SBP<130	HDL-C ≥ 40	0.299	0.898
14	TG<150	WC ≤ 94	**FPG ≥ 100**	HDL-C ≥ 40	*	0.046	0.138
3	TG<150	WC ≤ 94	*	*	*	0.015	0.045

TG = Triglycerides (mg/dl), WC = Waist Circumference (cm), FPG = Fasting Plasma Glucose (mg/dl), SBP = Systolic Blood Pressure (mmHg), HDL-C = High Density Lipoprotein Cholesterol (mg/dl), Age (years)
Bold values indicate that the predictor reached the MetS threshold within the AHA/NHLBI MetS Classification Criteria
* Indicates no further node splits within level
[1]Probability of MetS Classification
[2] MetS Index = Estimated probability of MetS compared to the overall prevalence of MetS in the NHANES cohort (33.1%)

Table 5: Male CART Decision Tree Model Performance.

classification criteria. Future research warrants the implementation and further validation of these pathways using a clinical sample. There still remains no clinically established criterion for pre-metabolic syndrome. These pathways show promise in developing a preliminary pre-metabolic syndrome classification tool to guide intervention before the onset of MetS using current models.

References

1. Alberti KGMM, Eckel RH, Grundy SM, Paul ZZ, James IC, et al. (2009) Harmonizing the metabolic syndrome: A joint interim statement of the international diabetes federation task force on epidemiology and prevention; National Heart, Lung, and Blood Institute; American Heart Association; World Heart Federation; International Atherosclerosis Society; and International Association for the Study of Obesity. Circulation 120: 1640-1645.

2. Grundy SM (2011) The metabolic syndrome. Atlas of atherosclerosis and metabolic syndrome 1: 1-26.

3. Ford ES, Li C, Zhao G (2010) Prevalence and correlates of metabolic syndrome based on a harmonious definition among adults in the US. Journal of Diabetes 2: 180-193.

4. Birnbaum HG, Mattson ME, Kashima S, Williamson TE (2011) Prevalence rates and costs of metabolic syndrome and associated predictor variables using employees' integrated laboratory data and health care claims. J Occup Environ Med 53: 27-33.

5. Boudreau D, Malone D, Raebel M (2009) Health care utilization and costs by metabolic syndrome predictor variables. Metabolic syndrome and related disorders 7: 305-314.

6. Miller B, Fridline M, Liu P, Marino D (2014) Use of CHAID decision trees to formulate pathways for the early detection of metabolic syndrome in young adults. Computational and mathematical methods in medicine.

7. Alberti KGM, Zimmet P, Shaw J (2005) The metabolic syndrome—a new worldwide definition. The Lancet 366: 1059-1062.

8. Kassi E, Pervanidou P, Kaltsas G, Chrousos G (2011) Metabolic syndrome: Definitions and controversies. BMC Med 9: 48.

9. Strazzullo P, Barbato A, Siani A, Cappuccio FP, Versiero M, et al. (2008) Diagnostic criteria for metabolic syndrome: A comparative analysis in an unselected sample of adult male population. Metab Clin Exp 57: 355-361.

10. Simmons R, Alberti K, Gale E, Colagiuri S, Tuomilehto Q, et al. (2010) The metabolic syndrome e: Useful concept or clinical tool? Report of a WHO expert consultation. Diabetologia 53: 600-605.

11. Liu J, Grundy SM, Wang W, Smith SC, Vega GL, et al. (2007) Ten-year risk of cardiovascular incidence related to diabetes, prediabetes, and the metabolic syndrome. Am Heart J 153: 552-558.

12. Edelenyi FS, Goumidi L, Bertrais S, Phillips C, Macmanus R, et al. (2008) Prediction of the metabolic syndrome status based on dietary and genetic parameters, using random forest. Genes & nutrition 3: 173-176.

13. Worachartcheewan A, Nantasenamat C, Isarankura-Na-Ayudhya C, Pidetcha P, Prachayasittikul V (2010) Identification of metabolic syndrome using decision tree analysis. Diabetes Res Clin Pract 90: e15-e18.

14. Stern SE, Williams K, Ferrannini E, DeFronzo RA, Bogardus C, et al. (2005) Identification of individuals with insulin resistance using routine clinical measurements. Diabetes 54: 333-339.

15. Gandomi AH, Fridline MM, Roke DA (2013) Decision tree approach for soil liquefaction assessment. The Scientific World Journal 8.

16. Kass GV (1980) An exploratory technique for investigating large quantities of categorical data. Applied statistics 119-127.

17. Biggs D, De Ville B, Suen E (1991) A method of choosing multiway partitions for classification and decision trees. Journal of Applied Statistics 18: 49-62.

18. Breiman L, Friedman J, Stone CJ, Olshen RA (1984) Classification and regression trees. CRC press.

19. Hosmer Jr DW, Lemeshow S, Sturdivant RX (2013) Applied logistic regression. John Wiley & Sons.

20. Camhi SM, Bray GA, Bouchard C, Greenway FL, Johnson WD, et al. (2011) The relationship of waist circumference and BMI to visceral, subcutaneous, and total body fat: Sex and race differences. Obesity 19: 402-408.

21. Hari P, Nerusu K, Veeranna V, Sudhakar R, Zalawadiya S, et al. (2012) A gender-stratified comparative analysis of various definitions of metabolic syndrome and cardiovascular risk in a multiethnic US population. Metabolic syndrome and related disorders 10: 47-55.

22. Despres JP, Lemieux I, Bergeron J, Pibarot P, Mathieu P, et al. (2008) Abdominal obesity and the metabolic syndrome: Contribution to global cardiometabolic risk. Arterioscler Thromb Vasc Biol 28: 1039-1049.

23. Connor BE (2013) Menopause, atherosclerosis, and coronary artery disease. Current opinion in pharmacology 13: 186-191.

3

Association of *PARL* Gene Rs3732581, Rs73887537 Polymorphisms with Type 2 Diabetes Mellitus, Insulin Resistance and Blood Lipid Levels

Jing Liu[1*], Xiao-feng Huang[2], Ju-xiang Liu[1], Jin-xing Quan[1], Li-min Tian[1], Xiao-juan Huang[3], Jia Liu[1], Yan-jia Xu[1], Qi Zhang[1], Shu-lan Zhang[2], Xiao-hui Chen[1] and Rui-lan Niu[2]

[1]*Department of Endocrinology, Gansu Provincial People's Hospital, 204 West Donggang Road, Lanzhou City 730000, Gansu Province, China*
[2]*The First Clinical College of Lanzhou University, Lanzhou City 730000, Gansu Province, China*
[3]*State Key Laboratory for Oxo Synthesis & Selective Oxidation, Lanzhou Institute of Chemical Physics, Chinese Academy of Sciences, Lanzhou 730000, China*

Abstract

Aim: The aim of the current study was to investigate the associations between rs3732581, rs73887537 of *PARL* gene with type 2 diabetes mellitus and its related phenotypes in Chinese T2DM case-control population.

Methods: We genotyped *PARL* gene rs3732581, rs73887537 polymorphisms in 543 T2DM patients and 384 healthy controls by using PCR-RFLP technique. Plasma glucose, insulin and lipid were measured by biochemical technique.

Results: rs73887537 polymorphism of *PARL* gene was not existed in the studied population. The genotype and allele distributions of rs3732581 polymorphism were not significantly different between T2DM and control groups (both $P>0.05$). However compared with carriers of C allele, the carriers of the GG genotype showed significantly higher levels of triglyceride, total cholesterol in the T2DM and control groups respectively.

Conclusion: rs73887537 polymorphism of *PARL* gene was not existed in the Chinese studied population. The rs3732581 polymorphism of *PARL* gene is not associated with the presence of T2DM. However, it is associated with blood lipid levels in T2DM and healthy Chinese population differently.

Keywords: *PARL* gene; Type 2 diabetes mellitus; Insulin resistance; Blood lipid levels; Polymorphisms

Introduction

Type 2 Diabetes Mellitus (T2DM) is a complex metabolic disorder, caused by multiple environmental and genetic factors. A considerable amount of research has been devoted to defining the genes involved in the aetiology of this widespread disease. Impairment of mitochondrial function is intrinsically related with diabetes and alterations in mitochondrial function are associated with both insulin resistance and loss of energy-dependent beta-cell insulin secretion [1]. Thus proteins regulating mitochondrial action and efficiency have become attractive candidate genes for diabetes susceptibility in the face of adverse environmental risk factors [2].

The presenilins-associated rhomboid-like (PARL) protein is an inner mitochondrial membrane rhomboid protease. Given the likely role of PARL in maintaining mitochondrial membrane integrity and function, and the known defects of mitochondria in diabetes [3-8]. The association of PARL and insulin resistance had been investigated. Walder K et al. reported that both in human and in animal subjects PARL expression is negatively correlated with blood glucose and plasma insulin levels [9]. The expression of the PARL homologue is reduced by 50% in skeletal muscle of obese, type 2 diabetic Psammomys obesus relative to lean glucose-tolerant animals. Exercise training, ameliorating symptoms of T2DM by reducing the plasma levels of glucose and insulin, also increased the levels of PARL in skeletal muscle [9]. Tang H et al. reported that the PARL mRNA level was lower in the insulin-resistant rats than in control animals, and is associated with low mitochondrial content and reduced mitochondrial enzyme activity in the skeletal muscle from the insulin-resistant rats [10]. These results suggest that high-fat-diet-induced insulin resistance is associated with

mitochondrial dysfunction in skeletal muscle, and may be the result of the decreased expression of the PARL gene [9,10]. It has been shown that PARL is a new candidate gene for obesity and T2DM [9].

Walder et al. reported that a SNP variant (Leu262Val) in PARL (dbSNP ID rs3732581 mapped to chromosome 3q27, a region reportedly linked to phenotypes associated with metabolic syndrome) was associated with insulin resistance in an age dependent manner in an American-Caucasian case–control study [9,11]. They believed that variation in PARL sequence may be an important new risk factor for T2DM and other components of the metabolic syndrome [9]. However, subsequent replicated studies failed to replicate the initial findings and disputed the association between this polymorphism and two measures of insulin resistance (fasting plasma insulin and blood glucose levels) [12-14]. T2DM is likely to be polygenic and multiple factors common disease of which genetic heterogeneity exists in different race and areas. The populations were recruited in the previous study are always European descents. Until now it is unclear whether this polymorphism is associated with T2DM and its related phenotypes in the Chinese population and due to the previous conflicting association results, the aim of the current study was to investigate the relationship between the rs3732581, rs73887537 variants and T2DM and its related phenotypes including fasting plasma insulin, glucose levels and BMI et al in Chinese T2DM case–control population.

*Corresponding author: Jing Liu, Department of Endocrinology, People's Hospital of Gansu Province, 204 West Donggang Road, Lanzhou city 730000, Gansu Province, China, E-mail: liujingwelcome@126.com

Materials and Methods

Subjects

A total of 927 Northwest Han Chinese individuals aged between 22 and 88 years in Gansu was recruited into this case–control study, among them 543 unrelated type 2 diabetic patients were recruited from the inpatients who were admitted to Gansu Provincial People's Hospital in 2008 and 2009. 384 controls who were ethnically age-and gender-matched unrelated healthy volunteers were selected randomly during the same period in Medical Examination Center (MEC) of the People's Hospital of Gansu Province. Identification of T2DM was based on the World Health Organization Definition (WHO) 1999 definition [15]. The controls and the patients were matched by age and sex. All subjects had no family history of diabetes and no history of significant concomitant diseases. T1DM, acute or chronic hepatopathy and nephropathy, severe ethanol abuse, cigarette abuse were excluded by clinical and laboratory examination. All the participants gave written informed consent, and the Ethics Committee of Lanzhou University approved all research protocols.

Measurement

Full history and physical examination was taken. Venous blood sample of 5 ml was drawn from all subjects into tubes containing ethylene diamine tetraacetic acid after an overnight fast. Plasma glucose concentrations were measured by the glucose oxidase-peroxidase method. Serum levels of insulin were measured by radioimmunoassay method. Serum concentrations of lipids including total cholesterol, triglyceride, high-density lipoprotein cholesterol, low-density lipoprotein cholesterol and HbA1c were measured using standard methods in Clinical Laboratory in Gansu Provincial People's Hospital. Insulin resistance and pancreatic B-cell function were assessed by homeostasis model assessment (HOMA-IR) as fasting glucose (mmol/l) × fasting insulin (μU/ml)/22.5 [16]. Height (m) and weight (kg) were

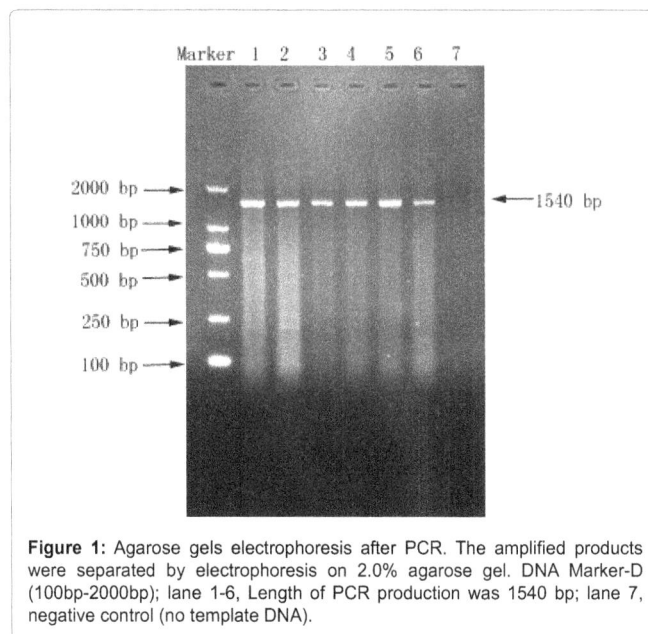

Figure 1: Agarose gels electrophoresis after PCR. The amplified products were separated by electrophoresis on 2.0% agarose gel. DNA Marker-D (100bp-2000bp); lane 1-6, Length of PCR production was 1540 bp; lane 7, negative control (no template DNA).

measured and body mass index was calculated as weight/height². Waist, hip circumferences (cm) were measured and waist-hip ratio and BMI were calculated. Anthropometric measurements from cases and control subjects were done in our ward in Medical Examination Center, respectively. The phenotypic characteristics of the study population are summarized in Table 1.

PCR amplification

Genomic DNA was extracted from peripheral blood leucocytes according to a standard protein K digestion and phenol/chloroform extraction method. Extracted DNA was dissolved in the appropriate volume of double distilled water. DNA concentration was measured with a nuclear acid analyzing instrument before preserving in -80°C. The reference sequence (i.e. wild type sequence) of PARL gene was extracted from the NCBI GenBank. We designed a set of primers using Primer 5.0 and Oligo 6.0 software to amplify a 1540-bp region that contains two single nucleotide polymorphism sites (rs3732581 and rs73887537 of PARL gene) by Polymerase Chain Reaction (PCR). The forward primer was 5'-ATAAGCCACCACCCCCAGTT-3', and the reverse primer was 5'-ACCACAAGCCCCAGAGTAGA-3'. (Primers were synthesized by Shanghai Sangon Biological Engineering Technology And Service Co., Ltd.). PCR was performed in a 50μl volume containing 2U of Taq Plus DNA polymerase, 5 μl of 10×Buffer, 2 μl of dNTP Mixture each 10 mM solution, 40 pM of each primer (forward and reverse), 40 ng of DNA and appropriate volume of sterile water.

The PCR conditions were as follows. Initial denaturing was performed at 94.0°C for 5min, and was followed by 35 cycles of denaturing at 94.0°C for 35 s, annealing at 63.5°C for 30 s, extension at 72.0°C for 1 min10s, and final extension at 72.0°C for 7 min. The PCR products were evaluated by electrophoresis in 2.0% agarose gel and visualized by ethidium bromide staining on an electrophoresis apparatus (FR-200A, Shanghai Furi 140 Science & Technology Co. Ltd) (Figure 1).

PCR-restriction fragment length polymorphisms

The PCR-amplified products were digested overnight with BstN I and Hpa II, as recommended by the manufacturer (Fermentas, Burlington, Ontario). After digestion, the restriction enzyme was inactivated at

Variable (units)	Controls	T2DM		P value
n	384	543		
Sex（M/F）	213/171	279/264		0.219
Age（Years）	55.75 ± 13.66	57.50 ± 11.80		0.230
Height（cm）	165.68 ± 7.55	164.68 ± 7.47		0.252
Weight（Kg）	68.46 ± 10.84	68.69 ± 12.49		0.866
Body mass index（Kg/m²）	24.86 ± 3.14	25.26 ± 3.93	Δ	0.277
Waist circumference (cm)	86.31 ± 8.35	89.14 ± 9.01		0.005**
Hip circumference (cm)	96.36 ± 9.52	94.94 ± 6.72		0.125
Waist and hips ratio	0.90 ± 0.07	0.94 ± 0.08		0.000**
Fasting glucose（mmol/L）	4.63 ± 0.50	10.69 ± 4.19	Δ	0.000**
Fasting insulin（mU/L）	8.21 ± 2.47	10.24 ± 4.28	Δ	0.000**
Hemoglobin A1c (%)	4.62 ± 0.75	8.36 ± 1.83	Δ	0.000**
HOMA-IR	1.70 ± 0.59	4.87 ± 2.88	Δ	0.000**
TC（mmol/L）	4.61 ± 0.87	4.83 ± 1.06		0.053
TG（mmol/L）	1.70 ± 0.79	2.19 ± 1.51	Δ	0.010*
LDL-C（mmol/L）	2.41 ± 0.67	2.71 ± 0.97		0.003**
HDL-C（mmol/L）	1.39 ± 0.30	1.07 ± 0.73		0.000**

Note: M: Male; F: Female; HOMA-IR: Homeostasis Model Assessment Insulin Resistance Index; TC: Total Cholesterol; TG: Triglyceride; LDL-C: High-Density Lipoprotein; HDL-C: Low-Density Lipoprotein. Sex Was Evaluated By X²-Test. Δ: Mann-Whitney U Test Compared with Control, *P<0.05, **P<0.01

Table 1: Baseline clinical characteristics of patients and controls. $\bar{x} \pm s$

65°C for 20 min. The digested products were separated by 2.0% agarose gel electrophoresis and visualized by ethidium bromide staining. All samples were successfully genotyped and a random selection of samples underwent sequencing. There was no discordance noted between the RFLP-PCR assays and sequencing methods. For the *PARL* rs3732581 polymorphism (BstN I), GG homozygous cases were represented by DNA bands of 65, 219, 451, and 805 bp. CC homozygous cases were represented by DNA bands of 65, 219, and 1256 bp. CG heterozygous cases displayed a combination of both alleles (65, 219, 451, 805 and 125 bp). For the *PARL* rs73887537 polymorphism (Hpa II), TT homozygous cases were represented by DNA bands of 52, 391, 480, and 617 bp (Figure 2). CC homozygous cases were represented by DNA bands of 52, 272, 345, 391 and 480 bp. TC heterozygous cases displayed a combination of both alleles (52, 272, 345, 391, 480 and 617 bp) (Figure 3).

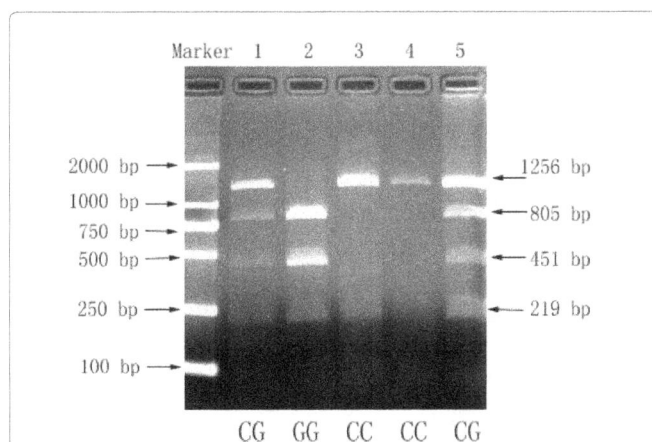

Figure 2: Genotyping analysis of the *PARL* rs3732581 polymorphism by PCR-RFLP analysis using BstN I digestion. DNA Marker-D (100bp-2000bp); lane 1, 5 CG heterozygous: 65, 219, 451, 805 and 125 bp; lane 2, GG homozygous: 65, 219, 451, and 805 bp; lane 3, 4 CC homozygous: 65, 219, and 1256 bp. The 65bp band had been run out of agarose gel.

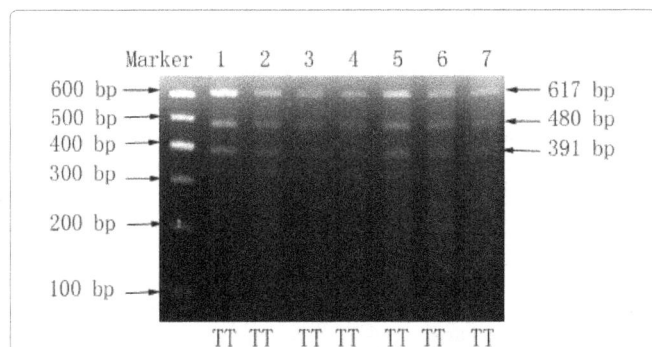

Figure 3: Genotyping analysis of the *PARL* rs73887537 polymorphism by PCR-RFLP analysis using Hpa II digestion. DNA MarkerGM331/2 (100bp-600bp); lane 1-7 TT homozygous: 52, 391, 480, and 617 bp. The 52bp band had been run out of agarose gel. We did not find rs73887537 polymorphism of PARL gene was existed in the studied population.

Statistical analysis

Genotype and allele frequencies were calculated by gene counting. Tests of Hardy-Weinberg equilibrium were performed using χ^2 test. Clinical characteristics were expressed as mean ± SD. Comparisons of genotype and allele frequencies between T2DM group and controls were performed using χ^2 test. To compare the means of the variables measured between the groups, the Student's *t*-test was used. One-way analysis of variance was used to test for differences in means of phenotypic characteristics between genotypes. For skewed distribution and homogeneity of variance the logarithmic transformation or nonparametric test was used. All *P*-values were two-tailed and Statistical significance was defined as *P<0.05*. Statistical analysis was performed using Statistical Package for the Social Sciences (SPSS, Version 11.5) for Windows.

Results

Compared with the control subjects, T2DM patients had significantly higher waist circumference, Waist-to-Hip Ratio (WHR), Fasting Plasma Glucose (FPG), Fasting Insulin (FINS), Hemoglobin A1c (HBA1c), Insulin Resistance Index (HOMA-IR), the plasma levels of Triglyceride (TG), Low-Density Lipoprotein Cholesterol (LDL-C) and Lower High-Density Lipoprotein Cholesterol (HDL-C) (*P<0.05*). However, there were no significant differences in age, height, weight, hip circumference, Body Mass Index (BMI), and the plasma levels of Total Cholesterol (TC) between the two groups. This is consistent with diabetic features (Table 1).

Genotyping of the *PARL* rs3732581 and rs73887537 variant was performed in 927 subjects, 543 with T2DM and 384 controls. We did not find rs73887537 polymorphism of *PARL* gene was existed in the studied Chinese population. *PARL* rs3732581 polymorphism genotype frequencies of GG, CG, and CC were 14.2%, 48.1%, 37.7% in T2DM group and17.4%, 46.9%, 35.7% in control group respectively, and allele frequencies of G, C were 38.2%, 61.8% in T2DM group and 40.9%, 59.1% in control group respectively. Genotype frequencies did not deviate from Hardy–Weinberg equilibrium in the combined study population and no significant difference was observed in the allele or genotype frequencies of *PARL* gene rs3732581 polymorphism between the T2DM and control groups (both *P<0.05*). The distributions of *PARL* gene rs3732581 polymorphism genotypes and alleles in the T2DM and control groups from a Chinese population are summarized in Table 2.

The subjects carrying GG genotype had higher plasma triglyceride level than that of the subjects carrying CG and CG+CC genotype (*P<0.05*) in T2DM group. The subjects carrying GG genotype had higher plasma triglyceride level than that of the subjects carrying CC and CG+CC genotype (*P<0.05*) and the subjects carrying GG genotype total cholesterol levels was higher than the subjects carrying CG and CG+CC genotype (*P<0.05*) in control group. Clinical characteristics by genotype are shown in Tables 3 and 4. However, there were no significant differences in other clinical characteristics in three genotypes in the two groups.

Groups	N	Genotype frequency n (%)			Allele frequency n (%)	
		GG	CG	CC	G	C
T2DM	543	77 (14.2)	261 (48.1)	205 (37.7)	415 (38.2)	671 (61.8)
Control	384	67 (17.4)	180 (46.9)	137 (35.7)	314 (40.9)	454 (59.1)
χ^2		1.876			1.346	
P value		0.391			0.246	

Table 2: Genotype and allele distribution of the PARL Leu262Val polymorphism in case and control groups.

Genotype	GG	CG	CC	CG+CC	P value
Age（Years）	57.92 ± 12.68	57.16 ± 11.53	57.79 ± 12.00	57.44 ± 11.71	
Height（cm）	164.27 ± 8.20	164.83 ± 7.15	164.64 ± 7.71	164.75 ± 7.38	
Weight（Kg）	69.25 ± 10.70	67.94 ± 13.50	69.42 ± 11.84	68.60 ± 12.76	
Body mass index（Kg/m²）	25.70 ± 3.85	24.92 ± 4.20	25.54 ± 3.60	25.20 ± 3.95	
Waist circumference (cm)	90.51 ± 9.20	89.34 ± 9.26	88.43 ± 8.69	88.94 ± 8.99	
Hip circumference (cm)	94.87 ± 5.32	94.19 ± 6.45	95.90 ± 7.40	94.95 ± 6.92	
Waist and hips ratio	0.96 ± 0.10	0.95 ± 0.07	0.92 ± 0.08	0.94 ± 0.08	
Fasting glucose（mmol/L）	11.06 ± 4.05	10.56 ± 3.69	10.73 ± 4.83	10.64 ± 4.22	
Hemoglobin A1c (%)	8.39 ± 1.42	8.44 ± 2.04	8.26 ± 1.69	8.36 ± 1.89	
Fasting insulin（mU/L）	10.70 ± 5.32	9.97 ± 3.91	10.41 ± 4.39	10.17 ± 4.12	Triglyceride:
HOMA-IR	5.17 ± 3.11	4.64 ± 2.36	5.05 ± 3.36	4.82 ± 2.85	GG/CG P=0.012◊
Total cholesterol（mmol/L）	5.17 ± 1.04	4.64 ± 1.05	4.94 ± 1.05	4.78 ± 1.06	GG/CG+CC P=0.015△
Triglyceride（mmol/L）	3.42 ± 2.48	1.88 ± 0.94	2.17 ± 1.45	2.01 ± 1.20	
LDL-C（mmol/L）	2.64 ± 0.79	2.65 ± 0.97	2.81 ± 1.03	2.72 ± 1.00	
HDL-C（mmol/L）	0.87 ± 0.30	1.18 ± 0.97	1.00 ± 0.36	1.10 ± 0.77	

HOMA-IR: homeostasis model assessment insulin resistance index; LDL-C: high-density lipoprotein; HDL-C: low-density lipoprotein. ◊: Kruskal-Wallis H test △: Mann-Whitney U test

Table 3: clinical characteristics of T2DM group by genotype. $\bar{x} \pm s$

Genotype	GG	CG	CC	CG+CC	P value
Age（Years）	59.04 ± 12.42	56.42 ± 13.87	53.05 ± 13.82	54.99 ± 13.88	
Height（cm）	166.19 ± 6.53	165.89 ± 8.29	165.11 ± 7.13	165.56 ± 7.79	
Weight（Kg）	68.42 ± 11.59	68.69 ± 12.04	68.16 ± 8.73	68.47 ± 10.72	
Body mass index（Kg/m²）	24.73 ± 3.84	24.80 ± 2.86	25.02 ± 3.15	24.90 ± 2.97	
Waist circumference (cm)	89.08 ± 8.01	87.44 ± 6.41	83.25 ± 9.98	85.67 ± 8.33	
Hip circumference (cm)	97.31 ± 6.31	97.60 ± 12.07	94.16 ± 6.24	96.14 ± 10.13	
Waist and hips ratio	0.92 ± 0.05	0.90 ± 0.06	0.88 ± 0.09	0.89 ± 0.08	
Fasting glucose（mmol/L）	4.65 ± 0.52	4.71 ± 0.48	4.51 ± 0.50	4.63 ± 0.50	
Hemoglobin A1c (%)	4.56 ± 0.89	4.62 ± 0.75	4.64 ± 0.67	4.63 ± 0.71	Total cholesterol:
Fasting insulin（mU/L）	7.78 ± 2.06	8.45 ± 2.62	8.13 ± 2.47	8.31 ± 2.55	GG/CC P=0.018
HOMA-IR	1.62 ± 0.52	1.77 ± 0.60	1.65 ± 0.62	1.72 ± 0.61	GG/CG P=0.036
Total cholesterol（mmol/L）	4.99 ± 1.14	4.55 ± 0.82	4.47 ± 0.74	4.52 ± 0.78	GG/CG+CC P=0.044▲ Triglyceride: GG/CC P=0.014
Triglyceride（mmol/L）	2.02 ± 0.89	1.70 ± 0.75	1.53 ± 0.72	1.63 ± 0.74	GG/CG+CC P=0.029
LDL-C（mmol/L）	2.61 ± 0.55	2.31 ± 0.72	2.45 ± 0.65	2.37 ± 0.69	
HDL-C（mmol/L）	1.35 ± 0.19	1.35 ± 0.31	1.47 ± 0.31	1.40 ± 0.32	

HOMA-IR: homeostasis model assessment insulin resistance index; LDL-C: high-density lipoprotein; HDL-C: low-density lipoprotein; ▲: T test after logarithmic transformation

Table 4: clinical characteristics of control group by genotype. $\bar{x} \pm s$

Discussion

The present study demonstrated that distributions of the PARL rs3732581 genotypes and alleles are not statistically different between the T2DM and control groups in a Chinese population (P=0.391, 0.246 respectively). The results showed that the PARL rs3732581 variant is not association with the presence of T2DM in Chinese population, despite it has been shown that PARL is a new candidate gene for obesity and T2DM [9]. In this study we also investigated the effect of the PARL rs3732581 genetic variant, on fasting plasma insulin and glucose levels, as well as BMI, in a healthy population and in a population diagnosed with T2DM. We found that the C allele is no significant effect neither on levels of fasting plasma insulin、glucose nor with BMI, despite the strong functional evidence that PARL is involved in regulating insulin levels [9]. Our data fail to replicate the previous result and these findings further support the works showing that the PARL rs3732581 variant has no effect on these parameters in population-based cohorts [12-14]. The differences in results could be explained by race and/or environmental differences between the studied populations.

Our results on the genotype and allele distribution of the PARL

rs3732581 variant in T2DM group of Chinese population were not similar to that reported for Irish population[13] (P=0.002, 0.016 respectively). Allele distribution in control group of Chinese population was not similar to that reported for Australia population (P=0.041) [14]. The difference could due to race differences. In addition, we did not find rs73887537 polymorphism of PARL gene was existed in the studied Chinese population.

Interestingly, in this study it was noted that the subjects carrying G allele of rs3732581 had higher plasma triglyceride level than that of the subjects carrying C allele (P<0.05) in T2DM group. The subjects carrying G allele had higher plasma triglyceride and total cholesterol levels than that of the subjects carrying C allele (both P<0.05) in control group. PARL appears to be one of the loci contributing to the chromosome 3 QTL cluster and a previous study reported a strong association of the genomic location of PARL (3q27) with phenotypes typically associated with MetS [11,17-20]. But there have been no studies published reporting on the functional effect this SNP has on metabolism. Our original findings required a better understanding of PARL gene and PARL structure, function, and mechanisms of regulation. The notable conserved core rhomboid domain of PARL is composed by 6 TMH (transmembrane helix), with the strictly conserved catalytic serine and histidine residues located in TMH-4 and TMH-6 respectively [21]. The *PARL* rs3732581 genetic variant is a common C→G SNP in exon 7 of PARL that encodes an amino acid substitution from leucine to valine in TMH-4 of PARL. While this substitution does not impact directly on the predicted catalytic sites of PARL, it could be reasonably expected to alter the conformation of the protein in the mitochondrial membrane, and may affect its activity [9]. On the other hand, it has been reported that *PARL* gene expression in skeletal muscle correlated with both citrate synthase expression, a marker of mitochondrial oxidative capacity in human subjects [9].

Mitochondria are highly dynamic organelles and undergo continuous fission and fusion events in physiological situations [22,23]. Mitochondrial structure and function are highly dependent on the processes of fusion and fission. PARL may involve in mitochondrial fusion [24]. Maintaining mitochondrial morphology is critical to normal cell function [25-33]. The imbalance in mitochondrial fusion and fission in metabolically active tissue such as skeletal muscle may result in defects associated with lipid metabolism [24]. There is substantial evidence that proteins participating in mitochondrial fusion or fission also have a role in metabolism [34-36]. Their expression is crucial in mitochondrial metabolism through the maintenance of the mitochondrial network architecture, and their reduced expression may explain some of the metabolic alterations associated with obesity. Kita et al. investigated the role of mitochondrial remodeling on Triacylglycerol (TG) accumulation in adipocytes and found that when the mitochondrial fusion was induced in adipocytes by silencing of mitochondrial fission proteins including Fis1 and Drp1, the cellular TG content was decreased [37]. In contrast, the silencing of mitochondrial fusion proteins including mitofusin 2 and Opa1 increased the cellular TG content followed by fragmentation of mitochondria [37]. They also found that Polyphenolic phytochemicals, negative regulators of cellular TG accumulation in adipocytes, have mitochondrial fusion activity [37]. These results strongly suggest that cellular TG accumulation is regulated, at least in part, via mitochondrial fusion and fission processes. On the other hand, it has been shown that deletion of PARL in the mouse resulted in premature postnatal death due to progressive cachexia and indications of increased apoptosis which correlated with reduced levels of cleaved Opa1. The antiapoptotic effects of Opa1 require PARL [38-40]. PARL positioned upstream of Opa1 in the control of apoptosis [38]. Opa1 has been shown to be involved in the regulation of the so-called "cristae remodeling" pathway of apoptosis and the regulation of mitochondrial fusion [38,39,41]. Cipolat et al. provide evidence that PARL may be required for the correct assembly of the Opa1-containing structures that regulate the integrity of the cristae junctions and that PARL and Opa1 interacted at the protein level as well [38]. So it is tempting to speculate that the PARL rs3732581 genetic variant could in some way influence the mitochondrial remodeling and metabolism of lipid through its interaction with Opa1 [38,42].

Moreover, it is also well known that nuclear genome has a leading role in the biogenesis of mitochondrial respiratory chain and that nuclear activity can be modulated by signals sent by mitochondria suggesting that dysregulated mitochondrial morphology could alter gene expression of proteins involved in lipid metabolism [43-45]. PARL is the only intramembrane-cleaving protease where the putative signaling moiety is also part of the protease itself. The β-cleavage of PARL releases within the mitochondrial matrix a 25 amino acid-long peptide termed Pβ-peptide which appears to execute mitochondrial retrograde signaling (MRS) [46-48]. MRS senses mitochondrial activities/dysfunctions and relay this information to the nucleus in

order to initiate appropriate physiological readjustments including metabolism [48]. Indeed, the release of the Pβ-peptide, the putative effectors molecule of the PARL signaling, is self-regulated. The β-cleavage is either executed by an unknown protease (PARLase) that is activated via a PARL-catalyzed cleavage or by PARL itself through an intermolecular reaction [46]. The proteolytic activity of PARL required for the β-cleavage of its N terminus could be supplied in trans [46]. So, it is tempting to speculate that the *PARL* rs3732581 genetic variant could in some way influence the MRS and metabolism of lipid through alter the conformation of the protein and its proteolytic activity.

It has been suggested that mitochondria ensure metabolite and mitochondrial DNA mixing and impaired fusion could result in lower mitochondrial content and impaired oxidative capacity, leading to a defective energy homeostasis. Given the prior evidence for a role for PARL in mitochondrial integrity and function, multivariant analysis was performed to assess the global effect of PARL sequence variation on mitochondrial content. The results showing that sequence variation in PARL have a significant influence on mitochondrial content ($P=0.00076$). But the association between the PARL rs3732581 variant and mitochondrial content level is not significant ($P=0.0701$) [49]. The PARL rs3732581 variant alone is unlikely to significantly influence metabolism of lipid through alter the mitochondrial content.

In summary, until now the role of PARL and/or the *PARL* rs3732581 genetic variant on metabolism of lipid is poorly understood. The mechanism of regulation of plasma triglyceride and total cholesterol levels by PARL and/or the *PARL* rs3732581 genetic variant remains to be determined. The different effects of the *PARL* rs3732581 genetic variant on plasma triglyceride and total cholesterol levels between the T2DM and control groups, suggesting that there might exist differences in the biological pathways of the two phenotypes between the case and control groups and further studies are required, although we cannot rule out the possibility that one or more of our results represent false positive findings. In conclusion, we did not find the rs73887537 polymorphism of *PARL* gene was existed in studied Chinese population and our results provided no evidence that the *PARL* rs3732581 variant had a role in T2DM susceptibility or was likely to be an important contributor to insulin resistance in Chinese population. However, we found that compared with carriers of C-allele the carriers of the GG genotype showed significantly higher levels of triglyceride and levels of triglyceride and total cholesterol in the T2DM and control groups respectively. The *PARL* rs3732581 variant may play a role in genetic predisposition to dyslipidemia which is a risk factor of diabetes in Chinese population. Our original findings were required to replicate in additional populations. A role for rs3732581 polymorphism of *PARL* gene in metabolic conditions could not be excluded and further comprehensive studies are required.

Acknowledgements

We acknowledge the excellent technical assistance of staff members working in Department of Endocrinology of Gansu Provincial People's Hospital and those working in MEC of Gansu Provincial People's Hospital. This study was supported by grants from the Natural Science Foundation of Gansu Province (No. 0803RJZA067).

Reference

1. Rolo AP, Palmeira CM (2006) Diabetes and mitochondrial function: role of hyperglycemia and oxidative stress. Toxicol Appl Pharmacol 212: 167-178.

2. Gloyn AL (2003) The search for type 2 diabetes genes. Ageing Res Rev 2: 111-127.

3. Vondra K, Rath R, Bass A, Slabochová Z, Teisinger J, et al. (1977) Enzyme activities in quadriceps femoris muscle of obese diabetic male patients. Diabetologia 13: 527-529.

4. Simoneau JA, Kelley DE (1997) Altered glycolytic and oxidative capacities of skeletal muscle contribute to insulin resistance in NIDDM. J Appl Physiol (1985) 83: 166-171.

5. Kelley DE, He J, Menshikova EV, Ritov VB (2002) Dysfunction of mitochondria in human skeletal muscle in type 2 diabetes. Diabetes 51: 2944-2950.

6. Björntorp P, Scherstén T, Fagerberg SE (1967) Respiration and phosphorylation of mitochondria isolated from the skeletal muscle of diabetic and normal subjects. Diabetologia 3: 346-352.

7. Simoneau JA, Colberg SR, Thaete FL, Kelley DE (1995) Skeletal muscle glycolytic and oxidative enzyme capacities are determinants of insulin sensitivity and muscle composition in obese women. FASEB J 9: 273-278.

8. Simoneau JA, Veerkamp JH, Turcotte LP, Kelley DE (1999) Markers of capacity to utilize fatty acids in human skeletal muscle: relation to insulin resistance and obesity and effects of weight loss. FASEB J 13: 2051-2060.

9. Walder K, Kerr-Bayles L, Civitarese A, Jowett J, Curran J, et al. (2005) The mitochondrial rhomboid protease PSARL is a new candidate gene for type 2 diabetes. Diabetologia 48: 459-468.

10. Tang H, Liu J, Niu L, He W, Xu Y (2009) Variation in gene expression of presenilins-associated rhomboid-like protein and mitochondrial function in skeletal muscle of insulin-resistant rats. Endocrine 36: 524-529.

11. Kissebah AH, Sonnenberg GE, Myklebust J, Goldstein M, Broman K, et al. (2000) Quantitative trait loci on chromosomes 3 and 17 influence phenotypes of the metabolic syndrome. Proc Natl Acad Sci U S A 97: 14478-14483.

12. Fawcett KA, Wareham NJ, Luan J, Syddall H, Cooper C, et al. (2006) PARL Leu262Val is not associated with fasting insulin levels in UK populations. Diabetologia 49: 2649-2652.

13. Hatunic M, Stapleton M, Hand E, DeLong C, Crowley VE, et al. (2009) The Leu262Val polymorphism of presenilin associated rhomboid like protein (PARL) is associated with earlier onset of type 2 diabetes and increased urinary microalbumin creatinine ratio in an Irish case-control population. Diabetes Res Clin Pract. 83: 316-319.

14. Powell BL, Wiltshire S, Arscott G, McCaskie PA, Hung J, et al. (2008) Association of PARL rs3732581 genetic variant with insulin levels, metabolic syndrome and coronary artery disease. Hum Genet 124: 263-270.

15. Alberti KG, Zimmet PZ (1998) Definition, diagnosis and classification of diabetes mellitus and its complications. Part 1: diagnosis and classification of diabetes mellitus provisional report of a WHO consultation. Diabet Med 15: 539-553.

16. Matthews DR, Hosker JP, Rudenski AS, Naylor BA, Treacher DF, et al. (1985) Homeostasis model assessment: insulin resistance and beta-cell function from fasting plasma glucose and insulin concentrations in man. Diabetologia 28: 412-419.

17. Francke S, Manraj M, Lacquemant C, Lecoeur C, Leprêtre F, et al. (2001) A genome-wide scan for coronary heart disease suggests in Indo-Mauritians a susceptibility locus on chromosome 16p13 and replicates linkage with the metabolic syndrome on 3q27. Hum Mol Genet 10: 2751-2765.

18. Luke A, Wu X, Zhu X, Kan D, Su Y, et al. (2003) Linkage for BMI at 3q27 region confirmed in an African-American population. Diabetes 52: 1284-1287.

19. Mori Y, Otabe S, Dina C, Yasuda K, Populaire C, et al. (2002) Genome-wide search for type 2 diabetes in Japanese affected sib-pairs confirms susceptibility genes on 3q, 15q, and 20q and identifies two new candidate Loci on 7p and 11p. Diabetes 51: 1247-1255.

20. Vionnet N, Hani EH, Dupont S, Gallina S, Francke S, et al. (2000) Genomewide search for type 2 diabetes-susceptibility genes in French whites: evidence for a novel susceptibility locus for early-onset diabetes on chromosome 3q27-qter and independent replication of a type 2-diabetes locus on chromosome 1q21-q24. Am J Hum Genet. 67: 1470-1480.

21. Koonin EV, Makarova KS, Rogozin IB, Davidovic L, Letellier MC, et al. (2003) The rhomboids: a nearly ubiquitous family of intramembrane serine proteases that probably evolved by multiple ancient horizontal gene transfers. Genome Biol 4: R19.

22. Bereiter-Hahn J, Vöth M (1994) Dynamics of mitochondria in living cells: shape changes, dislocations, fusion, and fission of mitochondria. Microsc Res Tech 27: 198-219.

23. Chan DC (2006) Mitochondrial fusion and fission in mammals. Annu Rev Cell Dev Biol 22: 79-99.

24. Civitarese AE, Ravussin E (2008) Mitochondrial energetics and insulin resistance. Endocrinology 149: 950-954.

25. Chen H, Detmer SA, Ewald AJ, Griffin EE, Fraser SE, et al. (2003) Mitofusins Mfn1 and Mfn2 coordinately regulate mitochondrial fusion and are essential for embryonic development. J Cell Biol 160: 189-200.

26. Chen H, Chomyn A, Chan DC (2005) Disruption of fusion results in mitochondrial heterogeneity and dysfunction. J Biol Chem 280: 26185-26192.

27. Okamoto K, Shaw JM (2005) Mitochondrial morphology and dynamics in yeast and multicellular eukaryotes. Annu Rev Genet 39: 503-536.

28. Alexander C, Votruba M, Pesch UE, Thiselton DL, Mayer S, et al. (2000) OPA1, encoding a dynamin-related GTPase, is mutated in autosomal dominant optic atrophy linked to chromosome 3q28. Nat Genet 26: 211-215.

29. Kijima K, Numakura C, Izumino H, Umetsu K, Nezu A, et al. (2005) Mitochondrial GTPase mitofusin 2 mutation in Charcot-Marie-Tooth neuropathy type 2A. Hum Genet 116: 23-27.

30. Frank S, Gaume B, Bergmann-Leitner ES, Leitner WW, Robert EG, et al. (2001) The role of dynamin-related protein 1, a mediator of mitochondrial fission, in apoptosis. Dev Cell 1: 515-525.

31. Bossy-Wetzel E, Barsoum MJ, Godzik A, Schwarzenbacher R, Lipton SA (2003) Mitochondrial fission in apoptosis, neurodegeneration and aging. Curr Opin Cell Biol 15: 706-716.

32. Olichon A, Baricault L, Gas N, Guillou E, Valette A, et al. (2003) Loss of OPA1 perturbates the mitochondrial inner membrane structure and integrity, leading to cytochrome c release and apoptosis. J Biol Chem 278: 7743-7746.

33. Arakaki N, Nishihama T, Kohda A, Owaki H, Kuramoto Y, et al. (2006) Regulation of mitochondrial morphology and cell survival by Mitogenin I and mitochondrial single-stranded DNA binding protein. Biochim Biophys Acta 1760: 1364-1372.

34. Bach D, Pich S, Soriano FX, Vega N, Baumgartner B, et al. (2003) Mitofusin-2 determines mitochondrial network architecture and mitochondrial metabolism. A novel regulatory mechanism altered in obesity. J Biol Chem 278: 17190-17197.

35. Bach D, Naon D, Pich S, Soriano FX, Vega N, et al. (2005) Expression of Mfn2, the Charcot-Marie-Tooth neuropathy type 2A gene, in human skeletal muscle: effects of type 2 diabetes, obesity, weight loss, and the regulatory role of tumor necrosis factor alpha and interleukin-6. Diabetes 54: 2685-2693.

36. Zorzano A, Liesa M, Palacín M (2009) Mitochondrial dynamics as a bridge between mitochondrial dysfunction and insulin resistance. Arch Physiol Biochem 115: 1-12.

37. Kita T, Nishida H, Shibata H, Niimi S, Higuti T, et al. (2009) Possible role of mitochondrial remodelling on cellular triacylglycerol accumulation. J Biochem 146: 787-796.

38. Cipolat S, Rudka T, Hartmann D, Costa V, Serneels L, et al. (2006) Mitochondrial rhomboid PARL regulates cytochrome c release during apoptosis via OPA1-dependent cristae remodeling. Cell 126: 163-175.

39. Frezza C, Cipolat S, Martins de Brito O, Micaroni M, Beznoussenko GV, et al. (2006) OPA1 controls apoptotic cristae remodeling independently from mitochondrial fusion. Cell 126: 177-189.

40. Delivani P, Martin SJ (2006) Mitochondrial membrane remodeling in apoptosis: an inside story. Cell Death Differ 13: 2007-2010.

41. Cipolat S, Martins de Brito O, Dal Zilio B, Scorrano L (2004) OPA1 requires mitofusin 1 to promote mitochondrial fusion. Proc Natl Acad Sci U S A 101: 15927-15932.

42. McQuibban GA, Saurya S, Freeman M (2003) Mitochondrial membrane remodelling regulated by a conserved rhomboid protease. Nature 423: 537-541.

43. Khalimonchuk O, Rödel G (2005) Biogenesis of cytochrome c oxidase. Mitochondrion 5: 363-388.

44. Liu Z, Butow RA (2006) Mitochondrial retrograde signaling. Annu Rev Genet 40: 159-185.

45. Scarpulla RC (2006) Nuclear control of respiratory gene expression in mammalian cells. J Cell Biochem 97: 673-683.

46. Sik A, Passer BJ, Koonin EV, Pellegrini L (2004) Self-regulated cleavage of the

mitochondrial intramembrane-cleaving protease PARL yields Pbeta, a nuclear-targeted peptide. J Biol Chem 279: 15323-15329.

47. Jeyaraju DV, Xu L, Letellier MC, Bandaru S, Zunino R, et al. (2006) Phosphorylation and cleavage of presenilin-associated rhomboid-like protein (PARL) promotes changes in mitochondrial morphology. Proc Natl Acad Sci U S A 103: 18562-18567.

48. Hill RB, Pellegrini L (2010) The PARL family of mitochondrial rhomboid proteases. Semin Cell Dev Biol 21: 582-592.

49. Curran JE, Jowett JB, Abraham LJ, Diepeveen LA, Elliott KS, et al. (2010) Genetic variation in PARL influences mitochondrial content. Hum Genet 127: 183-190.

4

Black Tea Polyphenols Suppress Postprandial Hyperglycemia *In Vivo* in Mice and Inhibit α-Glucosidase Activity *In Vitro*

Junki Yoshida[#], Akiko Tateishi[#], Yuko Fukui*, Mitsuhiro Zeida and Nobuyuki Fukui

Research Division, Suntory Global Innovation Center Limited (Suntory SIC), Seikadai, Seika-cho, Soraku-gun, Kyoto 619-0284, Japan
[#]Both the authors Contributed equally to the work.

Abstract

Black tea is reported to have various beneficial effects on health. Activated charcoal-treated black tea (ACBT) did not contain catechins nor caffeine and included small amount of theaflavins (TFs). We had further fractionated ACBT to obtain black tea polymerized polyphenols (BTPP), TFs-poor fraction and TFs-rich fraction and studied *in vitro* and/or *in vivo* effect of the fractions to elucidate the effect of ACBT. Sucrose-loading test in mice showed that ACBT and BTPP at the dose of, 1000 and 560 mg/kg, respectively, suppressed the increase of blood glucose level while secretion of insulin was not affected. We found that this effect is caused by inhibition of α-glucosidase activity. BTPP contained TFs, but the content was not at all enough to explain the activity of ACBT, ^{1}H NMR analysis of BTPP was carried and showed the existence of many benzotropolone ring containing substances as active compounds.

Keywords: Black Tea; α-Glucosidase; Sucrose; Postprandial Hyperglycemia; Benzotropolone Ring

Abbreviations: ACBT: Activated Charcoal-Treated Black Tea; AUC: Area Under the Curve; BMI: Body Mass Index; BTPP: Black Tea Polymerized Polyphenols; CMC·Na: Sodium Carboxymethyl Cellulose; DMSO: Dimethyl Sulfoxide; AcOEt: Ethylacetate; EC: (-)-Epicatechin; ECG: (-)-Epicatechin-3-O-Gallate; EGC: (-)-Epigallocatechin; EGCG: (-)-Epigallocatechin-3-O-Gallate; GLUT: Glucose Transporter; TF: Theaflavin; TF3G: Theaflavin-3-O-Gallate; TF3'G: Theaflavin-3'-O-Gallate; TF3, 3'diG: Theaflavin-3, 3'-di-O-Gallate

Introduction

Recently, overweight and obesity have become an increasingly serious problem in the world. From 1980 to 2013, their population increased in both underdeveloped and developed countries, regardless of gender, reaching 2.1 billion in 2013 [1]. Overweight and obesity are often accompanied by type II diabetes, ischemic heart disease, high blood pressure, various malignant tumors and other health problems [2]. It is necessary to solve these problems.

One of the most effective ways to prevent overweight or obesity is to suppress the degradation of sugars. Oral intake of carbohydrates are followed by digestion in stomach then in intestine, where α-glucosidase on the mucosal epithelia degrades them and produce glucose which is absorbed into the bloodstream. Acarbose, an inhibitor of α-glucosidase, is used to treat type II diabetes and reduce glucose absorption through delayed carbohydrate digestion. This drug therapy is to suppress rapid increase in blood glucose levels after eating, thereby preventing the glycotoxicity. Some studies showed that food ingredients such as salacia reticulata [3] and cacao liquor procyanidin [4] inhibited α-glucosidase (e.g., maltase and sucrase) activity. Therefore, regulation of sugar absorption and metabolism is useful for anti-obesity effects.

Tea, prepared from the leaves of *Camellia sinensis,* are popular beverages consumed all around the world. Teas are classified largely into three groups, green tea, oolong tea and black tea according to the fermentation degrees, non, semi and full fermentation, respectively. Recently, many studies have been done and reported on the effects of the teas and their fractionated products on health including obesity and various health area. Green tea was reported to reduce blood LDL cholesterol, suppress absorption of fat, enhance consumption and burning of energy in adipose tissue [5-7]. Oolong tea also has anti-obesity effects, e.g., inhibition of pancreatic lipase, delay of absorption of triglyceride from lymph duct and suppression of hypertriglyceridemia after meal [8,9]. In addition, anti-stress, anti-diabetes and anti-oxidation effects of the Oolong tea were also reported [10-15]. Black tea is consumed regularly for a long time in the world [6] and its ingredients are effective and beneficial for preventing obesity and hyperglycemia. Black tea was reported to enhance translocation of GLUT4 to cell membrane in muscle of C57BL/6J mice fed a high fat diet for 14 weeks [16]. Also, intake of black tea induced phosphorylation of phosphoinositide 3-kinase (PI3K) and its downstream Akt/protein kinase B was enhanced. PI3K/Akt-pathway and insulin independent AMP-activated protein kinase (AMPK) pathway were activated [17].

These findings suggest that black tea affects not only suppression of intestinal absorption of sugars but also glucose metabolism in muscle and other organs.

Black tea is composed of a few catechins (e.g., EC, ECG, EGC, and EGCG) and several polymerized polyphenols (e.g., TFs and thearubigins). Four major TFs in black tea, namely TF, TF3G, TF3'G and TF3, 3'diG have been identified. Although those amounts are only about 0.3~2% of dry weight of tea leaves [18], the TFs exhibited suppressive effects of the increasing blood glucose level [19]. However, the TFs was unstable because of oxidative polymerization and decomposition in the extract [18,20]. On the other hand, thearubigins were made by oxidative polymerization of TFs and/or polyphenols having benzotropolone ring and therefore have very complex structures.

To investigate the potential of the black tea ingredients, we isolated the Activated charcoal-treated black tea (ACBT), black tea polymerized polyphenols (BTPP) and their stable TFs by HPLC and NMR studies, and then these fractions were examined the suppression effect of α-glucosidase activity by *in vitro* and *in vivo* studies. Our results suggest that new fractions can be effective for preventing obesity and hyperglycemia.

*Corresponding author: Yuko Fukui, Ph.D., Research Division, Suntory Global Innovation Center Limited (Suntory SIC), 8-1-1 Seikadai, Seika-cho, Soraku-gun, Kyoto 619-0284, Japan, E-mail: Yuko_Fukui@suntory.co.jp

Materials and Methods

Chemicals

Theaflavin (TF), theaflavin-3-O-gallate (TF3G), theaflavin-3'-O-gallate (TF3'G), theaflavin-3, 3'-di-O-gallate (TF3, 3'diG) were from Nagara Science, Gifu, Japan.

Intestinal acetone powders from rat (SIGMA, St. Louis, MO, USA), glucose C II test Wako (Wako Pure Chemical Industries, Osaka, Japan), acarbose (SIGMA, St. Louis, MO, USA), distilled water (Otsuka Pharmaceutical Co, Tokyo, Japan), Glutest Neo Sensor (Sanwa Kagaku Kenkyusho, Aichi, Japan), ultra-sensitive mouse insulin ELISA kit (Morinaga Institute of Biological Science, Yokohama, Japan), DMSO-d_6 (Euriso Top, France), CMC·Na, maleic acid, sucrose, DMSO and all solvents for HPLC (Nacalai Tesque, Kyoto, Japan) were purchased from the companies shown in parentheses.

Preparation of ACBT: Two hundred grams of black tea leaves (*Camellia sinensis* (L.) Kuntze var. *assamica*) were extracted with 2 L of hot water for 10 min. After filtration, the extract was applied to an 80 ml of activated charcoal column (Kuraraychol, GW-H, Kuraray Chemical Co. Ltd.) whose temperature was kept at 65°C. The eluent in the fractions of 2 to 11 column volumes was concentrated and lyophilized yielding 39 g of ACBT.

Preparation of BTPP: Thirty grams of ACBT was applied to an HPLC column, Daiso SP-120-40/60 ODS-B (110 mm I.D. x 1000 mm), and eluted under monitoring of absorption at 280 nm, at a flow rate of 300 ml/min with 0.2% HCOOH in 15% CH_3CN/aq for 136 min. Elution was continued with 0.2% HCOOH in 80% CH_3CN/aq for 30 min to yield BTPP. The BTPP containing eluent was evaporated and lyophilized twice to remove HCOOH and yielded 8.4 g of dried matter, the yield was 28%.

Preparation of TFs-poor and TFs-rich fraction: Forty nine mg of BTPP was extracted with the mixture of water and ethyl acetate. The resulting aqueous layer yielded, 35.8 mg and the organic layer, 12.7 mg of dried matters. The aqueous layer was named TFs-poor fraction and the organic layer TFs-rich one, respectively.

HPLC analysis of TFs in ACBT, BTPP, TFs-poor and TFs-rich fractions: All fractions were dissolved with 50% CH_3CN and filtrated through 0.45 μm filter (Merck Millipore LH-4) and each was applied to an HPLC. HPLC was conducted using a Develosil ODS-MG-5 (Nomura Chemical, Japan, 4.6 mm I.D. x 150 mm) column and a flow rate of solvent at 1.0 ml/min; the isocratic solvent system used was as follows; 0.04% TFA in 76% H_2O, 21% CH_3CN, and 3% AcOEt. The HPLC was carried out with a photodiode array detector SPD-M10A (Shimadzu Co., Ltd., Japan) detecting absorbance at 375 nm and column temp at 40°C.

NMR analysis of BTPP: Five mg of BTPP was dissolved in 0.55 ml of DMSO-d_6 containing 10 μM of 4-bis (trimethylsilyl) benzene (Sigma-Aldrich) added as an internal standard in 5 mm I.D. NMR tube. ^1H NMR spectrum were obtained on AVANCE-3 HD-400 spectrometer (BRUKER BIOSPIN, Germany), with number of scans, 1024; relaxation delay (d1), 20 sec; acquisition time, 4.089 sec.

Measurement of α−glucosidase (sucrase) activity: Enzyme activity was measured essentially following the methods of Yoshikawa et al. [21-23] and Matsuda et al. [24,25]. We determined that intestinal expression of alpha glucosidase between rats and mice was the same from previous reports [26-28].

One gram of acetone powder from rat intestine was suspended in 45 ml of 0.1 M maleic acid buffer (pH 6.0), homogenized and centrifuged at 20,000 × G for 20 min at 4°C. The supernatant removed and diluted twice with the buffer was used as the crude enzyme. The sample in 25 μl of 50% DMSO was added to 50 μl of 74 mM sucrose substrate in 0.1 M maleic acid buffer (pH 6.0). After 3 min, reaction was stopped by adding 400 μl of distilled water and heating for 10 min in boiling water. After leaving on ice for 10 min, an aliquot of 100 μl was put into a well of a 96 well microplate, then 150 μl of glucose CII test Wako was added and left for 10 min to develop color. The amount of D-glucose formed was measured at 510 nm using a microplate reader Filter Max F5 (Molecular Devices, USA). A sample, substrate and crude enzyme were mixed and immediately put into boiling water and left for 10 min to inactivate the enzyme and to serve as a blank. Acarbose was used as a positive control.

Animals

Six-week-old male C57BL/6J mice were purchased from Japan SLC (Hamamatsu, Japan). Mice were maintained and acclimatized for a week in an air-conditioned room kept at 23 ± 1.5°C and 55 ± 10% humidity, under a constant 12 h light-dark cycle (light from 7:00 to 19:00). They were fed *ad libitum* on commercial laboratory chow, CE-2 (Clea, Japan) and water. All animal experiments were performed under the guidelines established by the Japanese Society of Nutrition and Food Science (Law No. 105 and Notification No.6 of the Japanese Government).

Sucrose loading experiment: Sucrose was dissolved in distilled water at the concentration of 0.2 g/ml and a dose of 2 g/kg body weight was administered to mice. To dissolve ACBT, a suspension of 1 g/ml of distilled water was heated at 50-60°C, then left at room temperature to cool before use. Solution of 0.5% CMC·Na was added to BTTP at the concentration of 280 or 560 mg/ml, heated at 50-60°C and cooled likewise. The test solutions were orally administered to mice weighing 19-21 g and had been fasted for 16 h. Oral sucrose loading immediately followed. Just before and after 15, 30, 60, 90, 120 min of the administration, ca. 25 μl of blood was obtained from tail vein and submitted to on-the-spot measurement of blood sugar level using Glutest Neo Sensor. Then the blood was centrifuged at 10,000 rpm for 5 min at 4°C and the resulting supernatant was collected and kept at -80°C before measuring insulin concentration using Ultra Sensitive Mouse Insulin ELISA Kit.

Statistical analysis: Values are the mean ± standard error (SEM). After t-test and one-way ANOVA, values were compared by Dunnett-type multiple comparison procedure. All analyses were done using SPSS statistics version 10.0 (SPSS Inc., Chicago, IL, USA). Differences were considered significant when probability values were less than 0.05.

Results

Analysis of TFs in ACBT, BTPP, TFs-poor and TFs-rich fractions

We prepared ACBT using an activated charcoal column and further fractionated it to obtain BTPP, TFs-poor and TFs-rich fractions as described in Materials and Methods. Amounts of four major black tea TFs in the fractions were analyzed by HPLC and shown in Table 1. Neither caffeine nor catechins were detected in those fractions. Apparently, TFs were not much lost, if any, at each fractionation step. Especially noteworthy is that more TF was recovered in TFs-poor fraction than in TFs-rich fraction. On the other hand, far more of other three TFs were found in TFs-rich fraction than in TFs-poor fraction as expected.

NMR analysis

Five mg of BTTP was submitted to NMR analysis as described in Materials and Methods. Signals from hydrogen-bonded OH groups of the benzotropolone ring (Figure 1b) were observed at around 15 ppm in full and expanded ¹H NMR spectra of BTPP (Figure 1a and 1c). Presence of six large and several smaller signals (Figure 1a) suggested that in addition to four TFs identified by HPLC, many compounds which have the benzotropolone ring should be present in BTPP.

Inhibition of α–glucosidase (sucrase) activity

Enzyme inhibition test was performed using crude sucrase preparation from rat intestinal acetone powder. Commercial TFs, e.g., TF, TF3G, TF3'G, TF3, 3'diG were shown to have sucrase inhibitory activity with IC_{50}. Black tea derived fractions, ACBT, BTPP, TFs-poor and TFs-rich fraction were also shown to inhibit sucrase with IC_{50} comparable to that of TFs. Apparently, BTPP and TFs-poor fraction showed similar but about twice stronger IC_{50} than ACBT. Also TFs-poor fraction had somewhat stronger activity than TFs-rich fraction. From the strength of activity and the amount of fraction, total activity unit and contribution of each fraction to the sucrase inhibitory activity of ACBT was calculated and shown (Table 2). It should be noted that, contribution of TFs-poor fraction was almost 4 times more than that of TFs-rich fraction and that four TFs combined together in each of ACBT, BTPP, TFs-poor and TFs-rich fraction contributed less than 1% of the inhibitory activity of each fraction (Tables 2 and 3).

These results clearly showed that although TFs had α–glucosidase (sucrase) inhibitory activity, contribution of TFs to the enzyme inhibitory activity of ACBT or BTPP was very low. Thus, presence of enzyme inhibitory substances other than TFs was strongly suggested. These and NMR results combined, benzotropolone ring containing thearubigins were suggested to be prime candidates for active substances.

Fraction	Weight (g)*	Content of TFs (mg)**				
		TF	TF3G	TF3'G	TF3, 3'diG	Total
ACBT	100	64.0	42.2	19.8	84.2	210.2
BTPP	28	59.5	44.6	20.0	87.8	211.9
TFs-poor	20.9	35.8	3.57	0.50	2.91	42.82
TFs-rich	7.1	25.7	61.9	26.7	127.1	241.39

*Weight of dried powder
**One mg of TFs were submitted to HPLC analysis as indicated in Materials and Methods and total amounts in each fraction were calculated.

Table 1: Fractions of black tea and content of tfs in each fraction.

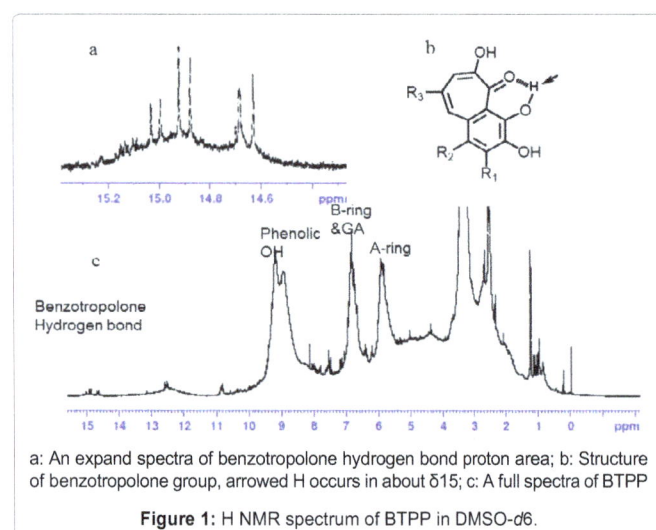

a: An expand spectra of benzotropolone hydrogen bond proton area; b: Structure of benzotropolone group, arrowed H occurs in about δ15; c: A full spectra of BTPP

Figure 1: H NMR spectrum of BTPP in DMSO-*d*6.

Fraction	Sucrase Inhibitory Activity		
	IC_{50} (mg/ml)	Total Activity Unit*	Contribution (%)
ACBT	0.516	194,000	100.0
BTPP	0.237	118,000	60.8
TFs-poor	0.239	87,400	45.1
TFs-rich	0.316	22,500	11.6

*Total activity unit is calculated by dividing amount of a material by IC_{50} value of the material.

Table 2: Sucrase inhibitory activity of black tea fractions.

TFs	IC_{50}(mg/ml)*	Total Activity Unit in Fractions of**			
		ACBT	BTPP	TFs-poor	TFs-rich
TF	0.479	134	124	75.0	54
TF3G	0.450	94	99	7.9	138
TF3'G	0.400	50	50	1.3	67
TF3, 3'diG	0.307	274	286	9.5	414
Total	—	552	559	93.7	673

*IC_{50} was measured using commercial TFs.
**Total activity unit is calculated as described in the legend of Table 2.

Table 3: Sucrase inhibitory activity of four tfs in black tea fractions.

Sucrose loading test

After 15 and 30 min of simultaneous oral administration of sucrose and ACBT (1000 mg/kg), the rise of blood glucose level was suppressed significantly (Figure 2). The suppression was 16.8% with ACBT when AUC for ACBT and control were compared (Figure 3). On the other hand, blood insulin level measured in the same experiment, was not affected significantly in ACBT group in both analyses (Figures 4 and 5).

BTPP derived from ACBT given at the dose of 560 mg/kg suppressed significantly the blood glucose level 15 and 30 min after the administration, while at the dose of 280 mg/ml, suppression occurred at 15 min (Figure 6). As for AUC, 560 mg/ml group showed significant 23% suppression while 280 mg/ml group showed suppression tendency by 12.2 % although not significant (Figure 7).

Discussion

It was shown that simultaneous administration of ACBT or BTPP and sucrose to C57BL/6J mice, suppressed the increase of blood glucose level, at the dose of 1000 mg/kg for ACBT (Figures 2 and 3) and 560 mg/kg for BTPP (Figures 6 and 7). On the other hand, no significant difference from control was observed in blood insulin level at any time point after the administration of ACBT at 1000 mg/kg (Figures 4 and 5). Insulin is a hormone known to be released upon increase of blood glucose level resulting from the absorption of glucose from intestine then suppress the blood glucose level. Accordingly, no increment of its blood level indicated that ACBT and BTPP suppressed the increase of blood glucose level by inhibiting the absorption of sugar from intestine. These results, i.e., suppression of blood glucose level without increasing insulin blood level strongly suggested that ACBT and BTPP could be effective in treating diabetics and pre-diabetics who are insulin resistant or insulin secretion incompetent [28].

We also showed that, *in vitro*, ACBT, BTPP and fractions derived thereof inhibited a rat intestine α-glucosidase, sucrase. Contribution of TFs-poor fraction was shown to be much more than TFs-rich fraction to the enzyme inhibitory activity of ACBT and BTPP (Table 2).

In the present study, we focused on sucrose and successfully showed that black tea fractionation products, suppressed absorption of sucrose by inhibiting sucrase. In the future studies, it would be interesting to

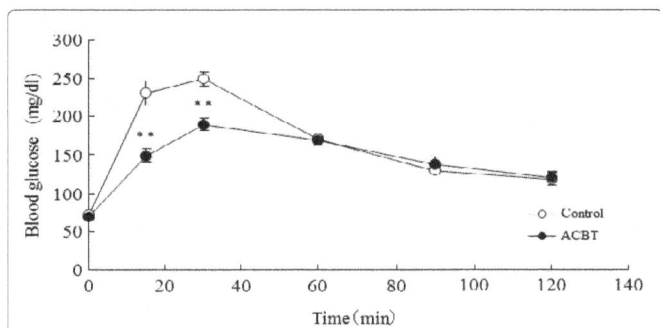

The mice (n = 8 per group) were administered water (control) or ACBT at a concentration of 1000 mg/kg body weight. Blood glucose levels were measured pre (0), 15, 30, 60, 90 and 120 min after sucrose loading. Values are presented as means ± SEM. ＊＊ p< 0.01, relative to the control by an unpaired t-test.

Figure 2: Effect of oral administration of ACBT on blood glucose after sucrose loading in C57/BL6 mice.

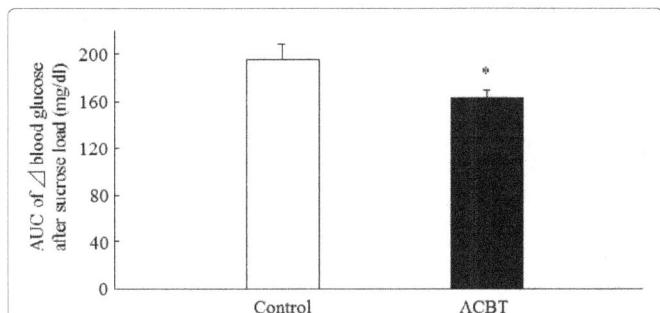

AUC of blood glucose in the experiment depicted in Figure 2 was calculated and shown. Values are presented as means ± SEM. *p < 0.05, relative to the control by an unpaired t-test.

Figure 3: Effect of oral administration of ACBT on blood glucose AUC after sucrose loading in C57/BL6 mice.

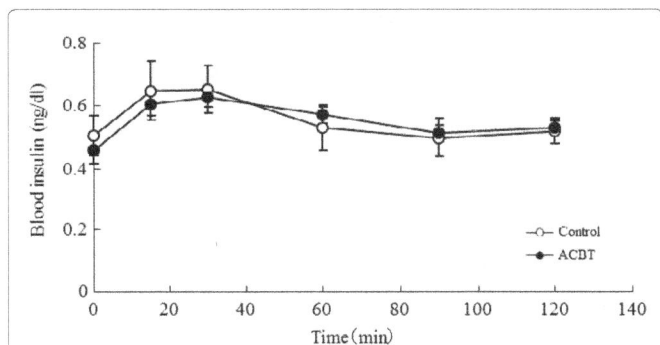

In the experiment depicted in Figure 2, blood insulin levels were measured pre (0), 15, 30, 60, 90 and 120 min after sucrose loading. Values are presented as means ± SEM.

Figure 4: Effect of oral administration of ACBT on blood insulin after sucrose loading in C57/BL6 mice.

test the effectiveness towards other sugars, e.g., starch, maltose and so on, which would lead to better understanding of the mode of action.

Resistant maltodextrin softens the rise of after-meal blood glucose level and thus, in metabolic syndrome patients if taken for 12 weeks with meals improved before-meal blood glucose level and the homeostasis model assessment ratio (HOMA-R), an index of insulin resistance, in comparison with placebo group [29]. Likewise, BTPP which we showed in the present study to suppress the rise of blood

glucose level induced by food intake, would affect before-meal blood glucose level and insulin resistance, if taken with each meal for a long time.

Many studies have been reported to show the relation between obesity and black tea extracts and polyphenols contained. Because many reports are on the effects of black tea extracts on lipid absorption through inhibition of fat degrading enzyme, lipase and on lipid metabolism, possibility that BTPP of our current interest might exert similar effects on after-meal lipids are suggested. Further studies are definitely needed to verify the possibility. As the active substances responsible for the above mentioned anti-obesity effects, catechins, e.g., EC, ECG, EGC and EGCG, TFs and other black tea specific polyphenols are listed [30-33].

Present study focused on sugars, especially sucrose and showed that while the active substances in BTPP were in TFs-poor fraction in addition to TFs, the contribution to the total enzyme inhibitory activity of BTPP was much more from the former than from the latter. TFs-poor fraction is a mixture of, in addition to TF, substances known as thearubigins whose structure is complex and several model compounds are proposed. From ^{1}H NMR analysis of BTPP, presence of many substances having flavan-3-ol and benzotropolone ring [32] was shown indicating the presence of benzotropolone ring containing substances other than TFs (Figure 1). In this respect, it is of interest to note that black tea extract and its fractions are known to have inhibitory activities over α-amylase and lipase, and polymer-like oxidation products are considered to be active compounds [32].

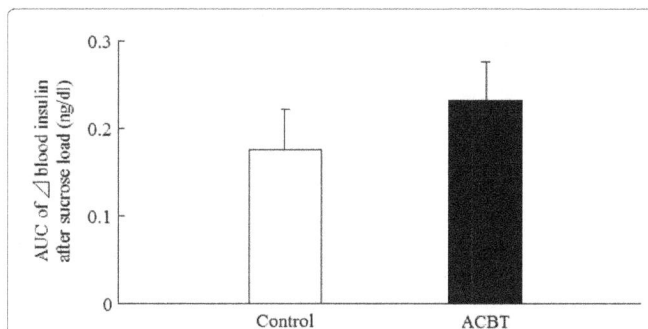

AUC of blood insulin in the experiment depicted in Figure 4 was calculated and shown. Values are presented as means ± SEM.

Figure 5: Effect of oral administration of ACBT on blood insulin AUC after sucrose loading in C57/BL6 mice.

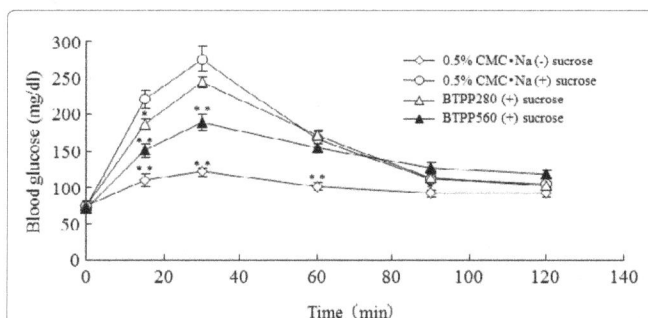

The mice (n = 8 per group) were administered 0.5% CMC·Na as control or BTPP at a concentration of 280, 560 mg/kg body weight. Blood glucose levels were measured pre (0), 15, 30, 60, 90 and 120 min after sucrose loading. Values are presented as means ± SEM. *p < 0.05, ＊＊ p< 0.01, relative to the control (one-way ANOVA followed by Dunnett's test).

Figure 6: Effect of oral administration of BTPP on blood glucose after sucrose loading in C57/BL6 mice.

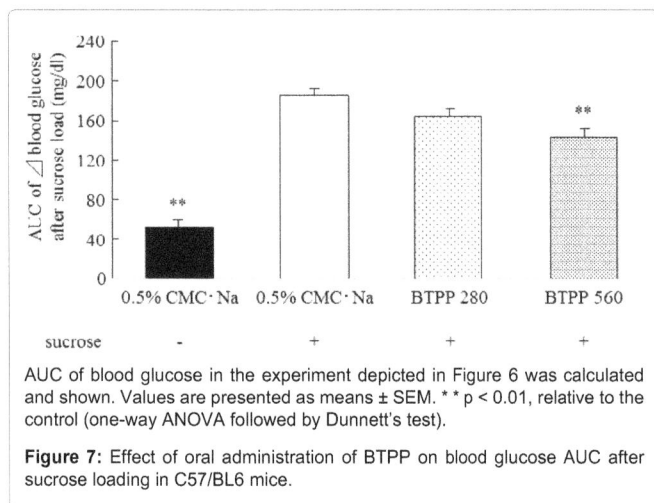

AUC of blood glucose in the experiment depicted in Figure 6 was calculated and shown. Values are presented as means ± SEM. * * p < 0.01, relative to the control (one-way ANOVA followed by Dunnett's test).

Figure 7: Effect of oral administration of BTPP on blood glucose AUC after sucrose loading in C57/BL6 mice.

In Figures 4 and 5 BTPP didn't affect insulinemia. However, blood glucose (as AUC) is about 20% reduced by its administration. Because insulin is released in proportion to the variation in blood glucose levels, insulin-independent glucose uptake is expected. Glucagon-like peptide-1 (GLP-1) is secreted from the small and large intestines in specialized intestinal L-cells. It increases following nutrient ingestion, stimulates glucose-dependent insulin release [34,35]. In addition, GLP-1 effects on peripheral tissues other than the pancreas, biological actions of GLP-1 or GLP-1 receptor agonists are mediated via direct (in pancreas, brain, kidney, and heart) or indirect (in stomach, liver, skeletal muscle, and adipose tissue) mechanisms [36]. In further research, we need to measure whether BTPP stimulates releasing GLP-1. In addition, poorly absorbed polyphenols such as flavan-3-ols, especially procyanidins have been reported that activate AMPK in skeletal or gastrocnemius muscle mediated vagal nerve [37]. BTPP may activate AMPK in the non-insulin-dependent manner, enhance translocation of GLUT4 to cell membrane. Further research is required in order to find out this mechanism.

Conclusion

ACBT inhibited sucrose-loading induced increase in blood glucose level, and majority of active substances were in BTPP. Main mechanism of the activity was the inhibition of sucrase resulting in glucose absorption suppression. Large contribution of TFs-poor fraction to the enzyme inhibitory activity and the presence of benzotropolone ring containing substances therein were shown.

Acknowledgements

We would like to thank Dr. H. Matsuda, Professor of Kyoto Pharmaceutical University, division of Medicinal Chemical Sciences - Pharmacognosy (Japan) and Dr. T. Iwashita, Suntory Foundation for Life Science (Japan) for valuable advices on measurement of α-glucosidase activity and on NMR study, respectively. We also thank to Mr. S. Nonaka and Ms. I. Misawa, Suntory Beverage & Food Ltd. for developing ACBT, to Mr. A. Ogaki, Mr. A. Mukai, Ms. N. Hiraki, Ms. S. Koido, Mr. T. Kondo and Mr. K. Kirimura, Suntory Global Innovation Center Limited. (Japan) for special support in in vitro and in vivo study, to Dr. T. Ohkuri, Suntory Global Innovation Center Limited. (Japan) for support in writing this paper.

References:

1. Ng M, Fleming T, Robinson M, Thomson B, Graetz N, et al. (2014) Global, regional, and national prevalence of overweight and obesity in children and adults during 1980–2013: a systematic analysis for the Global Burden of Disease Study 2013. Lancet 384: 766–781.

2. Haslam DW, James WP (2005) Obesity Lancet 366: 1197-1209.

3. Yoshikawa M, Pongpiriyadacha Y, Kishi A, Kageura T, Wang T, et al. (2003) Biological activities of Salacia chinensis originating in Thailand: the quality evaluation guided by alpha-glucosidase inhibitory activity. Yakugaku Zasshi 123: 871-880.

4. Yamashita Y, Okabe M, Natsume M, Ashida H (2012) Cacao liquor procyanidin extract improves glucose tolerance by enhancing GLUT4 translocation and glucose uptake in skeletal muscle. J Nutr Sci 1, e2: 1-9.

5. Cabrera C, Artacho R, Giménez R (2006) Beneficial effects of green tea--a review. J Am Coll Nutr 25: 79-99.

6. Westerterp-Plantenga MS (2010) Green tea catechins, caffeine and body-weight regulation. Physiol Behav 100: 42-46.

7. Zheng XX, Xu YL, Li SH, Liu XX, Hui R, et al. (2011) Green tea intake lowers fasting serum total and LDL cholesterol in adults: a meta-analysis of 14 randomized controlled trials. Am J Clin Nutr 94: 601-610.

8. Nakai M, Fukui Y, Asami S, Toyoda-Ono Y, Iwashita T, et al. (2005) Inhibitory effects of oolong tea polyphenols on pancreatic lipase in vitro. J Agric Food Chem 53: 4593-4598.

9. Toyoda-Ono Y, Yoshimura M, Nakai M, Fukui Y, Asami S, et al. (2007) Suppression of postprandial hypertriglyceridemia in rats and mice by oolong tea polymerized polyphenols. Biosci Biotechnol Biochem 71: 971-976.

10. Kurihara H, Fukami H, Koda H, Tsuruoka N, Sugiura N, et al. (2002) Effects of oolong tea on metabolism of plasma fat in mice under restraint stress. Biosci Biotechnol Biochem 66: 1955-1958.

11. Kurihara H, Fukami H, Asami S, Toyoda Y, Nakai M, et al. (2004) Effects of oolong tea on plasma antioxidative capacity in mice loaded with restraint stress assessed using the oxygen radical absorbance capacity (ORAC) assay. Biol Pharm Bull 27: 1093-1098.

12. Hosoda K, Wang MF, Liao ML, Chuang CK, Iha M, et al. (2003) Antihyperglycemic effect of oolong tea in type 2 diabetes. Diabetes Care 26: 1714-1718.

13. Chen QK, Chen ZM (1994) Tea and Health. In: Functional Foods of the East. CRC Press, Boca Raton, FL.

14. Benzie IF, Szeto YT (1999) Total antioxidant capacity of teas by the ferric reducing/antioxidant power assay. J Agric Food Chem 47: 633-636.

15. Kurihara H, Fukami H, Toyoda Y, Kageyama N, Tsuruoka N, et al. (2003) Inhibitory effect of oolong tea on the oxidative state of low density lipoprotein (LDL). Biol Pharm Bull 26: 739-742.

16. Nishiumi S, Bessyo H, Kubo M, Aoki Y, Tanaka A, et al. (2010) Green and black tea suppress hyperglycemia and insulin resistance by retaining the expression of glucose transporter 4 in muscle of high-fat diet-fed C57BL/6J mice. J Agric Food Chem 58: 12916-12923.

17. Yamashita Y, Wang L, Tinshun Z, Nakamura T, Ashida H (2012) Fermented tea improves glucose intolerance in mice by enhancing translocation of glucose transporter 4 in skeletal muscle. J Agric Food Chem 60: 11366-11371.

18. Haslam E (2003) Thoughts on thearubigins. Phytochemistry 64: 61-73.

19. Miyata Y, Tamaru S, Tanaka T, Tamaya K, Matsui T, et al. (2013) Theflavins and theasinensin A derived from fermented tea have antihyperglycemic and hypotriacylglycerolemic effects in KK-A(y) mice and Sprague-Dawley rats. J Agric Food Chem 61: 9366-9372.

20. Jhoo JW, Lo CY, Li S, Sang S, Ang CY, et al. (2005) Stability of black tea polyphenol, theaflavin, and identification of theanaphthoquinone as its major radical reaction product. J Agric Food Chem 53: 6146-6150.

21. Yoshikawa M, Murakami T, Shimada H, Matsuda H, Yamahara J, et al. (1997) Salacinol, potent antidiabetic principle with unique thiosugar sulfonium sulfate structure from the Ayurvedic traditional medicine Salacia reticulata in Sri Lanka and India. Tetrahedron Lett 38: 8367-8370.

22. Yoshikawa M, Murakami T, Yashiro K, Matsuda H (1998) Kotalanol, a potent alpha-glucosidase inhibitor with thiosugar sulfonium sulfate structure, from antidiabetic ayurvedic medicine Salacia reticulata. Chem Pharm Bull (Tokyo) 46: 1339-1340.

23. Yoshikawa M, Morikawa T, Matsuda H, Tnabe G, Muraoka O (2002) Absolute Stereostructure of Potent a-Glucosidase Inhibitor, Salacinol, with Unique Thiosugar Sulfonium Sulfate Inner Salt Structure from Salacia reticulate. Bioorganic & Medicinal Chemistry 10: 1547-1554.

24. Matsuda H, Murakami T, Yashiro K, Yamahara J, Yoshikawa M (1999) Antidiabetic principles of natural medicines. IV. Aldose reductase and alpha-glucosidase inhibitors from the roots of Salacia oblonga Wall. (Celastraceae):

structure of a new friedelane-type triterpene, kotalagenin 16-acetate. Chem Pharm Bull (Tokyo) 47: 1725-1729.

25. Matsuda H, Morikawa T, Yoshikawa M (2002) Antidiabetogenic constituents from several natural medicines. Pure Appl. Chem. 74(7): 1301-1308.

26. Goda T (2000) Regulation of the expression of carbohydrate digestion/absorption-related genes. Br J Nutr 84 Suppl 2: S245-248.

27. Honma K, Mochizuki K, Goda T (2007) Carbohydrate/fat ratio in the diet alters histone acetylation on the sucrase-isomaltase gene and its expression in mouse small intestine. Biochem Biophys Res Commun 357: 1124-1129.

28. Amy Hui-Mei Lina, Byung-Hoo Leeb, Wei-Jen Chang (2016) Small intestine mucosal a-glucosidase: A missing feature of in vitro starch digestibility. Food Hydrocoll. 53: 163-171.

29. Al-Goblan AS, Al-Alfi MA, Khan MZ (2014) Mechanism linking diabetes mellitus and obesity. Diabetes Metab Syndr Obes 7: 587-591.

30. Hashizume C, Kishimoto Y, Kanahori S, Yamamoto T, Okuma K, et al. (2012) Improvement effect of resistant maltodextrin in humans with metabolic syndrome by continuous administration. J Nutr Sci Vitaminol (Tokyo). 58: 423-430.

31. Uchiyama S, Taniguchi Y, Saka A, Yoshida A, Yajima H (2011) Prevention of diet-induced obesity by dietary black tea polyphenols extract in vitro and in vivo. Nutrition 27: 287-292.

32. Kobayashi M, Ichitani M, Suzuki Y, Unno T, Sugawara T, et al. (2009) Black-tea polyphenols suppress postprandial hypertriacylglycerolemia by suppressing lymphatic transport of dietary fat in rats. J Agric Food Chem 57: 7131-7136.

33. Kusano R, Andou H, Fujieda M, Tanaka T, Matsuo Y, et al. (2008) Polymer-like polyphenols of black tea and their lipase and amylase inhibitory activities. Chem Pharm Bull (Tokyo) 56: 266-272.

34. Fukui Y, Asami S, Maeda M (2010) Anti-Obesity Agent Comprising Compound Containing Benzotropolone Ring, WO2010/134595

35. Lovshin JA, Drucker DJ (2009) Incretin-based therapies for type 2 diabetes mellitus. Nat Rev Endocrinol 5: 262-269.

36. Tsuda T (2015) Possible abilities of dietary factors to prevent and treat diabetes via the stimulation of glucagon-like peptide-1 secretion. Mol Nutr Food Res 59: 1264-1273.

37. Matsumura Y, Nakagawa Y, Mikome K, Yamamoto H, Osakabe N (2014) Enhancement of energy expenditure following a single oral dose of flavan-3-ols associated with an increase in catecholamine secretion. PLoS One 9: e112180.

5

Carbonic Anhydrase: A New Therapeutic Target for Managing Diabetes

Ibrahim S Ismail*, Ameh D Amodu, Atawodi S Ene-ojoh and Umar I Alhaji

Department of Biochemistry, Ahmadu Bello University Zaria, Nigeria

Abstract

Background: Carbonic Anhydrase (CA) is a zinc metallo-enzyme that is critical to regulation of systemic acid-base homeostasis by facilitating urinary acidification. Inhibition of carbonic anhydrase results in metabolic acidosis which leads to decrease in pH.

Aim and objectives: The study aims to highlight the potential utility of erythrocyte carbonic anhydrase as therapeutic target for managing diabetes, by investigating changes of erythrocyte carbonic anhydrase activity in STZ induced diabetic rats.

Methods: Carbonic anhydrase activity was determined by the absorbance of p-nitrophenol at 345nm released from p-nitrophenyl acetate. HbA1c was determined by ion exchange method (Spectrum diagnostics). Biochemical parameters were determined by Accutrend GCT meters with cobias® test strips.

Results: The result revealed that inhibition of erythrocyte carbonic anhydrase results in significant increase in both blood lactate concentration and HbA1c level with significant reduction in blood glucose concentration. Metformin was found to reduce carbonic anhydrase activity and HbA1c level significantly and increased blood lactate concentration. The extract of Cadaba farinosa was found to reduce blood glucose concentration.

Conclusions: Inhibition of carbonic anhydrase can be associated with reduced circulating blood glucose level. Metformin may therefore reduce circulating blood glucose by inhibiting carbonic anhydrase. Increased level of HbA1c may probably be due to inhibition of erythrocyte carbonic anhydrase. Therefore Carbonic anhydrase can potentially serve as a therapeutic target for managing diabetes in combination as serving as valuable marker for lactic acidosis.

Keywords: Carbonic anhydrase; HbA1c; Lactate; Diabetes; Metformin; *Cadaba farinose*

Introduction

Carbonic anhydrases (CAs) are ubiquitous zinc metalloenzymes that primarily catalyze the reversible hydration of carbon dioxide to form bicarbonate and protons, a reversible reaction that occurs relatively slowly in the absence of a catalyst [1,2]. Several important physiological and pathological functions are played by the CA isozymes present in organisms, this includes transport of CO_2 and ions (such as H^+, Na^+ and Cl^-) along with pH-regulation in a variety of physiological processes ranging from respiration to intermediary metabolism at the cellular level [3,4]. These enzymes play very important role in providing bicarbonate as substrate for carboxylation in different essential metabolic pathways which include gluconeogenesis and synthesis of some amino acids (pyruvate carboxylase) lipogenesis (pyruvate carboxylase and acetyl coA carboxylase), ureagenesis (carbamoyl synthase I) and pyrimidine synthesis (Carbamoyl phosphate synthase II) [5]. Carbonic anhydrase is found in the blood of all vertebrates. Some early evidences suggest that the changes in carbonic anhydrases activities in erythrocytes may be an initial step of altered metabolism in diabetes mellitus [6]. However, the precise role of Carbonic anhydrase activity, in the development of diabetes mellitus, is currently unknown. It has been reported that inhibition of Carbonic anhydrase was found to impair proton secretion into the proximal tubule lumen and thereby decreased bicarbonate reabsorbtion and rate of acidification of urine, producing alkaline urine and eventually metabolic acidosis [7]. Carbonic anhydrase inhibitors are widely used in clinical practice as diuretics and antihypertensive drugs [8]. Recent studies showed that carbonic anhydrase inhibitors may provide a novel therapy for obesity, cancer, infection and Alzheimer's disease. However, as carbonic anhydrase are ubiquitous enzymes in vertebrates, carbonic anhydrase inhibition in organs other than the target may result in undesired side effects. The most frequent ones are: numbness and tingling of extremities; metallic taste; depression; fatigue; malaise; weight loss; decreased libido; gastrointestinal irritation; metabolic acidosis; renal calculi and transient myopia [9-12], which are all common among diabetic patients.

Metabolic acidosis is the most common serious acid-base disorder complicating diabetes mellitus. Metabolic acidosis is associated with increased mortality [13]. Lactic acidosis results in higher mortality than metabolic acidosis of a different etiology [14]. Lactic acidosis is an alarming metabolic signal of many pathological states, and endogenous clearance of lactate is a commonly used prognostic marker of illness [15]. When glucose disposal is stimulated with insulin, plasma lactate concentration increases and the concentration is positively correlated with the rate of glucose disposal [16]. In STZ induced diabetes (which is a model of type 1 diabetes) resting blood lactate is reported to be elevated [17,18], and STZ induced diabetes in rats has also been found to decrease skeletal muscle lactate transport [17]. Studies have shown that mono-carboxylate transporters (MCT) dependent lactate-H^+ flux is facilitated by bicarbonate transporters and carbonic anhydrase enzyme in various cells and tissue [19,20]. Accumulating evidence implicates changes in carbonic anhydrase activity in diabetes. This notion has not been adequately studied. Our present study aimed to study these changes and to highlight the potential usage of carbonic anhydrase as a new enzyme therapeutic target for managing diabetes;

*Corresponding author:** Ibrahim Salihu Ismail, Department of Biochemistry, Ahmadu Bello University Zaria, Nigeria, E-mail: salihuringim@yahoo.com

by analyzing changes in erythrocyte carbonic anhydrase activity in uncontrolled and treated STZ induced diabetic rats.

Materials and Methods

Preparation of extract of *cadaba farinosa* leaves

Cadaba farinosa leaves were collected and authenticated at the Biological science Department of Ahmadu Bello University Zaria, Nigeria. A voucher number was given as no. 2744 and was deposited at the herbarium of the department. The leaves were, washed, air-dried at room temperature, grinded to powder. The crude extract was obtained through successive soxhlet extraction by dissolving 800 g of powdered plant leaves in 2.5L of n-Hexane followed by ethyl acetate and finally methanol for 48 hours each in a soxhlet apparatus. The crude fractions were concentrated using rotary evaporator and stored in a dessicator until use.

Study animals

Male Wister albino rats of 180–220 grams weight were used for this study. Before initiation, the rats were allowed acclimatization period of 7 days in laboratory condition. Five rats each were housed in polycarbonate cages bedding with husk, 20 to 24°C temperature and relative humidity between 30 to 70 percent. The dark and light cycle of 12 hours each was maintained. Standard animal diet with pure water in glass bottles ad libitum were fed to the animals. The principles of laboratory animal care were followed according to the instructions by the Institutional Animal Ethics Committee.

Induction of diabetes: Diabetes was induced in all the rats except in the normal controls (Group I) by Streptozotocin(STZ) 60 mg per kg body weight, dissolved in ice cold citrate buffer (0.1 M, pH 4.5), through intraperitoneal route. Hyperglycemia was confirmed by elevated fasting glucose level >200 mg/dl in plasma, determined at 72 h after injection. Hyperglycemic rats were included for the study along with the normal control animals.

Study design: The animals were grouped into five groups of five rats each. Group I rats (Normal control); Group II (Diabetic control); Group III (Diabetic rats treated with Acetazolamide, 250 mg/kg/day for 28 days); Group IV (Diabetic rats treated with Metformin, 500 mg/kg/day for 28 days) and Group V (Diabetic rats treated with methanol extract of *Cadaba farinosa* leaves 1 g/kg/day for 28 days). Both animals were fed with standard animal feed mentioned above and distilled water. But Group I (Normal control) and Group II (Diabetic control) rats received only water at the time of treatment of other groups.

Collection and preparation of samples: The blood samples were collected by cardiac puncture in vials with EDTA and centrifuged at 3500 rpm for 10 minutes. The plasma was separated from the cells and buffy coat removed. The packed red cells were washed three times with normal saline (0.9% NaCl) and were lysed with ice cold water, yielding destroyed plasma membranes.

Biochemical analysis

Metabolic parameters: Blood glucose, lactate, cholesterol and triglycerides levels were measured using (Accutrend GCT Meter, Roche, Germany with Cobas test strips)

Glycosylated haemoglobin determination: HbA1c was estimated by ion exchange methods using standard reagent kits, according to the manufacturers' instruction, (Spectrum-diagnostics, Egypt).

Assay of carbonic anhydrase activity: Carbonic anhydrase activity was determined as mentioned by [21], with the modification described by [22] using spectrophotometer. In this assay, the esterase activity of carbonic anhydrase was determined from the hydrolysis rate of 3mM p-nitrophenyl acetate to p-nitrophenol. The assay system contained 100 µL hemolysate placed in 1 cm spectrometric cell containing 1.4 ml 0.05 M Tris- HCl buffer, pH: 7.4 and 1.5ml p-nitrophenyl acetate. The change in absorbance at 348 nm was measured over the period of 3 min before and after adding the sample. The absorbance was measured by a UV-Vis spectrophotometer (Shimadzu UV-2600 Spectrophotometer). One unit of enzyme activity was expressed as µmol of p-nitrophenol relased/min/µL from hemolysate at room temperature (25°C) [6,23].

Statistical analysis: Results were presented as mean ± standard Deviation (SD). Within and between groups, comparisons were performed by the analysis of variance (ANOVA) (using SPSS 20.0 for windows Computer Software Package). Significant differences were compared by Duncan's new Multiple Range test; a probability level of less than 5% ($P<0.05$) was considered significant.

Results

Acetazolamide reduces blood glucose; increases blood lactate and HbA1c level in STZ induced diabetic rats

We examined whether inhibition of carbonic anhydrase in STZ induced diabetic rats affects blood glucose, blood lactate and HbA1c level. Acetazolamide treated STZ induced diabetic rats at 250 mg/kg/day for 28 days resulted in 3 fold significant ($p<0.05$) increase in HbA1c when compared with normal control rats (Figure 1). Blood lactate was also significantly ($p<0.05$) increased 4 fold in STZ induced diabetic rats treated with Acetazolamide when compared with normal control (Figure 2). Blood glucose level reduced significantly ($p<0.05$) in STZ induced diabetic rats treated with acetazolamide when compared with normal control (Figure 3).

Metformin suppresses carbonic anhydrase activity; increases blood lactate and reduces HbA1c level in STZ induced diabetic rats

We treated STZ induced diabetic rats with Metformin 1000 mg/kg/day for 28 days. Significant ($p<0.05$) reduction in both blood glucose and HbA1c level was observed when compared with normal control (Figure 3). Metformin also significantly ($p<0.05$) reduces carbonic anhydrase activity when compared with normal control (Figure 4).

***Cadaba farinosa* extract lowers blood glucose and glycated hemoglobin (HbA1c) level in STZ induced diabetic rats:** To investigate the effect of crude methanol extract of *Cadaba farinosa* on STZ induced diabetic rats, the level of glucose and HbA1c were measured. The extract (1000 mg/kg/day for 28 days) significantly ($p<0.05$) reduces the level of blood glucose and HbA1c level when compared with diabetic control (Figure 2 and 3). Though, the reduction of HbA1c was not significant when compared with the diabetic control (Figure 1).

***Cadaba farinosa* extract affects carbonic anhydrase activity and blood lactate level in STZ induced diabetic rats:** We examined whether *cadaba farinosa* crude methanol extract affect carbonic anhydrase activity in the erythrocytes of STZ induced diabetic rats. The result showed a significant ($p<0.05$) reduction in carbonic anhydrase activity of the extract treated STZ induced diabetic rat when compared with normal control but a significant ($p<0.05$) increase in carbonic anhydrase activity was observed when compared with

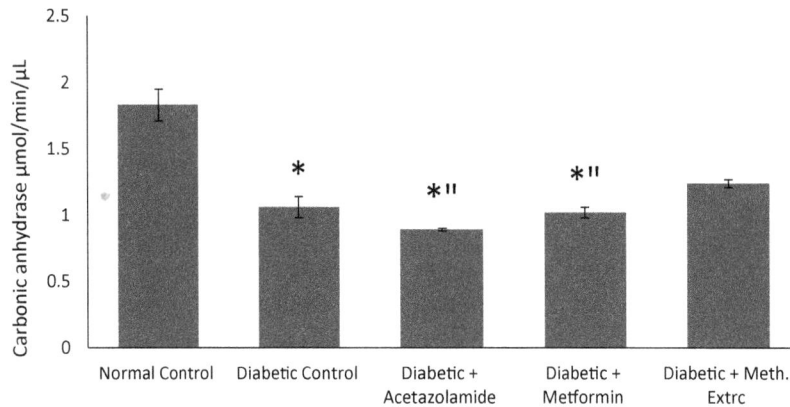

Figure 1: The effect of Acetazolamide, Metformin and Methanol extract of *Cadaba farinosa* on carbonic anhydrase activity levels in STZ induced diabetic rats treated at 250 mg/kg/day, 500 mg/kg/day and 1000 mg/kg/day doses for 28 days. *P<0.05 vs. Normal control; "P<0.05 vs. Diabetic control (n=5).

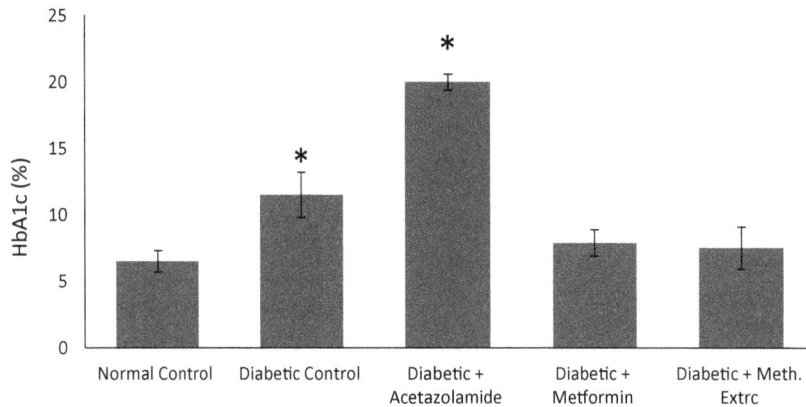

Figure 2: The effect of Acetazolamide, Metformin and Methanol extract of *Cadaba farinosa* on HBA$_{1c}$ levels in STZ induced diabetic rats treated at 250 mg/kg/day, 500 mg/kg/day and 1000 mg/kg/day doses for 28 days. *P <0.05 vs. Normal control; "P<0.05 vs. Diabetic control (n=5).

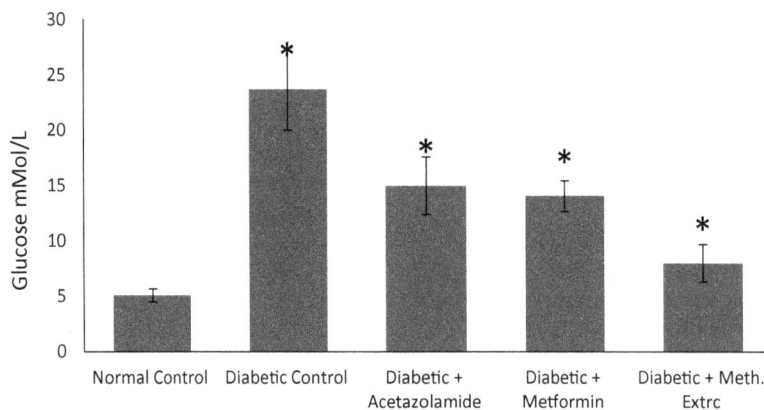

Figure 3: The effect of Acetazolamide, Metformin and Methanol extract of *Cadaba farinosa* on Glucose levels in STZ induced diabetic rats treated at 250 mg/kg/day, 500 mg/kg/day and 1000 mg/kg/day doses for 28 days. *P<0.05 vs. Normal control; "P<0.05 vs. Diabetic control (n=5).

uncontrolled diabetic control (Figure 4). Even though the change in lactate concentration was not significant when compared with both the normal and diabetic control, but lactate level increases in the extract treated diabetic group when compared with normal control and decreases when compared with diabetic control (Figure 2).

Acetazolamide, Metformin and *Cadaba farinosa* extract also affect blood cholesterol and Triglycerides levels in STZ induced diabetic rats

Figure 5 indicates, Acetazolamide and Metformin significantly (p<0.05) reduced blood cholesterol level (Figures 5 and 6), while blood

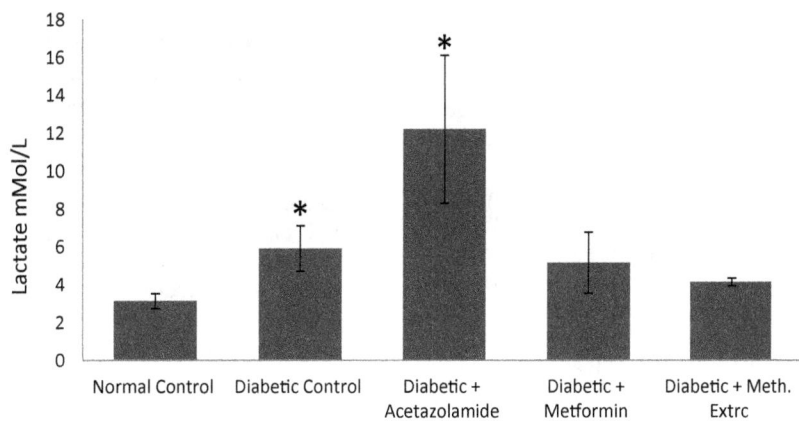

Figure 4: The effect of Acetazolamide, Metformin and Methanol extract of *Cadaba farinosa* on Lactate levels in STZ induced diabetic rats treated at 250 mg/kg/day, 500 mg/kg/day and 1000 mg/kg/day doses for 28 days. *P<0.05 vs. Normal control, (n=5).

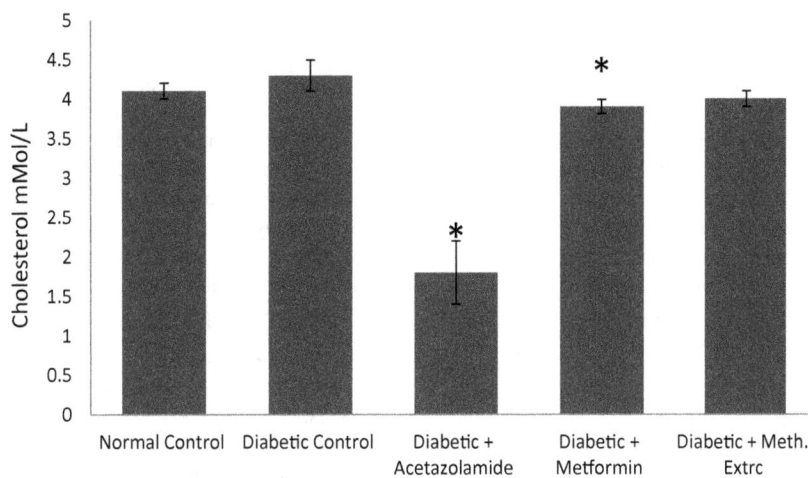

Figure 5: The effect of Acetazolamide, Metformin and Methanol extract of *Cadaba farinosa* on Cholesterol levels in STZ induced diabetic rats treated at 250 mg/kg/day, 500 mg/kg/day and 1000 mg/kg/day doses for 28 days. *P<0.05 vs. Normal control, (n=5).

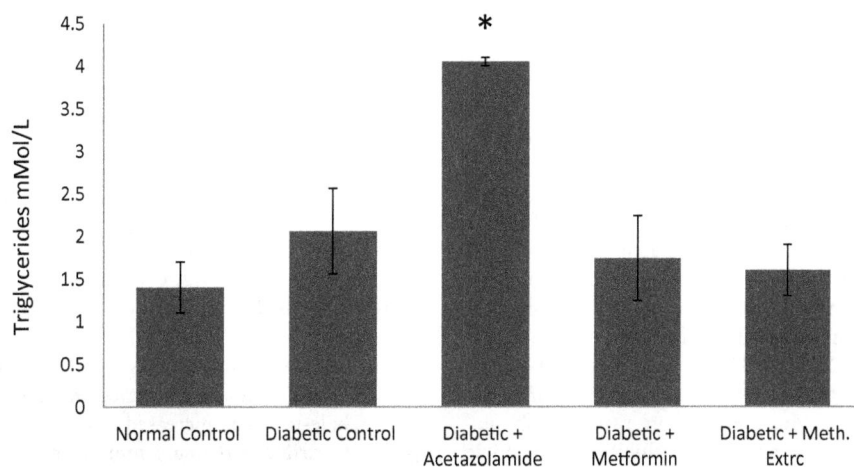

Figure 6: The effect of Acetazolamide, Metformin and Methanol extract of *Cadaba farinosa* on Triglycerides levels in STZ induced diabetic rats treated at 250 mg/kg/day, 500 mg/kg/day and 1000 mg/kg/day doses for 28 days. *P<0.05 vs. Normal control, (n=5).

triglycerides level increased significantly (p<0.05) under the effect of Acetazolamide (Figure 6).

Discussion

Our present research findings demonstrated that, prolonged untreated diabetes result in decreased carbonic anhydrase activity. [23] previously examined the changes in the activity of CA-III in hepatocytes of acute diabetic rats. Diabetes resulted in 50% reduction in the activity of CA-III. They also observed an approx. 98% reduction in CA-III content in the liver of chronic diabetes mellitus rats relative to controls. A 75% reduction in serum CA-III content was observed relative to control values after the administration of streptozotocin. The increased blood lactate level observed in the present study is consistent with the findings of [24,25] who showed that lactate is not only increased in the early stages of diabetes but has also been shown to predict its occurrence in the future. Forbath and De Meutter [26,27], had also reported that there is an increase in lactate production, in diabetic dogs and humans.

We investigated the role of carbonic anhydrase activity in diabetes by inhibiting the enzyme with a known inhibitor (Acetazolamide), and interestingly we found out that carbonic anhydrase inhibition in STZ induced diabetic rats' lowers blood glucose level. Previous published studies have provided mixed results regarding the potential of carbonic anhydrase inhibitors to modulate blood glucose levels. Acetazolamide and ethoxyzolamide were found to inhibit gluconeogenesis in vitro or after acute administration in rats [28-30]. [28] concluded that carbonic anhydrase is functionally important for gluconeogenesis in the male guinea pig liver when there is a requirement for bicarbonate as substrate. We may therefore suggest that carbonic anhydrase plays a crucial role in gluconeogenesis, due to the fact that carbonic anhydrase inhibition does not only lowers blood glucose level but increases blood lactate level as well. Many studies have demonstrated that suppression of hepatic gluconeogenesis is accompanied by increased blood lactate level as seen in metformin treatment of type II diabetes. High therapeutic metformin levels provoked a reduction in lactate uptake by the liver [31]. A potentially life-threatening complication of Metformin is the occurrence of lactic acidosis, metformin-associated lactic acidosis (MALA). To reproduce the result, we treated STZ induced diabetic rats with Metformin 500 mg/kg/day for 28 days in order to investigate the effect of Metformin on carbonic anhydrase activity and blood lactate level. For the first time our present study demonstrates that Metformin significantly (p<0.05) reduced carbonic anhydrase activity and increased blood lactate level.

However, the magnitude of the efflux of lactate into the bloodstream, which is the anionic form of lactic acid, may override the body's ability to utilize protons, hence converting hyperlactatemia into lactic acidosis. Indeed, it has been proposed that increased muscle release of lactate and alanine could be responsible for sustaining increased gluconeogenesis in NIDDM [32]. Since increased provision of lactate is of considerable importance for the increased gluconeogenesis found in diabetes. Similarly, carbonic anhydrase has been found to facilitate lactic acid transport in rat skeletal muscle fibers [33]. It's also reported that MCT1 and MCT4 transport activity is increased by interaction with carbonic anhydrase II (CAII) [20,34,35]. Since monocarboxylate (MCT) dependent lactate-H^+ flux is facilitated by bicarbonate transporters and carbonic anhydrase activity in various cells and tissues [33-37]. We may therefore report that inhibition of carbonic anhydrase may impair lactate flux across the MCT's in various cells and tissues. We may therefore suggest that the reported incidence of lactic acidosis that occur with Metformin therapy in type II diabetes might be the result of suppressed carbonic anhydrase activity.

It has been stated previously that the activity of carbonic anhydrase has reduced significantly in the liver of both acute and chronic streptozotocin induced diabetic rats. The ability of Metformin to inhibit carbonic anhydrase in diabetic rats points towards a negative change that indicates a powerful effect on aspects of the complex metabolic disturbance in diabetes. Therefore carbonic anhydrase could be a new enzymatic therapeutic target for managing diabetes.

The ability of metformin to lower circulating blood glucose levels in type II diabetic patients can be explained by various mechanisms, such as increased glucose uptake in liver and muscle, reduced gluconeogenesis, decreased lactate and alanine uptake, improved GLP-1 and reduced glucagon functions. Nevertheless, the molecular principles of metformin action remain debated.

The overall effect of the metformin action is that, metformin inhibits gluconeogenic enzymes and stimulates glycolysis by altering the activity of multiple enzymes in gluconeogenesis, glycogenolysis, ketogenesis and β-Oxidation pathways [38]. Gluconeogenesis accounts for 28-97% of overall hepatic glucose output depending on the feeding status in nondiabetic individuals, the rate being higher in patients with advanced type 2 diabetes mellitus [39]. Metformin was reported to reduce hepatic glucose output by up to 75% [40].

The uptake of gluconeogenic substrates, such as alanine and lactate, is reduced in the presence of metformin [41]. The effects of metformin on hepatic glycogen metabolism are not well-established; however, in vitro treatment of hepatocytes decreased glycogen synthesis [42]. With these various unestablished proposed mechanisms of metformin action, we may therefore propose that metformin reduces circulating blood glucose level due to inhibition of carbonic anhydrase, which facilitate lactate (a gluconeogenic substrate) uptake by the hepatocytes for the synthesis of glucose.

Metahonl leaf extract of Cadaba farinosa, lowers blood glucose level significantly (p<0.05) in STZ induced diabetic rats when compared with diabetic control. This similar trend has been observed with metformin treatment, an established hypoglycemic agent. Leaf extract of Cadaba farinosa is being used for the treatment of cancer and diabetes in some parts of northern Nigeria as folk medicine. We demonstrated for the first time that Cadaba farinosa methanol leaf extract has aminonitrile containing compounds from the FTIR spectra analysis, which showed absorption characteristic bands related to α-aminonitrile at 2226.31 cm^{-1} region which is tentatively assigned to Nitrile group (C≡N) (Data not shown here). Several amino nitriles have been developed as reversible inhibitors of dipeptidyl peptidase (DPP IV) for treating diabetes [43]. Vildagliptin is a recently released aminonitrile-containing antidiabetic drug that inhibits dipeptidyl peptidase IV (DPP-IV). We suggest that, the reduction in blood glucose level may be due to the presence of aminonitrile containing compounds in the leaves, but further research is required on the plant.

Moreover, our study also demonstrates relationship of carbonic anhydrase inhibition with dyslipidemia. Our results show significant decrease in total cholesterol (p<0.05), and significant increase in triglyceride (p<0.05) in STZ induced diabetic rats treated with Acetazolamide. Dyslipidemia is a common finding in diabetes mellitus. Diabetic dyslipidemia is associated with high plasma triglycerides, low HDL-Cholesterol and increased small dense LDL-Cholesterol particles [44]. Hypertriglyceridemia is more common in diabetics as compared to non-diabetics due to four (4) fold increase in VLDL triglyceride [45]. Our result is consistent with the findings above. Previous study reported the role of carbonic anhydrase in hepatic lipogenesis at the level of pyruvate carboxylation [46] and their role in providing bicarbonate as substrate for carboxylation in lipogenesis (pyruvate carboxylase and acetyl coA carboxylase), [5]. If truly carbonic anhydrase is associated with lipogenesis, it's therefore not surprising the changes seen in the level of cholesterol and triglyceride.

The results of the present study showed a 3 fold significant ($p<0.05$) increase in HbA1c level (Figure 2) in STZ induced diabetic rats treated with carbonic anhydrase inhibitor (Acetazolamide). This increase was exclusively as a result of direct inhibition of carbonic anhydrase *invivo*. Carbonic anhydrase has been associated with altered metabolism, because carbonic anhydrase is a pH-regulatory enzyme in most of the tissues including erythrocytes [22,47]. It has been reported that inhibition of carbonic anhydrase was found to impair proton secretion and eventually metabolic acidosis [7]. Metabolic acidosis results in decreased pH level. Several factors have been reported that can influence the rate of glycation of hemoglobin: which are pH [48-50], glucose concentration [48], carbonate [51] and catalysis by 2, 3-diphosphoglycerate [49,52,53] In 1958 [54] published a paper describing the heterogeneity of haemoglobin A. The hemoglobin fractions that eluted at more acidic pH on the anion exchanger carboxy methylcellulose and migrated more rapidly on electrophoresis were called minor haemoglobins or fast haemoglobins. Which could be sub fractionated into the species A (1a), A(1b), A(1c), A(1d). Later this fast haemoglobin was identified as Allen's HbA1c and the charge difference localised to the β chain [55]. Low intracellular pH (pHi) has been reported to increase glycation of hemoglobin as pH levels within the erythrocyte can increase (low erythrocyte pH) or decrease (high erythrocyte pH) HbA1c formation [56]. We may therefore suggest that, the increased HbA1c level seen in diabetes may be attributed to the increased anaerobic glycolysis in erythrocyte which produces lactate as the end product of glycolysis. Red blood cells produce lactic acid as a byproduct of the regeneration of ATP during anaerobic glycolysis but cannot use lactic acid [57]. The rate of production can increase 50-fold if either glucose or glycogen is required to generate ATP in the absence of oxygen [57]. Lactate is transported out of the cell via monocarboxylate transporters (MCT) in an electroneutral transport mode of 1 H^+: 1 Lactate [58].

H^+ transport system under conditions of exclusively aerobic metabolism is used by the cell to maintain a facilitation of CO_2 diffusion, whereas under conditions of dominating anaerobic glycolysis and low intracellular pH, it is mainly used to transport H^+ along with the lactate anion through the monocarboxylate transporters (MCT), a prerequisite for the elimination of lactic acid from the cell. Inhibition of carbonic anhydrase may result in increased intracellular lactate level as has been previously shown, which will lead to lactic acidosis and consequently decreased intracellular pH*i*. The presence of carbonic anhydrase significantly buffers pH*i*, on the other hand disruption of pH*i* via inhibition of Carbonic anhydrase may decrease lactate efflux and result in intracellular lactate accumulation which decreased pH*i*, and enhence increased HbA1c formation.

If what [56] reported is true, then we may conclude that inhibition of intracellular erythrocyte carbonic anhydrase will lead to accumulation of intracellular lactate and result in lactic acidosis which brings about decreased pH (pH*i*). At a low pH even glucose cannot be utilized anaerobically due to the fact that cellular energy production can be compromised in metabolic acidosis [59] as the activity of 6-phosphofructokinase, a critical enzyme in glycolysis, is pH dependent. The net effect is increased formation of HbA1c favored by low pH and continues supply of glucose to erythrocytes due to mass action effect; and also due to blockage of further oxidation of glucose to lactate to prevent further drop in pH.

We concluded that inhibition of carbonic anhydrase can be associated with reduced circulating blood glucose level. Metformin may therefore reduce circulating blood glucose by inhibiting carbonic anhydrase. Cadaba farinosa leaf extract reduces blood glucose level probably by its action on dipeptidyl peptidase IV due to the presence of aminonitrile containing compounds. Increased level of HbA1c may probably be due to inhibition of erythrocyte carbonic anhydrase which lead to decreased pH level.

Acknowledgments

We thank the staff of Animal house, Aliyu, and Salihu for their excellent technical help; and Dr. Auwal Ibrahim for editorial assistance.

References

1. Supuran CT (2007) Carbonic anhydrases as drug targets--an overview. Curr Top Med Chem 7: 825-833.

2. Carter MJ, Parsons DS (1971) The Isoenzymes of Carbonic Anhydrase: Tissue, subcellular Distribution and Functional Significance, with Particular Reference to the Intestinal Tract. J Physiol 215: 71-94.

3. Henry RP (1996) Multiple roles of carbonic anhydrase in cellular transport and metabolism. Annu Rev Physiol 58: 523-538.

4. Zanconato S, Cooper DM, Armon Y, Epstein S (1992) Effect of increased metabolic rate on oxygen isotopic fractionation. Respiration Physiology 89: 319-327.

5. Chegwidden WR, Dodgson SJ, Spencer IM (2000) The roles of carbonic anhydrase in metabolism, cell growth and cancer in animals. EXS: 343-363.

6. Gambhir KK, Oates P, Verma M, Temam S, Cheatham W (1997) High fructose feeding enhances erythrocyte carbonic anhydrase 1 mRNA levels in rat. Ann N Y Acad Sci 827: 163-169.

7. Hannedoeche T, Lazaro M, Delgado AG, Boitard C, Lacour B, et al. (1991) Feedback-mediated reduction in glomerular filtration during acetazolamide infusion in insulin-dependent diabetic patients. Clin Sci 81: 457-464.

8. Pastorekova S, Parkkila S, Pastorek J, Supuran CT (2004) Carbonic anhydrases: current state of the art, therapeutic applications and future prospects. J Enzyme Inhib Med Chem 19: 199-229.

9. Bartlett JD, Jaanus SD (1989) Clinical ocular pharmacology. Elsevier Inc, Butterworth, Boston, USA.

10. Maren TH (1992) Role of carbonic anhydrase in aqueous humor and cerebrospinal fluid formation. In: Barriers and Fluids of the Eye and Brain. Segal, MB (edn), MacMillan Press, London.

11. Maren TH (1995) The development of topical carbonic anhydrase inhibitors. J Glaucoma 4: 49-62.

12. Barboiu M, Supuran CT, Menabuoni L, Scozzafava A, Mincione F, et al. (1999) Carbonic anhydrase inhibitors. Synthesis of topically effective intraocular pressure lowering agents derived from 5-(w-aminoalkylcarboxamido)-1,3,4-thiadiazole-2- sulfonamide. J Enz Inhib 12: 23-46.

13. Celik U, Celik T, Avci A, Annagur A, Yilmaz HL, et al. (2009) Metabolic acidosis in a patient with type 1 diabetes mellitus complicated by methanol and amitriptyline intoxication. Eur J Emerg Med 16: 45-48.

14. Gunnerson KJ, Saul M, He S, Kellum JA (2006) Lactate versus non-lactate metabolic acidosis: a retrospective outcome evaluation of critically ill patients. Crit Care 10: R22.

15. Nguyen HB, Rivers EP, Knoblich BP, Jacobsen G, Muzzin A, et al. (2004) Early lactate clearance is associated with improved outcome in severe sepsis and septic shock. Crit Care Med 32: 1637-1642.

16. Yki-Järvinen H, Bogardus C, Foley JE (1990) Regulation of plasma lactate concentration in resting human subjects. Metabolism 39: 859-864.

17. Py G, Lambert K, Milhavet O, Eydoux N, Prefaut C, et al. (2002) Effects of streptozotocin induced diabetes on markers of skeletal muscle metabolism and monocarboxylate transporter 4 transporters. Metabolism 51: 807-813.

18. Enoki T, Yoshida Y, Hatta H, Bonen A (2003) Exercise training alleviates MCT1 and MCT4 reductions in heart and skeletal muscles of STZ-induced diabetic rats. J Appl Physiol (1985) 94: 2433-2438.

19. Becker HM, Deitmer JW (2004) Voltage dependence of H+ buffering mediated

by sodium bicarbonate cotransport expressed in Xenopus oocytes. J Biol Chem 279: 28057-28062.

20. Becker HM, Deitmer JW (2008) Nonenzymatic proton handling by carbonic anhydrase II during H+-lactate cotransport via monocarboxylate transporter 1. J Biol Chem 283: 21655-21667.

21. Verpoorte JA, Mehta S, Edsall JT (1967) Esterase activities of human carbonic anhydrases B and C. J Biol Chem 242: 4221-4229.

22. Parui R, Gambhir KK, Mehrotra PP (1991) Changes in carbonic anhydrase may be the initial step of altered metabolism in hypertension. Biochem Int 23: 779-789.

23. Dodgson SJ, Watford M (1990) Differential regulation of hepatic carbonic anhydrase isozymes in the streptozotocin-diabetic rat. Arch Biochem Biophys 277: 410-414.

24. Crawford SO, Hoogeveen RC, Brancati FL, Astor BC, Ballantyne CM, et al. (2010) Association of blood lactate with type 2 diabetes: the Atherosclerosis Risk in Communities Carotid MRI Study. Int J Epidemiol 39: 1647-1655.

25. Nicky K, Juan CM, Sean LM, Briana S, Tim C, et al. (2012) Methazolamide Is a New Hepatic Insulin Sensitizer That Lowers Blood Glucose In Vivo. Diabetes 61: 2146-2154.

26. Forbath N, Kenshole AB, Hetenyi G Jr (1967) Turnover of lactic acid in normal and diabetic dogs calculated by two tracer methods. Am J Physiol 212: 1179-1184.

27. De Meutter RC, Shreeve WW (1963) Conversion of DL-lactate-2-C14 or -3-C14 or pyruvate-2-C14 to blood glucose in humans: effects of diabetes, insulin, tolbutamide, and glucose load. J Clin Invest 42: 525-533.

28. Dodgson SJ, Forster RE 2nd (1986) Inhibition of CA V decreases glucose synthesis from pyruvate. Arch Biochem Biophys 251: 198-204.

29. Bode AM, Foster JD, Nordlie RC (1994) Glycogenesis from glucose and ureagenesis in isolated perfused rat livers. Influence of ammonium ion, norvaline, and ethoxyzolamide. J Biol Chem 269: 7879-7886.

30. Cao TP, Rous S (1978) Action of acetazolamide on liver pyruvate carboxylase activity, glycogenolysis and gluconeogenesis of mice. Int J Biochem 9: 603-605.

31. Radziuk J, Zhang Z, Wiernsperger N, Pye S (1997) Effects of metformin on lactate uptake and gluconeogenesis in the perfused rat liver. Diabetes 46: 1406-1413.

32. DeFronzo R, Golay A, Felber J (1985) Glucose and lipid metabolism in obesity and diabetes mellitus. In: J. Garrow, and D. Hallidaed (eds) Substrate and Energy Metabolism. Oxford University press, London, UK.

33. Wetzel P, Hasse A, Papadopoulos S, Voipio J, Kaila K, et al. (2001) Extracellular carbonic anhydrase activity facilitates lactic acid transport in rat skeletal muscle fibres. J Physiol 531: 743-756.

34. Becker HM, Hirnet D, Fecher-Trost C, Sültemeyer D, Deitmer JW (2005) Transport activity of MCT1 expressed in Xenopus oocytes is increased by interaction with carbonic anhydrase. J Biol Chem 280: 39882-39889.

35. Becker HM, Klier M, Deitmer JW (2010) Nonenzymatic augmentation of lactate transport via monocarboxylate transporter isoform 4 by carbonic anhydrase II. J Membr Biol 234: 125-135.

36. Svichar N, Chesler M (2003) Surface carbonic anhydrase activity on astrocytes and neurons facilitates lactate transport. Glia 41: 415-419.

37. Becker HM, Broer S, Deitmer JW (2004) Facilitated lactate transport by MCT1 when coexpressed with the sodium bicarbonate cotransporter (NBC) in Xenopus oocytes. Biophys J 86: 235-247.

38. Fulgencio JP, Kohl C, Girard J, Pégorier JP (2001) Effect of metformin on fatty acid and glucose metabolism in freshly isolated hepatocytes and on specific gene expression in cultured hepatocytes. Biochem Pharmacol 62: 439-446.

39. Consoli A, Nurjhan N (1990) Contribution of gluconeogenesis to overall glucose output in diabetic and nondiabetic men. Ann Med 22: 191-195.

40. Stumvoll M, Nurjhan N, Perriello G, Dailey G, Gerich JE (1995) Metabolic effects of metformin in non-insulin-dependent diabetes mellitus. N Engl J Med 333: 550-554.

41. Lutz TA, Estermann A, Haag S, Scharrer E (2001) Depolarization of the liver cell membrane by metformin. Biochim Biophys Acta 1513: 176-184.

42. Otto M, Breinholt J, Westergaard N (2003) Metformin inhibits glycogen synthesis and gluconeogenesis in cultured rat hepatocytes. Diabetes Obes Metab 5: 189-194.

43. Kuhn B, Hennig M, Mattei P (2007) Molecular recognition of ligands in dipeptidyl peptidase IV. Curr Top Med Chem 7: 609-619.

44. Mooradian AD (2009) Dyslipidemia in type 2 diabetes mellitus. Nat Clin Pract Endocrinol Metab 5: 150-159.

45. Arbeeny CM, Nordin C, Edelstein D, Stram N, Gibbons N, et al. (1989) Hyperlipoproteinemia in spontaneously diabetic guinea pigs. Metabolism 38: 895-900.

46. Biswas UK, Kumar A (2010) Study on Lipid Profile, Oxidation Stress and Carbonic Anhydrase Activity in Patients With Essential Hypertension. Journal of Clinical and Diagnostic Research 4: 3414-3420.

47. Botre F, Botre C (1991) Physiologic implication of carbonic anhydrase facilitated CO_2 diffusion: coupling to other biometabolic processes. In: Botre F, Gros G, Storey BT (eds) Carbonic Anhydrase from Biochemistry and Genetics to Physiology and Clinical Medicine. VCH Publishers Inc, Newyork, USA.

48. Higgins PJ, Bunn HF (1981) Kinetic analysis of the nonenzymatic glycosylation of hemoglobin. J Biol Chem 256: 5204-5208.

49. Lowrey CH, Lyness SJ, Soeldner JS (1985) The effect of hemoglobin ligands on the kinetics of human hemoglobin A1c formation. J Biol Chem 260: 11611-11618.

50. Gil H, Mata-Sagreda J, Schowen R (1991) Isotope Effects in the Nonenzymatic Glucation of Hemoglobin Catalyzed by Phosphate. Actual Fisico-quÂm Org 286-306.

51. Gil H, Vasquez B, Pena M, Uzcategui J (2004) Effect of Carbonate and Arsenate on the Kinetics of Glycation of Human Hemoglobin. J Phys Org Chem 17: 537-540.

52. Gil H, Uzcategui J (1993) Isotope Effects in the Nonenzymatic Glycation of Hemoglobin Catalyzed by DPG. Actual FÂsico-quÂm Org 109-121.

53. Baynes JW, Thorpe SR, Murtiashaw MH (1984) Nonenzymatic glucosylation of lysine residues in albumin. Methods Enzymol 106: 88-98.

54. Allen DW, Schroeder WA, Balog J (1958) Oberservations on the chromatographic heterogeneity of normal adult and fetal human hemoglobin: A study on the effectstallization and chromatography on the heterogeneity and isoleucine content. J Am Chem Soc 80: 1628-1634.

55. Rahbar S, Paulsen E, Ranney MR (1969) Studies of Hemoglobins in patients with diabtes mellitus. Diabetes 1: 332.

56. Speeckaert M, Van Biesen W, Delanghe J, Slingerland R, Wiecek A, et al.(2014) Are there better alternatives than haemoglobin A1c to estimate glycaemic control in the chronic kidney disease population?. Nephrol Dial Transplant 29: 2167-2177.

57. Luft FC (2001) Lactic acidosis update for critical care clinicians. J Am Soc Nephrol 12: S15-19.

58. Klier M, Fabian TA, Joachim WD, Holger MB (2014) Intracellular and Extracellular Carbonic Anhydrases Cooperate Non-enzymatically to Enhance Activity of Monocarboxylate Transporters. The Journal of Biological Chemistry. 289: 2765-2775.

59. Halperin FA, Cheema-Dhadli S, Chen CB, Halperin ML (1996) Alkali therapy extends the period of survival during hypoxia: studies in rats. Am J Physiol 271: R381-387.

6

A Rapid, Inexpensive and Non Invasive Screening for Metabolic Syndrome, Type 2 Diabetes Mellitus and Coronary Artery Disease in a Malaysian Population

Aye M[1]*, Cabot JSF[1] and Razak MSA[2]

[1]Department of Medicine, UniKL Royal College of Medicine, Perak, Malaysia
[2]State Health Department, Ministry of Health, Perak, Malaysia

Abstract

Introduction: The development of rapid, non-invasive and inexpensive tools to screen individuals at risk of developing metabolic syndrome and its consequences of type 2 diabetes and coronary artery disease is important from an epidemiologic and public health view.

Method: A cross sectional analysis was performed with 398 patients from January to November 2011 from records of an outpatient department of a district hospital in rural Malaysia, comprising all races, for prevalence of Metabolic Syndrome (MetS) according to different published criteria.

Result: The prevalence of MetS by different criteria was 49.0% by Hypertensive-Waist (HW), 32.7% Hyper triglyceridaemic-Waist (HTGW), 55.3% by International Diabetes Federation (IDF), 55.3% by Harmonized NCEPATP111 (HNCEPATP111), and 61% by Modified WHO (MWHO). Prevalence of type 2 Diabetes Mellitus (DM) by different criteria was 53.3, 55.4, 55.5, 56.3, 70.3 % respectively and that of Coronary Artery Disease (CAD) was: 21.0, 23.1, 22.7, 23.3 and 23.3% respectively. The agreement of IDF with HW, HTGW, Harmonized NCEPATP111, MWHO using Kappa index was 0.744, 0.560, 0.870 and 0.494 respectively.

Conclusion: HW is able to screen MetS better than HTGW and has better concordance with IDF, although its ability to screen for DM and CAD is somewhat less than HTGW. HW is therefore an excellent screening test for MetS as it is immediately available, non-invasive, requires no laboratory tests, has no appreciable cost, has better concordance with IDF than HTGW and is comparable to IDF and HNCEP for screening DM and CAD.

Keywords: Hypertensive-waist; Hypertriglyceridemic-waist; IDF; NCEPATPIII; Modified WHO; Metabolic syndrome

Introduction

Metabolic Syndrome (Mets) is a condition that substantially increases Coronary Artery Disease (CAD) and is characterized by a cluster of several metabolic abnormalities; centrally distributed obesity, decreased high density lipoprotein cholesterol (HDL-C), elevated triglycerides, hypertension, and hyperglycaemia [1-3]. Abdominal obesity is common in south Asians who, even in non-obese subjects, have a high percentage of body fat, thick subcutaneous adipose tissue, low muscular mass, hyperinsulinaemia and insulin resistance, a combination conducive to development of MetS even in the absence of hyperglycemia and elevated low density lipoprotein cholesterol [4-6]. 'Hypertriglyceridemic-Waist (HTGW) index', has been proposed as a simple and inexpensive tool to identify individuals at risk of developing CAD [7]. High concordance between IDF and HTGW was expected as both use values for waist circumference and fasting triglycerides levels. Gomez Huelgas et al. reported that HTGW showed a moderate agreement with metabolic syndrome defined by IDF and National Cholesterol Education Programme Adult Treatment Panel 111(Ncepatpiii) criteria [8]. The prevalence of MetS by HTGW was 19% in a Quebec cohort, 26.2% in France 11% in 137 American postmenopausal women and 19.7% in a Malaysian study [9-12]. The Malaysian study reported that it had a good correlation with IDF [12]. Prevalence of individual risk factors of MetS varies with ethnicity, with hypertension the most common chronic disease and co-morbidity in Malaysia and obesity also common in Malaysia population [13,14]. Hypertension appears to be a more frequent abnormality among the risk factors for MetS in Asian populations, than in Caucasians [15-18]. We studied Hypertensive-Waist (HW) in a Malaysian population as: 1) a tool to screen MetS, CAD and DM and compare HW with other established definitions of MetS such as IDF, Harmonised NCEPATP111 (HNCEPATP111), Modified World Health Organisation (MWHO), HTGW (Appendix); 2) compare the agreement of HW and other criteria to IDF [12].

Materials and Method

A cross sectional study of 398 patients was performed using the Epi Info version 6 (CDC) for population surveys. Sampling was selected by a clustered systematic randomized sampling with fifteen patients recruited every Thursday from the outpatient clinic. All ethnic groups (Malay, Indian and Chinese) were included, with age 20 years and above. Patients with known causes of hypertension, obesity and dyslipidemia such as Cushing's and Pseudo-Cushing's syndrome, chronic renal failure, nephrotic syndrome and hypothyroidism were excluded, as were smokers. HW had been reported comparable to IDF in detecting MetS and defined as systolic blood pressure ≥ 130 mmHg or diastolic blood pressure ≥ 85 mmHg or history of treated hypertension; plus a waist circumference ≥ 80 cm for women and ≥ 90 cm for men (we used 90 cm in lieu of 94 cm in reference as outlined under Material and Methods) [19,20]. We chose IDF to validate other definitions of MetS because: 1) it is ethnic specific; 2) WC is used as required criteria by IDF as it is for HW; 3) to have comparable data since most of local and other studies used IDF as a gold standard for agreement criteria [20].

*Corresponding author: Aye M, Department of Medicine, UniKL Royal College of Medicine, Perak, Malaysia, E-mail: mraaye@hotmail.com

The research purpose was explained to and consent obtained from all patients. Patients were interviewed and examined by the investigators and measurements of BMI (kg/m^2), Waist Circumference (WC) by cm and blood pressure (mmHg) were carried out by the same assigned staff nurse trained to measure WC. WC measurement was standardized using a measuring tape at the midpoint between the lower costal cartilage and the highest point of iliac crest at full expiration. Blood samples for fasting plasma sugar (FPG) (mmol/L), serum triglycerides (mmol/L) (TG) and high-density lipoprotein cholesterol (mmol/L) (HDL), total Cholesterol (TC). Low Density Lipoprotein-C (LDL-C) was taken in early morning after an overnight fast. Period of study was from January 15 to June 30, 2011. Cut-off points for definitions were adopted by the criteria of a Malay study in Appendix: Male waist circumference (WC) ≥ 90 cm, female ≥ 80 cm were assessed for MetS by IDF criteria when they had at least one of the following three criteria: BP ≥ 130/85 mmHg; TG ≥ 1.7 mmol/ L; HDL ≤ 1.29 mmol/ L for females and ≤ 1 mmol/ L for males and FBS ≥ 5.6 mmol/L [12]. Any three out of the five criteria for IDF was defined as MetS for HNCEPAPT111. Elevated FPG cut-off point for MWHO was >6.1mmol/L or DM and this plus any two of following : body mass index (BMI) ≥ 30 kg/m^2 , blood pressure 140/90 mmHg , HDL <I mmol /L for males and <0.9 mmol/L for females , high TG ≥ 1.7 mmol/L was defined as MetS according to MWHO criteria. The cut-off points for hypertension, WC and triglycerides and low HDL-C for HTGW, HW and IDF were the same. Fasting plasma glucose ≥ 7 mmol/L was defined as DM. Coronary Artery Disease (CAD) was defined by patients' record: coronary angiography, angioplasty, CABG, symptoms of angina or unstable angina plus ECG changes, cardiac biomarkers with or without echocardiogram changes and response to coronary vasodilators. Cut-off points for high TC and LDL-C were >5.2 mmol / L and 2.5 mmol /L respectively according to hospital protocol where the study was carried out. MetS was defined for

different criteria adopting the Table 1. WC was ≥ 90 cm for men and ≥ 80 cm for women in all definitions of MetS in this study [12]. Cut-off points for TG, HLD-C, systolic and diastolic BP, elevated fasting plasma glucose are the same in all criteria except WHO where cut-off points for systolic BP, diastolic BP, HDL-C were higher.

Statistical analyses were performed using the SPSS version 11.5 (SPSS Inc, Chicago, Il, USA). Student's t test was used to determine means; Chi Square test was used to determine association; Kappa index was used to determine agreement. Data were considered statistically significant with p-value < 0.05.

Results

194 males and 204 females were evaluated. The overall prevalence of MetS defined by HW = 44.8%; HTGW = 40.5%; IDF = 55.3%; HNCEPATPIII = 61.6%, MWHO = 38.9%. By gender and IDF criteria, males = 40% and females = 60%; by HNCEPATP111 and MWHO criteria = 44.5% and 55.5%, by HTGW criteria = 41.5% and 58.5% and by HW criteria = 40.5% and 59.5%. By ethnicity, highest prevalence of MetS was Indian by IDF criteria (43.2%); Malays by MWHO criteria (47.7%) and in Chinese by HNCEPAT111 criteria (18.4%). The prevalence of MetS was approximately equal among Malays and Indians with Chinese having the lowest prevalence by all criteria. By age MetS was highest in the age group 50-59 followed by age group ≥ 60, 40-49, 30-39 and 20-29 by all criteria definitions. Thus, there is a steady increase in the MetS prevalence with age up to 50-59 (Table 1).

Table 2 shows prevalence and association of DM and CAD by different definitions. DM by MWHO criteria was highest, followed by HNCEPATP111, IDF, HTGW and HW. This is because MWHO uses DM or elevated FPG was a major diagnostic criterion for MetS, and therefore MWHO criteria has highest odds ratio followed by the others.

Variable	Total Number (%)	IDF	HNCEP	Modified WHO	HTGW	HW
Metabolic syndrome	398	220 (55.3)	245(61.6)	155 (38.9)	130 (32.7)	195(49.0)
Age						
20-29		9 (4.1)	10 (4.1)	6 (3.9)	5 (3.8)	9 (4.6)
30-39		17 (7.7)	20 (8.2)	11 (7.1)	9(6.9)	13 (6.7)
40-49		53 (24.1)	56 (22.9)	36(23.2)	31 (23.8)	49 (25.1)
50-59		82 (27.3)	92 (37.6)	63(40.6)	49 (37.7)	73 (37.4)
≥ 60		59 (26.9)	67 (27.3)	39(25.2)	36 (27.7)	51 (26.2)
Gender						
Male	194 (48.8)	132 (60.0)	109 (44.5)	69(44.5)	54 (41.5)	79 (40.5)
Female	204 (51.2)	88 (40.0)	136 (55.5)	86(55.5)	76 (58.5)	116 (59.5)
Ethnicity						
Malay	139 (39.2)	88 (40.0)	101 (41.2)	74(47.7)	58 (44.6)	84 (43.1)
Indian	136 (38.3)	95 (43.2)	99 (40.4)	60(38.7)	50 (38.5)	79 (40.5)
Chinese	80(22.5)	37 (16.8)	45 (18.4)	21(13.5)	22 (16.9)	32 (16.4)

IDF: International Diabetes Federation; NCEPATP111: National Cholesterol Education Prevention Adult Treatment Panel 111; HTGW: high Triglyceride Waist; HW: Hypertensive Waist; HNCEP: HarmonizedNCEPATP111

Table 1: Distribution of demographic factors in study population with Metabolic Syndrome by different definitions   (percentage in parenthesis).

	IDF	HNCEP	Modified WHO	HTGW	HW
DM	122 (55.5) 4.44(2.85-6.91)	138 (56.3) 7.29(4.38-12.1)	109 (70.3) 8.70 (5.49-13.8)	72 (55.4) 2.50(1.63-3.84)	104 (53.3) 2.93(1.93-4.44)
CAD	50 (22.7) 1.89(1.11-3.22)	57 (23.3) 2.43(1.35-4.35)	36 (23.3) 1.63(0.98-2.71)	30 (23.1) 1.53(0.91-2.57)	41 (21.0) 1.37(0.83-2.28)

IDF: International Diabetes Federation; NCEPATP111: National Cholesterol Education Prevention Adult Treatment Panel 111; HTGW: High Triglyceride Waist; HW: Hypertensive Waist; HNCEP: Harmonizedncepatp111; CAD: Coronary Artery Disease; Figures In The Brackets Are Percentages, HNECPATP Is The Most Sensitive To Screen For Mets, DM And CAD

Table 2: Prevalence DM & CAD in patients with MetS and their association with MetS defined by different definitions.

The prevalence of CAD was highest by HNCEPATP111 and MWHO followed by HTGW IDF and HW. However, only HNCEPATP111 and IDF had significant association with CAD.

Table 3 shows mean: age, BMI, WC, Systolic BP (SBP), Diastolic BP (DBP), FPG, TG, HDL-C, TC, and LDL-C by all definitions.

Mean WC was highest with HW, and lowest with HNCEPATP 111. Mean systolic and diastolic BP was highest with HW definition with all other definitions having lower systolic and diastolic pressures than HW definition.

TG (normal value; 1.7 mmol/L for male and female) was highest by HTGW, followed by MWHO, HNCEPATP111, IDF, and lowest by HW. HDL-C (normal value: 1.30 mmol/L for females and normal value: 1.0 mmol for male) was lowest by MWHO, gradually increased by HNCEPATP111, IDF and highest by HW.

FPG (normal: 7 mmol/L) was highest by MWHO (as a required major criteria), followed by HTGW and comparable in the remaining three definitions.

TC mmol/L and LDL-C mmol/L was highest by HNCEPATP111 and HW and lower and comparable in the remaining three definitions.

Table 4 shows prevalence of MetS factors in different definitions of the syndrome. WC prevalence was high in HW, HTGW and IDF (as a required criterion) to diagnose MetS; and lower in MWHO and NCEPATP111.

Highest prevalence of elevated FPG was seen in MWHO (as a required criterion), followed by HNCEPATP111, IDF, HTGW, and HW.

Prevalence of high TG was highest in HTGW (as a required major criterion), followed by MWHO, IDF and HNCEPATP111 and HW.

Prevalence of low HDL-C was highest in MWHO, followed by HNCEPATP111 and IDF, HW and HTGW.

Hypertension prevalence was highest in HW (as a required criterion), followed by MWHO, HNCEPATP111 and IDF and HTGW.

Table 5 shows sensitivity and specificity, Kappa index and p values of MetS defined by HNCEPATPIII, MWHO, HTGW and HW vs. IDF.

	Hypertensive -waist	Hypertriglyceridemic-waist	IDF	H-NCEPATP 111	Modified WHO
Age	52.0 ± 12.6	53.1 ± 11.3	52.7 ± 11.4	52.9 ± 11.8	53.1 ± 11.3
BMI	31.1 ± 6.49	29.6 ± 5.79	30.4 ± 6.56	29.8 ± 6.55	30.6 ± 7.06
WC	101 ± 10.8	99.4 ± 9.85	100 ± 10.7	98.4 ± 11.4	98.8 ± 11.5
SBP	148 ± 13.7	143 ± 18.0	142 ± 16.7	142 ± 16.7	145 ± 14.0
DBP	87.4 ± 8.63	84.7 ± 9.83	85.2 ± 10.1	85.4 ± 9.96	86.7 ± 9.22
TG	1.81 ± 7.12	2.81 ± 2.04	2.15 ± 1.77	2.14 ± 1.71	2.30 ± 1.68
HDL-C	1.10 ± 0.39	1.04 ± 0.36	1.05 ± 0.34	1.04 ± 0.337	1.02 ± 0.33
FPG	7.41 ± 2.74	7.90 ± 3.15	7.73 ± 2.89	7.72 ± 2.80	8.53 ± 2.92
T C	5.59 ± 1.66	5.04 ± 1.32	5.09 ± 1.34	5.24 ± 1.53	5.04 ± 1.32
LDL-C	3.38 ± 1.51	3.14 ± 1.32	3.33 ± 1.33	3.35 ± 1.31	3.14 ± 1.24

BMI: Body Mass Index; WC: Waist Circumference; SBP: Systolic Blood Pressure; DBP: Diastolic Blood Pressure; TG: Triglycerides; HDL-C: High Density Lipoprotein-Cholesterol; FPG: Fasting Plasma Glucose; T:Total Cholesterol: LDL-C: Low Density Lipoprotein -Cholesterol

Table 3: Comparison of the baseline characteristics in subjects with MetS according to IDF, NCEPATPIII, MWHO, HTGW and HW.

Metabolic risks	Hypertensive -waist	Hypertriglyceridemic- waist	IDF	Harmonized NCEPATP111	Modified WHO
High WC	158 (100 %)	130 (100%)	220 (100%)	217 (88.6%)	134 (86.5%)
Raised FPG	112 (70.9%)	102 (78.5%)	174 (79.1%)	196 (80%)	152 (98.1%)
High TG	75 (47.5%)	130 (100%)	127 (57.7%)	144 (58.8%)	105 (67.2%)
Low HDLC	106 (67.1%)	89 (68.5%)	155 (70.5%)	175 (71.4%)	116 (74.8%)
High BP	158 (100%)	104 (80.0%)	186 (84.5%)	208 (84.9%)	137 (88.4%)

Table 4: Prevalence of metabolic risk factors of MS in the study cohort (n=398).

Definition	IDF Index					
	MetS	Normal	Sensitivity	Specificity	Kappa Index	p-Value
HW						
MetS (%)	182(93.3)	13 (6.7)	82.7%	92.6%	0.744	0.00
Normal (%)	38(18.7)	165(81.3)				
HTGW						
MS (%)	129(99.2)	1 (8)	58.6%	99.4%	0.560	0.00
Normal (%)	91(34.0)	177 (66.0)				
HNCEPATPIII						
MetS (%)	220 (89.8)	25 (10.2)	100%	85.9%	0.871	0.00
Normal (%)	0 (0)	153 (100)				
Mod. WHO						
MetS (%)	136(87.7)	19(12.3)	61.8%	89.3%	0.494	0.00
Normal (%)	84(34.6)	159 (65.4)				

Table 5: Agreement with IDF of other definitions which define metabolic syndrome.

Sensitivity and specificity of IDF vs. HNCEPATP111 was 100% and 85.9%; HW 82.7 and 92.6%, MWHO 61.8% and 89.3% and HTGW 58.6 and 99.4%.

The agreement (kappa index) between IDF definition and HNCEPATP111 was 0.817, MWHO was 0.494; HTGW was 0.560 and HW was 0.744 (p < 0.01) respectively. Therefore, there was excellent agreement between IDF and HNCEPATP111, good agreement with HW, and moderate agreement with HTGW and MWHO.

Discussion

Being hospital based, this study possibly may show a higher prevalence of MetS than the general population. In this cohort, the highest prevalence of MetS was defined by HNCEPATPIII, followed by IDF, HW, MWHO and HTGW. Since HNECEPATP111 does not include high WC, it diagnoses a somewhat different MetS group than does IDF. This finding is consistent with a report of a Korean study and others who claim WC should not be mandatory in definition of MetS as there are subjects without abdominal obesity who may still be at greater future risk of DM or CAD by having clustering of other risk factors [21,22]. This is also applicable to MWHO where elevated FPG is a required criterion to define MetS and therefore having lower prevalence of MetS in this and other Malaysian studies [12,21-23]. The prevalence of MetS is higher in IDF than NCEPATP111 in these studies possibly because of higher cut-off points of WC in two local studies to define NCEPATP111 [12,21-23]. In CURES-34 study IDF criteria was most sensitive to detect MetS followed by MWHO and NCEPATP111 [23-25].

IDF has very good agreement HNCEPATP111, moderately good agreement with HW and moderate agreement with HTGW and MWHO in our study, consistent with other studies [12,23,24]. The very good agreement with IDF and HNCEPATP111 is that both criteria have common risk factors for diagnosis of MetS, consisting of hypertension, elevated FPG, low HDLC and high TG.

Our study would suggest that it seems best to have fluid major criteria for the diagnosis of MetS. It also indicates that HNCEPATP111 appears suitable to diagnose MetS for Southeast Asians. This finding is consistent with reports from India, Sri Lanka and Korea [21,26,27].

The reason for reduced agreement of IDF with MWHO is probably because MWHO uses DM and/or raised fasting plasma glucose, greater cut off levels for systolic/diastolic blood pressures and low HDL to define MetS than the other definitions, accounting for reduced sensitivity of MWHO for MetS definition and hence the lowest detection rate. Likewise, the reason for reduced agreement with HTGW is that high TG is the least common risk factor among other definitions for developing MetS (Table 4). Therefore, when this risk factor and high WC are used to define MetS, it has lower sensitivity of MetS and poor agreement (second lowest agreement) with IDF, consistent with other reports of populations in Malaysia, Quebec, France and USA [9-12]. We agree that HTGW is not a good screening tool for MetS in Malaysia population.

There are very few studies that compare HW ability to screen for consequences of MetS such as DM and CAD with other definitions [28]. That study was also different from ours by use of different targets of study, higher cut-off points of WC and use of IDF to define MetS. HW has the ability to screen MetS, and has good agreement with IDF and HNCEPATP111. As MetS is associated with three fold higher risk of Type 2 DM and two to three fold higher risk of CAD, we believe HW to be a very simple, no cost, screening tool for DM for CAD [3]. Others report show WC is independently associated with hypertension and DM in African American women [28,29].

The lower prevalence of CAD and DM by HW than other definitions could be explained by several factors. IDF defined MetS cut-off point of WC for men as ≥ 94 cm, different from our study and Framingham Risk Score was used to define CVS risk in the study another [28]. Also there are many risk factors for developing CAD other than hypertension, especially dyslipidemia and elevated FPG, not measured by HW. The pattern of clustering of MetS factors varies among ethnic groups [13,14]. In South East Asias, hypertension and increased WC are the most common risk factor for developing MetS, with elevated TG the least associated risk factor [14,30,31]. Definitions that include high TG or elevated FPG as criteria to define MetS by HTGW and MWHO respectively would result in screening for a higher prevalence of DM and CAD. Low HDL-C and high TG lipid disorder is a virtual marker for DM, so HTGW gives a higher prevalence of DM and CAD [32]. HTGW is comparable to HNCEPATP111 and IDF and better than HW to screen for DM and CAD in this and other studies [8,33,34]. However in other studies, cut-off points for TG were lower than our study and thus the ability of HW as a tool to predict DM and CAD appears not less than HTGW which is claimed as a good tool to predict DM and CVS risks [8,33,34].

In our study HW was better than HTGW to detect MetS and has better agreement with IDF, and like HTGW, is comparable to IDF and HNCEPATP111 to screen DM and CAD. We agree with others that MetS and its components are associated with type 2 diabetes but have weak or no association with vascular risk in elderly populations, suggesting that attempts to define criteria that simultaneously predict risk for both cardiovascular disease and DM are not helpful [35]. Clinical focus should assess the optimum risk for each disease.

Therefore, we assert that HW is cheaper, easier, non-invasive and a more sensitive screening tool for MetS than HTGW. However, this may be applicable only in similar ethnic groups with similar clustering pattern of metabolic risk factors for MetS [13].

The prevalence of MetS was highest using the criteria of HNCEPATP111. IDF definition had very good agreement with HNCEPATPIII, and good agreement with HW. HW is a better screening test than HTGW for MetS, having comparable prevalence of DM and CAD with IDF and HNCEPATPIII and most importantly requires no blood work or time to identify most MetS patients who can then be more fully screened for potential complications. The screening and definition for MetS should be based on clustering pattern of metabolic risks in the study population. This is true of all ethnic Malaysians and should be confirmed in other ethnic groups as a good screen, especially in developing countries.

Acknowledgement

We would like to acknowledge Prof. Karuthan, Dept of Statistics and University Malaya for their statistical analysis, ethical and research committee of UniKLRCMP for permission and the research committee of UniKLRCMP for the research grant.

References

1. Choi KM, Kim SM, Kim YE, Choi DS, Baik SH, et al. (2007) Prevalence and cardiovascular disease risk of the metabolic syndrome using National Cholesterol Education Program and International Diabetes Federation definitions in the Korean population. Metabolism 56: 552-558.

2. Lemieux I, Poirier P, Bergeron J, Alméras N, Lamarche B, et al. (2007) Hypertriglyceridemic waist: a useful screening phenotype in preventive cardiology? Can J Cardiol 23: 23B-31B.

3. Zimmet P, M M Alberti KG, Serrano Ríos M (2005) [A new international diabetes federation worldwide definition of the metabolic syndrome: the rationale and the results]. Rev Esp Cardiol 58: 1371-1376.

4. Ahmed S, Ahmed SA, Ali N (2010) Frequency of metabolic syndrome in type 2 diabetes and its relationship with insulin resistance. J Ayub Med Coll Abbottabad 22: 22-27.

5. Yusuf S, Reddy S, Ounpuu S, Anand S (2001) Global burden of cardiovascular diseases: Part II: variations in cardiovascular disease by specific ethnic groups and geographic regions and prevention strategies. Circulation 104: 2855-2864.

6. Ravikiran M, Bhansali A, Ravikumar P, Bhansali S, Dutta P, et al. (2010) Prevalence and risk factors of metabolic syndrome among Asian Indians: a community survey. Diabetes Res Clin Pract 89: 181-188.

7. Lemieux I, Pascot A, Couillard C, Lamarche B, Tchernof A, et al. (2000) Hypertriglyceridemic waist: A marker of the atherogenic metabolic triad (hyperinsulinemia; hyperapolipoprotein B; small, dense LDL) in men? Circulation 102: 179-184.

8. Gomez-Huelgas R, Bernal-López MR, Villalobos A, Mancera-Romero J, Baca-Osorio AJ, et al. (2011) Hypertriglyceridemic waist: an alternative to the metabolic syndrome? Results of the IMAP Study (multidisciplinary intervention in primary care). Int J Obes (Lond) 35: 292-299.

9. Lemieux I, Alméras N, Mauriège P, Blanchet C, Dewailly E, et al. (2002) Prevalence of 'hypertriglyceridemic waist' in men who participated in the Quebec Health Survey: association with atherogenic and diabetogenic metabolic risk factors. Can J Cardiol 18: 725-732.

10. Czernichow S, Bruckert E, Bertrais S, Galan P, Hercberg S, et al. (2007) Hypertriglyceridemic waist and 7.5-year prospective risk of cardiovascular disease in asymptomatic middle-aged men. Int J Obes (Lond) 31: 791-796.

11. LaMonte MJ, Ainsworth BE, DuBose KD, Grandjean PW, Davis PG, et al. (2003) The hypertriglyceridemic waist phenotype among women. Atherosclerosis 171: 123-130.

12. Zainuddin LR, Isa N, Muda WM, Mohamed HJ (2011) The prevalence of metabolic syndrome according to various definitions and hypertriglyceridemic-waist in malaysian adults. Int J Prev Med 2: 229-237.

13. Sharifi F, Mousavinasab SN, Saeini M, Dinmohammadi M (2009) Prevalence of metabolic syndrome in an adult urban population of the west of Iran. Exp Diabetes Res 2009: 136501.

14. Nestel P, Lyu R, Low LP, Sheu WH, Nitiyanant W, et al. (2007) Metabolic syndrome: recent prevalence in East and Southeast Asian populations. Asia Pac J Clin Nutr 16: 362-367.

15. Ibrahim H, Yusoff MM (2007) Plant-based ethnic remedies for hypertension from Malaysia. Thieme.

16. Ismail MN, Chee SS, Nawawi H, Yusoff K, Lim TO, et al. (2002) Obesity in Malaysia. Obes Rev 3: 203-208.

17. Tan CE, Ma S, Wai D, Chew SK, Tai ES (2004) Can we apply the National Cholesterol Education Program Adult Treatment Panel definition of the metabolic syndrome to Asians? Diabetes Care 27: 1182-1186.

18. Alexander CM, Landsman PB, Teutsch SM, Haffner SM, Third National Health and Nutrition Examination Survey (NHANES III); National Cholesterol Education Program (NCEP) (2003) NCEP-defined metabolic syndrome, diabetes, and prevalence of coronary heart disease among NHANES III participants age 50 years and older. Diabetes 52: 1210-1214.

19. Hancu N, Roman G, Nita C, Negrean M (2004) Metabolic syndrome--practical approach. Rom J Intern Med 42: 237-245.

20. Nita C, Hancu N, Rusu A, Bala C, Roman G (2009) Hypertensive waist: first step of the screening for metabolic syndrome. Metabolic Syndrome Related Disorders 32: 227-233.

21. Lee WY, Park JS, Noh SY, Rhee EJ, Kim SW, et al. (2004) Prevalence of the metabolic syndrome among 40,698 Korean metropolitan subjects. Diabetes Res Clin Pract 65: 143-149.

22. Wasir JS, Misra A, Vikram NK, Pandey RM, Gupta R (2008) Comparison of definitions of the metabolic syndrome in adult Asian Indians. J Assoc Physicians India 56: 158-164.

23. Bee YT Jr, Haresh KK, Rajibans S (2008) Prevalence of Metabolic Syndrome among Malaysians using the International Diabetes Federation, National Cholesterol Education Program and Modified World Health Organization Definitions. Malays J Nutr 14: 65-77.

24. Mohamud WN, Ismail AA, Sharifuddin A, Ismail IS, Musa KI, et al. (2011) Prevalence of metabolic syndrome and its risk factors in adult Malaysians: results of a nationwide survey. Diabetes Res Clin Pract 91: 239-245.

25. Deepa M, Farooq S, Datta M, Deepa R, Mohan V (2007) Prevalence of metabolic syndrome using WHO, ATPIII and IDF definitions in Asian Indians: the Chennai Urban Rural Epidemiology Study (CURES-34). Diabetes Metab Res Rev 23: 127-134.

26. Misra A, Misra R, Wijesuriya M, Banerjee D (2007) The metabolic syndrome in South Asians: continuing escalation & possible solutions. Indian J Med Res 125: 345-354.

27. Chackrewarthy S, Gunasekera D, Pathmeswaren A, Wijekoon CN, Ranawaka UK, et al. (2013) A Comparison between Revised NCEP ATP III and IDF Definitions in Diagnosing Metabolic Syndrome in an Urban Sri Lankan Population: The Ragama Health Study. ISRN Endocrinol 2013: 320176.

28. Nita C, Rusu A, Bala C, Hancu N (2008) The Ability of Hypertensive Waist to Predict High Cardiovascular Risk in General Population. Applied Medical Informatics 23: 37-42.

29. Warren TY, Wilcox S, Dowda M, Baruth M (2012) Independent association of waist circumference with hypertension and diabetes in African American women, South Carolina, 2007-2009. Prev Chronic Dis 9: E105.

30. Aye M, Sazali M (2012) Waist circumference and BMI cut-off points to predict risk factors for metabolic syndrome among outpatients in a district hospital. Singapore Med J 53: 545-550.

31. Guagnano MT, Ballone E, Colagrande V, Della Vecchia R, Manigrasso MR, et al. (2001) Large waist circumference and risk of hypertension. Int J Obes Relat Metab Disord 25: 1360-1364.

32. Feeman WE Jr, Sattar N, OReilly DS, Packard CJ, Shepherd J, et al. (2004) Metabolic syndrome and diabetes mellitus. Circulation 109: E23.

33. Tanko LB, Bagger YZ, Qin G, Alexandersen P, Larsen PJ, et al. (2005) Enlarged waist combined with elevated triglycerides is a strong predictor of accelerated atherogenesis and related cardiovascular mortality in postmenopausal women. Circulation 111: 1883-1890.

34. Bailey DP, Savory LA, Denton SJ, Davies BR, Kerr CJ (2013) The hypertriglyceridemic waist, waist-to-height ratio, and cardiometabolic risk. J Pediatr 162: 746-752.

35. Sattar N, McConnachie A, Shaper AG, Blauw GJ, Buckley BM, et al. (2008) Can metabolic syndrome usefully predict cardiovascular disease and diabetes? Outcome data from two prospective studies. Lancet 371: 1927-1935.

7

Does Smoking and Alcohol Abuse Precipitate and Aggravate the Risk of Metabolic Syndrome?

María Eugenia Velasco-Contreras Grado*

Unit of Primary Attention of Health, Coordination of Comprehensive Health Care for the First Level of Care; Division of Information and Medical Support, Mexican Institute of Social Security, Mexico

Abstract

Objective: To know what is the degree of association between the presence of vascular complications in people with obesity, diabetes, hypertension and the different degree of consumption of tobacco or alcohol.

Methods: From March to December 2009 were 20,000 surveys to health workers and other occupational categories randomly selected in the 35 delegations of the IMSS, in each State. The study of variables included: affiliation, sex, age, job category, and registration of known diseases, smoking, nicotine addiction, and consumption of alcohol risk, addiction to alcohol, habits, physical exercise and eating habits. Analysis statistical, was held in the SPSS version 17 system, was obtained frequencies, point prevalence of the risk factors, smoking, prevalence of chronic diseases and Terminal vascular complications, chronic pulmonary damage, (COPD) liver cirrhosis and neoplasm's (cancer unspecified organ. Analysis bivariate estimate of the relative risk of Association of risk factors and addictions with obesity, and with chronic diseases and complications terminals, by estimating the right odds to the prevalence, CI=confidence interval; Chi-square of Mantel-Haenszel (Xmh)

Results: The consumption of more than five cigarettes per day in women associated with obesity RMP 1.43 IC (1.03-1.98) Xmh 2.1 and abusive consumption of alcohol is associated with obesity in men with 1.81 RMP IC (1.57-2.10) Xmh 8.0

With respect to vascular complications in women who smoke at least one cigarette a day's Association was found with cerebral vascular disease (EVC) 3.24 RMP IC (1.58-6.66) Xmh 3.38, with RMP cardiac infarct of 2.69 IC (1.66-4.38) Xmh 4.16; Women in large smokers for more than 5 cigarettes a day Association was found with EVC RMP 4.50 CI (1.37-14.8) Xmh 2.71; with infarct heart 3.07 IC (1.23-7.65) Xmh 2.53, diabetes, RMP 1.61 IC (1.05-2.46) Xmh 6.82 hypertension RMP 1.21 IC (1.00-1.74) Xmh 3.05 and Dyslipidemia RMP 1.22 IC (1.00-2.04) Xmh 2.29

Men in heavy smokers Association was established as follows: EVC, RMP 2.69 IC (2.22-14.61) Xmh 4.08; Cardiac infarct, RMP 2.68 IC (1.51 - 4.76) Xmh 3.48; diabetes, RMP 1.63 IC (1.20-2.20) Xmh 7.13; Hypertension, RMP 1.30 CI (1.00 - 1.69) Xmh 4.31.

With regard to the abusive consumption of alcohol in women Association was found with EVC, RMP 2.40 IC (1.08 - 5.31) Xmh 2.22.

In men with alcohol addiction Association was found to EVC, RMP 7.15 IC (1.65 - 31.01) Xmh 3.07, cardiac infarction, RMP 3.21 IC (1.16-8.92) Xmh 2.36, diabetes, RMP 1.96 IC (1.11-3.46) Xmh 2.35; arterial hypertension, RMP 1.75 IC (1.07-2.87) Xmh 2.26

In women with alcohol addiction Association was found to RMP 25.82 IC (7.46-98.40) cardiac infarct Xmh 7.68, diabetes, RMP 4.69 IC (1.71-12.80) Xmh 3.31; arterial hypertension, RMP 2.99 IC (1.17-7.66) Xmh 2.40

In hypertensive patients with more than 5 cigarettes a day smoking Association was found with EVC, RMP 85.6 IC (40.1-182.9) Xmh 12.6; Cardiac infarct, RMP 2.88 IC (2.50-3.33) Xmh 10.5. In hypertensive patients with alcohol addiction Association was found with EVC, RMP 45.9 IC (23.7-88.9) Xmh 9.13; Cardiac infarct, RMP 37.7 IC (22.5-62.1) Xmh 12.8. In large smoking diabetic patients Association was found with EVC, RMP 97.8 IC (36.4-262.5) Xmh 11.0, with RMP 50.8 IC (26.5-97.2) cardiac infarct Xmh 13.1. In diabetic patients with addiction alcohol Association was found with EVC, RMP 35.9 IC (15.1-85.4) Xmh 5.4, with cardiac infarct, RMP 26.9 IC (14.6-49.7) Xmh 8.1

Conclusions: The metabolic syndrome is identified clinically by obesity, associated with hypertension, diabetes mellitus and Dyslipidemia. This increases the risk of vascular complications even before having identified chronic diseases, diabetes and hypertension. In this study associated with vascular damage in women who smoke at least one cigarette in the day, both of EVC, and cardiac infarction. The increase of the Association is not much larger with more than 5 smoking a day, suggesting greater vascular lability in women who smoke without serious nicotine addiction. Analyze the Association of smoking of cigarettes more than 5 a day with other components of the metabolic syndrome is identified to increase the presence of diabetes 1.61 times higher in women and 1.63 in men, when compared with non-smokers, Increases 1.21-1.30 and women hypertension and 1.22 single dyslipidaemia in women. With respect to vascular complications, large men smoking their increase is one and a half times less than in women, but 2 and half times higher than in men non-smoking.

In hypertensive and diabetic heavy smokers compared patient's non-smoking increases by 85 and 100 times the risk of EVC respectively: for myocardial infarction 3-50 times more respectively. This suggests a clear difference in the coronary vascular damage generated by diabetes to hypertension.

In men, the abusive consumption of alcohol was clearly associated to obesity. In women compared with abstemias women the EVC associated with 2 and a half times more.

Addiction to alcohol in men increased 7 times more the presence of EVC. In men and women cardiac infarct, 3 and 25 times more, diabetes mellitus 2 and 5 and arterial hypertension 2 and 3 respectively when compared with abstainers men and women.

Keywords: Alcohol precipitate; Tobacco; Metabolic syndrome

Introduction

In recent decades non-communicable chronic diseases have become an epidemic, associated with unhealthy lifestyles. The set of diseases is integrated by increase of body fat in subcutaneous tissue and accumulate fat ectopic in internal organs: liver, pancreas, heart, muscles and probably kidney. Manifested by Overweight/obesity, steatosis liver, followed by high blood pressure, type 2 diabetes, dyslipidemias, cerebrovascular, renal, coronary disease, complicated by the epidemic of tobacco use and alcohol consumption give rise to chronic obstructive pulmonary disease, cirrhosis of the liver, and some types of cancer [1-6]. All give rise to major causes of disease, disability and premature death, which bring together the high cost for health, treatment and rehabilitation services [7-11]. The factors of risk more prevalent and with greater negative impact on global health is a lifestyle consisting of bad habits of nutrition, sedentary lifestyle, smoking and abusive consumption of alcohol [12] there is a body of information indicating that they are associated or generate metabolic syndrome; consisting of sobrepeso-obesidad, hypertension, hepatic steatosis, pre-diabetes, type 2 diabetes mellitus, Dyslipidemia; which explains, the global increase in morbidity and cardiovascular mortality, cancer, chronic lung damage, cirrhosis of the liver, and terminal kidney damage [7,8]. Sedentary; in 1994 who recognized it as an independent risk for diabetes mellitus type 2, osteoporosis, ischemic heart disease factor and estimated that by itself alone, double the risk of becoming ill or dying, compared with people who perform daily physical exercise [13,14]. Smoking- Who defined as a disease and public health of global magnitude problem; in 2006 reported that they died a day 14,500 people and 6 million a year from related diseases [15]. In developed countries causes 15% of total health care costs. In United States the annual cost of treatment of diseases attributable to tobacco is $50 billion dollars, with 47 billion losses in wages and productivity [10,11] disease control (CDC) defines to smoking, such as the consumption of at least 100 cigarettes during life and smoking at the present time. It is a disease that starts as a habit during adolescence and causes nicotine addiction in adults with physical and psychological dependence, difficult-to-treat for the suspension of smoking; due to the massive increase of Nicotinic Receptors in the central nervous system [16]. The national survey of 2007 addiction (ENA/2007), reported 26.4% of smokers and 25.6% of liabilities [17]. In health professionals smoking is higher than in the general population. In Mexico, the figures vary between 14% to 31%, depending on the institution, geographic area and population studied [18]. Smokers have more health problems, use more medical services, less physical exercise and have more depression. Has it been established according to the study of the global tobacco epidemic carried out by the whom that 50% of them have death before age 35. In relation to mortality: lung cancer is attributed 79%, obstructive pulmonary disease chronic myocardial infarction 78% to 48% and Cerebral Vascular disease 38%. In relation to the consumption of drinks with alcohol who defines alcoholism as a chronic disease characterized by disorders behavioral, mental and physical caused by compulsive consumption of alcoholic beverages. Addiction to alcohol is manifested by tolerance, dependence and withdrawal syndrome; with involvement of social, family, work and school life [19]. It is one of the main causes of the global burden of disease and disability. Its relationship with chronic diseases is clear since dependency, is associated with the chronic lack of control of hypertension, diabetes, has you been linked recently to cardiac infarct in cerebral vascular disease in men and women [19]. generates relatively long-term liver cirrhosis due to toxicity to the newspaper excessive consumption, and other individual the health

damage, such as physical injury from acute poisoning, death by accident of traffic, violence, homicides, suicides, family, generation of children and adolescents with chronic depression and high risk of alcoholism in adulthood [20] the official Mexican standard defines Overweight / obesity as a chronic disease accompanied by metabolic disturbances and deterioration in the State of health [21]. The prevalence of Overweight/obesity has increased in recent decades and is considered a pandemic for its contribution to the burden of disease. WHO estimates that there are 300 million obese worldwide, adding those who have overweighted the figure rises to 1000 million. In the last 20 years studies, have been conducted to define that obesity is always preceded by the overweight, that is not obesity, but neither is normal weight. Metabolic abnormality parameters increase exponentially to the extent of the subject moves away from its normal weight [22-26]. Much of its causality is considered by global increase in consumption of foods low in nutrients and very high in simple sugars, refined flour mixed with vegetable fats saturated, with reduction to zero consumption of fruits/vegetables and severe physical inactivity [27]. The obesity generates and is associated in most cases hypertension, glucose intolerance, diabetes type 2, coronary artery disease, lung disease, sleep apnoea sleep, joint diseases, vesicular diseases and several types of cancer. It is responsible for 40% of endometrial cancer, 25% of renal cancer and 10% of colon and breast cancers [28]. According to reports from several controlled studies published in the last decade changes in the habits of power through counseling can promote weight loss of 5 to 20 pounds in a year [27]. As primary treatment recommended the modification of behavior and ways of life in the way of eating and physical activity of moderate to intense daily minimum for 30 minutes [29]. In very small part have been studied the factors and determinants of chronic diseases that are part of the metabolic syndrome, with measuring isolated smoking and alcoholism no comprehensive assessment of the State of global health, and increased risk of morbidity and mortality for vascular complications such as cerebral vascular disease manifested as accident and aftermath, as well as a history of cardiac infarction myocardial infarction. We do not know if there is Association and as it increases the risk of vascular damage in obese patients with high probability of studying with metabolic syndrome with sedentary lifestyle, practice physical exercise of protection of health, with the consumption of legal drugs of high prevalence of global consumption such as tobacco and alcohol

The objective of this study is to know the prevalence of risk factors for the inappropriate eating habits in lifestyle, practice of physical exercise, use of legal drugs and his relationship with the presence of chronic diseases: obesity, hypertension, diabetes mellitus, Dyslipidemia, and its vascular complications: infarction cardiac, cerebral vascular disease or degenerative complications such as cancer, chronic obstructive pulmonary disease, and cirrhosis of the liver in health workers, compared with other job categories of the IMSS.

*Corresponding author: María Eugenia Velasco-Contreras Grado, Division of Information and Medical Support, Mexican Institute of Social Security, Insurgentes Sur 253, 5th floor. Colonia Roma Sur, delegation Cuauhtémoc, CP 06700, Mexico, E-mail: maria.velasco@imss.gob.mx

Methods

Study design

From March to December 2009 20,000 surveys were applied in the 35 delegations of the IMSS, in a sample of workers in ordinary regime, all labor categories, attached to the buildings that make up the infrastructure and organization of the Institute, State delegations and in the Federal District. A representative sample of the whole of the IMSS workers of all categories of both shifts according to the existing template was calculated at December 2008. (397,906), they were invited to participate through verbal consent, with anonymous registration of the survey. Sample was weighted by delegation and labor category, in the areas of administrative, social and medical benefits. The procedure for the selection, were allocated according to the proportion of each delegation IMSS.

Category

Health workers, Administrative and quartermaster of the total delegation sample.

Selection criteria

Workers of all labor categories who agree to participate. Exclusion criteria: what the worker does not accept participation criteria of elimination: surveys without registration of more than 50% of the requested data. The study of variables included: delegation, sex, marital status, age, work shift, service, job category, seniority, schooling, somatometría: current weight in kilos, height in cm, waist in cm, systolic, diastolic blood pressure, glucose, uric acid, hemoglobin, cholesterol, triglycerides, LDL, DHL, hereditary risk history, registration of known diseases, years of suffering from the disease, in the last year: number of consultations received, days of hospitalization, number of days of incapacity. Smoking away, this, exfumador, number of cigarettes per day, the addiction to nicotine, (Fagerstrom) assessment. Evaluation of the consumption of alcoholic beverages, abstemio, and risk alcohol consumption: responded in the affirmative that it has consumed in the last year more than 3 glasses, in less than 3 hours or more than 3 times.

Alcohol addiction

- **Tolerance:** You had the need to drink more to achieve the same effect.

- **Unit 1:** when you drink alcohol, ends up drinking more than what was initially planned.

- **Unit 2:** has tried to reduce the drinking quantity or stop drinking, but failed.

- **Unit 3:** in the days of baby, spends a number of considerable time to obtain alcohol or drink to recover from its effects.

- **Unit 4:** invest less time in work, enjoy a hobby, or be with others because of his fondness for drink.

- **Alcohol withdrawal syndrome:** when you stop drinking their hands tremble, sweat or feel restless and also drink to avoid these symptoms.

Pattern of physical exercise

Characteristics of the type of practiced physical exercise: frequency to the week, duration session and intensity. Indicator: 1) physical exercise practiced for 30 minutes or most days of the week. 2) Insufficient physical exercise 3) physical inactivity or sedentary lifestyle.

Eating pattern

Customary practice of an individual using a set of products in 3 sessions each day in order to meet the requirements of your body indicator: 1) pattern of habits and consumption of healthy food 2) pattern of inadequate food habits and consumption of unhealthy foods. Type of food it consumes, frequency per week and number of servings per occasion. Habits: add salt and sugar to your food, you make 3 meals a day, consume daily fruit and eat vegetables daily. Registration of diseases: condition of health given by chronic degenerative diseases and their complications: obesity, diabetes mellitus, arterial hypertension, cardiac infarct, cerebral vascular disease, obstructive pulmonary disease chronic (COPD), cancer, cirrhosis of the liver. Known by the worker as a result of medical care received as a diagnosis, treatment, regular consultations, hospitalization, disabilities and time evolution of the disease.

A questionnaire Likert-type and items with dichotomous choices, 78 questions, with 11 subscales were used: 1.-social and demographic; 2 Somatometría; 3. hereditary antecedents of risk; 4. pathologic personal antecedents; 5. disabilities; 6. tobacco use; 7. evaluation of the nicotine addiction; 8. evaluation of the consumption of alcoholic beverages; 9. detection of diseases; 10. Physical activity pattern; 11. Eating pattern. The instrument shows consistency or homogeneity, with an alpha of Cronbach 0.80. Surveys were sent to each delegation in number and distribution of categories of workers who should survey based on the number of workers by delegation in each category. With a responsible for performing distribution according to the guidelines for its application and invite the workers of randomly selected units of the delegation. Be informed directors of the units of the purpose of the survey, selection and training of personnel responsible for applying it. Workers who agreed to participate were cited in a classroom, Auditorium and multi-purpose room to record the survey in a single moment. The delegation head, sent surveys requested the coordination of integrated programs of health, the public health unit. They were validated for their capture in the optical reader system, responsible for the system developed reading template. It was cleaned and validated the database for processing and analysis.

Statistical analysis

Performed in the SPSS version 17 systems, the frequencies obtained is point prevalence of the risk factors, smoking, prevalence of chronic and Terminal vascular complications, chronic lung damage, liver cirrhosis and neoplasm's diseases. In analysis bivariate estimation the relative Association of risk factors, addictions with obesity, and those with chronic diseases and complications terminals.

Ethical aspects based on the regulation of the General Law of health in research in health, in the title 1, article 17 and category 1 is considered to this type of research as of minimal risk, minimal time investment, depends on truthful worker participation because it is an anonymous survey. The design is in keeping with the principles of the Declaration of Helsinki I, 1964, Declaration of Helsinki II, 1975, Tokyo, 1983 in Venice, 1989 Hong Kong. To ensure the confidentiality of the data of the study population, their right not to participate if it was not their will, when requesting consent was upheld, did not register his name and explained to his knowledge and clarity of the ethical aspects of the study, its purpose and further processing of the data collected.

Results

Sent 25 000 surveys with response rate of 79.5%, a total of 19,532 surveys were analyzed.

(Table 1) (Figure 1).

Sedentary lifestyle affects more than 85% of respondents, the highest prevalence is women in general with more than 90%, and the highest number was found in the men in the delegation from Zacatecas with 97%.

The consumption of foods with excess calories, junk, fast food and sweet bread in general affects 40% of the respondent.

With respect to the unhealthy habits like having fasting, not eat fruit and vegetables, add sugar and salt to food, is located at 30% (Table 2).

The frequency higher tobacco and alcohol addiction correspond to the male staff, with increased consumption of tobacco and alcohol of quartermaster personnel risk: 36.5% and 45.8% in men, 25.8% and

21.0% in women respectively. The consumption of more than five cigarettes a day, affecting a quarter of smokers, staff is the most affected with 9.2%. With respect to behaviors that indicate alcohol addiction, as often corresponds to the unit 1 which applies to drink more alcohol than was initially planned. Quartermaster staff does in 26.5% men and 17.4% women. Highlights the increased frequency of this same 1 dependence among medical 12.9% compared to doctors 9.0%, likewise was also higher frequencies compared between physicians and medical in addiction to alcohol with unit 3, 4 and alcoholic withdrawal syndrome. The Nuevo Leon delegation resulted in 3 occasions, higher for smoking and southern Veracruz for alcoholism on 4 occasions (Table 3).

The highest frequencies of chronic diseases correspond to the male staff, except for obesity, depression, and neoplasm's. It is doubled in men in Dyslipidemia, cardiac infarction and overweight have metabolic syndrome and is doubled in women in depression and neoplasm's. It is similar in both men and women for cerebral vascular complications. The doctors the frequency of dislipidemia is doubled when compared with the medical and in these double when compared with other job categories. The southern Veracruz delegation resulted in 4 times higher for overweight, obesity, hypertension, and Hidalgo in cirrhosis and metabolic syndrome (Table 4).

The likelihood of obesity was statistically significant in both men and women affected by habits of consumption of unhealthy foods, lack of consumption of healthy foods (fruits and vegetables), and in women with the bad habit of fasting. The highest Association occurred in the sedentary life in both sexes.

There was no statistical association with the habit of adding salt to

Demographic characteristics		Total		Age (years)		
		Number	%	Minimum value	Maximum value	Media
Sex	Man	7,347	37.6	18	79	40.7
	Woman	12,185	62.3	18	77	40.4
Labor category	Medical	3,603	18.4	22	75	44.1
	Administrative	4,264	21.8	18	74	41.2
	Quartermaster	2,581	13.2	18	68	33.6
	Other	9,084	46.5	18	73	41.6

Table 1: Demographic characteristics and categories of the IMSS workers.

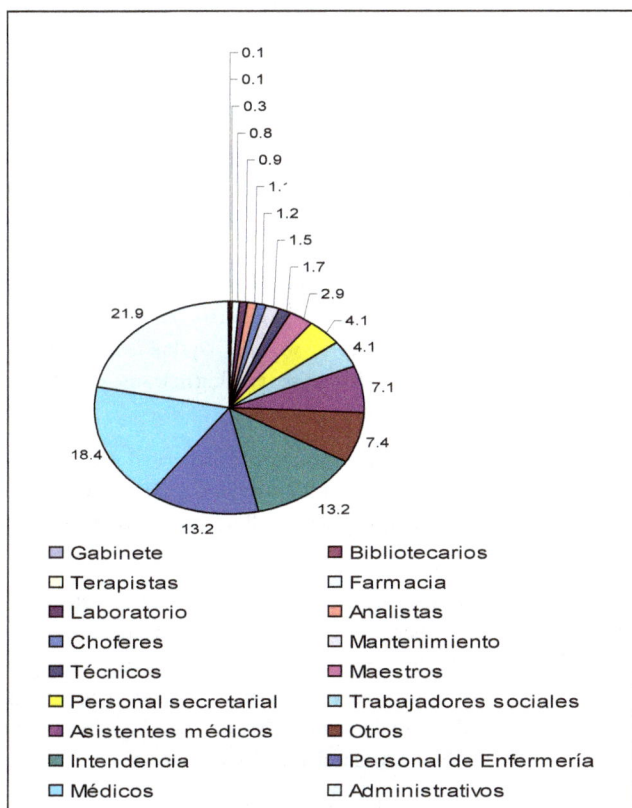

DELEGACION	TOTAL	Hombres	
		Edad promedio	Edad promedio
Aguascalientes	43	39	44
Baja California	40	40	40
Baja California Sur	39	35	42
Campeche	40	41	38
Coahuila	40	44	43
Colima	44	43	40
Chiapas	39	39	40
Chihuahua	41	41	41
Durango	40	39	41
Guanajuato	38	37	38
Guerrero	42	43	41
Hidalgo	39	39	40
Jajisco	38	39	37
Mexico Orient	38	37	39
Mexico Ponien	40	38	40
Michoacan	42	43	41
Morelos	37	40	37
Nayarit	40	40	41
Nuevo Leon	40	40	40
Oaxaca	42	42	42
Puebla	41	41	41
Queretaro	39	40	39
Quintana Roo	38	39	37
San Luis Potos	40	39	40
Sinaloa	40	39	40
Sonara	39	40	39
Tabasco	41	41	41
Tamaulipas	40	40	40
Tlaxcala	41	43	40
Veracruz Nort	42	43	41
Veracruz Sur	41	41	40
Yucatan	41	42	41
Zacatecas	42	41	42
DF Norte	41	40	41
DF Sur	40	41	40
NACIONAL	40	40	40

Pie chart values: 0.1, 0.1, 0.3, 0.8, 0.9, 1.1, 1.2, 1.5, 1.7, 2.9, 4.1, 4.1, 7.1, 7.4, 13.2, 13.2, 18.4, 21.9

Legend:
- Gabinete
- Bibliotecarios
- Terapistas
- Farmacia
- Laboratorio
- Analistas
- Choferes
- Mantenimiento
- Técnicos
- Maestros
- Personal secretarial
- Trabajadores sociales
- Asistentes médicos
- Otros
- Intendencia
- Personal de Enfermería
- Médicos
- Administrativos

Figure 1: Proportion by type of all labour categories and age average of men and women workers by delegation.

Habits of risk	Overall prevalence		Personal health				Other employment category		Higher prevalence	
			Medical		Nurses (I)		Men	Women	Men	Women
	Men	Women	Men	Women	Men	Women	Driver	Administrative	ZAC	NAY
+ Sedentary lifestyle	88.9	92.8	88.7	90.5	88.3	95.0	90.4	93.6	97.4	97.2
* Consumes							Quartermaster	Quartermaster	YUC	VERS
Excess calories	36.4	31.9	23.3	18.8	48.8	28.3	45.4	49.1	77.3	50.8
							Quartermaster	Quartermaster	YUC	YUC
Meals Fast	30.5	22.8	18.6	13.6	40.3	15.6	41.5	44.8	50.0	47.2
							Quartermaster	Quartermaster	YUC	YUC
Scrap	42.8	40.6	29.3	25.8	48.4	31.4	56.2	55.7	70.5	66
							Quartermaster	Quartermaster	MEXORO	MEXORO
Sweet bread	51.4	56.5	35.4	31.9	55.8	46.3	61.1	55.7	84.1	79.1
							Driver	Quartermaster	ZAC	NL
More than 5 tortillas per day	16.8	7.4	10.8	4.3	17.5	6.8	20.6	11.4	24.4	22.8
							Technical	Quartermaster	AGC	MOR
Add 2 or more c/sugar/day	28.9	26.7	20.4	17.1	28.9	26.3	34.8	36.1	45.5	36.6
							Quartermaster	Quartermaster	MOR	CAM
Add salt	52.9	53.6	42.7	41.3	50.0	50.7	63.3	65.7	66.3	62.2
							Quartermaster	Quartermaster	NL	YUC
Does not consume daily vegetable	39.4	34.0	26.4	21.6	35.9	28.8	46.6	47.4	48.8	49.1
							Driver	Quartermaster	NL	YUC
Does not consume fruit daily	39.5	30.0	26.4	21.6	36.2	22.3	47.2	42.9	54.9	51.7
							Administrative	Quartermaster	MEXPO	COAH
Does 3 Meals/day	30.0	31.6	31.1	28.5	29.8	31.2	34.0	35.8	44.6	48.6

Risk habits: behaviors or unhealthy habits that increase the probability of suffering from chronic diseases associated with obesity. +Sedentary lifestyle: Does physical exercise; *Consume for 4 to 7 days a week;
Excess calories: tamales, atoles, capeados, breaded, and fried.
Fast foods: hot dog, pizza, chicken style Kentucky.
Scrap: chips, cakes, biscuits, instant soups, soft drinks. Sweet bread 2 and more servings a day.
Unhealthy eating habits:
- Eating more than 5 tortillas a day.
- Add 2 and more tablespoons of sugar a day.
- Add salt to your food to consume them.
- Does not consume vegetables every day.
- Does not consume fruit every day.
- Does not 3 meals every day (he is fasting, only dinner)

Table 2: Practice of physical exercise and eating habits

consume their food in both sexes and in men although women with the consumption of fast foods, sweet bread and not make 3 meals or have fast men. In general, the Association of these factors with obesity was higher in women (Table 5).

Obesity is associated in men and women with smoking 5 or more cigarettes a day and is statistically significant. Respect to the Association of obesity with the consumption of alcohol risk and their addiction; It arose only in men with alcohol consumption risk, tolerance and dependence to alcohol from 1 to 4 and alcoholic withdrawal syndrome. There was no association with obesity in women who consume alcohol. (Table 6).

The likely to have chronic diseases was statistically significant in both men and women affected by obesity. There was no association with neoplasias. The strength of Association of obesity, with the presence of chronic diseases was higher in women than in men, except in cardiac infarction and cirrhosis of the liver. Chronic diseases in order of magnitude and strength of association with obesity are high blood pressure and diabetes mellitus, Dyslipidemia, and chronic obstructive pulmonary disease in women (Table 7).

Smoking at least one cigarette a day is associated with depression and was statistically significant in both men and women, with greater strength in women in whom also strongly with myocardial infarction and vascular disease (Table 8).

The Association of smoking more 5 cigarettes a day is strongly associated with depression in both sexes, with hypertension, diabetes mellitus, cardiac infarction, vascular disease brain; it was statistically significant, with higher strength of Association in men, except with chronic obstructive pulmonary disease, which was associated with greater strength in women. Dyslipidemia and neoplasms were only associated with intense smoking in women and liver cirrhosis associated with only in men (Table 9).

Alcohol consumption is associated with risk of depression in men and women with 4 times more force in them, as well as cerebral vascular disease only in them. Dyslipidemia is associated only in men (Table 10).

There is association with chronic disease and the consumption of alcohol with unit 4. They include hypertension, diabetes mellitus, and myocardial infarction with strong association in women and cirrhosis in both sexes. Depression is more strongly associated in men. There were only Association in men with neoplasms, lung disease and cerebral vascular disease. There were no cases of lung disease, or cerebral vascular disease in women.

Association of hypertension and diabetes mellitus risk factors with other chronic diseases addiction to tobacco, alcohol causes irreversible consequences (Table 11 and 12).

Does Smoking and Alcohol Abuse Precipitate and Aggravate the Risk of Metabolic...

45

| *Addiction | Overall prevalence | | Personal health | | | | Other employment category | | Higher prevalence | |
| | Men | Women | Medical | | Nurses (I) | | Men | Women | Men | Women |
			Men	Women	Men	Women				
Smoking	26.1	13.1	14.9	8.4	29.9	8.8	36.5	25.8	37.7	18.3
							Quartermaster	Quartermaster	NL	JAL
Smoking + 5 cigars Per day	6.5	2.2	4.0	2.0	5.2	0.9	9.2	4.8	9.2	4.8
							Technical	Quartermaster	NL	NL
Alcohol consumption Risk	40.3	12.7	34.4	9.9	39.6	9.0	45.8	21.0	51.7	24.5
							Quartermaster	Quartermaster	CHIH	COL
Unit 1	18.6	10.1	9.0	12.9	20.0	8.4	26.5	17.4	43.1	33.3
							Quartermaster	Quartermaster	VERS	VERS
Unit 2	16.7	8.2	7.1	4.9	19.8	5.3	26.8	12.7	44.8	29.0
							Quartermaster	Quartermaster	TLAX	VERS
Tolerance	12.3	4.5	5.8	3.4	14.2	3.0	16.9	8.1	24.4	16.7
							Quartermaster	Quartermaster	MEXPO	OAX
Unit 3	10.4	4.6	4.0	4.3	11.3	2.0	17.0	9.2	29.6	33.3
							Quartermaster	Quartermaster	VERN	VERS
Unit 4	3.4	1.2	0.8	1.6	4.7	0.4	5.2	1.7	10.3	6.6
							Quartermaster	Quartermaster	TLAX	TAB
Alcohol withdrawal syndrome	4.0	2.0	1.2	2.5	6.3	1.2	5.5	4.1	9.6	11.1
							Quartermaster	Quartermaster	COAH	OAX

*Addictions: Chronic diseases by periodic consumption of legal drugs: nicotine or alcohol. Risk alcohol consumption. In the past 12 months has drunk 3 or more alcoholic drinks in one period of less than 3 hours or more than 3 times.
Tolerance: You had the need to drink more to achieve the same effect.
Unit 1: when you drink alcohol, ends up drinking more than what was initially planned.
Unit 2: has tried to reduce the drinking quantity or stop drinking, but failed.
Unit 3: in the days of baby, spends a number of considerable times to obtain alcohol or drink to recover from its effects.
Unit 4: invest less time in work, enjoy a hobby, or be with others because of his fondness for drink.
Alcohol withdrawal syndrome: when you stop drinking their hands tremble, sweat or feel restless and also drink to avoid these symptoms.

Table 3: Addictions: Smoking and alcoholism.

| * Disease | Overall prevalence | | Personal health | | | | Other employment category | | Higher prevalence | |
| | Men | Women | Medical | | Nurses (I) | | Men | Women | Men | Women |
			Men	Women	Men	Women				
Overweight	36.5	36.4	37.7	38.5	29.9	42.8	40.5	40.8	49.5	51.9
							Master	Social work	VERS	COL
Obesity	11.4	12.9	12.1	11.9	13.4	14.7	13.9	15.7	18.4	19.1
							Technical	Social work	VERS	VERS
Hypertension	12.2	11.2	16.9	12.3	12.3	10.7	12.4	13.2	20.5	16.3
							Master	Master	VERS	COL
Dyslipidemia	8.5	5.1	19.2	10.0	6.2	6.3	5.0	6.5	14.9	15.0
							Technical	Social work	TAB	MEXPO
Diabetes	7.5	6.3	7.9	4.2	8.0	6.0	9.2	9.0	13.3	8.9
							Master	Master	OAX	SLP
Depression	2.6	4.6	2.5	4.0	2.2	3.7	5.0	6.6	5.6	5.4
							Driver	Master	NAY	COL
Cardiac infarct	1.3	0.7	2.0	0.7	1.1	0.4	1.5	2.1	4.1	1.9
							Therapists	Master	ARE	COL
Chronic obstructive pulmonary disease	1.0	0.8	0.8	0.6	1.1	0.5	2.0	1.0	2.3	1.9
							Master	Medical Assistant.	SLP	MICH
Neoplasm's	0.5	1.2	0.7	1.5	0.4	1.4	0.5	2.1	1.8	2.8
							Administrative	Master	WITHOUT	MOR
Cerebral vascular disease	0.4	0.4	0.4	0.3	0.4	0.6	0.7	1.4	1.3	1.0
							Master	Master	PUE	MEXPO
Cirrhosis of the liver	0.3	0.2	0.4	0.3	0.7	0.1	0.2	0.7	2.7	1.0
							Quartermaster	Medical Assistant.	HGO	VERN

							Driver	Medical Assistant.	HGO	BCS
Overweight and metabolic syndrome	0.5	0.2	1.2	0.6	0.0	0.2	1.4	0.5	1.8	1.3
							Quartermaster	Social work	HGO	AGC
Metabolic syndrome and obesity	0.3	0.2	0.9	0.6	0.0	0.2	0.2	0.3	2.7	1.22

*Diagnostic acquainted with registration: evolution time, number of consultations per year, hospitalizations and disability days in the past year. SM=metabolic syndrome: Overweight/obesity, hypertension, diabetes and Dyslipidemia

Table 4: Frequency of chronic diseases.

Table of contingency, degree of Association and statistical significance

Risk factor	Obesity in men 11.4%					Obesity in women 12.9%				
	Prevalence in exposed	RMP	IC		Xmh	+ P <.05	Prevalence in exposed	RMP	IC		Xmh	+ P <.05
Sedentary lifestyle	14.3	1.83	1.58	2.13	8.05	+	15.9	2.17	1.92	2.45	12.58	+
Eat: Excess calories	12.1	1.68	1.33	2.11	4.47	+	13.5	1.55	1.31	1.84	5.09	+
Fast foods	11.7	1.15	0.97	1.38	1.60		13.3	1.15	1.02	1.3	2.22	+
Scrap	11.8	1.27	1.04	1.55	2.39	+	13.7	1.61	1.37	1.88	5.91	+
Sweet bread	11.4	1.05	0.86	1.29	0.45		13.2	1.23	1.06	1.44	2.67	+
More than 5 tortillas per day	11.4	1.21	0.61	2.42	0.54		13.1	1.43	1.44	4.11	3.43	+
More than 2 c/sugar day	13.3	1.3	1.12	1.52	3.35	+	16.3	1.48	1.32	1.65	6.72	+
Add salt	11.8	1.1	0.96	1.28	1.34		12.6	0.95	0.85	1.05	-1.03	
Does not consume vegetables	13.4	1.38	1.19	1.6	4.36	+	15.2	1.34	1.2	1.49	5.19	+
Does not consume fruit	13.8	1.43	1.23	1.66	4.74	+	15.8	1.39	1.24	1.56	5.69	+
Do 3 meals	12.5	1.16	0.99	1.37	1.81		14.5	2.08	1.36	3.29	6.72	+

*Global prevalence of obesity in men and women. PE=prevalence in exposed (with the risk factor) RMP=reason for the prevalence odds, CI=confidence interval; Xmh = Chi-square of Mantel-Haenszel.

Table 5: Association of obesity with poor diet and sedentary lifestyle habits.

Risk factors	Table of contingency, degree of Association and statistical significance										
	Obesity in men 11.4%					Obesity in women 12.9%				
	Prevalence in exposed	RMP	IC		Xmh	+ P <.05	Prevalence in exposed	RMP	IC		Xmh	+ P <.05
Smoking	11.9	1.08	0.91	1.29	0.81		13.9	1.10	0.95	1.29	1.20	
You smoke more than five cigarettes a day	15.3	1.44	1.11	1.88	2.71	+	17.4	1.43	1.03	1.98	2.17	+
Consumption of Alcohol in Risk	15.8	1.81	1.57	2.10	8.00	+	13.3	1.04	0.89	1.23	0.52	
Tolerance	20.2	2.08	1.61	2.69	5.67	+	15.6	1.25	0.70	2.21	0.75	
Deprivation syndrome Alcoholic	23.6	2.46	1.61	3.75	4.31	+	10.8	0.82	0.29	2.31	-0.38	
Unit 1	15.1	1.43	1.12	1.82	2.91	+	12.0	0.92	0.59	1.44	-0.35	
Unit 2	15.4	1.46	1.13	1.88	2.93	+	10.7	0.81	0.47	1.38	-0.77	
Unit 3	14.6	1.36	0.98	1.87	1.85		8.9	0.65	0.30	1.43	-1.075	
Unit 4	20.4	2.03	1.25	3.29	2.91	+	9.5	0.71	0.17	3.05	-0.46	

Smoking: Chronic disease by the consumption of nicotine in cigarettes. Risk alcohol consumption. In the past 12 months has drunk 3 or more alcoholic drinks in one period of less than 3 hours or more than 3 times.
Tolerance: You had the need to drink more to achieve the same effect.
Unit 1: when you drink alcohol, ends up drinking more than what was initially planned.
Unit 2: has tried to reduce the drinking quantity or stop drinking, but failed.
Unit 3: in the days of baby, spends a number of considerable time to obtain alcohol or drink to recover from its effects.
Unit 4: invest less time in work, enjoy a hobby, or be with others because of his fondness for drink.
Alcohol withdrawal syndrome: when you stop drinking their hands tremble, sweat or feel restless and also drink to avoid these symptoms.
RMP=reason for the prevalence odds, CI=RMP confidence interval, Xmh=Chi-square of Mantel-Haenszel

Table 6: Association of obesity with smoking and alcoholism

Disease	Table of contingency, degree of Association and statistical significance									
	Obesity in men 11.4%					Obesity in women 12.9%				
	Prevalence in exposed	RMP	IC		Xmh	+ P <.05	Prevalence in exposed	RMP	IC		Xmh	+ P <.05
High blood pressure	23.0	2.77	2.33	3.31	11.70	+	23.8	2.40	2.09	2.75	12.70	+
Diabetes mellitus	21.7	2.36	1.90	2.93	7.97	+	27.2	2.75	2.32	3.26	12.17	+
Dyslipidemia	22.5	2.52	2.06	3.10	9.16	+	25.0	2.39	1.98	2.89	9.31	+
Depression	19.5	1.93	1.34	2.78	3.57	+	18.6	1.58	1.27	1.97	4.11	+
Neoplasm's	16.2	1.52	0.63	3.64	0.93		15.2	1.22	0.78	1.90	0.86	
Disease Pulmonary OBS. Chronic	22.5	2.30	1.31	4.03	2.98	+	36.9	4.00	2.41	6.63	5.79	+
Cardiac infarct	33.0	3.95	2.56	6.11	6.65	+	22.2	1.94	1.15	3.28	2.51	+
Cerebral Vascular disease	31.8	3.67	1.49	9.02	3.03	+	32.4	3.24	1.58	6.67	3.38	+
Cirrhosis of the liver	47.8	7.24	3.18	16.46	5.52	+	37.9	4.15	1.96	8.80	4.02	+

RMP = reason for the prevalence odds, CI = RMP confidence interval, Xmh = Chi-square ofMantel-Haenszel

Table 7: Association of obesity with chronic diseases of the metabolic syndrome.

Table of contingency, degree of Association and statistical significance									
Disease	* Men 24.1%					* 12.9% women				
	Prevalence in exposed	RMP	IC		Xmh	+ P <.05	Prevalence in exposed	RMP	IC		Xmh	+ P <.05
High blood pressure	19.1	0.72	0.60	0.86	-3.70		11.5	0.86	0.73	1.03	-1.99	
Diabetes mellitus	24.2	1.01	0.82	1.24	0.09		15.0	1.21	0.98	1.48	1.78	
Dyslipidemia	22.0	0.88	0.72	1.08	-1.24		11.0	0.82	0.64	1.07	-1.47	
Depression	34.2	1.67	1.23	2.26	3.31	+	18.8	1.60	1.28	1.99	4.21	+
Neoplasms	24.3	1.01	0.48	2.15	0.04		17.2	1.41	0.92	2.15	1.57	
Disease Pulmonary Chronic obstructive	33.8	1.62	0.99	2.66	1.92		16.9	1.37	0.72	2.63	0.96	
Cardiac infarct	22.3	0.91	0.56	1.48	-0.39		28.4	2.69	1.66	4.38	4.16	+
Disease Vascular brain	31.8	1.47	0.60	3.62	0.85		32.4	3.24	1.58	6.66	3.38	+
Cirrhosis of the liver	30.4	1.38	0.57	3.36	0.71		10.3	0.78	0.24	2.57	-0.41	

* Prevalence of smoking in men and women. + currently smoke at least one cigarette every day. .
RMP = reason for the prevalence odds, CI = RMP confidence interval, Xmh = Chi-square ofMantel-Haenszel

Table 8: Association of chronic diseases with smoking.

Table of contingency, degree of Association and statistical significance									
Disease	Men * 6.2%					Women * 2.1%				
	Prevalence in exposed	RMP	IC		Xmh	+ P <.05	Prevalence in exposed	RMP	IC		Xmh	+ P <.05
High blood pressure	7.7	1.30	1.00	1.69	4.31	+	2.5	1.21	0.84	1.74	3.05	+
Diabetes mellitus	9.4	1.63	1.20	2.20	7.13	+	3.3	1.61	1.06	2.46	6.82	+
Dyslipidemia	6.1	0.97	0.69	1.37	-0.33		2.6	1.22	0.73	2.04	2.29	+
Depression	14.2	2.58	1.70	3.92	10.28	+	3.9	1.97	1.26	3.07	9.16	+
Neoplasms	10.8	1.83	0.64	5.18	1.15		4.6	2.27	1.05	4.90	2.15	+
Disease Pulmonary Chronic obstructive	16.9	3.11	1.66	5.82	3.72	+	9.2	4.77	2.04	11.15	3.98	+
Cardiac infarct	14.9	2.68	1.51	4.76	3.48	+	6.2	3.07	1.23	7.65	2.53	+
Cerebral Vascular disease	27.3	5.69	2.22	14.61	4.08	+	8.8	4.50	1.37	14.80	2.71	+
Cirrhosis of the liver	30.4	6.65	2.72	16.25	4.80	+	6.9	3.43	0.81	14.50	1.78	

* Prevalence of smoking in men and women. + Currently smoke 5 cigarettes a day.
RMP=reason for the prevalence odds, CI=RMP confidence interval, Xmh=Chi-square ofMantel-Haenszel,

Table 9: Association of chronic diseases with smoking 5 cigarettes a day.

Table of contingency, degree of Association and statistical significance

Disease	Men * 38.4%						Women * 11.4%					
	Prevalence in exposed	RMP	IC		Xmh	+ P <.05	Prevalence in exposed	RMP	IC		Xmh	+ P <.05
High blood pressure	39.6	1.06	0.92	1.22	0.78		8.9	0.74	0.60	0.89	-3.09	
Diabetes mellitus	37.4	0.96	0.80	1.15	-0.46		10.6	0.92	0.72	1.16	-0.72	
Dyslipidemia	43.4	1.26	1.07	1.48	2.70	+	12.8	1.15	0.90	1.46	1.10	
Depression	48.4	1.53	1.14	2.04	2.89	+	22.2	2.33	1.90	2.87	8.21	+
Neoplasms	35.1	0.87	0.44	1.71	-0.40		11.9	1.05	0.64	1.73	0.20	
Disease Pulmonary Chronic obstructive	46.5	1.40	0.88	2.24	1.41		15.4	1.42	0.72	2.78	1.01	
Cardiac infarct	34.0	0.83	0.54	1.27	-0.86		14.8	1.35	0.73	2.51	0.97	
Cerebral Vascular disease	54.5	1.93	0.83	4.48	1.56		23.5	2.40	1.08	5.31	2.22	+
Cirrhosis of the liver	47.8	1.48	0.65	3.35	0.94		13.8	1.24	0.43	3.58	0.40	

Table 10: Association of chronic diseases with risk alcohol consumption.

Table of contingency, degree of Association and statistical significance

Disease	Men * 1.4%						Women * 0.2%					
	Prevalence in exposed	RMP	IC		Xmh	+ P <.05	Prevalence in exposed	RMP	IC		Xmh	+ P <.05
High blood pressure	2.2	1.75	1.07	2.87	2.26	+	0.4	2.99	1.17	7.66	2.40	+
Diabetes mellitus	2.5	1.96	1.11	3.46	2.35	+	0.7	4.69	1.71	12.80	3.31	+
Dyslipidemia	1.4	1.04	0.52	2.06	0.10		0.2	0.92	0.12	6.88	-0.80	
Depression	5.8	4.72	2.48	8.97	5.21	+	0.7	4.92	1.65	14.68	3.17	+
Neoplasms	8.1	6.36	1.92	21.06	3.47	+	0.7	4.00	0.53	30.03	1.46	
Disease Pulmonary Obstructive. Chronic	4.2	3.17	0.98	10.23	2.03	+	0.0	0.00	0.00	0.00	0.00	
Cardiac infarct	4.3	3.21	1.16	8.92	2.36	+	3.7	25.82	7.46	98.40	7.68	+
Disease. Vascular brain	9.1	7.15	1.65	31.01	3.07	+	0.0	0.00	0.00	0.00	0.00	
Cirrhosis of the liver	17.4	15.36	5.13	45.99	6.53	+	3.4	21.67	2.81	167.06	4.25	+

* Prevalence of alcohol-dependent 4: invest time to get alcohol and drink or drinks to recover from its effects

RMP = reason for the prevalence odds, CI=RMP confidence interval, Xmh=Chi-square ofMantel-Haenszel,

Table 11: Association of chronic diseases with 4 alcohol dependence

Risk factors	Workers with hypertension 2252						Workers withDiabetes mellitus 1329					
	Prevalence in exposed	RMP	IC		Xmh	+ P <.05	Prevalence in exposed	RMP	IC		Xmh	+ P <.05
Add sugar	16.1	**1.36**	1.16	1.61	2.0	+	15.8	2.63	2.01	3.44	3.48	+
Sedentary lifestyle	15.0	**1.34**	1.13	1.59	1.7		7.4	1.15	0.86	1.56	0.35	
Overweight	13.2	**1.14**	0.96	1.36	0.7		7.1	0.99	0.74	1.32	-0.03	
Smoking	15.4	**1.31**	1.11	1.55	1.7.		10.7	1.65	1.25	2.17	1.49	
Consumption of alcohol of risk	13.5	**1.12**	0.96	1.36	0.68		7.5	104	0.78	1.39	0.10	
DISEASES	Associated diseases											
Obesity	22.5	**2.11**	1.8	2.47	5.5	+	13.5	2.16	1.65	2.83	2.5	+
Diabetes / Hypertension	37.0	**3.70**	3.18	4.31	12.6	+	21.6	4.15	3.16	5.46	5.84	+
Dyslipidemia	25.5	**2.26**	1.94	2.64	6.6	+	13.1	1.89	1.46	2.46	2.19	+
Depression	21.0	**1.74**	1.49	2.04	4.1	+	11.4	1.59	1.22	2.08	1.5	+
Neoplasms (cancer)	23.4	**1.9**	1.63	2.21	5.16	+	28.1	4.01	3.17	5.08	7.5	+
COMPLICATIONS	Associated irreversible sequelae and complications											
Cardiac infarct	56.0	**5.06**	4.4	5.81	20.9	+	41.7	6.16	4.9	7.76	12.4	+
Disease Vascular Brain	48.2	**4.19**	3.64	4.82	17.1	+	24	3.36	2.65	4.26	5.9	+

Disease											
Pulmonary Obstructive chronic	34.8	**2.93**	2.54	3.38	10.6	+	25	3.5	2.76	4.44	6.3	+
Liver cirrhosis	44.2	**3.7**	3.28	4.34	15.1	+	46.1	6.65	5.3	8.33	13.9	+
SMOKING	Complications and irreversible consequences associated with smoking more than 5 cigarettes a day										
Cardiac infarct	34.6	2.88	2.5	3.33	10.5	+	37.5	50.8	26.5	97.2	13.1	+
Disease Vascular Brain	26.8	85.6	40.12	182.9	12.6	+	31.2	97.8	36.4	262.5	11.0	+
Disease Pulmonary Obstructive chronic	34.4	55.9	32.9	95.8	16.1	+	44.1	70.3	34.9	141.5	15.8	+
Neoplasms (cancer)	25.5	27.05	17.3	42.1	11.7	+	26.9	31.4	17.7	57.8	9.3	+
ALCOHOLISM	Complications and irreversible consequences associated with alcohol consumption with unit 4										
Cardiac infarct	27.5	37.7	22.85	62.1	12.8	+	23.2	26.9	14.6	49.7	8.1	+
Disease Vascular Brain	19.5	45.9	23.7	88.9	9.13	+	15.6	35.9	15.1	85.4	5.4	+
Liver cirrhosis	39.1	193.08	76.6	487.5	18.6	+	37.5	177.1	53.3	594.2	13.3	+
Neoplasms (cancer)	16.2	16.8	10.4	26.3	7.2	+	23	23.7	13.3	42.3	7.8	+

Table 12: Table of contingency, degree of Association and statistical significance.

Discussion

IMSS staff presents a frequency of risk factors causing damage to her health similar to the population open to the extent that it resembles their level of schooling, designated by his category work in personnel administration, compared with nurses and medical staff. This situation arises both in sedentary lifestyle, bad eating habits and very prominent in the consumption of legal drugs tobacco and alcohol. Sedentary lifestyle in this study was identified by a criterion of physical exercise moderate to severe for 30 minutes or most days of the week, so its prevalence was above 90% with greater involvement of women in general. There is an area of important opportunity because in the clinic is perceived which is considered not sedentary people who performed hiking to move or during their daily activities under this heading. To get the benefit for the health of the physical exercise it is required for a minimum time of 20 minutes and to achieve changes in heart rate with increase of 80% of the maximum heart rate for age. This generates increased due to the increase in mitochondrial oxygen consumption in muscles, increase of glucose transporters, increase the sensitivity of receptors to insulin, decrease blood pressure, endorphins increase, decrease of hepatic fat and decrease in visceral fat in general [29] the bad habits of power in this study were identified by the frequency of 4 to 7 days a week of food consumption with excess calories: tamales, atoles, capeados, breaded, and fried. Fast foods: hot dog, pizza, chicken style kentoky. Scrap: chips, cakes, biscuits, instant soups, soft drinks. Sweet bread 2 and more servings a day. More than 5 a day, 2 and more tablespoons of sugar a day. Add salt to your food to consume them. Not eat vegetables every day. Not eat fruit every day. Not make 3 meals every day, be fasting, only dinner. These everyday habits cause metabolic changes that translate into response Glycemic with abrupt rise of the glucose derived from the consumption of sugar refined with leap of the insulin response with proportional oscillations to the glycemic index of foods high glycemic index all the identified here, (its consumption is an undesirable habit of power.) who are studying with high levels of insulin, which in turn increase the risk of cardiovascular disease and characterized metabolic syndrome by: elevation of insulin, overweight, obesity, lifting of 100 mg/dl fasting glucose or higher, postprandial of 140 mg/dl or higher, elevation of blood pressure of 130/85 or greater, triglycerides of 150 mg/dl or higher, uric acid 5 mg/dl or greater, waist 80cm and 90cm in men or older women. Decrease of less than 40 high-density lipoprotein cholesterol mg/dl in men of 50 mg/dl in women [3] respect of the habit of not consuming vegetables and fruit, has been included as a risk factor for the presence of type 2 diabetes mellitus in an index of risk for early identification of pre-diabetes published by Dr. Tuomilehto J in 2002. In this study is clearly associated to obesity in men and women. It is based on adding a point of increased risk of diabetes who not integrated into your daily diet vegetables and fruits, rich in antioxidants, vitamins, enzymes and other nutrients that promote balance Endocrine-Metabolic [30] quartermaster staff presents the higher frequencies in the consumption of unhealthy food and lack of consumption of vegetables and fruit with 10 percentage points higher than the average value, both in men and in women. This is related to their increased frequency of obesity compared with health workers. In our study analyzed the Association of cigarette smoking at least a day associated with depression 3-4 times in men and women respectively. Women also associated with the presence of myocardial infarction 4 times more and 3 times more cerebral vascular disease, compared with women non-smokers, this suggests greater sensitivity to vascular damage generated by at least one smoking a day for women to compare this result in men smokers in this study. In the smokers of more than five cigarettes a day, was associated to obesity, twice in both sexes and was statistically significant. Studies have been conducted to identify the brain areas involved in addiction, the effect is shared in certain food addiction and nicotine [31] the smoking was associated clearly greater than 5 cigarettes a day with hypertension, diabetes mellitus, depression, cardiac infarct, cerebral vascular disease, was statistically significant in both sexes, with greater strength in men; except with chronic obstructive pulmonary disease, which was associated with greater strength in women. When comparing workers with obesity, more nicotine addiction doubles the risk of developing hypertension, diabetes and its complications in terminal damage to organs with greater impact on women, highlighting the presence of cerebral vascular disease followed by cardiac infarct in obese women smokers. Neoplasms are associated in women smokers more 5 cigarettes a day; not so in obese non-smokers. With this result the most damage to health with respect to the dose of nicotine (and other components of the cigar) consumed per day, and which reveal the series of alterations physiopathological which have been linked to the consumption of cigarettes with more than 4 thousand substances including nicotine, including more than

40 factors and carbon monoxide is evident, by different mechanisms generate hypertension, diabetes, Dyslipidemia, (metabolic syndrome) vascular, pulmonary, liver damage and cancer [32].

Risk (CAR) alcohol and behavior of consumption with varying degrees of addiction, until syndrome withdrawal alcoholic uncomplicated (SDA) (syndrome of severe deprivation and seizures)

The CAR was 40% in men and 12% in women; again the quartermaster staff presents the prevalence but high, 45.8% in men and 21.0% for females. With respect to conduct of alcohol dependence, the increased frequency was 1: drink more alcohol then planned initially, 26.5% men and 17.4% women. Highlights the higher frequency among medical 12.9 doctors 9.0% %, was also higher in unit 3, 4 and SDA. This result alerts us to apply these questions as part of early detection first consumption of alcohol risk and subsequently tolerance until 1-4 dependence on men and women and identify the behaviors of different degree of alcohol addiction, and promptly inform them about the medium-term risk and accumulated daily alcohol consumption for "acute" damage associated with high mortality and morbidity as the EVC and infarction heart, with irreversible consequences such as liver and vascular complications associated with metabolic syndrome and liver damage by periodic abusive consumption of alcohol [32]. With regard to the Association of obesity - metabolic syndrome with CAR; it arose only in men. There was no association with obesity in women who consume alcohol. Note that in the causation of obesity in men alcohol use plays an important role, by comparing it with the presence of obesity in women who consume unhealthy food and other inadequate habits in your daily diet as they are fasting presented 6 times more in obese women. The probability of depression was statistically significant in both men and women affected by alcohol consumption risk, with greater strength in women. Is alert to female staff who have CAR, because alcohol addiction associated with the presence of the myocardial infarction in women, diabetes and high blood pressure, this suggests damage specific periodic daily alcohol consumption to alter the production of hormones such as catecholamines, steroids with pancreatic dysfunction in the production of insulin and presence of diabetic status. We highlight the most cardiovascular damage in women and neoplasms in males, their physiopathological mechanisms have been associated with the elevation of catecholamines, hypertension and massive production of oxidants, they begin the degenerative cellular damage included the breast cancer in women and prostate in men to be most frequent in the Mexican population [33].

The frequency of registration of chronic disease and its complications was higher in men. We believe that this may be ultimately to greater involvement of men by the consumption of legal drugs alcohol and tobacco, 38%-11% in women for alcohol and 26 against 12% for women with regard to tobacco, this situation is the best evidence that the vascular complications of metabolic syndrome can be initiated and precipitated by the consumption of tobacco and alcohol. Here it should be noted affecting risk factors most frequently quartermaster personnel. That should alert physicians of promotion and prevention of health to intervene with education to eat healthy foods, exercise and give timely attention of addictions with priority from the open population, as its future health Outlook is not encouraging.

Conclusions

The likelihood of obesity, chronic diseases and complications was statistically significant in both men and women affected by unhealthy eating habits, sedentary lifestyle and consumption of legal drugs tobacco and alcohol. . In general, the strength of Association of these risk factors with obesity was higher in women this is absolutely indispensable to promote a Decalogue of healthy eating habits for the entire population, practice of daily physical exercise and enjoy your life without drugs.

1. Do 3 meals a day and if it is possible in addition 2 snacks of fruit/vegetable.

2. Drink 3 glasses of cool water or fruits without sugar, in addition to vegetable soups.

3. Include vegetables and fruit at all times

4. Consummated on the 3 main meals: meat of chicken or fish, or pork, or beef, or seafood or veal, eat 2 pieces of bread or 2 integral tortillas a day, made with cooked whole grains

5. 3 times a week 2 whole eggs

6. Eat 3 times per week nuts or peanuts or almonds

7. Do not eat food in via public

8. Does not consume soft drinks, or Light soft drinks, cookies, snacks, fried, sweet biscuits, if you are overweight: don't eat tortillas or bread, do not add sugar or salt.

9. Carried out in 4 to 7 days a week 30 minutes of moderate to intense physical exercise: jogging, aerobics, weightlifting, pilates, spinning, dancing.

10. Stop smoking and seek the help of urgent when it is greater than 5 cigarette consumption per day. Suspend risk alcohol consumption (placed in a visible sign that is risk alcohol consumption and upon affirmative answer any of the questions associated with tolerance or dependence, seek help in a group AA if you have any degree of alcohol addiction).

References

1. Isomaa B, Almgren P, Tuomi T, Forsén B, Lahti K, et al. (2001) Cardiovascular morbidity and mortality associated with the metabolic syndrome. Diabetes Care 24: 683-689.

2. Lakka HM, Laaksonen DE, Lakka TA, Niskanen LK, Kumpusalo E, et al. (2002) The metabolic syndrome and total and cardiovascular disease mortality in middle-aged men. JAMA 288: 2709-2716.

3. Grundy SM, Cleeman JI, Merz CN, Brewer HB Jr, Clark LT, et al. (2004) Implications of recent clinical trials for the National Cholesterol Education Program Adult Treatment Panel III guidelines. Circulation 110: 227-239.

4. Katzmarzyk PT, Church TS, Janssen I, Ross R, Blair SN (2005) Metabolic syndrome, obesity, and mortality: impact of cardiorespiratory fitness. Diabetes Care 28: 391-397.

5. Fan AZ, Russell M, Naimi T, Li Y, Liao Y, et al. (2008) Patterns of alcohol consumption and the metabolic syndrome. J Clin Endocrinol Metab 93: 3833-3838.

6. Bijnen FC, Caspersen CJ, Mosterd WL (1994) Physical inactivity as a risk factor for coronary heart disease: a WHO and International Society and Federation of Cardiology position statement. Bull World Health Organ 72: 1-4.

7. Global status report on noncommunicable disaeses 2010 . Geneva, World Health Organization.

8. Global atlas on cardiovascular disease prevention and control. Geneva, World Health Organization, 2011.

9. Mathers CD, Loncar D (2006) Projections of global mortality and burden of disease from 2002 to 2030. PLoS Med 3: e442.

10. Lim SS, Vos T, Flaxman AD, Danaei G, Shibuya K, et al. (2012) A comparative risk assessment of burden of disease and injury attributable to 67 risk factors and risk factor clusters in 21 regions, 1990-2010: a systematic analysis for the Global Burden of Disease Study 2010. Lancet 380: 2224-2260.

11. The global burden of disease: 2004 update. Geneva, World Health Organization, 2008.

12. Rehm J and colab. (2002) Alcohol as a Risk Factor for Burden of Disease. World Health Organization.

Does Smoking and Alcohol Abuse Precipitate and Aggravate the Risk of Metabolic...

51

13. Schrauwen-Hinderling VB1, Hesselink MK, Meex R, van der Made S, Schär M, et al. (2010) Improved ejection fraction after exercise training in obesity is accompanied by reduced cardiac lipid content. J Clin Endocrinol Metab 95: 1932-1938.

14. Tuomilehto J, Lindström J, Eriksson JG, Valle TT, Hämäläinen H, et al. (2001) Prevention of type 2 diabetes mellitus by changes in lifestyle among subjects with impaired glucose tolerance. N Engl J Med 344: 1343-1350.

15. Tobacco free initiative (2006) World Health organization. Geneva.

16. Neuroscience of psychoactive substance use and dependence (2004) ISBN 92 4 156235 8. World Health Organization.

17. National survey of 2007 addiction (ENA/2007)

18. Ministry of health, General Directorate of epidemiology, National Institute of Psychiatry. National addictions survey. Tobacco. Mexico DF: SSA, 2008

19. Rehm J and colab (2002) alcohol as a risk factor for burden of disease. World Health Organization.

20. Alcoholism. Scientific evidence-based clinical guidelines: Socidroga-alcohol 2008,(2rdedn),

21. Standard Oficial Mexicana NOM-174-SSA1-1998, for the comprehensive management of obesity. México D.F. 2000

22. Haffner SM, Mykkänen L, Festa A, Burke JP, Stern MP (2000) Insulin-resistant prediabetic subjects have more atherogenic risk factors than insulin-sensitive prediabetic subjects: implications for preventing coronary heart disease during the prediabetic state. Circulation 101: 975-980.

23. Bonora E, Kiechl S, Willeit J, Oberhollenzer F, Egger G, et al. (1998) Prevalence of insulin resistance in metabolic disorders: the Bruneck Study. Diabetes 47: 1643-1649.

24. Dandona P, Aljada A, Chaudhuri A, Mohanty P, Garg R (2005) Metabolic syndrome: a comprehensive perspective based on interactions between obesity, diabetes, and inflammation. Circulation 111: 1448-1454.

25. Sonnenberg GE, Krakower GR, Kissebah AH (2004) A novel pathway to the manifestations of metabolic syndrome. Obes Res 12: 180-186.

26. Jennie C Brand-Miller Karola, Stockman, Fiona Atkinson, Peter Petocs, et al. (2009) Glycemic index, postprandial glycemia, and the shape of the curve in healthy subjets: analysis of a database of more than 1000 foods. Am j Clin Nutr 89: 97-105

27. Tuomilehto J, Lindström J, Eriksson JG, Valle TT, Hämäläinen H, et al. (2001) Prevention of type 2 diabetes mellitus by changes in lifestyle among subjects with impaired glucose tolerance. N Engl J Med 344: 1343-1350.

28. The practical guide to the identification, evaluation and treatment of overweight and obesity in adults (2000) NHLBI Obesity Education Initiative.

29. Schrauwen-Hinderling VB, Hesselink MK, Meex R, van der Made S, Schär M, et al. (2010) Improved ejection fraction after exercise training in obesity is accompanied by reduced cardiac lipid content. J Clin Endocrinol Metab 95: 1932-1938.

30. Tuomilehto J, Lindström J, Eriksson JG, Valle TT, Hämäläinen H, et al. (2001) Prevention of type 2 diabetes mellitus by changes in lifestyle among subjects with impaired glucose tolerance. N Engl J Med 344: 1343-1350.

31. Neuroscience of Psychoactive Substance Use and Dependence (2004). ISBN 92 4 156235 8 World Health Organization.

32. Lim SS, Vos T, Flaxman AD, Danaei G, Shibuya K, et al. (2012) A comparative risk assessment of burden of disease and injury attributable to 67 risk factors and risk factor clusters in 21 regions, 1990-2010: a systematic analysis for the Global Burden of Disease Study 2010. Lancet 380: 2224-2260.

33. Aalto M, Pekuri P, Seppä K (2001) Primary health care nurses' and physicians' attitudes, knowledge and beliefs regarding brief intervention for heavy drinkers. Addiction 96: 305-311.

8

C358A Polymorphism of the Endocannabinoid Degrading Enzyme Fatty Acid Amide Hydrolase (FAAH) Influence On Metabolic Parameters a High Protein/Low Carbohydrate versus a Standard Hypocaloric Diet

R Aller, O Izaola, R Bachiller, E Romero and DA de Luis*

Center of Investigation of Endocrinology and Nutrition, Medicine School and Department of Endocrinology and Investigation, Hospital Clinico Universitario, University of Valladolid, Valladolid, Spain

Abstract

Background and aim: The C385A polymorphism of FAAH gene (rs324420C>A) has been associated with obesity. We investigate the role of this polymorphism on cardiovascular risk factors and weight loss secondary to a high protein/ low carbohydrate vs. a standard hypocaloric diets (1000 kcal/day) during 9 months.

Methods: A sample of 284 subjects with obesity (body mass index (BMI) >30) was enrolled. These subjects were randomly allocated to one of two diets for a period of nine months Diet S (standard protein hypocaloric diet) vs. Diet HP (high protein-low carbohydrate hypocaloric diet).

Results: After both diets and in both genotype groups (CC vs. CA+AA), body mass index (BMI), weight, fat mass, waist circumference and systolic blood pressure decreased. With the diet type HP and in non A carriers, glucose (-5.3 ± 1.2 mg/dl vs. -1.8 ± 2.1 mg/dl; p<0.05), insulin levels (-3.1 ± 1.9UI/L vs. -1.1 ± 2.0 UI/L; p<0.05), HOMA-R (-0.9 ± 0.8 units vs. -0.3 ± 1.0 units; p<0.05), total cholesterol (-11.9 ± 8.2 mg/dl vs. -0.1 ± 3.1mg/dl; p<0.05), and LDL- total cholesterol (-9.8 ± 4.2 mg/dl vs. -1.0 ± 2.1mg/dl; p<0.05) decreased. After diet S and in patients with both genotypes, total cholesterol (-6.0 ± 3.1 mg/dl vs. -10.0 ± 8.2mg/dl; ns), triglycerides (-8.1 ± 7.1 mg/dl vs. -13.1 ± 8.9 mg/dl; ns) and LDL- total cholesterol (-5.9 ± 3.0 mg/dl vs. -9.1 ± 5.8mg/dl; p<0.05) decreased.

Conclusion: Non carriers of the allele A385 of FAAH showed an improvement on insulin and HOMA-R levels with a high protein hypocaloric diet after weight loss during 9 months. A standard hypocaloric diet produced a similar improvement in lipid profile in both genotypes.

Keywords: FAAH; Hypocaloric diet; Metabolic parameters; Polymorphism

Abbreviations: BMI: Body Mass Index; HOMA-R: Homeostasis Model Assessment; IR: Insulin Resistance; WC: Waist Circumference; FFM: Fat Free Mass; FM: Fat mass; WHR: Waist to hip ratio; SBP: Systolic Blood pressure; DBP: Diastolic blood pressure

Introduction

Obesity is major public health problems that are estimated to affect >50% of the population and have been linked as risk factors for many common diseases [1]. One of the pathways related with obesity is the endocannabinoid system, which is involved in the control of food intake and body weight. This endocannabinoid system comprises of a number of proteins involved in endocannabinoid synthesis, degradation, and signaling and has been demonstrated to play a role in appetite and body weight, as above mentioned [2]. One of these proteins is Fatty acid amide hydrolase (FAAH), this enzyme inactive the orexigenic effect of the endocannabinoid N-arachidonoylethanolamine (andamide) by a rapid hydrolysis to ethanolamine and arachidonic acid [3].

One polymorphism of this enzyme (cDNA 385 C->A) (rs324420) has been described [4]. SNPs are estimated to participate in 90% of the disparities between individuals and consist in a replacement in a single nitrogenous base that occurs in at least 1% of population [5]. Some of these SNPs may affect the synthesis and functions of proteins and, therefore, may alter the nutritional requirements and nutrient metabolism [6,7], as well as elicit important roles in individual's risk of developing diseases [8]. Some studies have shown an interaction between this polymorphism and the metabolic response after weight loss secondary to different hypocaloric diets [9-11]. Perhaps, the percentage of macronutrients in these hypocaloric diets and the type of dietary fat may influence the heterogeneous metabolic responses secondary to weight loss as a function of this polymorphism. A recent meta-analysis of clinical trials with low-carbohydrate/high protein diets has shown that such diets have favorable effects on weight reduction and other major cardiovascular risk factors [12]. As far as we know, no studies have evaluated the effect of this polymorphism on response to diets of this type.

In attempting to understand the role of (rs324420) variant of Fatty acid amide hydrolase in obese patients, we decide to investigate the role of this polymorphism on cardiovascular risk factors and weight loss secondary to a high protein/low carbohydrate vs. a standard hypocaloric diets (1000 kcal/day) during 9 months.

Subjects and Methods

Subjects

A sample of 284 subjects (75 males/209 females) with obesity (body mass index (BMI) >30) was enrolled in a prospective way. These subjects

Corresponding author: Dr. D. A de Luis, Professor Associated of Nutrition, Executive Director of Institute of Endocrinology and Nutrition, Medicine School, Valladolid University, C/Los perales 16, Simancas 47130, Valladolid, Spain
E-mail: dadluis@yahoo.es

were randomly allocated to one of two diets for a period of nine months Diet S (standard protein hypocaloric diet) vs. Diet HP (high protein-low carbohydrate hypocaloric diet). Local ethical committee (CEIC-HURH) approved the protocol (4-2014 CEIC HURH) and patients approved the use of their genetic material for this study. This study was conducted according to the guidelines laid down in the Declaration of Helsinki a. All patients were recruited in a Nutrition Clinic Unit and signed an informed consent. Exclusion criteria included; total cholesterol > 300 mg/dl, triglycerides > 300 mg/dl, blood pressure > 140/90 mmHg, fasting plasma glucose >110 mg/dl, as well as the use of drugs with potential metabolic effects as statins, fibrates, metformin, sulphonilurea, thiazolidinedions, insulin, glucocorticoids, antineoplastic agents, angiotensin receptor blockers, angiotensin converting enzyme inhibitors and psychoactive medications.

Procedures and dietary intervention

Weight, height, body mass index, fat mass (bioimpedance), waist circumference, blood pressure, basal glucose, c-reactive protein (CRP), insulin, total cholesterol, LDL-cholesterol, HDL-cholesterol, triglycerides blood and adypokines (leptin, adiponectin and resistin) levels were measured within the start of the trial and repeated after 3 months and 9 months of both dietary intervention. 284 obese subjects were randomly allocated to one of two diets for a period of nine months. Diet S (standard protein hypocaloric diet) consisted in a diet of 1093 cal/day, 53% carbohydrates (144.3 g/day), 27% fats (32.6 g), and 20% proteins (55.6 g/day). The distribution of fats was; 20.9% of saturated fats, 67.4% of monounsaturated fats and 11.6% of polyunsaturated fats. Diet HP (high protein-low carbohydrate hypocaloric diet) consisted in a diet of 1050 cal/day, 33% of carbohydrates (86.1 g/day), 33% of fats (39.0 g/day) and 34% of proteins (88.6 g/day). The distribution of fats was; 23.5% of saturated fats, 63.8% of monounsaturated fats and 12.6% of polyunsaturated fats. The exercise program consisted of an aerobic exercise at least 3 times per week (60 min each). The adherence of these diets was assessed each 7 days with a phone call by a dietitian in order to improve compliment of the calorie restriction and macronutrient distribution. National composition food tables were used as reference [13].

Genotyping of FAAH gene polymorphism

Oligonucleotide primers and probes were designed with the Beacon Designer 4.0 (Premier Biosoft International®, LA, CA). The polymerase chain reaction (PCR) was carried out with 50 ng of genomic DNA, 0.5 uL of each oligonucleotide primer (primer forward: 5'-ATG TTG CTG GTT ACC CCT CCT C -3'; primer reverse: 5'-CAG GGA CGC CAT AGA GCT G-3'), and 0.25 uL of each probes (wild probe: 5'-Fam-CTG TCT CAG GCC CCA AGG CAG G-BHQ-1-3') and (mutant probe: 5'-Hex-CTG TCT CAG GCC ACA AGG CAG G -BHQ-1-3') in a 25 uL final volume (Termociclador iCycler IQ (Bio-Rad®), Hercules, CA). DNA was denaturized at 95°C for 3 min; this was followed by 50 cycles of denaturation at 95°C for 15 s, and annealing at 59.3° for 45 s. The PCR were run in a 25 uL final volume containing 12.5 uL of IQTM Supermix (Bio-Rad®, Hercules, CA) with hot start Taq DNA polymerase. Hardy Weinberg equilibrium was assessed.

Assays

Plasma glucose levels were determined by using an automated glucose oxidase method (Glucose analyser 2, Beckman Instruments, Fullerton, California), coefficients of variation of intra-assay (IACV) (1.5%) and inter-assay (IECV) (2.1%). Insulin was measured by RIA (RIA Diagnostic Corporation, Los Angeles, CA) with a sensitivity of 0.5mUI/L (normal range 0.5-30 mUI/L), coefficients of variation of

intra-assay (IACV) (1.8%) and inter-assay (IECV) (2.5%) [14], and the homeostasis model assessment for insulin resistance (HOMA-R) were calculated using these values [15]. CRP was measured by immunoturbimetry (Roche Diagnostics GmbH, Mannheim, Germany), with a normal range of (0-7 mg/dl) and analytical sensitivity 0.5 mg/dl with a coefficients of variation of intra-assay (IACV) (2.1%) and inter-assay (IECV) (2.3 Plasma hormone levels were evaluated using the multiplex Biorad© 10 plex assay following manufacturer's instructions (Bio-Rad®, Hercules, CA). This system allows for quantitative measurement of different hormones, while consuming a small amount of biological material; resistin, leptin and adiponectin. Limits of detection were as follows (pg/ml): leptin (1.8), resistin (1.4) and adiponectin (3.8).

Serum total cholesterol and triglyceride concentrations were determined by enzymatic colorimetric assay (Technicon Instruments, Ltd., New York, N.Y., USA), while HDL cholesterol was determined enzymatically in the supernatant after precipitation of other lipoproteins with dextran sulfate-magnesium. LDL cholesterol was calculated using Friedewald formula [16].

Anthropometric measurements and blood pressure

Body weight was measured to an accuracy of 0.1 Kg and body mass index computed as body weight/(height²). Waist (narrowest diameter between xiphoid process and iliac crest) and hip (widest diameter over greater trochanters) circumferences to derive waist-to hip ratio (WHR) were measured, too. Blood pressure was measured twice after a 10 minutes rest with a random zero mercury sphygmomanometer and a large cuff size was, and averaged. Tetrapolar body electrical bioimpedance (EFG, Akern, It) was used to determine body composition with an accuracy of 50 g [17]. Resistance and reactance were used to calculate total body water, fat and fat-free mass. The same investigator measured patients. Precautions taken to insure valid BIA measurements were; no alcohol within 24 hours of taking the test, no exercise or food for four hours before taking the test.

Statistical analysis

Sample size was calculated to detect differences over 3 kg in body weight with 90% power and 5% significance (n=140 in each dietary intervention). The distribution of variables was analyzed with Kolmogorov-Smirnov test. Quantitative variables were analyzed with a 2-way ANOVA model with genotype as the intergroup factor and intervention as the intragroup intervention. Qualitative variables were analyzed with the chi-square test, with Yates correction as necessary, and Fisher's test. A Chi square test was used to evaluate the Hardy–Weinberg equilibrium. The statistical analysis was performed for the combined C385A and A385A as a group and C385C as second group (dominant model). A p-value under 0.05 was considered statistically significant.

Results

Two hundred and eighty four patients gave informed consent and were enrolled in the study. The mean age was 50.2 ± 10.2 years and the mean BMI 35.0 ± 3.4, with 75 males (26.4%) and 209 females (73.6%). One hundred and ninety seven patients (48 males/149 females) (69.4%) had the genotype CC and 87 (30.7%) patients (27 males/60 females) CA (n=84, 29.6%) or AA (n=3, 1.1%) (A allele carriers). The Hardy Weinberg equilibrium was fulfilled p=0.37. Sex distribution was similar in groups, males (24.4% vs. 30.1%) and females (75.6% vs. 69.9%). Age was similar in both groups (CC genotype: 51.1 ± 10.1 years vs. A carriers group: 49.9 ± 12.8 years: ns).

Anthropometric characteristics of participants at baseline and at 3-9 months of intervention are shown in Table 1. With the diet type HP (high protein hypocaloric diet) and in both genotype groups (CC vs. CA+AA), body mass index (BMI) (-2.4 ± 1.0 kg/m^2 vs. -2.3 ± 1.3 kg/m^2: ns), weight (-7.4 ± 2.1 kg vs. -8.1 ± 4.2 kg:ns), fat mass (-5.4 ± 3.0 kg vs. -5.9 ± 3.1 kg: ns), waist circumference (-7.4 ± 5.1 cm vs. -7.9 ± 4.5 cm: ns) and systolic blood pressure (-4.2 ± 2.1 mmHg vs. -4.9 ± 1.9 mmHg:ns) decreased. There were not significant differences between the effects (on weight, BMI, waist circumference, systolic blood pressure and fat mass) in either genotype group. With the diet type S (Standard hypocaloric diet) and in both genotypes, BMI (-2.9 ± 1.1 kg/m^2 vs. -2.0 ± 1.0 kg/m^2:ns), weight (-9.6 ± 5.0 kg vs. -6.8 ± 3.9 kg ns), fat mass (-6.2 ± 3.2 kg vs. -5.1 ± 3.1 kg: ns), systolic blood pressure (-6.0 ± 1.1 mmHg vs. -5.9 ± 1.8 mmHg:ns) and waist circumference (-7.5 ± 4.1 cm vs. -7.1 ± 3.8 cm: ns) decreased. There were no significant differences between the effects in either genotype group with diet S. The effects of both diets on weight, BMI, waist circumference, systolic blood pressure and fat mass were similar.

In the 140 subjects (97 CC genotype and 43 A allele carriers) treated with diet HP, basal assessment of nutritional intake with a 3 days written food record showed a basal calorie intake of 2009.2 ± 331.9 kcal/day, a carbohydrate intake of 213.31 ± 20.9 g/day (40.9% of calories), a fat intake of 90.1 ± 23.1 g/day (41.0% of calories) and a protein intake of 80.8 ± 53.1 g/day (27.1% of calories). During the intervention, these subjects reached the recommendations of diet; 1008.4 ± 90.1 calories (33.2% of carbohydrates, 32.7% of lipids and

37.1% of proteins). The 144 subjects (100 CC genotype and 44 A allele carriers) treated with diet S, basal assessment of nutritional intake with a 3 days written food record showed a basal calorie intake a calorie intake of 2018.2 ± 321.9 kcal/day, a carbohydrate intake of 213.8 ± 21.2 g/day (42.9% of calories), a fat intake of 90.0 ± 11.1 g/day (38.3% of calories) and a protein intake of 89.9 ± 10.9 g/day (19.8% of calories). During the intervention, these patients reached the recommendations of diet; 1013.1 ± 92.1 calories (51.6% of carbohydrates, 29.5% of lipids and 18.9% of proteins).

Table 2 shows the cardiovascular risk factors. With the diet type HP and in non A carriers, glucose (-5.3 ± 1.2 mg/dl vs. -1.8 ± 2.1 mg/dl; p<0.05), insulin levels (-3.1 ± 1.9UI/L vs. -1.1 ± 2.0 UI/L; p<0.05), HOMA-R (-0.9 ± 0.8 units vs. -0.3 ± 1.0 units; p<0.05), total cholesterol (-11.9 ± 8.2 mg/dl vs. -0.1 ± 3.1mg/dl; p<0.05), and LDL- total cholesterol (-9.8 ± 4.2 mg/dl vs. -1.0 ± 2.1mg/dl; p<0.05) decreased. All these parameters remained unchanged in patients with A allele. With the diet S and in patients with both genotypes, total cholesterol (-6.0 ± 3.1 mg/dl vs. -10.0 ± 8.2mg/dl; ns), triglycerides (-8.1 ± 7.1 mg/dl vs. -13.1 ± 8.9 mg/dl; ns) and LDL- total cholesterol (-5.9 ± 3.0 mg/dl vs. -9.1 ± 5.8mg/dl; p<0.05) decreased.

Table 3 shows levels of adipocytokines. With the diet HP and in both genotypes, leptin levels (-16.9 ± 9.1 ng/ml vs. -19.4 ± 11.0 ng/ml: ns) decreased. With the diet S, leptin levels (-18.5 ± 5.3 ng/ml vs. -20.1 ± 4.9 ng/ml: ns) decreased in both genotypes, too. The amount of leptin decrease was similar with both diets. Adiponectin and resistin levels remained unchanged after both diets in all groups.

Characteristics	±						DIET S (n=144)					
	CC(n=97)			CA+AA (n=43)			CC(n=100)			CA+AA (n=44)		
	0 time	At 3 mths	At 9 mths	0 time	At 3 mths	At 9 mths	0 time	At 3 mths	At 9 mths	0 time	At 3 mths	At 9 mths
BMI	34.8 ± 5.1	33.7 ± 4.1*	32.4 ± 4.1*	34.1 ± 5.5	32.5 ± 5.0*	31.8 ± 5.0*	35.3 ± 5.6	33.7 ± 4.4*	32.2 ± 5.1*	34.9 ± 4.2	33.5 ± 4.0*	33.1 ± 5.0*
Weight (kg)	91.7 ± 17.6	86.5 ± 13.0*	84.3 ± 10.0*	92.1 ± 17.4	87.8 ± 12.1*	82.8 ± 12.4*	91.8 ± 19.6	88.2 ± 16.1*	81.8 ± 11.2*	90.6 ± 11.3	85.8 ± 9.3*	84.9 ± 9.0*
Fat mass (kg)	36.3 ± 7.0	32.9 ± 7.2*	30.9 ± 8.2*	35.2 ± 11.1	31.8 ± 10.1*	28.8 ± 11.0*	36.8 ± 7.4	33.6 ± 8.1*	30.6 ± 8.2*	37.1 ± 9.1	34.4 ± 8.1*	33.1 ± 10.1*
WC (cm)	111.8 ± 12.6	106.6 ± 10.7*	104.6 ± 9.1*	112.4 ± 9.2	107.4 ± 9.1*	104.3 ± 11.1*	112.6 ± 10.8	107.7 ± 9.0*	105.1 ± 10.3*	109.9 ± 10.8	106.2 ± 8.0*	104.8 ± 7.1*
WHR	0.95 ± 0.07	0.92 ± 0.06	0.94 ± 0.1	0.97 ± 0.01	0.95 ± 0.1	0.94 ± 0.02	0.95 ± 0.07	0.93 ± 0.09	0.94 ± 0.06	0.95 ± 0.1	0.93 ± 0.09	0.92 ± 0.10
SBP (mmHg)	127.2 ± 11.8	123.6 ± 13.7*	123.1 ± 14.9*	129.7 ± 10.3	126.1 ± 11.1*	124.1 ± 10.2*	127.8 ± 10.1	124.1 ± 9.1	121.8 ± 11.8*	125.2 ± 10.1	122.9 ± 12.2	120.0 ± 8.0*
DBP (mmHg)	82.1 ± 10.5	79.5 ± 8.1	79.1 ± 11.0	82.8 ± 9.1	78.1 ± 8.0	78.2 ± 9.0	81.1 ± 10.1	79.6 ± 6.1	79.9 ± 6.1	79.8 ± 5.2	79.0 ± 8.2	79.1 ± 7.1

HP: high protein/low carbohydrate. S: standard. DBP: Diastolic blood pressure. Mths: Months SBP: Systolic blood pressure. WHR: Waist to hip ratio. WC: Waist circumference. (*) p<0.05, in each genotype group with basal values. No statistical differences between genotypes with CC vs. CA+AA carriers in each diet.

Table 1: Changes in Anthropometric Variables (Mean ± S.D).

Characteristics	DIET HP (n=140)						DIET S (n=144)					
	CC(n=97)			CA+AA (n=43)			CC(n=100)			CA+AA (n=44)		
	0 time	At 3 mths	At 9 mths	0 time	At 3 mths	At 9 mths	0 time	At 3 mths	At 9 mths	0 time	At 3 mths	At 9 mths
Glucose (mg/dl)	104.6 ± 9.2	99.2 ± 11.1*	99.3 ± 9.1*	104.5 ± 12.2	103.9 ± 10.0	101.5 ± 9.1	102.2 ± 11.1	99.7 ± 9.4	100.5 ± 9.1	99.9 ± 9.1	96.8 ± 6.1	97.3 ± 7.0
Total chol. (mg/dl)	209.4 ± 20.8	196.1 ± 20.1*	200.5 ± 21.7*	203.4 ± 20.1	204.7 ± 30.0	204.1 ± 10.1	203.8 ± 30.9	197.6 ± 31.4*	197.9 ± 11.4*	217.6 ± 20.2	206.1 ± 18.1*	202.1 ± 12.3*
LDL-chol. (mg/dl)	131.8 ± 20.2	120.3 ± 20.1*	122.2 ± 10.1*	126.6 ± 21.2	127.4 ± 20.1	128.1 ± 10.1	124.4 ± 20.5	119.9 ± 21.2*	118.8 ± 15.1*	133.7 ± 11.1	125.3 ± 12.9*	121.9 ± 19.8*
HDL-chol. (mg/dl)	55.3 ± 10.5	54.7 ± 9.1	55.1 ± 8.1	56.4 ± 10.0	56.1 ± 9.1	55.3 ± 8.2	56.6 ± 11.2	53.8 ± 9.2	52.9 ± 13.0	55.2 ± 10.1	54.8 ± 8.2	55.3 ± 10.2
TG (mg/dl)	128.3 ± 49.1	112.3 ± 31.4*	107.2 ± 21.2*	108.6 ± 30.1	110.8 ± 31.2	109.9 ± 19.3	126.1 ± 42.1	122.4 ± 34.1	119.2 ± 31.1	130.0 ± 41.3	105.3 ± 11.3*	104.9 ± 21.9*
Insulin (mUI/L)	11.6 ± 5.4	8.9 ± 5.1*	7.5 ± 5.0*	10.8 ± 7.0	10.4 ± 9.0	8.8 ± 7.1	11.1 ± 5.0	10.2 ± 5.9	9.7 ± 3.2	10.1 ± 5.1	7.8 ± 4.1	7.0 ± 5.0
HOMA	2.4 ± 0.9	2.0 ± 0.9*	1.5 ± 1.1*	2.8 ± 1.0	2.7 ± 2.0	2.4 ± 1.3	2.2 ± 1.1	2.5 ± 1.0	2.3 ± 1.3	2.2 ± 1.0	1.6 ± 0.8	1.9 ± 1.1
CRP (mg/dl)	5.0 ± 3.1	4.4 ± 3.2	3.9 ± 3.0	4.0 ± 3.1	5.1 ± 3.0	4.9 ± 3.2	4.9 ± 3.0	4.3 ± 4.1	4.8 ± 4.0	5.2 ± 4.0	5.3 ± 3.1	5.4 ± 3.1

HP: high protein/low carbohydrate. S: standard. Chol: Cholesterol. TG: Triglycerides CRP: c reactive protein. HOMA: Homeostasis model assessment. Mths: months (*) p<0.05, in each group with basal values. No statistical differences between genotypes with CC vs. CA+AA carriers in each diet.

Table 2: Clasical Cardiovascular Risk Factors (Mean ± S.D).

Characteristics	DIET HP (n=140)						DIET S (n=144)					
	CC(n=97)			CA+AA (n=43)			CC(n=100)			CA+AA (n=44)		
	0 time	At 3 mths	At 9 mths	0 time	At 3 mths	At 9 mths	0 time	At 3 mths	At 9 mths	0 time	At 3 mths	At 9 mths
Adiponectin (ng/ml)	10.1 ± 6.0	9.7 ± 5.2	10.0 ± 7.0	10.2 ± 5.0	11.0 ± 9.1	10.8 ± 7.3	11.1 ± 4.0	10.9 ± 3.0	10.8 ± 4.1	9.8 ± 5.0	10.1 ± 4.3	10.3 ± 4.1
Resistin (ng/ml)	7.1 ± 3.0	7.0 ± 5.0	6.9 ± 4.8	7.30 ± 3.1	7.1 ± 3.1	7.2 ± 3.3	8.0 ± 2.5	7.9 ± 3.1	7.8 ± 2.9	7.0 ± 3.2	7.3 ± 4.1	6.9 ± 3.0
Leptin (ng/ml)	31.8 ± 17.4	21.9 ± 13.1*	15.3 ± 10.1*	38.1 ± 10.1	20.1 ± 9.0*	18.4 ± 9.1*	33.5 ± 12.0	20.4 ± 7.0*	15.0 ± 5.1*	41.8 ± 10.2	22.9 ± 8.3*	21.4 ± 7.1*

(*) p<0.05, in each group with basal values. No statistical differences between genotypes with CC vs. CA+AA carriers in each diet.

Table 3: Circulating Adypocitokines (Mean ± S.D).

Discussion

The main finding of our study is the association of the C385C genotype with an additional improvement on lipid profile, glucose, insulin and HOMA-R levels after a high protein hypocaloric diet. A standard hypocaloric diet produced a similar improvement in lipid profile in both genotypes. A significant decrease of weight, fat mass, waist circumference, total cholesterol and LDL-cholesterol were observed in subjects with both diets in all genotype groups. These relevant data are interesting because there are few intervention studies in this topic area. Five studies reported that carriers of the A allele of rs324420 had different changes in several biochemical parameters after weight loss secondary to a dietary intervention. Aberle et al. [9] have shown that carriers of the A allele had a significantly greater improvement in cholesterol profile compared to non-carriers of A allele when following a low fat diet during a short intervention trial of 6 weeks. De Luis et al. [10] have shown with a standard hypocaloric diet during 3 months (52% of carbohydrates, 25% of lipids and 23% of proteins) that carriers of the A allele was associated with higher improvements in HDL cholesterol and glucose levels than non A allele carriers. In other study with two branches of intervention of 12 weeks [11], the allele A385 of FAAH was associated with a lack of improvement on metabolic parameters after a low fat hypocaloric diet and a low carbohydrate hypocaloric diet. However, in this study [11], the type of diet interacts with the genotype and the low fat diet produce a significant decrease of glucose, HOMA-R, and insulin levels. The type of dietary fat in hypocaloric diet has shown a relevant roll in the metabolic reponse. For example, in a study during 3 months with a high monounsaturaded hypocaloric diet [18], subjects with C385C genotype showed a higher improvement on insulin and HOMA-R levels than non-carriers. However, in a similar design with an enriched monounsaturated fat hypocaloric diet during 12 weeks subjects with C385C genotype had a significant improvement on insulin and HOMA-R levels with a better response of weight, fat mass and waist circumference than A carriers [19]. Besides these adults' works, Knoll et al. [20] have been carried out a study in children. Knoll et al. did not detect evidence for an association of FAAH genotypes with weight reduction in overweight and obese children and adolescents.

In order to explain these contradictories results, we can hypothesize several theories. Firstly, the distribution of macronutrients in the prescribed diets may influence on secondary metabolic responses to weight loss as a function of this polymorphism. For example, distribution of macronutrients and percentage of dietary fat were not reported in one study [9]. In other study [10], percentage of monounsaturated fat acids was 30% of all dietary fat with 1520 kcal. The percentage of polyunsaturated fatty acids was around 10%, this data was similar than 11-12% of our present study. In other study (23%) the percentage was higher than previously reported [18]. Secondly, age and initial average weight of populations are two factors that influence in the interaction of FAAH genotype and weight response. In the pediatric study [20], a young overweight population (average 10-11

years) was evaluated. In the other studies [9-11,18,19], a middle age obese population (average 45-50 years) was included. Finally, duration of dietary intervention may influence secondary metabolic responses to weight loss as a function of this polymorphism. The duration of interventions has been around 6-12 weeks [9-11,18,19]. The study of Knoll et al. [20] lasted 1 year. Recently, a study after biliopancreatic diversion [21] showed that the allele A358 of fatty acid amide hydrolase was associated with a better initial percentage of excess weight loss 9 and 12 months after biliopancreatic diversión. However, biochemical changes were similar in both genotypes after 12 months of follow-up. In order to understand all these previous data, we must consider that the endocannabioid system is a complex redundant system, in this way the mesolimbic addition and reward/craving circuit including the medial forebrain bundle projections to the *nucleus accumbens* shows a high correlation of FAAH enzyme expression and CB1 receptor density [22]. Time of intervention, age average of population and type of diet intervention could influence in the metabolic responses with an interaction with this SNPs.

Recently, some interesting studies have shown the importance of rs324420 in metabolism and weight. Monteleone et al. [23] have shown that 385C/A SNP of the FAAH gene may predispose subjects to get a clinically meaningful weight gain after antipsychotic exposure. Finally, Ando et al. [24] have reported that the minor 385A allele was less frequent in the AN participants than in the controls (allele-wise, odds ratio = 0.799, 95% confidence interval [CI] 0.653-0.976).

In conclusion, non-carriers of the allele A385 of FAAH showed an improvement on insulin and HOMA-R levels with a high protein hypocaloric diet after weight loss during 9 months. A standard hypocaloric diet produced a similar improvement in lipid profile in both genotypes. Secondary weight loss after diet was similar in both genotypes. Further studies are needed to explore the right macronutrient distribution and type of dietary fats to evaluate this interaction gene-environment.

Acknowledgement

D. A de Luis designed the study and wrote the article, R. Aller recruitedpatients, made dietary evaluation and wrote the article, E Romero realized laboratory test, O Izaolarecruited patients and made dietary evaluation, R Bachiller recruited patients andmade dietary evaluation

References

1. Nguyen DM, El-Serag HB (2010) The epidemiology of obesity. Gastroenterol Clin North Am 39: 1-7.

2. Ameri A (1999) The effects of cannabinnoids on the brain. Prog Neurobiol 58: 315-348.

3. McKinney MK, Cravatt BF (2005) Structure and function of Fatty Acid Amide hydrolase. Annu Rev Biochem 74: 411-432.

4. Sipe JC, Chiang K, Gerber AL, Beutler E, Cravatt BF (2002) A Missense mutation in human fatty acid amide hydroxylase associated with problem drug abuse. Proc Natl Acad Sci USA 99: 8394-8399.

5. Trujillo E, Davis C, Milner J (2006) Nutrigenomics, Proteomics, Metabolomics, and the Practice of Dietetics. J Am Diet Assoc 106: 403-413.

6. Mooser V, Ordovas JM (2003) 'Omic' approaches and lipid metabolism: are these new technologies holding their promises? Curr Opin Lipidol 14: 115-119.

7. Kaput J, Rodriguez RL (2004) Nutritional genomics: The next frontier in the postgenomic era. Physiol Genomics 16: 166-177.

8. Grody VW (2003) Molecular genetic risk screening. Annu Rev Med 54: 473-490.

9. Aberle J, Fedderwitz I, Klages N, George E, Beil FU (2007) Genetic variation in two proteins of the endocannabinoid system and their influence on body mass index and metabolism under low fat diet. Horm Metab Res 39: 395-397.

10. De Luis DA, Gonzalez Sagrado M, Aller R, Izaola O, Conde R (2012) Effects of C385A missense polymorphism of the endocannabinoid degrading enzyme fatty acid amide hydrolase on weight loss after a hypocaloric diet. Metabolism Clin Exper 60: 730-734.

11. De Luis DA, Gonzalez Sagrado M, Aller R, Izaola O, Conde R (2010) Effects of C385A missense polymorphism of the degrading enzyme fatty acid amide hydrolase on weight loss, adipocytokines and insulin resistance after 2 hypocaloric diets. Metabolism Clin Exper 59: 1387-1392.

12. Santos FL, Esteves SS, da Costa Pereira A, Yancy WS Jr, Nunes JP (2012) Systematic review and meta-analysis of clinical trials of the effects of low carbohydrate diets on cardiovascular risk factors. Obes Rev 13: 1048-1066.

13. Mataix J, Mañas M (2003) Tablas de composición de alimentos españoles. University of Granada.

14. Duart MJ, Arroyo CO, Moreno JL (2002) Validation of an insulin model for the reactions in RIA. Clin Chem Lab Med 40: 1161-1167.

15. Mathews DR, Hosker JP, Rudenski AS, Naylor BA, Treacher DF, et al. (1985) Homeostasis model assessment: insulin resistance and beta cell function from fasting plasma glucose and insulin concentrations in man. Diabetologia 28: 412-414.

16. Friedewald WT, Levy RJ, Fredrickson DS (1972) Estimation of the concentration of low-density lipoprotein cholesterol in plasma without use of the preparative ultracentrifuge. Clin Chem 18: 499-502.

17. Lukaski H, Johson PE, Bolonchuk VW, Lykken GI (1985) Assessment of fat-free mass using bioelectrical impedance measurements of the human body. Am J Clin Nutr 41: 810-817.

18. De Luis DA, Izaola O, Aller R, de La Fuente B, Pacheco D (2013) Effects of C358A polymorphism of the endocannabinoid degrading enzyme fatty acid amide hydrolase (FAAH) on weight loss, adipocytokines levels, and insulin resistance after a high polyunsaturated fat diet in obese patients Endocrinol Invest 36: 965-969.

19. De Luis D, Aller R, Izaola O, Conde R, de la Fuente B, et al. (2013) Genetic variation in the endocannabinoid degrading enzyme fatty acid amide hydrolase (FAAH) and their influence on weight loss and insulin resistance under a high monounsaturated fat hypocaloric diet. J Diabetes Complications 27: 235-239.

20. Knoll N, Volckmar AL, Putter C, Scherag A, Kleber M, et al. (2012) The FAAH gene variant rs324420 AA/CA is not associated with weight loss in a 1 year lifestyle intervention for obese children and adolescents. Horm Metab Res 44: 75-77.

21. De Luis DA, Sagrado MG, Pacheco D, Terroba MC, Martin T, et al. (2010) Effects of C358A missense polymorphism of the endocannabinoid degrading enzyme fatty acid amide hydrolase on weight loss and cardiovascular risk factors 1 year after biliopancreatic diversion surgery. Surg Obes Relat Dis 6: 516-520.

22. Di Marzo V, Goparaju SK, Wang L, Liu J, Batkai S, et al. (2001) Leptin-regulated endocannabinoids are involved in maintaining food intake. Nature 410: 822-825.

23. Monteleone P, Milano W, Petrella C, Canestrelli B, Maj MJ (2010) Endocannabinoid Pro129Thr FAAH functional polymorphism but not 1359G/A CNR1 polymorphism is associated with antipsychotic-induced weight gain. J Clin Psychopharmacol 30: 441-445.

24. Ando T, Tamura N, Mera T, Morita C, Takei M, et al. (2014) Association of the c.385C>A (p.Pro129Thr) polymorphism of the fatty acid amide hydrolase gene with anorexia nervosa in the Japanese population. Mol Genet Genomic Med 2: 313-318.

9

Effects of a High Protein/Low Carbohydrate Versus a Standard Hypocaloric Diet on Weight and Cardiovascular Risk Factors, Role of a Lys656asn Polymorphism of Leptin Receptor Gene

Daniel de Luis[1,2]*, Rocío Aller[1], Olatz Izaola[1,2], Primo D[1] and Romero E[1,2]

[1]Center of Investigation of Endocrinology and Nutrition, Medicine School, Spain
[2]Department of Endocrinology and Nutrition, Hospital Clínico Universitario, Spain

Abstract

Background: The SNP of the leptin receptor (Lys656Asn) has been related with metabolic parameters. The aim of our design was to evaluate the influence of Lys656Asn variant of Leptin receptor gene on weight loss and metabolic parameters secondary to a high protein/low carbohydrate vs. a standard hypocaloric diets.

Design: A total of 280 obese subjects were randomly allocated to one of two diets during 9 months (Diet HP (high protein-low carbohydrate hypocaloric diet) and Diet S (standard protein hypocaloric diet)).

Results: After both diets and in both genotypes, body mass index (BMI), fat mass, weight, systolic blood pressure and waist circumference decreased, without differences between both diets. With the diet type HP and in both genotypes, triglycerides decreased. In subjects with Lys656Lys genotype, glucose, insulin levels, HOMA-R, total cholesterol and LDL- total cholesterol decreased after HP diet. No statistical changes were detected in Asn allele carriers. After diet S and in patients with Lys656Lys genotypes, only total cholesterol, triglycerides and LDL- total cholesterol decreased, without changes in Asn allele carriers.

Conclusion: Obese subjects with Asn656 allele have a different metabolic response than Lys656Lys genotype subjects, secondary to the same weight loss with two different hypocaloric diets.

Keywords: High protein/low carbohydrate; Standard hypocaloric diet; LYS656ASN; LEPR; Leptin

Abbreviations: BMI: Body Mass Index; HOMA: Homeostasis Model Assessment; IR: Insulin Resistance; LEPR: Leptin Receptor; WC: Waist Circumference; FFM: Fat Free Mass; FM: Fat Mass; WHR: Waist to Hip Ratio; SBP: Systolic Blood Pressure; DBP: Diastolic Blood Pressure

Introduction

The incidence of obesity is increasing all Western Countries. This dramatically increasing in obesity prevalence has led to an important increase of investigation on adipose tissue and its role in metabolism, inflammation and other physiologic processes [1]. Obesity has a low grade systemic inflammation and adipose tissue is considered an active secretory organ of a new family of molecules called adipokines (for example, leptin). Leptin is a protein containing 167 amino acids, demonstrates structural similarities with cytokines and is mainly produced by white adipose tissue. Some studies have confirmed that other tissues express leptin, including ovaries, placenta, stomach, pituitary, skeletal muscle and liver [2]. This adipokine acts as an afferent satiety signal, regulating appetite in humans. Obese patients may be leptin resistant and are characterized by high, rather than low, levels of leptin [3]. Considering everything previously mentioned, the role of leptin in the obesity is an area of important investigation.

Some genetic variant (polymorphisms) in leptin receptor gene have been studied with contradictory results [4]. One of them is the SNP on codon 656, this change produce a modification in electric charge with a possibility to be functional. Patients with rs8179183 variant of LEPR gene have a different metabolic response than wild type after weight loss secondary to different diets [5-7]. In these previous studies, only leptin levels had a significant decrease in wild group. However, although dietary intakes are the main tool to decrease weight in obese subjects, responded to diet was heterogeneous, and a role for genetic turned determinants in the inter individual variation is postulated [8].

A recent meta-analysis with low-carbohydrate/high protein diets has shown that such diets have benefit effects on weight loss, metabolic parameters and cardiovascular risk factors [9]. As far as we know, no interventional designs have been realized in order to evaluate the effect of this polymorphism on response to diets of this type.

The aim of our study was to evaluate the effect of this polymorphism on metabolic parameters and weight loss secondary to a high protein/ low carbohydrate vs. a standard hypocaloric diets (1000 kcal/day) during 9 months.

Methods and Subjects

Subjects

A sample of 280 obesity non diabetic outpatients was analyzed in a prospective way. Written informed consent was fulfilled from all subjects. Exclusion criteria included history of stroke or cardiovascular disease during the previous 12 months, total cholesterol > 275 mg/dl, triglycerides > 350 mg/dl, fasting plasma glucose >110 mg/dl, blood pressure > 140/90 mmHg, as well as the use of treatments to diabetes mellitus (insulin, sulphonilurea, dypeptidil type IV inhibitors drugs, thiazolidinedions) , glucocorticoids, antineoplasic agents, angiotensin

***Corresponding author:** Dr. Daniel de Luis, Professor of Endocrinology and Nutrition, Executive Director of Center of Investigation of Endocrinology and Clinical Nutrition, Medicine School, Valladolid University, Valladolid, Spain
E-mail: dadluis@yahoo.es

receptor blockers, angiotensin converting enzyme inhibitors, psychoactive medications, statins and other lipid drugs. This study was conducted according to the guidelines laid down in the Declaration of Helsinki and all procedures involving human subjects were approved by the Local Ethical Committee.

Procedure

Basal fasting glucose, total cholesterol, c-reactive protein (CRP), insulin, insulin resistance (HOMA-IR), LDL-cholesterol, HDL-cholesterol, plasma triglycerides concentration and adipokines (leptin, resistin, adiponectin) levels were determined within the start of the trial and repeated after 3 months and 9 months of both dietary intervention. Weight, height, and blood pressure measures were determined within the start of the trail and repeated 3 and 9 months of intervention. A tetrapolar bioimpedance was realized in order to measure fat mass. These measures were realized at same time of the day (morning). Genotype of Lys656Asn variant of Leptin receptor gene was studied.

280 obese patients were randomly allocated to one of two diets. Diet HP (a hypocaloric diet, high protein-low carbohydrate) consisted in a diet of 1050 cal/day, 33% of fats (39.0 g/day), 33% of carbohydrates (86.1 g/day) and 34% of proteins (88.6 g/day). The distribution of fats was; 63.8% of monounsaturated fats, 23.5% of saturated fats and 12.6% of polyunsaturated fats. Diet S (hypocaloric diet, standard protein) consisted in a diet of 1093 cal/day, 27% fats (32.6 g), 53% carbohydrates (144.3 g/day) and 20% proteins (55.6 g/day). The distribution of fats was; 67.4% of monounsaturated fats, 20.9% of saturated fats, and 11.6% of polyunsaturated fats. The exercise program was an aerobic physical activity at least 3 times per week (60 min each). The adherence of these diets was recorded each 7 days with a phone call in order to improve both diets. National composition food tables were used as reference [10].

Genotyping of LEPR gene polymorphism

Probes and oligonucleotide primers were designed with the Beacon Designer 4.0 (Premier Biosoft International ®, LA, CA). The polymerase chain reaction (PCR) was realized with 250 ng of genomic DNA, 0.5 µL of each primer (primer forward: 5'-GCA GTT CCT ATG AGA GGA CC-3'; primer reverse: 5'-AAA TTG GGA ATA CCT TCC AAA GT-3'), and 0.25 uL of each probes wild probe: (5'-Fam-AGT GAC ATT TTT CTC CTT TTT CAT AGT ATC-Tamra-3' and mutant probe: 5'-Hex-AGT GAC ATT TTT CTC GTT TTT CAT AGT AT- Tamra -3´) in a 25 µL final volume (Termociclador iCycler IQ (Bio-Rad®), Hercules, CA). DNA was denaturated at 95ºC for 3 min; this was followed by 50 cycles of new denaturation at 95ºC for 15 s, and annealing at 59.3ºC for 45 s). The PCR were run in a 25 µL final volume containing 12.5 µL of IQTM Supermix (Bio-Rad®, Hercules, CA) with hot start Taq DNA polymerase. The Hardy Weinberg equilibrium was examined with p value>0.05.

Anthropometric measurements and blood pressure

Weight was measured to an accuracy of 0.1 Kg and BMI was calculated as body weight/(height^2). Hip (widest diameter over greater trochanters) and waist (narrowest diameter between xiphoid process and iliac crest) circumferences to derive waist-to hip ratio (WHR) were determined, too. Body electrical bio impedance was used to determine body composition [11] (Biodynamics Model 310e, Seattle, WA, USA).

Blood pressure was measured twice after a 10 minutes rest with a random zero mercury sphygmomanometer and averaged.

Biochemical assays

Cholesterol and triglyceride concentrations were measured by enzymatic colorimetric assay (Technicon Instruments, Ltd., New York, N.Y., USA), while HDL cholesterol was measured enzymatically in the supernatant after precipitation of other lipoproteins with dextran sulphate-magnesium. Low-density lipoprotein cholesterol was determined using Friedewald formula.

Plasma glucose levels were determined by using an automated glucose oxidase method (Glucose analyser 2, Beckman Instruments, Fullerton, California). Insulin was determined by enzymatic colorimetric (Insulin, WAKO Pure-Chemical Industries, Osaka, Japan) [12] and the homeostasis model assessment for insulin resistance (HOMA-IR) was determined using these values [13]. CRP was determined by immunoturbimetry (Roche Diagnostics GmbH, Mannheim, Germany), with a normal range of (0-7 mg/dl) and analytical sensivity 0.5 mg/dl.

Plasma hormone levels were measured using the multiplex Biorad© 10 plex assay following manufacturer's instructions (Bio-Rad®, Hercules, CA). This system lets for quantitative measurement of different molecules, while consuming a small amount of material; resistin, leptin and adiponectin. Limits of detection were as follows (pg/ml): resistin (1.4), leptin (1.8), and adiponectin (3.8).

Statistical analysis

Sample size was calculated to observed differences over 10% in leptin levels with 90% power and 5% significance (n=130). The distribution of variables was analyzed with Kolmogorov-Smirnov test. Quantitative variables with normal distribution were analyzed with a two-tailed, paired Student's-t test. A Chi square test was used to evaluate the Hardy–Weinberg equilibrium. Non-parametric parameters were analyzed with the Wilcoxon test. A mixed model has been used within and between subjects to test the interaction between the polymorphism groups and outcome variables, due to the repeated measures study design. Qualitative parameters were analyzed with the chi-square test, with Yates correction as necessary, and Fisher's test. The statistical analysis was realized for the combined Lys656/Asn656 and Asn656/Asn656 as a group and genotype Lys656/Lys 656 as other group (dominant model). A p-value under 0.05 was considered statistically significant.

Results

280 patients gave signed consent and were included in the study. The mean age was 49.5 ± 11.2 years and the mean body mass index 37.8 ± 3.2, with 75 males (26.8%) and 205 females (73.2%). One hundred and eighty eight patients (54 males/134 females) (67.1%) had the genotype Lys656/Lys656 and 92 (32.9%) patients (21 males/71 females) Lys656/Asn656 (n=81, 28.9%) or Asn656/Asn656 (n=11, 3.9%) (Asn allele carriers). The Hardy Weinberg equilibrium was fulfilled p=0.23. Sex frequency was equal in both groups, males (22.7% vs 23.6%) and females (77.3% vs 76.4%). Age was equal in both groups (Lys656Lys genotype: 49.7 ± 10.2 years vs Asn carriers group: 48.9 ± 12.7 years:ns).

In the 139 subjects (94 Lys656Lys genotype and 45 Asn allele carriers) randomized to diet HP, basal determination of dietary intake with a 3 days written food register detected a basal calorie intake of 2099.8 ± 432.6 kcal/day, a fat intake of 90.0 ± 29.3 g/day (41.1% of calories), a carbohydrate intake of 219.38 ± 30.9 g/day (40.8% of calories) and a protein intake of 81.2 ± 59.1 g/day (27.1% of calories). During the trial, these patients attained the recommendations of diet; 1010.4 ± 91.1 calories (34.2% of carbohydrates, 32.6% of lipids and

36.2% of proteins). The 141 subjects (94 Lys656Lys genotype and 47 Asn allele carriers) randomized to diet S, basal assessment of dietary intake with a 3 days written food register showed a basal calorie intake a calorie intake of 2028.4 ± 394.1 kcal/day, a fat intake of 91.0 ± 13.1 g/day (38.4% of calories), a carbohydrate intake of 213.9 ± 28.3 g/day (42.7% of calories), and a protein intake of 90.9 ± 11.9 g/day (19.9% of calories). During the trial, these patients reached the recommendations of diet; 1008.8 ± 97.1 calories (51.8% of carbohydrates, 29.4% of lipids and 18.8% of proteins).

Anthropometric parameters of patients at baseline and at 3-9 months of intervention are shown in Table 1. With the diet type HP (high protein hypocaloric diet) and in both genotype groups (Lys656Lys vs Lys656Asn+Asn656Asn), body mass index (BMI) (-2.2 ± 1.1 kg/m² vs -1.9 ± 1.3 kg/m²: ns), weight (-6.1 ± 2.0 kg vs -6.7 ± 4.0 kg:ns), fat mass (-5.2 ± 3.1 kg vs -5.1 ± 3.0 kg: ns), systolic blood pressure (-4.1 ± 2.0 mmHg vs -3.1 ± 1.9 mmHg:ns) and waist circumference (-6.1 ± 5.0 cm vs -6.3 ± 4.5 cm: ns) decreased. There were not significant differences between the changes (on weight, waist circumference, BMI, systolic blood pressure and fat mass) in either genotype group. With the diet type S (Standard hypocaloric diet) and in both groups, body mass index (-1.3 ± 1.0 kg/m² vs -1.1 ± 0.9 kg/m²:ns), weight (-4.8 ± 3.0 kg vs -5.1 ± 3.2 kg ns), fat mass (-4.3 ± 3.1 kg vs -4.0 ± 3.0 kg: ns), blood pressure (-4.0 ± 1.9 mmHg vs -4.4 ± 1.9 mmHg:ns) and waist circumference (-5.2 ± 4.0 cm vs -6.0 ± 3.9 cm: ns) decreased. There were no statistical differences between the effects in either genotype group with diet S. Table 2 shows the metabolic parameters. With the diet type HP and in both genotypes, triglycerides (-19.0 ± 8.1 mg/dl vs -13.1 ± 7.9 mg/dl;ns) decreased. Only in patients with Lys656Lys genotype, glucose (-4.1 ± 1.1 mg/dl vs -1.1 ± 2.5 mg/dl; p<0.05), insulin levels (-2.6 ± 2.0 UI/L vs -0.9±2.0 UI/L;p<0.05), HOMA-IR (-0.5 ± 1.0 units vs -0.1 ± 1.1 units; p<0.05), total cholesterol (-12.0 ± 8.1 mg/dl vs -5.1 ± 6.1 mg/dl; p<0.05), and LDL- total cholesterol (-6.8 ± 4.1 mg/dl vs -2.9 ± 3.1 mg/dl;p<0.05) decreased. All these parameters remained

Characteristics	DIET HP (n=139)								DIET S (n=141)							
	LysLys(n=94)				LysAsn+ AsnAsn (n=45)				LysLys (n=94)				LysAsn+ AsnAsn (n=47)			
	0 time	At 3 months	At 9 months	p value	0 time	At 3 months	At 9 months	p value	0 time	At 3 months	At 9 months	p value	0 time	At 3 months	At 9 months	p value
BMI	34.7 ± 5.3	33.0 ± 4.0*	32.4 ± 4.0*	0.01	34.9 ± 6.0	33.2 ± 6.0*	33.0 ± 5.1*	0.01	34.6 ± 5.9	34.1 ± 4.2*	33.9 ± 5.0 *	0.01	35.1 ± 4.1	34.2 ± 5.0*	34.0 ± 5.1*	0.02
Weight (kg)	91.7 ± 14.6	87.5 ± 13.1*	85.6 ± 10.1*	0.02	91.2 ± 16.4	86.8 ± 16.1*	83.5 ± 12.4*	0.01	90.9 ± 19.6	89.6 ± 10.1*	86.1 ± 10.2*	0.02	91.8 ± 15.3	87.7 ± 10.3*	86.3 ± 9.1*	0.01
Fat mass (kg)	35.7 ± 7.0	32.5 ± 7.1*	30.5 ± 8.2*	0.01	36.9 ± 11.1	33.8 ± 10.1*	31.8 ± 10.0*	0.02	36.6 ± 6.4	33.1 ± 8.1*	31.9 ± 9.2*	0.01	37.1 ± 9.1	34.2 ± 10.1*	33.9 ± 10.0*	0.04
WC (cm)	111.4 ± 11.6	107.9 ± 11.7*	105.1 ± 9.2*	0.01	111.4 ± 9.2	106.4 ± 9.7*	104.2 ± 10.1*	0.03	110.8 ± 10.8	106.8 ± 9.1*	105.6 ± 11.3*	0.03	106.3 ± 10.9	106.8 ± 10.0*	105.3 ± 8.1*	0.04
WHR	0.96 ± 0.07	0.94 ± 0.06	0.94 ± 0.1	0.34	0.94 ± 0.01	0.93 ± 0.1	0.94 ± 0.03	0.49	0.95 ± 0.07	0.94 ± 0.06	0.94 ± 0.08	0.67	0.95 ± 0.1	0.94 ± 0.09	0.92 ± 0.10	0.57
SB (mmHg)	126.0 ± 11.8	122.7 ± 13.7*	122.2 ± 10.9*	0.01	128.7 ± 12.3	126.4 ± 13.1*	125.9 ± 11.2*	0.03	126.1 ± 10.1	122.3 ± 10.1*	122.8 ± 12.8*	0.03	131.2 ± 10.8	126.5 ± 12.1*	125.0 ± 9.0*	0.02
DB (mmHg)	81.1 ± 10.5	78.2 ± 8.1	78.1 ± 12.0	0.48	82.3 ± 9.1	80.1 ± 8.1	78.8 ± 9.1	0.53	80.4 ± 10.2	75.9 ± 6.4	78.9 ± 6.0	0.24	80.7 ± 5.2	79.8 ± 8.1	79.2 ± 7.0	0.45

H: High Protein/Low Carbohydrate; S: Standard; DB: Diastolic Blood Pressure; Mths: Months; SB: Systolic Blood Pressure; WHR: Waist to Hip Ratio; WC: Waist Circumference; (*) <0.05, in each genotype group with basal values. No statistical differences between genotypes with Lys/lys vs Lys/Asn+Asn/Asn carriers in each diet. Quantitative variables with normal distribution were analyzed with a two-tailed, aired Student's-t test (weight, fat mass, BMI). Non-parametric parameters were analyzed with the Wilcoxon test (WC, WHR, SB, DB).

Table 1: Changes in Anthropometric Variables (Mean ± S.D).

Characteristics	DIET H (n=139)								DIET S (n=141)							
	LysLys(n=94)				LysAsn+ AsnAsn (n=45)				LysLys (n=94)				LysAsn+ AsnAsn (n=47)			
	0 time	At 3 months	At 9 months	p value	0 time	At 3 months	At 9 months	p value	0 time	At 3 months	At 9 months		0 time	At 3 months	At 9 months	p value
Glucose (mg/dl)	103.2 ± 10.2	99.1 ± 13.1˙	98.1 ± 10.1˙	0.01	100.9 ± 12.2	99.9 ± 13.0	98.5 ± 9.8	0.22	101.4 ± 11.1	98.7 ± 9.2	99.5 ± 9.1	0.34	98.9 ± 9.4	96.8 ± 6.3	98.3 ± 7.1	0.45
Total ch. (mg/dl)	209.1 ± 19.8	197.8 ± 21.1˙	198.5 ± 30.7˙	0.02	206.6 ± 21.1	200.7 ± 31.0	207.4 ± 10.2	0.38	211.8 ± 40.9	199.0 ± 30.4˙	198.3 ± 18.4˙	0.03	203.6 ± 21.2	196.4 ± 19.1	193.8 ± 12.9	0.34
LDL-ch. (mg/dl)	127.9 ± 20.1	119.7 ± 20.9˙	120.2 ± 13.1˙	0.01	126.9 ± 27.2	123.4 ± 21.1	129.1 ± 12.1	0.41	125.2 ± 18.5	118.1 ± 23.2˙	117.8 ± 18.0˙	0.01	124.6 ± 18.1	120.2 ± 20.9	119.9 ± 19.8	0.09
HDL-ch. (mg/dl)	54.5 ± 10.5	53.7 ± 8.1	55.1 ± 7.1	0.78	56.8 ± 10.0	56.3 ± 9.0	55.8 ± 8.1	0.68	56.2 ± 11.2	53.2 ± 9.4	52.7 ± 11.0	0.55	55.0 ± 11.1	53.8 ± 8.1	55.1 ± 11.2	0.23
TG (mg/dl)	125.8 ± 43.1	114.1 ± 30.4˙	106.1 ± 22.2˙	0.01	120.3 ± 20.1	112.8 ± 33.2˙	107.9 ± 20.3˙	0.03	130.1 ± 42.6	119.4 ± 33.1˙	118.1 ± 30.1˙	0.01	121.0 ± 40.3	119.9 ± 18.3	117.9 ± 30.9	0.56
Insulin (mUI/L)	10.8 ± 5.4	9.0 ± 5.2˙	8.2 ± 5.0˙	0.03	11.6 ± 7.1	10.4 ± 9.1	9.8 ± 7.4	0.18	10.9 ± 5.0	9.1 ± 4.9	9.4 ± 4.2	0.09	10.7 ± 5.0	10.5 ± 4.2	8.9 ± 7.0	0.45
HOMA	2.2 ± 0.9	2.0 ± 0.8˙	1.7 ± 1.1˙	0.02	2.6 ± 1.1	2.7 ± 2.1	1.9 ± 1.3	0.09	2.3 ± 1.1	2.0 ± 1.0	2.1 ± 1.1	0.28	2.3 ± 1.2	2.2 ± 2.0	2.4 ± 1.6	0.34
CR (mg/dl)	4.8 ± 3.1	4.7 ± 3.2	2.6 ± 3.0	0.03	4.4 ± 3.1	5.1 ± 4.0	3.9 ± 3.2	0.19	5.0 ± 4.0	5.3 ± 4.1	4.9 ± 4.0	0.16	5.2 ± 4.0	5.1 ± 3.9	5.3 ± 3.1	0.45

H: High Protein/Low Carbohydrate; S: Standard; Chol: Cholesterol; TG: Triglycerides; CR: C Reactive Protein; HOMA: Homeostasis Model Assessment; Mths: Months (*) <0.05, in each group with basal values. No statistical differences among genotypes in each diet or in different diet groups. Quantitative variables with normal distribution were analyzed with a two-tailed, aired Student's-t test (glucose, Insulin, HOMA-IR, HDL cholesterol, C reactive protein). Non-parametric parameters were analyzed with the Wilcoxon test (total cholesterol, LDL cholesterol, trygliceride).

Table 2: Clasical Cardiovascular Risk Factors (Mean ± S.D).

Characteristics	DIET H (n=139)								DIET S (n=141)							
	LysLys(n=94)				LysAsn+ AsnAsn (n=45)				LysLys (n=94)				LysAsn+ AsnAsn (n=47)			
	0 time	At 3 months	At 9 months	p value	0 time	At 3 months	At 9 months	p value	0 time	At 3 months	At 9 months	p value	0 time	At 3 months	At 9 months	p value
Adionectin (ng/ ml)	10.2 ± 6.0	9.6 ± 5.1	10.3 ± 8.0	0.23	10.8 ± 7.0	11.1 ± 9.0	10.9 ± 7.2	0.34	11.0 ± 4.1	10.8 ± 4.0	9.9 ± 4.3	0.34	9.9 ± 5.1	10.6 ± 4.9	10.8 ± 4.1	0.43
Resistin (ng/ ml)	7.4 ± 3.2	7.2 ± 5.0	6.9 ± 4.3	0.45	7.3 ± 3.1	7.0 ± 3.2	7.1 ± 3.1	0.45	8.0 ± 2.5	7.9 ± 3.1	7.7 ± 2.8	0.45	8.0 ± 3.1	7.1 ± 4.0	6.9 ± 4.0	0.31
Letin (ng/ml)	31.8 ± 17.4	21.9 ± 13.1*	15.3 ± 10.1*	0.01	39.1 ± 10.9	20.8 ± 9.2*	18.5 ± 9.5*	0.01	31.9 ± 13.0	20.3 ± 8.0*	15.0 ± 6.1*	0.01	41.9 ± 10.1	22.7 ± 9.3*	21.6 ± 8.1*	0.02

(*) <0.05, in each group with basal values. No statistical differences among genotypes in each diet or in different diet groups. Quantitative variables with normal distribution were analyzed with a two-tailed, aired Student's-t test (resistin). Non-parametric parameters were analyzed with the Wilcoxon test (leptin and adiponectin).

Table 3: Circulating Adyocitokines (mean ± S.D).

unchanged in patients with Asn allele carriers. With the diet S and in patients with Lys656Asn genotypes, only total cholesterol (-13.2 ± 7.1 mg/dl vs -5.1 ± 8.2 mg/dl;p<0.05), triglycerides (-12.1 ± 7.1 mg/ dl vs -4.1 ± 7.9 1 mg/dl; p<0.05) and LDL- total cholesterol (-5.7 ± 3.1 mg/dl vs -2.1 ± 5.1 mg/dl; p<0.05) decreased. Lipid profile remained unchanged in patients with Asn allele genotype.

Table 3 reports levels of adipokines. With the diet HP and in both group of genotypes, leptin levels (-16.3 ± 12.1 ng/ml vs. -20.0 ± 11.1 ng/ ml: ns) decreased. With the diet S, leptin levels (-16.9 ± 5.2 ng/ml vs. -21.1 ± 4.3 ng/ml: ns) decreased in both groups, too. The decrease of leptin levels was similar with diet HP and S.

Discussion

Findings from our study suggest that, in obese patients following a high protein hypocaloric diet, carriers of the Asn 656 allele of the LEPR gene do not respond with a decrease of LDL cholesterol, insulin levels and HOMA-IR after a significant weight loss. These obese patients (Asn carriers) do not show a decrease of triglyceride and LDL cholesterol levels after a significant weight loss with a normal hypocaloric diet. After 9 months of two type of hypocaloric diets significantly reduced BMI, weight, fat mass, waist circumference and systolic blood pressure in obese subjects with different genotypes.

Several population-based studies have been realized to study the effects of this SNP in the leptin receptor gene (LEPR) on BMI. A meta-analysis of linkage and association of LEPR SNPs with BMI reported that, although certain genotypic effects could be population-specific, there was no evidence that any allele (Lys109Arg, Gln223Arg, Lys656Asn) is associated with body mass index or waist circumference [14]. Our results (basal and post treatment) are in agreement with the literature.

Interventional designs with this SNP are limited. Rossum et al. [15] did not show relation between Lys656Asn SNP and weight regain in a cohort in The Netherlands. Other study [5] demonstrated the different changes in weight loss and leptin response secondary to a hypocaloric diet with a 25% of calories from fats and with <20% of monounsaturated fats in relation with Lys656Asn SNP. In other design of our group, the weight loss secondary to a high polyunsaturated fatty acid (PUFA) diet produced, in carriers of ASn656 allele, a different change than non-Asn allele carriers, with a lack of improvement in insulin, leptin levels, and HOMA-IR. Therefore, obese subjects with this mutant allele have a better lipid profile after weight loss [7]. This better metabolic response in obese subjects without Asn allele has been detected with a high monounsaturated fatty acid (PUFA) diet, too [16]. In a randomized clinical trial [6] with 2 different hypocaloric diets (a low fat versus a low carbohydrate diet), a different metabolic response was observed, too.

Only leptin levels have a significant decrease in subjects with genotype Lys656Lys secondary to weight loss with both diets. The changes in serum leptin concentration due to 2 months' intervention with low fat are higher than with a low carbohydrate diet (low fat diet: 30.3%; p <0.05) and (low carbohydrate diet: 15.5%; p< 0.05).

A limitation of previous studies is the short term intervention (2-3 months), in our present study dietary intervention has been realized during 9 months. The longest intervention study in the literature was one year after the realization of a biliopancreatic derivation [17]. In both genetic groups, BMI, weight, glucose, triglyceride, total cholesterol, LDL cholesterol, and blood pressure decreased. Initial weight percent loss at 1 year of follow-up was higher in mutant group than in wild-type group (38.9% vs 29.9%; p<0.05). In our present study, after a high protein hypocaloric diet, subjects with Lys656Lys genotype of the LEPR gene showed a decrease of LDL cholesterol, insulin levels and HOMA-IR after weight loss. These obese subjects showed a decrease of LDL cholesterol and triglyceride levels after standard hypocaloric diet. 9 months of both diets significantly reduced weight, body mass index, waist circumference, fat mass and systolic blood pressure in obese subjects with both genotypes, with poorer biochemical response in patients carrying the allele Asn. The decrease of leptin levels was similar in both diets and in both genotypes.

Other authors have obtained association between SNP on codon 656 and obesity parameters. In postmenopausal females with intolerance of glucose (ITG), relationships were found with Lys656Asn for fasting insulin, as well as in response to an oral glucose test. In premenopausal females with ITG, associations were detected with Lys656Asn for overall glucose response to the glucose load [18]. In other studies, differences in substrate oxidation rates were found. In fasting conditions, Lys656Lys showed a trend to oxidize more carbohydrates and less fat than Asn656 carriers [19].

These different metabolic responses could be related with inclusion criteria and heterogeneity of subjects in the intereventional studies, distribution of nutrients of the hypocaloric diets, time course of dietary intervention and interaction with other polymorphisms in LEPR gene. For example Xenachis et al. [20] have study the response to a hypocaloric diet in the LEPR gene polymorphism, but in a different polymorphisms (Thr343Ser). The overweight women carried the Ser allele lost more weight in response to low calorie diet than non carriers. At last, other theories could be explained through an association of genetic variation in this receptor with the functionality of Leptin receptor and, therefore, influenced the leptin response and weight lost to energy restriction. Mars et al. [21] had observed heterogeneity of metabolic responses with the Lys109Arg, Gln223Arg and Lys656Asn SNPS in the initial decline in leptin after a hypocaloric diet with a 21.5% of fats.

In conclusion, carries of ASn656 allele have a different metabolic change than wild genotype obese, with a lack of decrease of HOMA-IR, insulin levels, total cholesterol and LDL cholesterol after a high protein hypocaloric diet and a lack of decrease of HOMA-IR, insulin, total cholesterol, LDL cholesterol and triglycerides after a standard hypocaloric diet. This polymorphism did not influence in terms of weight loss.

Authors Contribution

Daniel Antonio de Luis designed the study an wrote the article. R Aller realized nutritional evaluation. O IZaola realized nutritional evaluation. D Primo realized laboratory analysis. E Romero designed the study an wrote the article.

References

1. Meier U, Gressner AM (2004) Endocrine regulation of energy metabolism: review of pathobiochemical and clinical chemical aspects of leptin, ghrelin, adiponectin and resistin. Clin Chem 50: 1511-1525.

2. de Luis DA, Castrillon JLP, Dueñas A (2009) Leptin and Obesity. Minerva Med 100: 229-236.

3. Considine RV, Sinha MK, Heiman ML, Kriauciunas A, Stephens TW, et al. (1996) Serum immunorective-leptin concentrations in normal-weight and obese humans. N engl J Med 334: 292-295.

4. Heo M, Leíble RL, Boyer BB, Cheng WK, Koulu M, et al. (2001) Pooling analisis of genetic data: The assocation of leptin receptor (LEPR) polymorphisms with variables related to human adiposity. Genetics 159: 1163-1178.

5. de Luis Roman D, de la Fuente RA, Sagrado MG, Izaola O, Vicente RC (2006) Leptin receptor Lys656Asn polymorphism is associated with decreased leptin response and weight loss secondary to a lifestyle modification in obese patients. Arch Med Res 37: 854-859.

6. de Luis DA, Aller R, Izaola O, Sagrado MG, Conde R (2008) Influence Of Lys656Asn polymorphism of leptin receptor gene on leptin response secondary to two hypocaloric diets: a randomized clinical trial. Ann Nutr Metab 52: 209-214.

7. de Luis DA, Aller R, Izaola O, Sagrado MG, Conde R, et al. (2015) Effect of Lys656Asn Polymorphism of Leptin Receptor Gene on Cardiovascular Risk Factors and Serum Adipokine Levels after a High Polyunsaturated Fat Diet in Obese Patients. J Clin Lab Anal 29: 432-436.

8. de Luis DA, Aller R, Izaola O, Sagrado MG, Conde R (2008) Influence of ALA54THR polymorphism of FABP-2 on weight loss and insulin levels secondary to two hypocaloric diets: a randomized clinical trial. Diabetes Res Clin Pract 82: 113-118.

9. Santos FL, Esteves SS, da Costa Pereira A, Yancy WS Jr, Nunes JP (2012) Systematic review and meta-analysis of clinical trials of the effects of low carbohydrate diets on cardiovascular risk factors. Obes Rev 13: 1048-1066.

10. Mataix J, Mañas M (1998) Tablas de composición de alimentos españoles. Ed: University of Granada.

11. Lukaski HC, Johnson PE, Bolonchuk WW, Lykken GI (1985) Assessment of fat-free mass using bioelectrical impedance measurements of the human body. Am J Clin Nutr 41: 810-817.

12. Mathews DR, Hosker JP, Rudenski AS, Naylor BA, Treacher DF, et al. (1985) Homesotasis model assessment: insulin resistance and beta cell function from fasting plasma glucose and insulin concentrations in man. Diabetologia 28: 412-414.

13. Duart MJD, Arroyo CO, Frígols JLM (2002) Validation of a insulin model for the reactions in RIA. Clin Chem Lab Med 40: 1161-1167.

14. Heo M, Leibel RL, Fontaine KR, Boyer BB, Chung WK, et al. (2002) A meta-analytic investigation of linkage and association of common leptin receptor (LEPR) polymorphism with body mass index and waist circumference. Int J Obes Relat Metab Disord 26: 640-646.

15. Rossum CTM, Hoebee B, van Baak M, Mars M, Saris WHM, et al. (2003) Genetic variation in the leptin receptor gene, leptin, and weight gain in young Dutch Adults. Obes Res 11: 377-386.

16. de Luis DA, Aller R, Izaola O, Conde R, Bouza JE (2013) Lys656Asn polymorphism of leptin receptor gene is related with leptin changes after a high monounsaturated fat diet in obese patients. J Investig Med 61: 286-290.

17. de Luis DA, Aller R, Sagrado MG, Izaola O, Terroba MC, et al. (2010) Influence of lys656asn polymorphism of leptin receptor gene on surgical results of biliopancreatic diversion. J Gastrointest Surg 14: 899-903.

18. Wauters M, Mertens I, Rankinen T, Chagnon C, Bouchard C, et al. (2001) Leptin receptor gene polymorphisms are associated with insulin in obese women with impaired glucose tolerance. J Clin Endocrinol Metab 86: 3227-3232.

19. Wauters M, Considine R, Chagnon M, Mertens I, Rankinen T, et al. (2002) Leptin levels, leptin receptor gene polymorphisms, and energy metabolism in women. Obes Res10: 394-400.

20. Xenachis C, Samojlik E, Raghuwanshi MP, Kirschner MA (2001) Leptin, insulin and TNF-alpha in weight loss. J Endocrinol Invest 24: 865-870.

21. Mars M, Van Rossum C, de Graaf C, Hoebee B, de Groot L, et al. (2004) Leptin responsiveness to energy restriction: Genetic variation in the leptin receptor gene. Obes Res 12: 442-446.

10

Bioactivity in Whey Proteins Influencing Energy Balance

Liam McAllan[1,2], Paul D Cotter[1,3], Helen M Roche[4], Riitta Korpela[5] and Kanishka N Nilaweera[1]*

[1]Teagasc Food Research Centre, Moorepark, Fermoy, Cork, Ireland

[2]Department of Pharmacology and Therapeutics, University College Cork, Cork, Ireland

[3]Alimentary Pharmabiotic Centre, University College Cork, Cork, Ireland

[4]UCD Conway Institute of Biomolecular & Biomedical Research, & UCD Institute of Food & Health, University College Dublin, Belfield Dublin 4, Ireland

[5]Institute of Biomedicine, Biomedicum Helsinki, P.O. Box 63, FI-00014 University of Helsinki, Finland

Abstract

Obesity develops due to energy (food) intake exceeding energy expenditure. Nutrients that reduce the positive energy balance are thus being considered as therapies to combat obesity. Here, we review the literature related to the physiological, cellular and endocrine effects of intake of whey proteins, namely α-lactalbumin, β-lactoglobulin, glycomacropeptide and lactoferrin. Moreover, we discuss how dietary composition and obesity may influence whey protein effects on the above parameters. Evidence suggests that intake of whey proteins causes a decrease in energy intake, increase in energy expenditure, influence insulin sensitivity and glucose homeostasis and alter lipid metabolism in the adipose, liver and muscle. These physiological changes are accompanied by alterations in the plasma levels of energy balance related hormones (cholecystokinin, ghrelin, insulin and glucagon-like peptide-1) and the expression of catabolic and anabolic genes in the above tissue in the direction to cause a negative energy balance.

Keywords: Nutrition; Diet; Metabolic syndrome; Human; Rodent

Abbreviations: CCK: Cholecystokinin; FAS: Fatty Acid Synthase; GLP-1: Glucagon-Like Peptide-1; TAG: Triacylglycerol

Introduction

Obesity is a major health problem in the world because it increases the risk of development of several clinical conditions including cardiovascular disease, stroke, hypertension and type 2 diabetes [1]. The weight gain occurs due to storage of energy consumed in excess of daily requirement, as triacylglycerol (TAG) in the adipose tissue. The resulting increase in the mass of the adipose tissue causes the gain of weight, and it may even lead to the development of obesity [2]. The prevalence of obesity and associated co-morbidities has reached epidemic proportions globally. Hence, it is no surprise that there is a growing interest to identify therapies in particular those involving nutrients that could reduce weight gain and thus the development of obesity.

Whey is the milk serum that remains after precipitation of casein during cheese production, and it contains proteins, vitamins, minerals and trace amounts of fat. Whey associated proteins include α-lactalbumin, β-lactoglobulin, glycomacropeptide and lactoferrin [3]. There is accumulating evidence suggesting that whey protein intake influences the balance between energy (food) intake and energy expenditure, insulin sensitivity and glucose homeostasis as well as lipid metabolism in tissues in particular in the adipose tissue. Here, we review data from *in vivo* (human and rodent) and *in vitro* studies related to the above effects of α-lactalbumin, β-lactoglobulin, glycomacropeptide and lactoferrin and briefly discuss in the last section the actions of recently identified minor whey proteins. Furthermore, we discuss how dietary composition and obesity could influence the actions of these dietary proteins. Because authors of some of the studies mentioned below have not stated whether the whey proteins were provided as a concentrate or isolate, we have used the term "whey proteins" where this classification has not been specified.

Food (Energy) Intake

Studies conducted in humans have shown that intake of 20 to 50 g of whey proteins reduces short term *ad libitum* food intake. Akhavan

et al. showed that whey protein concentrate (20-40 g) dose dependently reduces subsequent (30 min) *ad libitum* pizza meal energy intake in lean subjects, with 40g having the greatest impact compared to the water control [4]. This effect extends up to 2 h in lean subjects [5]. In comparison to casein, whey proteins (48 g) delay the desire to eat a subsequent meal by up to 180 mins in lean subjects [6], suggesting that the whey proteins induce satiety in comparison to casein intake. The results of rodent studies with regard to the effects of whey proteins on food (energy) intake are largely in agreement with that observed in humans. The suggestion that whey proteins induce satiety has been further confirmed in mice by showing that whey protein isolate providing 30% energy increased intermeal interval (satiety) compared to soy protein during the 7 day period of the study [7]. Similar findings have been reported from a long term study lasting 10 weeks [8]. These data are consistent with the findings from human studies that whey proteins reduce food intake by inducing satiety in the lean state. However, a functional relationship between whey proteins and food intake has not been consistently reported. For instance, although Hall et al. showed that whey proteins reduce food intake compared to casein in humans [6], this response was not observed in rats given a whey protein isolate in comparison to casein diet (300 g/kg diet) for 7 weeks, despite the fact that the rats on the whey protein isolate diet showed a significantly reduced weight gain compared to the rats on the casein diet [9]. It is possible that physiological and neuroendocrine differences that exist between the species (humans vs. rats) may have given rise to the inconsistent effects of whey protein and casein on food intake. There is evidence that macronutrient composition in the diet could also impact upon the effect of whey proteins on food intake. Veldhorst et al. showed that a diet containing proteins, carbohydrates and fat providing 10, 55 and 35% energy, respectively, reduces hunger in humans if whey

*Corresponding author: Kanishka Nilaweera, Teagasc Food Research Centre, Moorepark, Fermoy, County Cork, Ireland
E-mail: kanishka.nilaweera@teagasc.ie

proteins were included in comparison to either soy and casein [10]. Similar results have been obtained from a study conducted in rats, which showed that whey protein concentrate with energy content of 55% reduced cumulative energy intake compared to whole milk protein if the former protein had been supplied in a diet with either 35% and 10% energy from carbohydrates and lipids, respectively, or in a diet with 45% energy solely from lipids [11]. No differences in cumulative energy intake were observed if the proteins were provided in diets with 15% and 30% energy from carbohydrates and fats, respectively. These data highlights the importance of the carbohydrate composition in the diet on whey protein effects on food intake. In addition to dietary composition, weight gain also seems to influence the effect of whey proteins on short term food intake. This is revealed by the finding that intake of whey protein isolate (50 g) reduced subsequent pizza intake in normal weight but not in obese subjects [12]. Similar findings have been reported by another human study [13] and in high fat diet induced obese mice [14]. In the latter case, diet induced obese mice that drank water supplemented with whey protein isolate at 100 g/L for 11 weeks show similar energy intake to obese mice on un-supplemented water, despite the former group showing a significant decrease in body weight [14]. Thus, in addition to protein source, quality and time of consumption mentioned by Anderson et al. [5], both macronutrient composition in the diet and state of energy balance (lean vs. obese), should be considered as important factors influencing the whey protein effects on food intake.

A number of studies have attempted to identify the individual whey proteins present in the concentrate or isolate that might be causing the reduction in food intake in humans and rodents. Because glycomacropeptide has been shown to stimulate the production of the satiety hormone cholecystokinin (CCK) [15], a role for this whey protein in the regulation of food intake has been suggested. The findings of Veldhorst et al. support the latter suggestion, since it was shown that ingestion of a breakfast diet with whey protein providing 10% energy reduced lunchtime energy intake in lean subjects more than intake of a whey protein associated breakfast diet without glycomacropeptide [16]. This suggests that glycomacropeptide may reduce energy intake possibly by inducing satiety, as previously reported. This finding is not in agreement with data from several other studies performed on lean subjects with diets containing whey protein without glycomacropeptide (providing 44% energy) [17] and whey protein diets with added glycomacropeptide (21% w/w) [18]. To explore the possibility that the discrepancies in the data on the effects of glycomacropeptide on food intake might be due to the variations in the degree of protein glycosylation, Keogh et al. provided 50 g of minimal glycosylated or glycosylated glycomacropeptide as well glycomacropeptide depleted whey protein concentrate to obese and overweight subjects and found that their subsequent lunch time meal intake was not affected by the dietary challenges [19]. The data suggest that the degree of glycosylation studied in the glycomacropeptide is not critical for the actions of this whey protein on food intake. As the above study was performed on obese or over-weight individuals that as described above appear to be less sensitive to whey protein effects on food intake, it would be interesting to find out whether the outcome on food intake would be different with lean individuals. However, taking in to account the data from human studies described above, and data from a rat study which revealed that glycomacropeptide does not impact on food intake [9], it could be argued that this whey protein does not have a significant effect on this physiological process. Utilising a similar approach as in their previous studies, Veldhorst et al. showed that breakfast diets with α-lactalbumin providing 10% or 25% energy reduces lunch time energy intake in lean subjects compared to a breakfast diet with casein, soy or

whey without glycomacropeptide [20]. This data is in agreement with the results of another study [21], which together suggest an important role for α-lactalbumin in suppression of food intake in lean humans. In addition to this whey protein, β-lactoglobulin has also been shown to influence energy intake. The study by Pichon et al. that showed data highlighting the importance of dietary composition on whey protein effects on energy intake, also tested the effects of β-lactoglobulin on energy intake in rats and found that β-lactoglobulin reduced energy intake compared to whole milk proteins [11]. In summary, consumption of whey proteins as an isolate or concentrate appears to reduce food (energy) intake in humans and rodents by inducing satiety compared to casein, soy or carbohydrates. This effect is influenced by the macronutrients in the whey protein diet and by development of obesity. In the former case, a high carbohydrate composition appears to favour the actions of whey proteins. Of the whey proteins that have been studied, data suggests an important role(s) for α-lactalbumin and β-lactoglobulin in the regulation of food (energy) intake, with no significant regulatory role for glycomacropeptide in this physiological process.

Lipid Metabolism

In over-weight or obese humans and rodents, whey proteins have been shown to improve lipid metabolism, particularly elevated plasma, adipose and hepatic TAG levels. Recently Pal et al. demonstrated that intake of whey protein isolate (27 g) twice daily for 12 weeks causes a reduction in fasting TAG levels in over-weight and obese subjects compared to casein intake [22]. A similar effect has also been observed in obese rats with intake of whey protein concentrate at 32% (wt/wt) compared to 8% (wt/wt) [23]. Even at a reduced whey protein isolate content (24% wt/wt providing 18% energy), these dietary proteins reduce high fat (providing 60% energy) diet induced weight gain and body fat in mice compared to casein intake [24]. The reduction in body weight and fat content observed by the latter study was not due to a difference in the intestinal fat absorption in the two groups. The authors thus investigated whether whey protein isolate may affect adipocyte lipid metabolism [25]. By providing the same high fat diets containing either whey protein isolate or casein for 21 weeks, it was shown that the adipocyte cross sectional area was reduced in mice fed with whey proteins compared to casein. This suggests that whey proteins influence lipid metabolism in adipocytes much more than casein, although the extent of the reduction in adipocyte size may have been influenced by the fact that the diets contain calcium, which is known to influence lipid metabolism in this tissue [26]. Given that the liver is also important for regulation of lipid metabolism, the same authors assessed in a separate study how the same dietary challenge may impact upon the lipid metabolism in the liver of high fat diet-induced obese mice subjected to a 7 week calorie restriction [27]. Compared to calorie restricted obese mice on the casein diet, calorie restricted obese mice on the whey protein isolate diet had reduced TAG levels in the liver. The specificity with which whey protein isolate influences hepatic lipid content has been further demonstrated (in the absence of calorie restriction) by the study by Shertzer et al. [14]. In the studies mentioned above, except for the latter, the observed effects of whey protein on lipid metabolism were shown relative to casein. Interestingly, in contrast, soy proteins at 24% (wt/wt) in the diet of rats had a similar effect on body weight and abdominal fat as whey proteins [8]. This data could be interpreted to suggest that whey protein effects on lipid metabolism are detectable only when casein is used as the control protein, or that the lack of an effect on lipid metabolism in comparison to soy might be due to the fact that the above study assessed dietary protein effects on lean rats as oppose to obese rodents, which are known to have a higher body weight and body fat content and thus, are likely to be more susceptible to whey protein effects on lipid metabolism. A number of studies have attempted to determine how each individual whey protein affects lipid metabolism. Two human studies show date related to the actions of lactoferrin and glycomacropeptide. By providing overweight human subjects with enteric coated lactoferrin (100 mg/d) or placebo tablets for a period of 8 weeks, it has been found that lactoferrin reduces body weight, visceral fat mass as well as hip circumference [28]. In contrast, ingestion of glycomacropeptide-enriched whey protein diet (with 15 g of proteins) twice daily replacing two daily meals for 6 months or once daily for further 6 months, had no significant effect on body weight or plasma TAG concentrations compared to skim milk powder diet [29]. It would be interesting to further define whether the outcome would have been different if a higher glycomacropeptide content was used, given also that data from a rodent study described below suggests an important role for this whey protein in the regulation of lipid metabolism. It has been shown that rats ingesting whey protein isolate diet supplemented with glycomacropeptide at 100 and 200 g/kg reduces carcass fat compared to rats on a whey protein isolate diet or casein diet [9]. Because there were no differences in food intake between the groups, the data suggests a food intake-independent effect of glycomacropeptide on lipid metabolism (fat content) in these animals. With the view to assessing how other whey proteins, namely α-lactalbumin, β-lactoglobulin and lactoferrin may influence body weight and body fat content in rodents, Pilvi et al. subjected high fat diet induced obese mice to a 70% energy restricted diet containing whey protein isolate or each of the whey proteins mentioned above (18% energy) for a period of 7 weeks to induce weight loss [30], and subsequently allowed *ad libitum* access to the diets for further 7 weeks to allow weight gain. Results suggest that α- lactalbumin is the most beneficial whey protein in terms of causing fat loss when provided as part of an energy restricted diet or fed *ad libitum*. Although lactoferrin caused the most weight loss and had a similar effect on percentage fat content to α-lactalbumin in the initial 7 weeks, during the *ad libitum* feeding period however, lactoferrin caused the most gain in total fat content. In contrast, the human study mentioned above found that lactoferrin reduces body weight and fat content [28]. In further support for a role for lactoferrin in reducing adiposity, it has been shown *in vitro* that this whey protein specifically inhibits adipogenesis and lipid accumulation in adipocytes [31,32]. Although Pilvi et al. study showed that β-lactoglobulin was the least effective whey protein for inducing weight loss and for preventing weight gain [30], Pichon et al. found that β-lactoglobulin (55% energy) causes the least weight gain when supplemented in a diet containing only fat providing 45% of energy in comparison to a diet containing 35% and 10% energy from carbohydrates and fat or in a diet with 15% and 30% energy from the same macronutrients, respectively [11]. The data again highlights the importance of macronutrient composition on whey proteins effects on energy balance. Note here that the macronutrient composition providing the maximum whey protein effects on body weight and body fat content appear to differ from the composition that seemed to provide a greater reduction in food intake mentioned previously; in both cases however, a diet with carbohydrate and fat providing 35% and 10% energy respectively appear to be effective to bring about both changes in food intake and body weight/lipid metabolism. In summary, whey protein isolate appears to reduce body weight and lipid metabolism both in obese humans and in rodents in comparison to casein intake, with specific effects observed in the adipocytes and in the liver, although these effects appear to be influenced by macronutrient composition in the diet. Available data suggest an important role(s) for α-lactalbumin, β-lactoglobulin, lactoferrin and glycomacropeptide in the regulation of lipid metabolism in humans and/or in rodents.

Insulin Sensitivity and Glucose Homeostasis

In healthy and overweight humans and rodents whey protein intake has been shown to cause an acute insulinotropic response. This has been shown by supplementation of whey proteins into glucose drinks or test meals, which augments postprandial insulin release, resulting in an enhancement of glucose disposal in both healthy [33,34] and type-2 diabetic [35] subjects. Similar effects have been seen in anesthetised mice, where gastic gavage of whey protein (75 mg) and glucose (75 mg) together augmented the insulin response 3-fold and increased glucose disposal by 31% in comparison to glucose alone [36]. In addition to acute responses, prolonged whey protein intake also improves insulin sensitivity in the obese state in both rodents [14,23,27,37,38] and humans [22]. Of the whey proteins that have been tested, both α-lactalbumin and glycomacropeptide have been found to increase the postprandial insulin release (in comparison to casein protein intake) with glycomacropeptide having a greater effect than whey protein isolate or α-lactalbumin [16]. Long-term glycomacropeptide intake has also been shown to improve fasting blood insulin levels in both humans [29] and rats [9]. Similarly a high protein diet (55% kcal) with β-lactoglobulin as it source of protein was shown by Pichon et al. [11] to reduce insulin resistance and improve fasting blood insulin levels in rats to a greater extent than that of comparable high whey protein concentrate diet. The actions of α-lactalbumin and β-lactoglobulin on insulin sensitivity and glucose homeostasis may be due to the bioactive peptides in the proteins, since several dipeptides from α-lactalbumin and β-lactoglobulin have been found to increase glucose uptake in L6 myotubes and isolated skeletal muscles *in vitro* [39]. A role for lactoferrin in the regulation of glucose homeostasis has also been suggested based on the findings that circulating levels of lactoferrin correlate negatively with hyperglycemia and positively with insulin sensitivity [40], and that intake of a lactoferrin rich whey protein isolate supplemented high fat diet improves glucose tolerance in mice in comparison to high fat diet containing casein [38]. In summary, whey protein intake appears to stimulate insulin release and could improve glucose tolerance and insulin sensitivity long term, even when accompanied by high fat feeding. The available data also suggest that this effect may be a common feature of α-lactalbumin, β-lactoglobulin, lactoferrin and glycomacropeptide, with the latter being more potent than α-lactalbumin.

Energy Expenditure

Whey protein (18 g) intake prior to a bout of heavy resistance training increases post-training resting energy expenditure in humans compared to carbohydrate intake [41]. Interestingly, this effect diminishes if the whey protein meal was ingested after the resistance exercise, even if the protein content in the diet was at 30 g [42]. The data suggest that the timing of the dietary challenge is crucial for detecting whey protein induced changes in resting energy expenditure. Intake of whey proteins also appears to increase thermogenesis, possibly because of its higher thermic effect compared to soy or casein [33]. This may possibly be due to the whey protein induced increased protein metabolism in tissues [43]. To our knowledge, of the whey proteins associated with regulation of energy balance, only α-lactalbumin has been shown to influence energy expenditure. The study by Hursel et al. which reported an effect of α-lactalbumin (41% energy from the protein) ingestion on lunchtime meal intake in the healthy humans, also found that this whey protein significantly increases diet-induced thermogenesis compared to intake of whole milk protein rich diet [21]. Whether α-lactalbumin, or any other whey protein, could influence energy expenditure in obese humans remains to be determined, although data from a rodent study clearly suggests such an effect; it has been shown that diet-induced obese mice drinking water supplemented with whey proteins (100 g/L) have increased O_2 consumption compared to obese mice drinking unsupplemented water [14]. In summary, compared to carbohydrates, soy and casein, intake of whey proteins appears to increase energy expenditure in lean and obese states by influencing thermogenesis and resting energy expenditure. In the latter case, the timing of the dietary challenge might be important, in particular when associated with exercise, for obtaining an effective change in this parameter linked to energy expenditure. It is tempting to suggest that the effect of whey proteins on energy expenditure might be due to the actions of α-lactalbumin present in the whey protein isolate or concentrate, however, this may be premature given that there are no data showing whether other whey proteins could influence energy expenditure to the same extent.

Cellular Activity and Endocrine System

It is well established that the hormones CCK, ghrelin, insulin and glucagon-like peptide-1 (GLP-1) play important roles in energy balance regulation by inhibiting (CCK, insulin and GLP-1) and stimulating (ghrelin) food (energy) intake and/or by inducing a catabolic (GLP-1) and anabolic (ghrelin and insulin) responses on lipid metabolism in tissues [44,45]. Given the effects of whey proteins on food intake and body weight, it is no surprise that whey proteins modulate these hormones. A study by Bowen et al. showed that whey protein induced decrease in energy intake in humans, is accompanied by an increased plasma level of CCK and GLP-1 and reduces levels of ghrelin [46]. These changes were noted as early as 15 mins and continued up to 180 mins after the dietary challenge, suggesting potential acute and chronic effects of whey proteins on hormonal levels. In the case of insulin, whey proteins appear to acutely increase hormone levels, but over a time, there is a notable decline. Similar effects on hormone levels have been observed in studies conducted with only lean [6] and obese subjects [13], suggesting that whey proteins modulate hormone levels independent of weight gain and that the changes are consistent with an attempt to increase catabolism. Similar data have been obtained from rodent studies. Zhou et al. showed that the reduction in food intake in lean rats on a diet supplemented with 24% (wt/wt) whey protein concentrate, is accompanied by an increased GLP-1 level in the plasma [8]. Given that both α-lactalbumin and β-lactoglobulin have been shown to influence food (energy) intake, it would be interesting to find out whether these proteins are responsible for the observed changes in hormone levels detected in human and rodent studies.

An advantage of conducting rodent studies in comparison to human studies is that in the former case, it is possible to dissect and analyse tissues of interest to identify specific changes in expression of energy balance related genes. To our knowledge, such investigations have not been conducted to assess the impact of whey proteins on gene expression in centres of the brain important for regulation of energy balance. In contrast, there is data to suggest that whey proteins influence gene expression related to lipid metabolism in the adipocytes and in the liver cells. The study by Pilvi et al. mentioned above performed a detailed microarray analysis of gene expression in the (reduced) adipocytes of obese mice that had ingested whey proteins [25]. This analysis revealed an increased expression of several genes involved in insulin signalling pathway in the whey protein group compared to the control casein group. The microarray data also revealed an increased expression of genes for leptin and β_3-adrenergic receptor. Since the mass of the adipose tissue and leptin gene expression has previously been shown to be closely linked [47], the significance of the increased expression of leptin gene in adipocytes with reduced cross sectional area remains to be determined. In contrast, a potential functional

relationship could exist between the reduction in the adipose tissue and increased β_3-adrenergic receptor expression, given that the receptor activation is known to increase hormone sensitive lipase-mediated hydrolysis of fat, increase fat oxidation and induce uncoupling protein-mediated thermogenesis [48,49], all of which are likely to reduce mass of the adipose tissue. This also indicates a potential mechanism by which whey proteins could reduce adiposity. With regard to the rat liver, whey proteins have been found to reduce activity of several lipogenic enzymes including fatty acid synthase (FAS) compared to casein intake [50]. In contrast, in the muscle, FAS expression and activity was increased in response to whey protein challenge [50], possibly to reduce hepatic production of lipids and to promote synthesis of lipids in the muscle so that these could be oxidised in the mitochondria in the muscle cells to generate energy in the form of adenosine 5' triphosphate. With regard to the above mentioned changes in the cellular activity observed in the adipose, muscle and liver, it is important to further define how they arise by investigating the impact of the whey proteins implicated in lipid metabolism, namely α-lactalbumin, β-lactoglobulin, lactoferrin and glycomacropeptide. In summary, in comparison to casein and carbohydrates (glucose and fructose), whey proteins appear to drive endocrine and cellular changes consistent with a catabolic effect. This is achieved by up-regulation of the production of catabolic hormones (CCK, GLP-1 and insulin), by reduction in the production of anabolic hormone ghrelin and by modulation of the expression or activity of lipogenic, lipolytic and fat oxidation related genes in the liver, adipose and in the muscle. The decrease in insulin levels observed over time with whey protein intake might be a mechanism to reduce anabolic effects of this hormone on adipocytes [45].

Minor Whey Proteins

In addition to the above mentioned whey proteins, many other lower-abundance proteins have been found within the whey fraction. Due to recent advances in milk proteomics [51,52], this list of minor whey proteins is increasing. In fact, a recent proteomic investigation of the whey fraction has found 293 unique gene products, 176 of which were newly identified in whey [52]. Although the potential energy balance related roles of these minor whey proteins have yet to be investigated, it is interesting that some of these proteins such as lipoprotein lipase, perilipin-2 and fatty acid binding proteins 3 and 5, have defined roles in lipid metabolism and storage. Recently, a study assessed the impact of a novel whey protein isolate rich in lactoperoxidase on high fat diet induced obesity [38] and found that this diet dose-dependently reduced bodyweight, fat mass gain, hepatic lipid accumulation and improved glucose tolerance [38]. These findings again raise the energy balance related impact of minor whey proteins.

Summary and Conclusions

Overall the data suggest that whey proteins (α-lactalbumin and β-lactoglobulin) decrease food intake, possibly by altering the plasma levels of hormones (CCK, GLP-1, ghrelin and insulin) important for energy balance regulation. In addition, whey proteins (α-lactalbumin, β-lactoglobulin, lactoferrin and glycomacropeptide) also alter lipid metabolism. This may be achieved by (1) decreasing FAS gene expression and hence TAG production in the liver, (2) by increasing lipogenesis in the muscle possibly for oxidation, and (3) by increasing β_3-adrenergic receptor expression in the adipocytes, possibly to decrease FAS expression in this tissue. Whey protein intake (α-lactalbumin, β-lactoglobulin, lactoferrin and glycomacropeptide) improves insulin sensitivity and glucose tolerance, preventing high fat diet induced insulin resistance. With regard to energy expenditure, whey proteins (α-lactalbumin) increases this energy balance related parameter possibly by increasing protein anabolism in the tissues. As the macro- and micro-nutrient (calcium) composition in the diet and obesity all influence the mechanisms involved in the regulation of energy balance, one could envisage that any changes in these mechanisms could greatly impact upon the ability of whey proteins to influence the balance between energy intake and energy expenditure. A better understanding of how specific whey proteins influence energy balance may help in the formulation of dietary interventions that could prevent or reduce obesity.

Acknowledgement

The on-going work in the area of whey protein effects on energy balance is funded by Teagasc, Ireland. The authors have no conflicts of interest. Each author listed contributed by reviewing the literature and/or by critically reviewing the manuscript.

References

1. Schelbert KB (2009) Comorbidities of obesity. Prim Care 36: 271-285.

2. Hajer GR, van Haeften TW, Visseren FL (2008) Adipose tissue dysfunction in obesity, diabetes, and vascular diseases. Eur Heart J 29: 2959-2971.

3. Krissansen GW (2007) Emerging health properties of whey proteins and their clinical implications. J Am Coll Nutr 26: 713S-723S.

4. Akhavan T, Luhovyy BL, Brown PH, Cho CE, Anderson GH (2010) Effect of premeal consumption of whey protein and its hydrolysate on food intake and postmeal glycemia and insulin responses in young adults. Am J Clin Nutr 91: 966-975.

5. Anderson GH, Tecimer SN, Shah D, Zafar TA (2004) Protein source, quantity, and time of consumption determine the effect of proteins on short-term food intake in young men. J Nutr 134: 3011-3015.

6. Hall WL, Millward DJ, Long SJ, Morgan LM (2003) Casein and whey exert different effects on plasma amino acid profiles, gastrointestinal hormone secretion and appetite. Br J Nutr 89: 239-248.

7. Yu Y, South T, Huang XF (2009) Inter-meal interval is increased in mice fed a high whey, as opposed to soy and gluten, protein diets. Appetite 52: 372-379.

8. Zhou J, Keenan MJ, Losso JN, Raggio AM, Shen L, et al. (2011) Dietary whey protein decreases food intake and body fat in rats. Obesity (Silver Spring) 19: 1568-1573.

9. Royle PJ, McIntosh GH, Clifton PM (2008) Whey protein isolate and glycomacropeptide decrease weight gain and alter body composition in male Wistar rats. Br J Nutr 100: 88-93.

10. Veldhorst MA, Nieuwenhuizen AG, Hochstenbach-Waelen A, van Vught AJ, Westerterp KR, et al. (2009) Dose-dependent satiating effect of whey relative to casein or soy. Physiol Behav 96: 675-682.

11. Pichon L, Potier M, Tome D, Mikogami T, Laplaize B, et al. (2008) High-protein diets containing different milk protein fractions differently influence energy intake and adiposity in the rat. Br J Nutr 99: 739-748.

12. Bellissimo N, Desantadina MV, Pencharz PB, Berall GB, Thomas SG, et al. (2008) A comparison of short-term appetite and energy intakes in normal weight and obese boys following glucose and whey-protein drinks. Int J Obes (Lond) 32: 362-371.

13. Bowen J, Noakes M, Clifton PM (2007) Appetite hormones and energy intake in obese men after consumption of fructose, glucose and whey protein beverages. Int J Obes (Lond) 31: 1696-1703.

14. Shertzer HG, Woods SE, Krishan M, Genter MB, Pearson KJ (2011) Dietary whey protein lowers the risk for metabolic disease in mice fed a high-fat diet. J Nutr 141: 582-587.

15. Pedersen NL, Nagain-Domaine C, Mahe S, Chariot J, Roze C, et al. (2000) Caseinomacropeptide specifically stimulates exocrine pancreatic secretion in the anesthetized rat. Peptides 21: 1527-1535.

16. Veldhorst MA, Nieuwenhuizen AG, Hochstenbach-Waelen A, Westerterp KR, Engelen MP, et al. (2009) Effects of complete whey-protein breakfasts versus whey without GMP-breakfasts on energy intake and satiety. Appetite 52: 388-395.

17. Burton-Freeman BM (2008) Glycomacropeptide (GMP) is not critical to whey induced satiety, but may have a unique role in energy intake regulation through cholecystokinin (CCK). Physiol Behav 93: 379-387.

18. Lam SM, Moughan PJ, Awati A, Morton HR (2009) The influence of whey protein and glycomacropeptide on satiety in adult humans. Physiol Behav 96: 162-168.

19. Keogh JB, Woonton BW, Taylor CM, Janakievski F, Desilva K, et al. (2010) Effect of glycomacropeptide fractions on cholecystokinin and food intake. Br J Nutr 104: 286-290.

20. Veldhorst MA, Nieuwenhuizen AG, Hochstenbach-Waelen A, Westerterp KR, Engelen MP, et al. (2009) A breakfast with alpha-lactalbumin, gelatin, or gelatin + TRP lowers energy intake at lunch compared with a breakfast with casein, soy, whey, or whey-GMP. Clin Nutr 28: 147-155.

21. Hursel R, van der Zee L, Westerterp-Plantenga MS (2010) Effects of a breakfast yoghurt, with additional total whey protein or caseinomacropeptide depletedalpha-lactalbumin-enriched whey protein, on diet-induced thermogenesis and appetite suppression. Br J Nutr 103: 775-780.

22. Pal S, Ellis V, Dhaliwal S (2010) Effects of whey protein isolate on body composition, lipids, insulin and glucose in overweight and obese individuals. Br J Nutr 104: 716-723.

23. Belobrajdic DP, McIntosh GH, Owens JA (2004) A high-whey-protein diet reduces body weight gain and alters insulin sensitivity relative to red meat in wistar rats. J Nutr 134: 1454-1458.

24. Pilvi TK, Korpela R, Huttunen M, Vapaatalo H, Mervaala EM (2007) High-calcium diet with whey protein attenuates body-weight gain in high-fat-fed C57Bl/6J mice. Br J Nutr 98: 900-907.

25. Pilvi TK, Storvik M, Louhelainen M, Merasto S, Korpela R, et al. (2008) Effect of dietary calcium and dairy proteins on the adipose tissue gene expression profile in diet-induced obesity. J Nutrigenet Nutrigenomics 1: 240-251.

26. Zemel MB (2004) Role of calcium and dairy products in energy partitioning and weight management. Am J Clin Nutr 79: 907S-912S.

27. Pilvi TK, Seppanen-Laakso T, Simolin H, Finckenberg P, Huotari A, et al. (2008) Metabolomic changes in fatty liver can be modified by dietary protein and calcium during energy restriction. World J Gastroenterol 14: 4462-4472.

28. Ono T, Murakoshi M, Suzuki N, Iida N, Ohdera M, et al. (2010) Potent anti-obesity effect of enteric-coated lactoferrin: decrease in visceral fat accumulation in Japanese men and women with abdominal obesity after 8-week administration of enteric-coated lactoferrin tablets. Br J Nutr 104: 1688-1695.

29. Keogh JB, Clifton P (2008) The effect of meal replacements high in glycomacropeptide on weight loss and markers of cardiovascular disease risk. Am J Clin Nutr 87: 1602-1605.

30. Pilvi TK, Harala S, Korpela R, Mervaala EM (2009) Effects of high-calcium diets with different whey proteins on weight loss and weight regain in high-fatfed C57BL/6J mice. Br J Nutr 102: 337-341.

31. Yagi M, Suzuki N, Takayama T, Arisue M, Kodama T, et al. (2008) Lactoferrin suppress the adipogenic differentiation of MC3T3-G2/PA6 cells. J Oral Sci 50: 419-425.

32. Moreno-Navarrete JM, Ortega FJ, Ricart W, Fernandez-Real JM (2009) Lactoferrin increases (172Thr)AMPK phosphorylation and insulin-induced (p473Ser)AKT while impairing adipocyte differentiation. Int J Obes (Lond) 33: 991-1000.

33. Acheson KJ, Blondel-Lubrano A, Oguey-Araymon S, Beaumont M, Emady-Azar S, et al. (2011) Protein choices targeting thermogenesis and metabolism. Am J Clin Nutr 93: 525-534.

34. Nilsson, M, Holst JJ, Bjorck IM (2007) Metabolic effects of amino acid mixtures and whey protein in healthy subjects: studies using glucose-equivalent drinks. Am J Clin Nutr 85: 996-1004.

35. Frid AH, Nilsson M, Holst JJ, Bjorck IM (2005) Effect of whey on blood glucose and insulin responses to composite breakfast and lunch meals in type 2 diabetic subjects. Am J Clin Nutr 82: 69-75.

36. Gunnarsson PT, Winzell MS, Deacon CF, Larsen MO, Jelic K, et al. (2006) Glucose-induced incretin hormone release and inactivation are differently modulated by oral fat and protein in mice. Endocrinology 147: 3173-3180.

37. Huang XF, Liu Y, Rahardjo GL, McLennan PL, Tapsell LC, et al. (2008) Effects of diets high in whey, soy, red meat and milk protein on body weight maintenance in diet-induced obesity in mice. Nutr Diet 65: S53-S59.

38. Shi J, Tauriainen E, Martonen E, Finckenberg P, Ahlroos-Lehmus A, et al. (2011) Whey protein isolate protects against diet-induced obesity and fatty liver formation. Int Dairy J 21: 513-522.

39. Morifuji M, Koga J, Kawanaka K, Higuchi M (2009) Branched-chain amino acid-containing dipeptides, identified from whey protein hydrolysates, stimulate glucose uptake rate in L6 myotubes and isolated skeletal muscles. J Nutr Sci Vitaminol (Tokyo) 55: 81-86.

40. Moreno-Navarrete JM, Ortega FJ, Bassols J, Ricart W, Fernandez-Real JM (2009) Decreased circulating lactoferrin in insulin resistance and altered glucose tolerance as a possible marker of neutrophil dysfunction in type 2 diabetes. J Clin Endocrinol Metab 94: 4036-4044.

41. Hackney KJ, Bruenger AJ, Lemmer JT (2010) Timing protein intake increases energy expenditure 24 h after resistance training. Med Sci Sports Exerc 42: 998-1003.

42. Benton MJ, Swan PD (2007) Effect of protein ingestion on energy expenditure and substrate utilization after exercise in middle-aged women. Int J Sport Nutr Exerc Metab 17: 544-555.

43. Boirie Y, Dangin M, Gachon P, Vasson MP, Maubois JL, et al. (1997) Slow and fast dietary proteins differently modulate postprandial protein accretion. Proc Natl Acad Sci U S A 94: 14930-14935.

44. Cummings DE, Overduin J (2007) Gastrointestinal regulation of food intake. J Clin Invest 117: 13-23.

45. Nogueiras R, Lopez M, Dieguez C (2010) Regulation of lipid metabolism by energy availability: a role for the central nervous system. Obes Rev 11: 185-201.

46. Bowen J, Noakes M, Clifton PM (2006) Appetite regulatory hormone responses to various dietary proteins differ by body mass index status despite similar reductions in ad libitum energy intake. J Clin Endocrinol Metab 91: 2913-2919.

47. Galic S, Oakhill JS, Steinberg GR (2010) Adipose tissue as an endocrine organ. Mol Cell Endocrinol 316: 129-139.

48. Weyer C, Gautier JF, Danforth E Jr. (1999) Development of beta 3-adrenoceptor agonists for the treatment of obesity and diabetes--an update. Diabetes Metab 25: 11-21.

49. Holm C (2003) Molecular mechanisms regulating hormone-sensitive lipase and lipolysis. Biochem Soc Trans 31: 1120-1124.

50. Morifuji M, Sakai K, Sanbongi C, Sugiura K (2005) Dietary whey protein downregulates fatty acid synthesis in the liver, but upregulates it in skeletal muscle of exercise-trained rats. Nutrition 21: 1052-1058.

51. Hettinga K, van Valenber H, de Vries S, Boeren S, van Hooijdonk T, et al. (2011) The host defense proteome of human and bovine milk. PLoS One 6: e19433.

52. Le A, Barton LD, Sanders JT, Zhang Q (2011) Exploration of bovine milk proteome in colostral and mature whey using an ion-exchange approach. J Proteome Res 10: 692-704.

11

Antidiabetic Effects of Ginseng in Humans and Rodents

Zhanxiang Wang[1]* and Hongji Zhang[2]

[1]Herman B Wells Center for Pediatric Research, Basic Diabetes Group, Department of Pediatrics, Indiana University School of Medicine, USA

[2]Department of Urology, Indiana University School of Medicine, USA

Abstract

Ginseng, one of the most commonly used herbs worldwide, has known anti-hyperglycemic effects. Twenty-eight (28) studies on diabetic mice and rats from 7 research centers (in 6 different nations) indicate that both Asian ginseng (*Panax ginseng*) and American ginseng (*Panax quinquefolius*) are effective anti-hyperglycemic supplements, putatively acting via improvements in insulin secretion, insulin sensitivity, islet protection, obesity reduction, anti-oxidation, energy expenditure, and fat absorption. Investigations in clonal beta-cells (MIN6, RINmF, INS-1, HIT-T15) and non-beta-cells (3T3-L1, C1C12, HepG2) further confirm that ginseng may protect against pancreatic beta-cell apoptosis and promote insulin secretion and glucose uptake. Among 18 human trials from 4 independent groups, 15 are single dose trials; whereas, 4 are long-term trials, with treatment periods lasting longer than 4 weeks. Eleven of the single dose trials observed anti-diabetic effects, while 4 observed no improvements. In the long-term studies, two-thirds of the studies on type 2 diabetic (T2D) patients observed anti-hyperglycemic effects. Based upon the sound evidence from cell lines and animal models, along with the improvements from the majority of human subject trials, ginseng appears to be a potent anti-diabetic supplement. Regardless, more long-term trials on T2D patients are required before ginseng can be safely recommended as a broadly-used anti-diabetic agent.

Keywords: MDA; Ginseng; Ginsenoside; Diabetes

Introduction

Type 2 diabetes (T2D) is a worldwide epidemic disease. Because commonly prescribed anti-diabetic drugs are riddled with safety concerns and/or have limited efficacy, management of T2D can be challenging. Therefore, alternative medicines, derived from natural products which have very little to no side-effects, offer exciting possibilities for the development of successful anti-diabetic therapies.

Originally used as a stress-reducing tonic for several thousand years in Asia, Ginseng is one of the most popular herbal supplements in the world [1]. In support of ancient Asian wisdom, a number of contemporary researchers have suggested that pharmacological doses of ginseng positively affect the cardiovascular, immune, and central nervous systems [2,3]. The primary active components of ginseng are the ginsenosides (ginseng saponins) that comprise 3-6% of ginseng. Based on their structure, the ginsensosides can be classified into 3 groups: the panaxadiol group (Rb1, Rb2, Rb3, Rc, Rd, Rg3, Rh2); the panaxatriol group (Re, Rf, Rg1, Rg2, Rh1); and the oleanolic group (Ro) [2,4]. In China, herbs are routinely used in combination with conventional anti-diabetic therapies to improve hyperglycemia. For single-herb prescriptions, ginseng is the most commonly-used herb: for example, ginseng is one of the top 10 most frequently-prescribed herbs, among the 30 anti-diabetic formulas currently approved by the Chinese government [5]. Intriguing results from basic research have demonstrated that ginseng improves diabetes by enhancing insulin sensitivity, stimulating insulin secretion, protecting pancreatic islets and inhibiting intestinal absorption of carbohydrates [6]. In addition to reliable *in vitro* and *in vivo* evidence (Table 1), the majority of reports in human trials also indicate that ginseng administration does indeed have anti-diabetic effects [7-20], though some controversy does exist [16,21,22]. In this review, we focus on the anti-diabetic effects of ginseng from both animal and randomized, controlled human studies, discuss possible reasons for the discrepancies among human trials and provide topics for future investigations.

Animal Studies

Mice

A number of independent research groups have shown that ginseng has hypoglycemic effects. The majority of the reports are from the Kimura group (Japan), Chung group (South Korea), Yuan group (USA), and Cheng group (Taiwan).

Early in the 1980s, Kimura et al. [23] revealed that ginseng radix (root) extract (10-50 mg/kg) decreased blood glucose and increased blood insulin concentrations in alloxan-induced diabetic mice. Insulin antisera injections abolished these effects, indicating that ginseng-stimulated insulin release is critical for the observed anti-hyperglycemic effects [23]. A 3-h treatment of ginseng extract (0.5 mg/ml) stimulated insulin biosynthesis in islets from KK-CAy mice [24]. The Kimura group further observed that the anti-hyperglycemic effect of ginseng was diminished in diabetic KK-CAy and alloxan-induced diabetic mice, if ginseng was combined with anemarrhena or licorice (two additional herbs commonly used in traditional Asian medicine) [25], indicating potential interaction of ginseng with other drugs.

Investigations from Chung and colleagues from South Korea also demonstrated that ginseng has anti-diabetic effects that synergize with the anti-diabetic drug, metformin. Oral administration of white ginseng radix and rootlet for 4 weeks in KKAy mice significantly reduced fasting blood glucose levels, presumably by blocking intestinal glucose absorption [26]. In high fat (HF) diet-fed ICR mice, the Chung group showed that wild ginseng ethanol extract (WGEE, 250 and 500 mg/kg) significantly inhibited body weight gain, fasting blood glucose, triglyceride and free fatty acid levels in a dose-dependent manner. WGEE also improved the insulin resistance index (>55%) and decreased white and brown adipocyte diameter (>46%) compared to HF-fed controls [27]. A vinegar-processed, as well as non-processed, form of ginseng radix (500 mg/kg/day for 8 weeks) both have significant anti-metabolic

*Corresponding author: Zhanxiang Wang, MD, PhD, 635 Barnhill Dr, MS2031, Herman B Wells Center for Pediatric Research, Department of Pediatrics, Indianapolis, IN 46202, USA, E-mail: wangz@iupui.edu

Groups	Nation	Cell	Ginseng type	Outcome
Luo	USA	INS	American Ginseng	Protect apoptosis[66]
Chung	Korea	HIT-T15	Compound K*	Increase GSIS[29]
		HIT-T15	RG3	Increase GSIS[31]
		RINmF	Fermented ginseng	Protect apoptosis/Increase GSIS[67]
		MIN6	Rb1, Rg1	Protect apoptosis/Increase GSIS[68]
Kim	Korea	MIN6	Ginseng extract	Protect apoptosis[69]
Yuan	USA	MIN6	Ginseng extract	Protect apoptosis/Increase GSIS[70]
Shang	China	3T3-L1	Rb1	Increase glucose uptake[71]
		3T3-L1 /C2C12	Rb1	Increase glucose uptake[72]
Zhang	China	3T3-L1	Re	Activate insulin signaling[73]
Jun	Korea	3T3-L1	Rb1,Rg1	Increase glucose uptake[68]
Lee	Korea	3T3-L1	Rg3,Re	Increase glucose uptake[74]
Kwon	Korea	C2C12	Rc	Increase glucose uptake[75]
Chung	Korea	HepG2	Compound K*	Lipid metabolism[76]
		HepG2	Rg1	Inhibited liver glucose production[77]
Yuan	USA	C2C12	IH-901*	Stimulation of glucose uptake[78]

*: intestine metabolites of ginsenoside

Table 1: Summary of Cell Studies.

syndrome effects in HF-fed ICR mice, with >81% decrease in insulin resistance, >67% reduction in white adipocytes and a marked inhibition of weight gain (approx. >53%), compared to the HF-fed control animals [28]. Further, in male db/db mice treated for 8 weeks, Compound K (CK), a major intestinal ginsenoside metabolite from the ginseng radix, also exhibited an anti-hyperglycemic effect through increases in insulin secretion, similar to that of sulfonylureas, potent insulin secretagogues. Importantly, the CK (10 mg/kg) + metformin (150 mg/kg) group had the lowest insulin resistance index indicating synergistic effects of the drug combination [29]. In a long-term study using C57BL/KsJ db/ db mice, CK improves oral glucose tolerance, increases insulin release and protects against the destruction of pancreatic islets. CK shifted hepatic glucose metabolism from production to utilization and improved insulin sensitivity by elevating plasma adiponectin levels and up-regulating genes for the glucose transporter and adipogenesis in the adipose tissue [30]. In ICR mice, ginsenoside Rg3 suppressed blood glucose levels by enhancing insulin secretion [31]. In the same ICR mice model, ginseng extract (IH-901 at 25 mg/kg) lowered plasma glucose, triglyceride, cholesterol and free fatty acid levels approximately 20.7-41.6%. Plasma insulin levels were significantly increased between 2.2 and 3.4-fold. Furthermore, histological observation show preserved architecture of the pancreatic islet.

Interesting work from the Yuan group (United States) validated that ginseng berries and leaves are also effective anti-diabetic supplements; juice prepared from the ginseng berry or a water extract of American ginseng can also achieve this goal. Daily intraperitoneal injections of *Panax ginseng* berry extract (150 mg/kg) in db/db mice for 5 consecutive days significantly decreased fasting blood glucose (FBG) levels (180.5 ± 10.2 mg/dl vs. control 226.0 ± 15.3 mg/dl). After 12 days of treatment, the db/db mice returned to fasting normoglycemia (134.3 ± 7.3 mg/dl), while FBG concentrations in vehicle-treated mice remained high (254.8 ± 24.1 mg/dl). Ginseng-treated mice also lost a significant amount of weight between days 5 and 12. Lean littermates treated with the same dose of ginseng berry extract also lost weight but did not have comparable reductions in FBG [32]. Similar to the db/db mouse study, obese-diabetic ob/ob mice treated with the ginseng berry extract presented with significant weight loss, reductions in both food intake and plasma

cholesterol and increases in energy expenditure and body temperature, compared to lean littermate controls. The ginsenoside Re plays an important role in the anti-hyperglycemic action of ginseng [33,34]. The same dose of ginseng berry extract (150 mg/kg) exhibits more potent anti-hyperglycemic activity, compared to ginseng root extract and only ginseng berry shows marked anti-obesity effects in ob/ob mice [35]. As a more convenient, safe, and practical means of delivery, the Yuan group prepared ginseng berry juice that can be provided orally. Ob/ob mice given ginseng berry juice preparation (0.6 ml/kg) for 10 consecutive days had significantly lower FBG levels and notable improvements in both glucose tolerance and body weight, which all persisted for at least 10 d following cessation of the treatment [36]. Daily intraperitoneal injections of extracts from the American ginseng leaf (50 or150 mg/kg) in diabetic ob/ob adult mice significantly increased glucose disposal, decreased body weight, and increased body temperature by day 12 of treatment [37]. In ob/ob mice, daily intraperitoneal injections for 12 days of American ginseng root extract (300 mg/kg), prepared by a simple water extraction procedure, significantly improves FBG levels and glucose tolerance, while simultaneously reducing body weight [38]. A research group from Taiwan reported that the hypoglycemic effect of ginseng was only produced in pentobarbital-anesthetized BALB/c and C57BL/6 mice; however, in conscious mice this effect could be achieved only if guanethidine was provided at a sufficient dose to block sympathetic tone [39].

Ginseng also has an inhibitory effect on the absorption of dietary fat in male Balb/c mice [40]. Aerobic exercise plus ginseng appears to lower serum lipid, regulate lipid metabolism, promote anti-oxidation, and enhance immune activity in a mouse model of hyperlipidemia through feeding of a high cholesterol diet [41]. However, *in vivo* administration of ginseng extract and ginsenosides may cause significant impairment of PPAR α-dependent activation of genes involved in the fatty-acid β-oxidation, suggesting that the use of ginseng be limited under certain pathophysiological conditions, such as hypercholesterolemia [42].

Rats

Using the rat as research model, a number of independent groups have demonstrated that ginseng has obvious hypoglycemic effects; in a 40-week study ginseng treatment delayed the development of diabetes. Studies with rats are primarily from four independent groups in Korea, one group from the United States, one from Japan and the Cheng group from Taiwan.

An early report from a Japanese group showed that Ginseng radix fraction (10-50mg/kg) increased liver glycogen content, inhibited epinephrine-induced transient hyperglycemia and reduced free fatty acid release from rat epididymal fat pad [43]. Later four independent Korean groups demonstrate that ginseng has anti-obesity effects, which may have beneficial effects on the pathobiology of diabetes. Kim et al. [44] showed that administration of crude saponin from Korean red ginseng (200 mg/kg, ip) for 3 weeks in obese, male Sprague-Dawley rats (HF diet-induced) significantly reduced body weight, food intake and fat content to levels comparable to that of normal weight, chow-fed rats. The hypothalamic NPY expression and serum leptin levels were also reduced in the ginseng-treated HF-fed rats [44]. The results further implicate that the anti-obesity effects of ginseng may result from energy expenditure and normalizing hypothalamic neuropeptides and serum biochemicals related to the control of obesity [45]. Another group from Korea observed that ginseng attenuated the development of overt diabetes. Oral administration of Korean red ginseng (KRG) (200 mg/kg/d) in Otsuka Long-Evans Tokushima Fatty (OLETF) rats for 40 weeks reduced weight gain and visceral fat mass (without altering food intake), improved insulin sensitivity and significantly preserved glucose tolerance comparable to control animals for up to 50 weeks of age. KRG promoted fatty acid oxidation in skeletal muscle and cultured C2C12 muscle cells by the AMPK medicated up-regulation of PPAR-gamma coactivator-1 alpha, nuclear respiratory factor-1, and glucose transporter 4 (GLUT4) [46]. More recent research from the Chung group in Korea further confirmed ginseng's anti-diabetic effect: ginseng provided via an oral or injection route lowers hyperglycemia induced by streptozotocin (STZ) in Sprague Dawley rats. Oral administration of 250 or 500 mg/kg of fermented ginseng for 20 days (starting one week before STZ injection) reduces plasma glucose level and elevates plasma insulin levels by 266% and 334%, respectively. STZ-induced destruction of pancreatic islets was hindered, through mechanisms involving reductions of nitric oxide synthase (iNOS) and cyclooxygenase-2 (COX-2) [47].

Research completed by Liu et al. [48] from Taiwan indicates that ginseng may reverse the development of insulin resistance. In rats with insulin resistance induced by the consumption of a high fructose diet, oral administration of *Panax ginseng* root (125.0 mg/kg, thrice daily for 3 days) reduced the elevated glucose-insulin index. The plasma glucose concentrations were significantly lower than those of the vehicle-treated group. Importantly, the plasma glucose-lowering response of tolbutamide was markedly prolonged in *Panax ginseng* root treatment group, suggesting that oral administration of *Panax ginseng* could be a suitable adjuvant therapy for those with insulin resistance [48]. Liu et al. also showed that in high-fat fed Wistar rats plasma glucose is decreased and plasma insulin and C-peptide levels are increased by 60 min following an intravenous injection of ginsenoside Rh2 (0.1-1.0 mg/kg). Rh2 also enhanced insulin secretion mediated by the pancreatic nerve [49]. Intravenous infusion of Rh2 over 120 min in STZ-diabetic rats decreased plasma glucose in a dose-dependent manner, while also increasing gene expression of GLUT 4 in soleus muscle [50]. Single intravenous injections of ginsenoside Rh2 in rats with high-fructose diet-induced insulin resistance decreased plasma glucose concentrations, ultimately improving insulin sensitivity [51].

Researchers from the United States recently observed that either acute or chronic administration of ginsenoside Rb1 is safe and effective in rats. Acute intraperitoneal injections of Rb1 dose-dependently (>5 mg/kg) suppressed food intake mediated by central mechanisms (without eliciting signs of toxicity). Additionally, 4-week administration of ginsenoside Rb1 (10 mg/kg) significantly reduced food intake, body weight gain, and body fat content and increased energy expenditure in HFD-induced obese rats. Rb1 also significantly decreased fasting blood

glucose and improved glucose tolerance. These effects were greater than those in pair-fed rats, suggesting that the anti-hyperglycemic effect of Rb1 is only partially attributable to reduced food intake and body weight. Importantly, at an effective dose, acute intraperitoneal administration of Rb1 dose-dependently suppressed food intake that was not caused by taste aversion (Table 2) Rb1-treated obese rats also had no obvious health problems, e.g. diarrhea. Additionally, no chronic non-specific toxic effects were observed (assessed by end-study plasma ALT, AST, and creatinine concentrations) [52].

Human Subjects Trials

Studies investigating the anti-diabetic properties of ginseng in humans have only recently appeared. In this review, we only discuss 18 human trials that are double (or single)-blinded placebo-controlled studies. The majority of these reports indicate that ginseng does indeed have anti-diabetic potential.

In 1995, as a result of their research involving 36 diabetic patients, Sotaniemi et al. [7] suggested that ginseng would be a useful therapeutic adjunct in the management of T2D. Oral ginseng (100 or 200 mg/day) for 8 weeks normalized HbA1c levels, reduced fasting blood glucose concentrations, and reduced body weight, while simultaneously elevating mood and improving psychophysical performance and physical activity [7].

Later, several reports from a group in the United Kingdom confirmed ginseng's effects in regulation of blood glucose in human subjects. In their 3 single-dose trials, involving more than 87 healthy individuals, 200 mg and 400 mg of orally-provided ginseng significantly reduced blood glucose at all three of the post-treatment follow-ups [8-10]. However, the authors were unable to find a long-term effect on glucose regulation when non-diabetic participants (n=31) were provided *Panax ginseng* for 8 weeks, suggesting against the chronic use of ginseng in individuals with normal glucose control [11].

Multiple reports from a research group in Canada observed that American ginseng (AG) and Korean red ginseng (KRG; *Panax ginseng* that has been heated) affect postprandial glycemia in humans; the exception being null effects from one batch of AG that had marked decrements in total ginsenosides. In their first report, including 10 non-diabetic subjects, significant reductions in area under the glycemic curve (18 ± 31%) were observed when ginseng (3 g) was taken orally 40 min before the glucose challenge; there were no differences in effect if the ginseng and glucose were administered together. In 9 diabetic patients,

Groups	Nation	Model	Ginseng type	Research outcome (year)
Kimura	Japan	Mice(Alloxan diabetic)	Ginseng extract	+(1980)[23] +(1981)[43] +(1981)[24] +(1999)[25]
Chung	Korea	Diabetic mice (KKAy, ICR, db/db, C57BL/KsJ) Rat(STZ treated)	Ginseng, Rg3, compound K,	+(2001)[26] +(2004)[27] +(2007)[28] +(2007)[29] +(2007)[30] +(2008)[31] +(2011)[78] +(2010)[47]
Yuan	USA	Diabetic mice (db/db, ob/ob)	American Ginseng extract, berry/leaf/ root	+(2002)[32] +(2002)[33] +(2002)[34] +(2003)[35] +(2004)[37] +(2007)[36] +(2009)[38]
Cheng	Taiwan	Mice(STZ treated)	Ginseng	+(2010)[39]
		Rat(insulin resistant, or STZ treated)	Ginseng, Rh2	+(2005)[48] +(2006)[49] +(2006)[50] +(2007)[51]
Kim	Korea	Rat(fatty,Dawley)	Korea red Ginseng	+(2005)[44] +(2009)[45]
Lee	Korea	Rat(fatty,Long-Evans)	Korea red Ginseng	+(2009)[46]
Liu	USA	Rat(obese)	Rb1	+(2010)[52]

+: indicating antidiabetic effects.

Table 2: Summary of Animal Studies.

Groups	Nation	Human subjects	Ginseng type and dose	Outcome(year)
Sotaniemi	Finland	T2D(30)	Ginseng(100-200mg,8 week oral)	+(1995)[7]
Reay	UK	Norm(30)	Ginseng(1 dose, 200-400mg oral)	+(2005)[8]
		Norm(57)	Ginseng(1 dose)	+(2006)[9] [10]
		Norm(41)	Ginseng(200mg, 8 week oral)	- (2009)[11]
Vuksan	Canada	T2D(9)	American Ginseng(1 dose)	+(2000)[12]
		T2D(19)	Korean red Ginseng(6g/d,12 week oral)	+(2008)[19]
		Norm(10)	American Ginseng(1 dose)	+(2000)[12]
		Norm(10)	American Ginseng(1 dose)	+(2000)[13]
		Norm(10)	American Ginseng(1 dose)	+(2000)[14]
		Norm(12)	Asian Ginseng(1 dose)	+(2001)[15]
		Norm(12)	Asian ginseng(1 dose)	+(2004)[16]
		Norm(19)	Korean red Ginseng (1 dose)	+(2006)[18]
		Norm(12)	Asian Ginseng(1 dose)	+(2007)[17]
		Norm(13)	Korean red Ginseng(1 dose)	+(2011)[20]
		Norm(12)	Asian Ginseng(1 dose)	- (2004)[16]
		Norm(12)	Asian ginseng(1 dose)	- (2003)[53]
		Norm(22)	Asian ginseng(1 dose)	- (2003)[54]
Reed	USA	T2D(14)	Korea red ginseng/Re (3-8g/d, 4 week oral)	- (2011)[22]
Others	Japan Korea		Ginseng extract	+*[55] [56] [57]

*: lipid metabolism; T2D = type 2 diabetes, Norm = healthy people, number of individuals in bracket; 1 dose = 1 single dose experiment. +: positive in antidiabetic effect; -: null in antidiabetic effect.

Table 3: Summary of Human Trials.

AG attenuated postprandial glycemia by similar amount (19 ± 22% and 22 ± 17%, respectively), regardless if the ginseng administration was before or at same time as the glucose challenge [12]. They further demonstrated that 3 g AG was sufficient to achieve maximal glucose reduction. AG reduced postprandial glycemia at 30 min irrespective of dose and time of administration [13]. In non-diabetic individuals, 3, 6, or 9 of AG (taken 40, 80, or 120 minutes before a glucose challenge) similarly improved glucose tolerance; all treatments reduced area under the incremental glucose curve (26.6%-38.5%) [14]. While 1, 2, or 3 g of AG are equally effective in reductions in glycemia (around 10%), the blood glucose concentration during the last hour of the test was significantly lower when ginseng was administered 40 min before the challenge, rather than 0, 10, or 20 min pre-glucose challenge [15]. Among the 8 commonly-used ginseng sources (American, American-wild, Asian, Asian-red, Vietnamese-wild, Siberian, Japanese-rhizome, and Sanchi ginseng), only American ginseng and Vietnamese ginseng lowered plasma glucose at 90 min in 12 healthy participants given 3 g of ginseng, while the other species of ginseng had opposite effects, actually elevating glucose levels [16]. American ginseng (9 g) administered 40 min before a 2-h OGTT, also significantly reduced glycemia by 27.7% and insulin increase by 23.8%, relative to the non-treated control [17]. However, in 2 additional trials, normal subjects were provided Asian ginseng or a different batch of AG (6 g, 40 min prior to a 75 g OGTT). In these studies, there was no significant effect on the incremental plasma glucose, incremental plasma insulin, or the insulin sensitivity index. However, they found marked decrements in total ginsenosides and Rb1/Rg1 ratio in those batches of AG, which might be an explanation for the contradictory results [53,54].

When evaluating the different forms of ginseng, Sievenpiper et al. demonstrated that 2 g of KRG-rootlets (40 min prior to oral glucose test) is sufficient to achieve reproducible reductions (29%) in postprandial glycemia [18]. Long-term outcomes (efficacy and safety) of KRG are also encouraging. Nineteen well-controlled type 2 diabetics (sex: 11 M, 8 F; age: 64 ± 2 years) took 2 g KRG (total 6 g/day) 40 min prior to each meal for 12 weeks as an adjunct to their usual anti-diabetic therapy (diet and/or medications). Improvements in glycemic control were observed; although HbA1c did not improve, plasma glucose was reduced by 8-11%, fasting and OGTT plasma insulin was increased y 33-38%, and insulin sensitivity increased by 33%, compared with placebo-treated controls [19]. Interestingly, the KRG rootlets

had >6-fold more total ginsenosides than the KRG-body, but did not significantly affect postprandial glucose. However, despite this reduced ginsenoside profile, KRG-body lowered postprandial glucose levels at 45, 60, 90, and 120 min during the glucose tolerance test, rendering an overall reduction of 27% (AUC) compared to the control (p < 0.05). This suggests a potential therapeutic dose range for ginsenosides [20].

However, more recent research from a group in the United States observed no anti-diabetic effect from AG. Fifteen overweight or obese subjects (sex: 14 F, 1 M; BMI = 34 ± 1; age = 46 ± 3 yr) with impaired glucose tolerance or newly diagnosed T2D were randomized to 30 days of treatment with ginseng root extract (8 g/day), ginsenoside Re (250-500 mg/day), or placebo. Beta cell function was assessed as the disposition index (DI); oral glucose tolerance test and insulin sensitivity (IS) were also monitored. Values for DI and IS were not different among the placebo, ginseng, and ginsenoside Re-treated groups. Ginsenosides Re, Rb$_1$, and Rb$_2$ were not detectable in plasma after treatment with ginseng root extract or ginsenoside Re (Table 3). They argued that poor systemic bioavailability might be responsible for the absence of a therapeutic effect [22].

In addition to blood glucose regulatory effect, oral administration of ginseng has also been observed to have effects on lipid metabolism in human [55-57].

Discussion

In the development of T2D, both islet beta-cell dysfunction and muscle insulin resistance play important roles [58,59]. Evidence from cell studies indicates that ginseng (both Asian ginseng [*Panax ginseng*] and American ginseng [*Panax quinquefolius*]) could protect islet beta-cell function and enhance glucose uptake, both supportive of ginseng being a potent anti-diabetic supplement. Twenty-eight animal studies from seven different international research groups confirm these effects and suggest ginseng may delay diabetes progression. *In vivo* anti-hyperglycemia mechanisms of ginseng involve increased insulin secretion, insulin sensitization and islet protection with additional anti-obesity, anti-oxidation, energy expenditure and glucose absorption effects. Interestingly, ginseng is found to synergize with metformin but may have adverse interactions with other herbs. Positive outcomes from long-term studies (>40 weeks) indicate ginseng may be beneficial for chronic use in diabetic individuals. Overall, evidence-based data acquired from animal studies support the anti-diabetic effects of ginseng.

In human studies, among 18 trials (299 human subjects) from four research groups, only 4 trials (74 cases) are T2D patients, with most being non-diabetic volunteers; In addition, only 4 studies are long-term (>4 weeks) trials. The majority, if not all, of one dose trials observed anti-hyperglycemic effects for both American ginseng and *Panax ginseng*. In three long-term independent trials with T2D patients, two trials demonstrated positive effects (invovling 30 patients) [7], while one showed no effects (involving 14 patients) [19]. The failure to observe anti-diabetic effects in some of the human trials may be due to the difference in batches of Ginseng used, of which ginsenoside levels may differ. Yet, the genetic and metobolic differences of human subjets among the trial groups should also be considerd. Since drug pharmacokinetic and pharmacodynamic differences exist among different populations [60,61] and between genders [61,62]. Different response rates to specific drugs also exist [63], even the gut microbiome (important for human health) could be different due to genetic background, gender [64] and diet habits [65]. Thus, different populations may absorb/metaoblize ginseng differently, which would affect the bioavailability of the effective compounds in Ginseng. Therefore in the future, while more T2D patients and research centers are inclined to participte in ginseng trials, it is also necessary to investigate the pharmacodynamic differences of ginseng among different populations. In Chinese medicine, ginseng is primarily administered in low doses in combination with other herbs for synergistic effects, therefore it will also be necessary to define how ginseng synergizes with other natural dietary supplements or with routinely used anti-diabetic drugs in diabetes treatment.

Acknowledgement

Zhanxiang Wang analyzed data and wrote the manuscript; Hongji Zhang collected and analyzed data, as well as helped in discussion. We thank Dr. Stephanie Yoder for critical reading of the manuscript. This study is partially supported by grant from the National Institutes of Health (CTSI-KL2 RR025760 to ZW).

References

1. Bahrke MS, Morgan WP, Stegner A (2009) Is ginseng an ergogenic aid? Int J Sport Nutr Exerc Metab 19: 298-322.

2. Attele AS, Wu JA, Yuan CS (1999) Ginseng pharmacology: multiple constituents and multiple actions. Biochem Pharmacol 58: 1685-1693.

3. Yuan CS, Wu JA, Osinski J (2002) Ginsenoside variability in American ginseng samples. Am J Clin Nutr 75: 600-601.

4. Xiang YZ, Shang HC, Gao XM, Zhang BL (2008) A comparison of the ancient use of ginseng in traditional Chinese medicine with modern pharmacological experiments and clinical trials. Phytother Res 22: 851-858.

5. Xie W, Zhao Y, Zhang Y (2011) Traditional chinese medicines in treatment of patients with type 2 diabetes mellitus. Evid Based Complement Alternat Med 726723.

6. Yin J, Zhang H, Ye J (2008) Traditional chinese medicine in treatment of metabolic syndrome. Endocr Metab Immune Disord Drug Targets 8: 99-111.

7. Sotaniemi EA, Haapakoski E, Rautio A (1995) Ginseng therapy in non-insulin-dependent diabetic patients. Diabetes Care 18: 1373-1375.

8. Reay JL, Kennedy DO, Scholey AB (2005) Single doses of Panax ginseng (G115) reduce blood glucose levels and improve cognitive performance during sustained mental activity. J Psychopharmacol 19: 357-365.

9. Reay JL, Kennedy DO, Scholey AB (2006) The glycaemic effects of single doses of Panax ginseng in young healthy volunteers. Br J Nutr 96: 639-642.

10. Reay JL, Kennedy DO, Scholey AB (2006) Effects of Panax ginseng, consumed with and without glucose, on blood glucose levels and cognitive performance during sustained 'mentally demanding' tasks. J Psychopharmacol 20: 771-781.

11. Reay JL, Scholey AB, Milne A, Fenwick J, Kennedy DO (2009) Panax ginseng

12. Vuksan V, Sievenpiper JL, Koo VY, Francis T, Beljan-Zdravkovic U, et al. (2000) American ginseng (Panax quinquefolius L) reduces postprandial glycemia in nondiabetic subjects and subjects with type 2 diabetes mellitus. Arch Intern Med 160: 1009-1013.

13. Vuksan V, Stavro MP, Sievenpiper JL, Koo VY, Wong E, et al. (2000) American ginseng improves glycemia in individuals with normal glucose tolerance: effect of dose and time escalation. J Am Coll Nutr 19: 738-744.

14. Vuksan V, Stavro MP, Sievenpiper JL, Beljan-Zdravkovic U, Leiter LA, et al. (2000) Similar postprandial glycemic reductions with escalation of dose and administration time of American ginseng in type 2 diabetes. Diabetes Care 23: 1221-1226.

15. Vuksan V, Sievenpiper JL, Wong J, Xu Z, Beljan-Zdravkovic U, et al. (2001) American ginseng (Panax quinquefolius L.) attenuates postprandial glycemia in a time-dependent but not dose-dependent manner in healthy individuals. Am J Clin Nutr 73: 753-758.

16. Sievenpiper JL, Arnason JT, Leiter LA, Vuksan V (2004) Decreasing, null and increasing effects of eight popular types of ginseng on acute postprandial glycemic indices in healthy humans: the role of ginsenosides. J Am Coll Nutr 23: 248-258.

17. Dascalu A, Sievenpiper JL, Jenkins AL, Stavro MP, Leiter LA, et al. (2007) Five batches representative of Ontario-grown American ginseng root produce comparable reductions of postprandial glycemia in healthy individuals. Can J Physiol Pharmacol 85: 856-864.

18. Sievenpiper JL, Sung MK, Di Buono M, Seung-Lee K, Nam KY, et al. (2006) Korean red ginseng rootlets decrease acute postprandial glycemia: results from sequential preparation- and dose-finding studies. J Am Coll Nutr 25: 100-107.

19. Vuksan V, Sung MK, Sievenpiper JL, Stavro PM, Jenkins AL, et al. (2008) Korean red ginseng (Panax ginseng) improves glucose and insulin regulation in well-controlled, type 2 diabetes: results of a randomized, double-blind, placebo-controlled study of efficacy and safety. Nutr Metab Cardiovasc Dis 18: 46-56.

20. De Souza LR, Jenkins AL, Sievenpiper JL, Jovanovski E, Rahelic D, et al. (2011) Korean red ginseng (Panax ginseng C.A. Meyer) root fractions: Differential effects on postprandial glycemia in healthy individuals. J Ethnopharmacol 137: 245-250.

21. Sievenpiper JL, Arnason JT, Vidgen E, Leiter LA, Vuksan V (2004) A systematic quantitative analysis of the literature of the high variability in ginseng (Panax spp.): should ginseng be trusted in diabetes? Diabetes Care 27: 839-840.

22. Reeds DN, Patterson BW, Okunade A, Holloszy JO, Polonsky KS, et al. (2011) Ginseng and ginsenoside Re do not improve beta-cell function or insulin sensitivity in overweight and obese subjects with impaired glucose tolerance or diabetes. Diabetes Care 34: 1071-1076.

23. Kimura M, Waki I, Chujo T, Kikuchi T, Hiyama C, et al. (1981) Effects of hypoglycemic components in ginseng radix on blood insulin level in alloxan diabetic mice and on insulin release from perfused rat pancreas. J Pharmacobiodyn 4: 410-417.

24. Waki I, Kyo H, Yasuda M, Kimura M (1982) Effects of a hypoglycemic component of ginseng radix on insulin biosynthesis in normal and diabetic animals. J Pharmacobiodyn 5: 547-554.

25. Kimura I, Nakashima N, Sugihara Y, Fu-jun C, Kimura M (1999) The antihyperglycaemic blend effect of traditional chinese medicine byakko-ka-ninjin-to on alloxan and diabetic KK-CA(y) mice. Phytother Res 13: 484-488.

26. Chung SH, Choi CG, Park SH (2001) Comparisons between white ginseng radix and rootlet for antidiabetic activity and mechanism in KKAy mice. Arch Pharm Res 24: 214-218.

27. Yun SN, Moon SJ, Ko SK, Im BO, Chung SH (2004) Wild ginseng prevents the onset of high-fat diet induced hyperglycemia and obesity in ICR mice. Arch Pharm Res 27: 790-796.

28. Yun SN, Ko SK, Lee KH, Chung SH (2007) Vinegar-processed ginseng radix improves metabolic syndrome induced by a high fat diet in ICR mice. Arch Pharm Res 30: 587-595.

29. Yoon SH, Han EJ, Sung JH, Chung SH (2007) Anti-diabetic effects of compound K versus metformin versus compound K-metformin combination therapy in diabetic db/db mice. Biol Pharm Bull 30: 2196-2200.

30. Han GC, Ko SK, Sung JH, Chung SH (2007) Compound K enhances insulin

secretion with beneficial metabolic effects in db/db mice. J Agric Food Chem 55: 10641-10648.

31. Park MW, Ha J, Chung SH (2008) 20(S)-ginsenoside Rg3 enhances glucose-stimulated insulin secretion and activates AMPK. Biol Pharm Bull 31: 748-751.

32. Xie JT, Zhou YP, Dey L, Attele AS, Wu JA, et al. (2002) Ginseng berry reduces blood glucose and body weight in db/db mice. Phytomedicine 9: 254-258.

33. Attele AS, Zhou YP, Xie JT, Wu JA, Zhang L, et al. (2002) Antidiabetic effects of Panax ginseng berry extract and the identification of an effective component. Diabetes 51: 1851-1858.

34. Xie JT, Aung HH, Wu JA, Attel AS, Yuan CS (2002) Effects of American ginseng berry extract on blood glucose levels in ob/ob mice. Am J Chin Med 30: 187-194.

35. Dey L, Xie JT, Wang A, Wu J, Maleckar SA, et al. (2003) Anti-hyperglycemic effects of ginseng: comparison between root and berry. Phytomedicine 10: 600-605.

36. Xie JT, Wang CZ, Ni M, Wu JA, Mehendale SR, et al. (2007) American ginseng berry juice intake reduces blood glucose and body weight in ob/ob mice. J Food Sci 72: S590-S594.

37. Xie JT, Mehendale SR, Wang A, Han AH, Wu JA, et al. (2004) American ginseng leaf: ginsenoside analysis and hypoglycemic activity. Pharmacol Res 49: 113-117.

38. Xie JT, Wang CZ, Li XL, Ni M, Fishbein A, et al. (2009) Anti-diabetic effect of American ginseng may not be linked to antioxidant activity: comparison between American ginseng and Scutellaria baicalensis using an ob/ob mice model. Fitoterapia 80: 306-311.

39. Lee KS, Yu WJ, Wang MJ, Wu HT, Chang CH, et al. (2010) Autonomic regulation of insulin secretion is changed by pentobarbital in mice. Neurosci Lett 479: 6-9.

40. Karu N, Reifen R, Kerem Z (2007) Weight gain reduction in mice fed Panax ginseng saponin, a pancreatic lipase inhibitor. J Agric Food Chem 55: 2824-2828.

41. Yang Y, Wu T, He K, Fu ZG (1999) Effect of aerobic exercise and ginsenosides on lipid metabolism in diet-induced hyperlipidemia mice. Zhongguo Yao Li Xue Bao 20: 563-565.

42. Yoon M, Lee H, Jeong S, Kim JJ, Nicol CJ, et al. (2003) Peroxisome proliferator-activated receptor alpha is involved in the regulation of lipid metabolism by ginseng. Br J Pharmacol 138: 1295-1302.

43. Kimura M, Waki I, Tanaka O, Nagai Y, Shibata S (1981) Pharmacological sequential trials for the fractionation of components with hypoglycemic activity in alloxan diabetic mice from ginseng radix. J Pharmacobiodyn 4: 402-409.

44. Kim JH, Hahm DH, Yang DC, Kim JH, Lee HJ, et al. (2005) Effect of crude saponin of Korean red ginseng on high-fat diet-induced obesity in the rat. J Pharmacol Sci 97: 124-131.

45. Kim JH, Kang SA, Han SM, Shim I (2009) Comparison of the antiobesity effects of the protopanaxadiol- and protopanaxatriol-type saponins of red ginseng. Phytother Res 23: 78-85.

46. Lee HJ, Lee YH, Park SK, Kang ES, Kim HJ, et al. (2009) Korean red ginseng (Panax ginseng) improves insulin sensitivity and attenuates the development of diabetes in Otsuka Long-Evans Tokushima fatty rats. Metabolism 58: 1170-1177.

47. Yuan HD, Chung SH (2010) Fermented ginseng protects streptozotocin-induced damage in rat pancreas by inhibiting nuclear factor-kappaB. Phytother Res 24: S190-S195.

48. Liu TP, Liu IM, Cheng JT (2005) Improvement of insulin resistance by panax ginseng in fructose-rich chow-fed rats. Horm Metab Res 37: 146-151.

49. Lee WK, Kao ST, Liu IM, Cheng JT (2006) Increase of insulin secretion by ginsenoside Rh2 to lower plasma glucose in Wistar rats. Clin Exp Pharmacol Physiol 33: 27-32.

50. Lai DM, Tu YK, Liu IM, Chen PF, Cheng JT (2006) Mediation of beta-endorphin by ginsenoside Rh2 to lower plasma glucose in streptozotocin-induced diabetic rats. Planta Med 72: 9-13.

51. Lee WK, Kao ST, Liu IM, Cheng JT (2007) Ginsenoside Rh2 is one of the active principles of Panax ginseng root to improve insulin sensitivity in fructose-rich chow-fed rats. Horm Metab Res 39: 347-354.

52. Xiong Y, Shen L, Liu KJ, Tso P, Wang G, et al. (2010) Antiobesity and

53. Sievenpiper JL, Arnason JT, Leiter LA, Vuksan V (2003) Variable effects of American ginseng: a batch of American ginseng (Panax quinquefolius L.) with a depressed ginsenoside profile does not affect postprandial glycemia. Eur J Clin Nutr 57: 243-248.

54. Sievenpiper JL, Arnason JT, Leiter LA, Vuksan V (2003) Null and opposing effects of Asian ginseng (Panax ginseng C.A. Meyer) on acute glycemia: results of two acute dose escalation studies. J Am Coll Nutr 22: 524-532.

55. Kim SH, Park KS (2003) Effects of Panax ginseng extract on lipid metabolism in humans. Pharmacol Res 48: 511-513.

56. Yamamoto M, Uemura T, Nakama S, Uemiya M, Kumagai A (1983) Serum HDL-cholesterol-increasing and fatty liver-improving actions of Panax ginseng in high cholesterol diet-fed rats with clinical effect on hyperlipidemia in man. Am J Chin Med 11: 96-101.

57. Yamamoto M, Kumagai A, Yamamura Y (1983) Plasma lipid-lowering action of ginseng saponins and mechanism of the action. Am J Chin Med 11: 84-87.

58. DeFronzo RA (2010) Current issues in the treatment of type 2 diabetes. Overview of newer agents: where treatment is going. Am J Med 123: S38-S48.

59. Marchetti P, Lupi R, Del Guerra S, Bugliani M, Marselli L, et al. (2010) The beta-cell in human type 2 diabetes. Adv Exp Med Biol 654: 501-514.

60. Takahashi H, Wilkinson GR, Nutescu EA, Morita T, Ritchie MD, et al. (2006) Different contributions of polymorphisms in VKORC1 and CYP2C9 to intra- and inter-population differences in maintenance dose of warfarin in Japanese, Caucasians and African-Americans. Pharmacogenet Genomics 16: 101-110.

61. Donovan MD (2005) Sex and racial differences in pharmacological response: effect of route of administration and drug delivery system on pharmacokinetics. J Womens Health (Larchmt) 14: 30-37.

62. Anderson GD (2005) Sex and racial differences in pharmacological response: where is the evidence? Pharmacogenetics, pharmacokinetics, and pharmacodynamics. J Womens Health (Larchmt) 14: 19-29.

63. Ripley E, King K, Sica DA (2000) Racial differences in response to acute dosing with hydrochlorothiazide. Am J Hypertens 13: 157-164.

64. Kovacs A, Ben-Jacob N, Tayem H, Halperin E, Iraqi FA, et al. (2011) Genotype is a stronger determinant than sex of the mouse gut microbiota. Microb Ecol 61: 423-428.

65. Wu GD, Chen J, Hoffmann C, Bittinger K, Chen YY, et al. (2011) Linking long-term dietary patterns with gut microbial enterotypes. Science 334: 105-108.

66. Luo JZ, Luo L (2006) American ginseng stimulates insulin production and prevents apoptosis through regulation of uncoupling protein-2 in cultured beta cells. Evid Based Complement Alternat Med 3: 365-372.

67. Yuan HD, Chung SH (2010) Protective effects of fermented ginseng on streptozotocin-induced pancreatic beta-cell damage through inhibition of NF-kappaB. Int J Mol Med 25: 53-58.

68. Park S, Ahn IS, Kwon DY, Ko BS, Jun WK (2008) Ginsenosides Rb1 and Rg1 suppress triglyceride accumulation in 3T3-L1 adipocytes and enhance beta-cell insulin secretion and viability in Min6 cells via PKA-dependent pathways. Biosci Biotechnol Biochem 72: 2815-2823.

69. Kim HY, Kim K (2007) Protective effect of ginseng on cytokine-induced apoptosis in pancreatic beta-cells. J Agric Food Chem 55: 2816-2823.

70. Lin E, Wang Y, Mehendale S, Sun S, Wang CZ, et al. (2008) Antioxidant protection by American ginseng in pancreatic beta-cells. Am J Chin Med 36: 981-988.

71. Shang W, Yang Y, Jiang B, Jin H, Zhou L, et al. (2007) Ginsenoside Rb1 promotes adipogenesis in 3T3-L1 cells by enhancing PPARgamma2 and C/EBPalpha gene expression. Life Sci 80: 618-625.

72. Shang W, Yang Y, Zhou L, Jiang B, Jin H, et al. (2008) Ginsenoside Rb1 stimulates glucose uptake through insulin-like signaling pathway in 3T3-L1 adipocytes. J Endocrinol 198: 561-569.

73. Zhang Z, Li X, Lv W, Yang Y, Gao H, et al. (2008) Ginsenoside Re reduces insulin resistance through inhibition of c-Jun NH2-terminal kinase and nuclear factor-kappaB. Mol Endocrinol 22: 186-195.

74. Lee OH, Lee HH, Kim JH, Lee BY (2011) Effect of ginsenosides Rg3 and Re on glucose transport in mature 3T3-L1 adipocytes. Phytother Res 25: 768-773.

75. Lee MS, Hwang JT, Kim SH, Yoon S, Kim MS, et al. (2010) Ginsenoside Rc,

antihyperglycemic effects of ginsenoside Rb1 in rats. Diabetes 59: 2505-2512.

an active component of Panax ginseng, stimulates glucose uptake in C2C12 myotubes through an AMPK-dependent mechanism. J Ethnopharmacol 127: 771-776.

76. Kim do Y, Yuan HD, Chung IK, Chung SH (2009) Compound K, intestinal metabolite of ginsenoside, attenuates hepatic lipid accumulation via AMPK activation in human hepatoma cells. J Agric Food Chem 57: 1532-1537.

77. Kim SJ, Yuan HD, Chung SH (2010) Ginsenoside Rg1 suppresses hepatic glucose production via AMP-activated protein kinase in HepG2 cells. Biol Pharm Bull 33: 325-328.

78. Yuan HD, Kim SJ, Chung SH (2011) Beneficial effects of IH-901 on glucose and lipid metabolisms via activating adenosine monophosphate-activated protein kinase and phosphatidylinositol-3 kinase pathways. Metabolism 60: 43-51.

12

Effects of Atorvastatin and Niacin, Alone and in Combination, On Lowering Serum LDL-Cholesterol and Lipoprotein (a) in Hyperlipidemia Patients

Jhuma KA[1]*, Giasuddin ASM[2], Haq AMM[3], Huque MM[3] and Mahmood N[4]

[1]*Department of Biochemistry, Medical College for Women & Hospital, Plot-4, Road-9, Sector-1, Uttara Model Town, Dhaka-1230, Bangladesh*
[2]*Department of Medical Laboratory Science, State College of Health Sciences & Adjunct Professor, State University of Bangladesh, Dhanmondi, Dhaka-1209, Bangladesh*
[3]*Department of Medicine, Medical College for Women & Hospital, Plot-4, Road-9, Sector-1, Uttara Model Town, Dhaka-1230, Bangladesh*
[4]*Department of Medicine, (Nephrology Unit), Medical College for Women & Hospital, Plot-4, Road-9, Sector-1, Uttara Model Town, Dhaka-1230, Bangladesh*

Abstract

Background & objectives: Effects of statins on serum lipids in hyperlipidemia are not well defined. We compared the effects of atorvastatin and niacin, alone and combination, on lowering serum LDL-C and Lp (a) and increasing HDL-C in hyperlipidemia patients.

Patients and methods: A total of 150 adult patients (Group-A) with hyperlipidemia and 100 normal adults controls (Group-B) were included in the study. The fasting blood samples were taken and serum (I°) were stored frozen until analysed for TG, TC, LDL-C, HDL-C, and Lp (a). The 50 patients (Group A1) were prescribed Atorvastatin (10 mg once daily for 3 months), 50 patients (Group A2) were prescribed Niacin (50 mg twice daily for 3 months) and 50 patients (Group A3) were prescribed combination of the two drugs with same doses for 3 months. Blood samples were taken again at follow up and serum (II°) was stored frozen until analysed for lipids by biochemical methods.

Results: Lipid parameters (mg/dl), i.e. TG, TC, LDL-C, & Lp(a), were raised and HDL-C was reduced in patients (Group-A) compared to controls (Group-B); Atovastatin (10 mg/ day) and Niacin (50 mg/2day) significantly lowered TG,TC, LDL-C & Lp(a) and raised HDL-C in Group A1 and Group A2 respectively; Combination therapy (atorvastatin: 10 mg/day + Niacin : 50 mg*2/day) was much more effective in lowering TG, TC, LDL-C & LP(a) and raising HDL-C in Group A3.

Conclusions: The effects of combination therapy of the two drugs were much higher than their effects alone and therefore, can be adopted in hyperlipidemia patients.

Keywords: Atorvastatin; Niacin; LDL-Cholesterol; HDL-Cholesterol; Lipoprotein(a); Hyperlipidemia

Introduction

Atherosclerosis of the coronary and peripheral vasculature due to hyperlipidemia is the leading cause of death among men and women in the USA and rest of the world [1-4]. Recent evidences support the role of Low-Density Lipoprotein Cholesterol (LDL-C) in the pathogenesis of atherosclerosis and the risk of Coronary Artery /Heart Disease (CAD/CHD) events [5-7]. The development of the "statins" class of drugs provided a momental leap in the management by pharmacotherapy of hyperlipidemia and CHD risk reduction. Randomised clinical trials have provided strong evidence that lowering plasma cholesterol with statins reduces the risk of cardiovascular/CHD events [5-7].

The recent update of the National Cholesterol Education Programme (NCEP) is the most aggressive approach to date for reducing CHD risk. A focal element of the report is the modification of LDL-C goal in high-risk patients to <70 mg/dL. This therapeutic option is valid (in high-risk patients) even if baseline LDL-C is <100 mg/dL. The report addressed high-risk patients with elevated total Triglycerides (TG) or lower High-Density Lipoprotein Cholesterol (HDL-C). It is recommended that patients in this category be given a combination of folic acid derivative or nicotinic acid in addition to an LDL-C lowering agent. When drug therapy is initiated in high-risk or moderately high-risk patients, the report recommends that such therapy be intensified to achieve reductions in LDL-C levels by at least 30–40%, if feasible [7,8].

In cases of exceptionally elevated LDL-C levels, a statin treatment alone may be insufficient to achieve optional LDL-C reduction. In such cases, a combination therapy such as statin plus exetimibe, statin plus niacin and statin plus cholestyramine may be considered keeping in mind intolerable adverse effects or drug interactions [7]. Although the principal focus is on plasma/serum LDL-C currently more rationale approach would be to reduce the concentrations of all cholesterol-bearing lipoproteins that contain apoprotein B. The lipoprotein (a) [Lp(a)] is the most important and relevant one in this regard [5-7].

Lp(a) has become a focus of research interest owing to the results of case-control and prospective studies linking elevated plasma levels of this lipoprotein with the development of CAD [9-11]. Lp (a) contains a Low-Density Lipoprotein (LDL)-like moiety, in which the apolipoprotein B-100 component is covalently linked to the unique glycoprotein Apolipoprotein (a) [Apo(a)]. Apo (a) is composed of repeated loop-shaped units called kringles, the sequences of which are highly similar to a kringle motif present in the fibrinolytic proenzyme plasminogen [10,12,13]. Based on the similarity of Lp(a) to both LDL and plasminogen, it has been hypothesized that the function of this unique lipoprotein may represent a link between the fields of

*Corresponding author: Khadija Akther Jhuma, Associate Professor of Biochemistry, Department of Biochemistry, Medical College for Women & Hospital, Plot-4, Road-9, Sector-1, Uttara Model Town, Dhaka-1230, Bangladesh, E-mail: jhuma1991@yahoo.com

atherosclerosis and thrombosis [9-13]. Serum Lp(a) levels are reported to be elevated in Diabetes Mellitus (DM) and an independent risk factor for CAD in DM, particularly non-insulin dependent DM (NIDDM) patients [9,10,14]. Elevated serum concentrations of Lp(a) (>30 mg/dl) were reported to confer an increased risk of CAD and, because of this association, the measurement of plasma Lp(a) is requested increasingly as part of CAD risk assessment [14-16].

However, it appears that the report of NCEP did not give due consideration about the role of Lp(a) in atherosclerosis. Does statins alone or in combination reduce the plasma levels of Lp(a)? The probable beneficial effects of lowing serum Lp(a) levels in CHD risk reduction by statins have not been considered which remained to be evaluated [7,8]. Although Lp(a) has been shown to accumulate in atherosclerotic lesions, its contribution to the development of atheromas is unclear. Regarding studies on Lp(a) with Bangladeshi patients only limited reports are available. One study on serum Lp(a) level in patients with Cerebrovascular Disease (CVD) was reported earlier [17]. Recently, another study showing elevation of serum Lp(a) level in patients with DM was reported [18]. Literature survey has indicated that no study about the effects of statins on serum Lp(a) and LDL-C levels in Bangladeshi patients has been reported. In the light of the NCEP report, we therefore planned the present study about the effects of pharmacotherapy with atorvastatin (statin) and niacin (vitamin), alone and in combination, in lowering serum LDL-C and Lp(a) levels and increasing HDL-C, in Bangladeshi patients with hyperlipidemia. The study is expected to reveal the probable role of Lp(a) in monitoring the lipid-lowering effects of atorvastatin and niacin and hence their efficacy in reducing risk for CAD events in patients with hyperlipidemias.

Patients and Methods

A total of 150 adult patients (Group-A) (Gender: males: 76, females: 74; Age range: 32-65 yrs; Mean age ± SD: 48.5 ± 10.5 yrs) with

Parameter (mg/dl)	Subjects		Student's t-test* (A vs B)
	Group-A (n=150)	Group-B (n=100)	
TG	Range: 110-375 Mean ± SD: 170 ± 50	50-170 90 ± 15	t = 15.384, df =248 p<0.001
TC	Range: 170 – 250 Mean ± SD: 210 ± 16	135-200 150 ± 15	t = 12.723, df =248 p<0.001
LDL-C	Range: 80-150 Mean ± SD: 105 ± 15	70-125 80 ± 11	t = 2.524, df =248 p<0.005
HDL-C	Range: 15-60 Mean ± SD: 38 ± 10	32-66 48 ± 12	t = 2.681, df =248 p<0.025
Lp(a)	Range: 35.5-95.5 Mean ± SD: 55.4 ± 16.3	9.5 – 41.5 23.7 ± 10.4	t = 12.613, df =248 p<0.001

Table 1: Lipid parameters in patients (Group-A) before intervention with atorvastatin and niacin and in normal control (Group-B) and their statistical analysis by Student's t-test.

hyperlipidemia and 100 healthy adults (Group-B) (Gender: males: 54, females: 46; Age range: 30-65 yrs; Mean age ± SD: 45.5 ± 11.5) as normal controls (NCs) were included in the case-control prospective interventional study. The study was carried out at the Medical Research Unit (MRU), Medical College for Women & Hospital (MCW&H), Uttara, Dhaka-1230 and Bangladesh. The study was approved by the Ethical Review Committee (ERC) of MRU, MCW&H, Dhaka and BMRC, Dhaka, Bangladesh.

The patients were diagnosed as having hyperlipidemia without diabetes, hypertension, infections and thyroid diseases according to standard clinical and laboratory criteria [10,19-21]. After obtaining consent, clinical details and findings were recorded as per proforma designed for each patient. The fasting blood samples were taken as 1st degree samples (I^0), serum separated were aliquoted and stored frozen until analysed for serum lipid profile, i.e. TG, total cholesterol (TC), LDL-C, HDL-C, and Lp(a). The 50 patients (Group- A1) were prescribed Atorvastatin (10 mg once daily for 3 months), 50 patients (Group-A2) were prescribed Niacin (50mg twice daily for 3 months) and 50 patients (Group-A3) were prescribed combination of the two drugs with same doses for 3 months. Then 2nd degree blood samples (II^0) were taken at the end of 3 months period when patients reported for follow up. Our patients were not receiving any other lipid lowering drugs. The serum separated (II^0) were aliquoted and stored frozen, less than 3 months, until analyzed for the same lipid profile to see the effects of interventions on them. The lipid parameters were estimated by biochemical methods using research kits obtained from reputed commercial companies. Atorvastatin was chosen as it was reported to be the safest statin in terms of toxicity, particularly hepatotoxicity, nephrotoxicity, gastrointestinal upset, muscle aches, etc and secondly, atorvastatin was shown to have the highest effects in lowering serum TG and LDL-C concentrations [6-8]. Niacin was chosen as it was cheaper and readily available to the patients free of cost from our hospital (MCW&H); Secondly, Niacin is expected to facilitate in reducing atorvastatin dose. The results were analyzed statistically using standard statistical tests in computer [22,23].

Results

Table 1 shows the lipid parameters and their statistical analyses in patients (Group A) before intervention with atorvastatin and niacin and in normal controls (Group-B). Among the lipid parameters, TG, TC, LDL-C and Lp(a) were elevated and HDL-C was reduced in patients significantly (p<0.05). The effects of atorvastatin alone (10 mg/day) in patients with hyperlipidemia are stated in Table 2. TG, TC, LDL-C and LP (a) levels were lowered by 30%, 30% and 29% respectively, while HDL-C was raised by 15%, which were significant by Paired t test (P<0.05). Table 3 shows the effects of niacin alone (50 mg* 2/day) in patients with hyperlipidemia. TG, TC LDL-C and Lp(a)

Parameter (mg/dl)	Patient (Group-A1)		Percent Reduction	Paired t-test* (A1-I0 vs A1-II0)
	A1-I0(n=50)	A1-II0(n=50)		
TG	Range: 115-350 Mean ± SD: 170 ± 55	110-301 150 ± 45	30%	t = 2.332, df =49 p<0.025
TC	Range: 175-240 Mean ± SD: 205 ± 15	170 – 230 180 ± 16	15%	t = 12.128, df =49 p<0.05
LDL-C	Range: 80-150 Mean ± SD: 101 ± 20	68-135 71 ± 14	30%	t = 2.475, df =49 p<0.025
HDL-C	Range: 20-65 Mean ± SD: 40 ± 12	28-70 46 ± 12	15%↑	t = 2.115, df =49 p<0.05
Lp(a)	Range: 38.5 – 90.5 Mean ± SD: 58.5 ± 18	30.4-70.5 45.6 ± 15	20%	t = 2.214, df =49 p<0.05

* P ≤ 0.05: Significant; P > 0.05: Not Significant

Table 2: Effects of atorvastatin alone (10 mg/day) on lipid parameters in patients (Group-A1) with hyperlipidemia and their statistical analysis by Paired t- test.

were lowered significantly by 25%, 25%, 25% respectively, (P<0.05). However, reduction of Lp(a) by 10% and increase of HDL-C by 10% were not significant by paired t-test (p>0.05). Table 4 shows the effects of combination therapy (atorvastatin 10 mg/day + Niacin 50 mg* 2/ day) on lipid parameters in patients with hyperlipidemia. Interestingly the combination therapy was much more effective in reducing Lp(a) by 30% and increasing HDL-C by 25% compared to treatments singly by paired t-test (p<0.01). Table 5 shows the comparison by Z-test of the

Parameter (mg/dl)	Patient (Group-A2)		Percent Reduction	Paired t-test* (A2-I0 vs A2-IIo)
	A2-I0(n=50)	A2- II0 (n=50)		
TG	Range: 120-375 Mean ± SD: 185 ± 55	100-305 140 ± 22	25%	t = 2.229, df =49 p<0.05
TC	Range: 180-235 Mean ± SD: 210 ± 15	140 – 205 165 ± 17	25%	t = 2.208, df = 49 p<0.05
LDL-C	Range: 80-150 Mean ± SD: 110 ± 15	72-120 88 ± 12	25%	t = 2.214, df = 49 p<0.05
HDL-C	Range: 16-60 Mean ± SD: 40 ± 11	22-72 45 ± 10	10%↑	t = 2.014, df = 49 p<0.05
Lp(a)	Range: 38 – 98 Mean ± SD: 60 ± 18	32-75 51 ± 15	10%	t = 2.012, df = 49 p>0.05

* P ≤ 0.05: Significant; P > 0.05: Not Significant

Table 3: Effects of niacin alone (50 mg×2/day) on lipid parameters in patients (Group-A2) with hyperlipidemia and their statistical analysis by Paired t-test.

Parameter (mg/dl)	Patient (Group-A3)		Percent Reduction	Paired t-test* (A3-Io vs A3-IIo)*
	A3-I0(n=50)	A3- II0(n=50)		
TG	Range: 110-375 Mean ± SD: 175 ± 45	100-300 130 ± 35	30%	t = 2.423, df = 49 p=<0.025
TC	Range: 170-250 Mean ± SD: 210 ± 17	140 – 230 160 ± 20	25%	t = 2.534, df = 49 p=<0.025
LDL-C	Range: 80-150 Mean ± SD: 115 ± 16	60-115 78 ± 14	3%	t = 2.612, df = 49 p=<0.025
HDL-C	Range: 15-60 Mean ± SD: 35 ± 12	30-80 45 ± 14	25%↑	t = 2.456, df = 49 p=<0.025
Lp(a)	Range: 40 – 98 Mean ± SD: 62 ± 18	22-70 44 ± 12	30%	t = 2.724, df = 49 p=<0.010

* P ≤ 0.05: Significant; P > 0.05: Not Significant

Table 4: Lipid lowering effects of combination therapy with Atorvastatin: (10 mg/day) & Nacin (50 mg×2/day) in patients (Group-A3) with hyperlipidemia and their statistical analysis by Paired t-test.

Parameter (mg/dl)	Effects according to intervention % reduction (↓); %Increase (↑)			Z-test for proportion
	Group-A1	Group-A2	Group-A3	
TG	30% (↓)	25% (↓)	30% (↓)	A1 vs A2 Z = 1.35 (< 1.96); NS (p>0.05) A2 vs A3 Z = 1.35 (< 1.96); NS (p>0.05) A3 vs A1 Z = 0.00 (< 1.96); NS (p>0.05)
TC	15% (↓)	25% (↓)	25% (↓)	A1 vs A2 Z = 3.32 (> 3.0); HS (p<0.005 A2 vs A3 Z = 0.00 (< 1.96); NS (p>0.05) A3 vs A1 Z = 3.32 (> 3.0); HS (p<0.005)
LDL-C	30% (↓)	25% (↓)	31% (↓)	A1 vs A2 Z = 1.35 (< 1.96); NS (p>0.05) Gr A2 vs Gr A3 Z = 1.76 (< 1.96); NS (p>0.05) A3 vs A1 Z = 0.28 (< 1.96); NS (p>0.05)
HDL-C	15% (↑)	10% (↑)	25% (↑)	A1 vs A2 Z = 1.66 (< 1.96); NS (p>0.05) A2 vs A3 Z = 6.01 (> 3.0); HS (p<0.005) A3 vs A1 Z = 3.84 (> 3.0); HS (p<0.005)
Lp(a)	20% (↓)	10% (↓)	30% (↓)	A1 vs A2 Z = 3.84 (> 3.0); HS (p<0.005) A2 vs A3 Z = 7.65 (> 3.0); HS (p<0.005) A3 vs A1 Z = 2..1 (> 1.96); S (p>0.05)

A1: Patients treated with atorvastatin alone (10 mg/day); A2: Patients treated with niacin alone (50 mg×2/day); A3: Patients treated with atorvastatin (10 mg/day) plus niacin (50 mg×2/day); NS: Not significant; S: significant; HS: Highly significant.

Table 5: Comparison by Z- test for proportion of the effects on reducing or increasing the individual components of the lipid profile according to intervention.

percentages (proportions) of the effects on reducing or increasing the individual components of the lipid profile according to intervention.

Discussion

Statins are well known to reduce adverse cardiovascular outcomes in patients with cardiovascular disease (CVD) and slow the progression of coronary atherosclerosis in proportion to their ability to reduce LDL-C. However, residual cardiovascular risk persists despite the achievement of target LDL-C levels with statin therapy in patients with established CVD [24,25]. The recent update of the NCEP is the most aggressive approach to date for reducing CHD risk [7,8]. When drug therapy is initiated in high risk or moderately high risk patients, the report recommended that such therapy be intensified to achieve reduction in LDL-C levels by at least 30-40% if feasible [7,8]. Secondly, a combination therapy such as statin plus ezetimibe, statin plus niacin and statin plus cholestyramine may be considered keeping in mind intolerable adverse effects or drug interaction [7].

The present study showed that TG, TC, LDL-C and Lp(a) were elevated, while HDL-C was reduced significantly (p< 0.05) indicating hyperlipidemia in our patients (Table 1). Either atorvastatin (10 mg/ day) alone or niacin (50 mg×2/day) alone reduced TG (25-30%), TC (15-25%), LDl-C (25-30%) and Lp(a) (10-20%) and raised HDL-C (10-15%) significantly (P<0.05) (Tables 2 and 3). Our interventional study revealed that combination therapy with atorvastatin (10 mg/day) plus niacin (50 mg×2/ day) was much better in reducing the lipid levels, ie. TG (30%), TC (25%), LDL-C (30%) and Lp(a) (30%) and in elevating HDL-C (25%) significantly (p<0.05) (Tables 4 and 5). Atorvastatin was chosen as it was reported to be the safest statin in terms of toxicity, particularly hepatotoxicity, nephrotoxicity, gastrointestinal upset, muscle aches, etc and secondly, atorvastatin was shown to have the highest effects in lowering serum TG and LDL-C concentrations [6-8].

Our findings were interesting particularly in relation to reducing LDL-C and Lp(a) and elevating HDL-C. It appears that the report of NCEP did not give proper consideration about the role of Lp(a) in atherosclerosis [8,9]. Lp(a) has become a focus of research interest owing to the results of case-control and prospective studies linking elevated plasma levels of this lipoprotein with the development of CAD [9-11]. Two long term follow-up studies reported that the combination therapy with statin (simvastatin) to niacin and statin (simvastatin) to fenofibrate did not reduce the rate of fatal cardiovascular events, nonfatal myocardial infarction or nonfatal stroke as compared with simvastatin alone [24,25]. These non-incremental clinical benefits for addition of niacin to statin therapy during a 36 months follow-up period were observed, despite significant improvements in the LDL-C and HDL-C levels [24-26]. Our findings as well as other reports clearly suggested that some other factor or factors are responsible for continued clinically fatal events. One of the most important contenders for this factor is possibly Lp (a). As Lp(a) has structures similar to both LDL and plasminogen, it has been hypothesized that the function of Lp(a) may represent a link between the field of atherosclerosis and thrombosis [11-13]. The fact that plasma Lp(a) levels are largely genetically determined and vary widely among different ethnic groups, adds scientific interest to the ongoing study of this enigmatic molecule. Only limited studies have been reported on serum levels of Lp(a) in some populations including Indian subcontinent [14,27,28]. Further studies are warranted with combination therapy involving other statins also and following-up for a longer period to evaluate in terms of occurrence of fatal and non-fatal cardiovascular and other related events. Meanwhile, combination therapy with atorvastatin and niacin for hyperipidemias, particularly with CHD/CAD, can be adopted keeping in mind the tolerance and acceptability by patients.

Acknowledgements

The authors gratefully acknowledge Bangladesh Medical Research Council (BMRC), Mohakhali, Dhaka-1212, Bangladesh for financing the study through Research Project Grant.

The authors appreciate Mr. Moniruzzaman and Mr. Mizanur Rahman at MRU, MCW&H, Plot-4 Road-9 Sector-1, Uttara Model Town, Dhaka-1230, Bangladesh for internet browsing and composing the manuscript.

References

1. Rosamond WD, Chambless LE, Folsom AR, Cooper LS, Conwill DE, et al. (1998) Trends in the incidence of myocardial infarction and in mortality due to coronary heart disease, 1987 to 1994. N Engl J Med 339: 861-867.

2. Murray CJ, Lopez AD (1997) Mortality by cause for eight regions of the world: Global Burden of Disease Study. Lancet 349: 1269-1276.

3. Coresh J, Kwiterovich PO Jr (1996) Small, dense low-density lipoprotein particles and coronary heart disease risk: A clear association with uncertain implications. JAMA 276: 914-915.

4. American Heart Association (2005) Heart Disease and Stroke Statistics Update. Dallas, Texas.

5. Havel RJ, Rapaport E (1995) Management of primary hyperlipidemia. N Engl J Med 332: 1491-1498.

6. Knopp RH (1999) Drug treatment of lipid disorders. N Engl J Med 341: 498-511.

7. Balbisi EA (2006) Management of hyperlipidemia: new LDL-C targets for persons at high-risk for cardiovascular events. Med Sci Monit 12: RA34-39.

8. Grundy SM, Cleeman JI, Merz CNB, Brewer Jr HB, Clark LT, et al. (2004) Implications of recent clinical trials for the National Cholesterol Education Program Adult Treatment Panel III guidelines. Circulation 110: 227-239.

9. Danesh J, Collins R, Peto R (2000) Lipoprotein(a) and coronary heart disease. Meta-analysis of prospective studies. Circulation 102: 1082-1085.

10. Fujiwara F, Ishii M, Taneichi H, Miura M, Toshihiro M, et al. (2005) Low incidence of vascular complications in patients with diabetes mellitus associated with liver cirrhosis as compared with type 2 diabetes mellitus. Tohoku J Exp Med 205: 327-334.

11. Marcovina SM, Koschinsky ML (1998) Lipoprotein(a) as a risk factor for coronary artery disease. Am J Cardiol 82: 57U-66U.

12. BERG K (1963) A NEW SERUM TYPE SYSTEM IN MAN--THE LP SYSTEM. Acta Pathol Microbiol Scand 59: 369-382.

13. Scanu AM, Fless GM (1990) Lipoprotein (a). Heterogeneity and biological relevance. J Clin Invest 85: 1709-1715.

14. Devanapalli B, Lee S, Mahajan D, Bermingham M (2002) Lipoprotein (a) in an immigrant Indian population sample in Australia. Br J Biomed Sci 59: 119-122.

15. Gaw A, Brown EA, Gourlay CW, Bell MA (2000) Analytical performance of the Genzyme LipoPro Lp(a) kit for plasma lipoprotein(a)-cholesterol assay. Br J Biomed Sci 57: 13-18.

16. Barghash NA, Elewa SM, Hamdi EA, Barghash AA, El Dine R (2004) Role of plasma homocysteine and lipoprotein (a) in coronary artery disease. Br J Biomed Sci 61: 78-83.

17. Hoque MM, Sultana P, Arslan MI (2005) Lipoprotein-a: a laboratory tool for clinical categorization of CVD. Mymensingh Med J 14: 75-79.

18. Giasuddin ASM, Jhuma KA, Mujibul Haq AM (2008). Lipoprotein(a) status in Bangladeshi patients with diabetes mellitus. J Med Coll Women Hosp 6: 74-82.

19. Alberti KG, Zimmet PZ (1998) Definition, diagnosis and classification of diabetes mellitus and its complications. Part 1: diagnosis and classification of diabetes mellitus provisional report of a WHO consultation. Diabet Med 15: 539-553.

20. Chobanian AV, Bakris GL, Black HR, Cushman WC, Green LA, et al. (2003) The Seventh Report of the Joint National Committee on Prevention, Detection, Evaluation, and Treatment of High Blood Pressure: the JNC 7 report. JAMA 289: 2560-2572.

21. Rifai N, Bachorik PS, Albers JJ (2001) Lipids, Lipoproteins and Apolipoproteins. In: Burtis CA, Ashwood ER, (eds.), Tielz Fundamentals of Clinical Chemistry, (5thedn), Saunders Company, Philadelphia, USA, 462-493.

22. Kirkwood BR, Sterne JAC (2008). Essential Medical Statistics (2ndedn) Oxford: Blackwell Science Ltd.

23. Prabhakara GN (2008). Biostatiscs (1stedn) Jaypee Brothers, Medical publishers, New Delhi, India.

24. ACCORD Study Group, Ginsberg HN, Elam MB, Lovato LC, Crouse JR 3rd, et al. (2010) Effects of combination lipid therapy in type 2 diabetes mellitus. N Engl J Med 362: 1563-1574.

25. AIM-HIGH Investigators, Boden WE, Probstfield JL, Anderson T, Chaitman BR, et al. (2011) Niacin in patients with low HDL cholesterol levels receiving intensive statin therapy. N Engl J Med 365: 2255-2267.

26. Nicholls SJ, Ballantyne CM, Barter PJ, Chapman MJ, Erbel RM, et al. (2011) Effect of two intensive statin regimens on progression of coronary disease. N Engl J Med 365: 2078-2087.

27. Scanu AM (2003) Lp(a) lipoprotein--coping with heterogeneity. N Engl J Med 349: 2089-2090.

28. Scanu AM (2003) Lipoprotein(a) and the atherothrombotic process: mechanistic insights and clinical implications. Curr Atheroscler Rep 5: 106-113.

13

Biomarkers of Oxidative Stress in Syndrome Metabolic Patients

Francisco Avilés-Plaza[1], Juana Bernabé[2], Begoña Cerdá[2], Javier Marhuenda[2*], Pilar Zafrilla[2], Tânia O. Constantino[3], Juana Mulero[2], Cristina García-Viguera[4], Diego A. Moreno[4], José Abellán[5] and Soledad Parra-Pallarés[1]

[1]Clinical Analysis Service, Biochemical Section of University Hospital Virgen de la Arrixaca, Murcia, Spain
[2]Department of Food Technology and Nutrition, Catholic University of San Antonio, Murcia, Spain
[3]Faculty of Pharmacy, University of Porto, Porto, Portugal
[4]CSIC, CEBAS, Department of Food Sci & Technol, Res Group Qual Safety & Bioactiv Plant Food, Murcia, Spain
[5]Chair of Cardiovascular Risk, Catholic University of San Antonio, Murcia, Spain

Abstract

Background: Owing to the proposal of the increase of oxidative stress (OxS) as an early event in the development of the metabolic syndrome (MetS), the aim of the present study was to evaluate certain OxS biomarkers in patients with MetS compared to healthy people age-matched and younger to assess the relevance of aging in OxS and MetS.

Methods: A total of 72 patients, 32 who fulfilled the Adult Treatment Panel III criteria for the MetS and 40 individuals without MetS, 20 age-matched to the MetS patients (Control I) and 20 younger subjects (Control II) were studied. We measured several anthropometric and serum parameters and two kinds of molecules related to OxS: modified molecules by reactive oxygen species (ROS) such as oxidized LDL (oxLDLc), and consumed or inducted molecules (enzymes or antioxidants such as Glutathione reductase GR,) associated with ROS metabolism. The statistical analysis was performed using SPSS v18.0.

Results: Only significant differences were observed in the values of GR between the MetS patients and Control I (50.31 ± 8.15 U/L vs 59.50 ± 9.98 U/L). We found significantly higher levels in the MetS patients compared to Control II of oxLDLc (96.77 ± 23.05 U/L vs 60.17 ± 16.28 U/L), F_2-isoprostanes (3.17 ± 1.78 µg/g creatinine vs 2.04 ± 0.80 µg/g creatinine) and protein cabonils (PC) (0.56 ± 0.26 nmol/mg vs 0.29 ± 0.13 nmol/mg).

Conclusions: Results have shown that MetS patients don't present a superior OxS in comparison to age-related healthy individuals. Finally, aging is more relevant to OxS than MetS *per se*.

Keywords: Metabolic syndrome; Oxidative stress biomarkers; Aging; Oxidized low density lipoprotein; Reactive oxygen species; Antioxidant enzymes

Introduction

During the last years, metabolic syndrome (MetS) has consistently increased worldwide. It is becoming a public health concern and a clinical condition highly related to increasing obesity incidence, sedentary lifestyle, and excessive caloric intake. The National Cholesterol Education Program's Adult Treatment Panel III report (ATP III) identified the MetS as a multiplex risk factor for cardiovascular disease (CVD). The componets of MetS are: impaired glucose tolerance, hypertriglyceridemia, low high-density lipoprotein (HDL) levels, raised blood pressure, and obesity (particularly visceral adiposity) [1]. A lifestyle summarized as a lack of physical activity and moderate-to-high intake of calories seems to be one of the most important causes of rapidly increasing prevalence of the MetS [2].

Oxidative stress is defined as an imbalance between oxidants (ROS) and the antioxidant defense in the organism in favor of oxidants. These oxidants can interact with proteins, phospholipidis or nucleic acids. During oxidation, diferent compounds are formed so may serve as biomarkers of oxidative stress (OxS) process in humans [3]. Increased OxS has been suggested as an early event in the development of the MetS and might contribute to disease progression [4,5]. Therefore, OxS occurs predominantly in people with MetS than among those without it, although not all authors have found this [6,7].

The association between the MetS and a high prevalence of ox-LDL was reported the first time for Paul Holvoet [8,9]. They supported the predictive value of the MetS for coronary heart disease (CHD) and

suggested that baseline levels of oxLDL add prognostic information concerning future risk for myocardial infarction (MI) [10]. These findings, along with previous research into the association of LDL oxidation with atherosclerosis and CHD, provide evidence that LDL oxidation is a common basis for the MetS and CHD or, more particularly, for inducing atherothrombotic coronary disease [11,12]. Tsimikas et al. [13] also demonstrated the temporal increases of circulating oxLDL in association with acute coronary syndromes. In aggregate, these data supported the hypothesis that an increase in oxLDL reflects plaque instability although the oxidation of LDL takes place in the arterial wall and not in the circulation [14].

Aging is a biological state related with progressive decline of organ functions and the development of age-related diseases. The causes of aging remain unknown, probably being related to a multifactorial process. To date, the free radical and mitochondrial theories seem to be the two most noticeable theories on aging [15]. They related OxS and mitochondria, so damaged mitochondria can produce an increso of ROS, leading to progressive increase of the potential damage in the organism. Aging is a gradual and adaptive process characterized by a diminished homeostatic response resulting from accumulated physiologic, biochemical; psychological and social wear on an organism

*Corresponding author: Javier Marhuenda Hernández, Department of Food Technology and Nutrition, Catholic University of San Antonio, Murcia, Spain, E-mail: jmarhuenda@ucam.edu

[16,17]. Even being considered as normal physiological process, it can be boost in presence of high levels of OxS or by chronic inflammatory processes (CIP) [18].

Owing to the increase of OxS derived by aging, the aim of this study was to evaluate certain OxS biomarkers in patients with MetS compared to healthy people of similar age and younger, in order to determine whether the OxS is modified in MetS patients owing to its relationship with aging.

Materials and Methods

Study population

The study included a total of 72 patients, 32 who fulfilled the Adult Treatment Panel III criteria for the MetS: obesity (waist circumference $\geq$ 102 cm in men or $\geq$ 88 cm in women), blood pressure of 130/85 mmHg or higher, fasting glucose of 110 mg/dL or more, TG of 150 mg/dL or more and HDLc below 40 mg/dL for men or 50 mg/dL for women. The MetS was defined as present when subjects had $\geq$ 3 of the risk factors.

We also studied 40 individuals without MetS, 20 age-related to the MetS patients (Control Group I) and 20 younger subjects (Control Group II). Both patients groups with MetS (n=32) and the Control Group I (n=20) were recruited at the cardiovascular risk unit in Primary Care of Murcia. The Control Group II was composed by younger healthy volunteers.

The inclusion criteria of all the patients were: no vitamin supplements consumption; alcohol consumption $\leq$ 30 g/day. No renal, hepathic or gastrointestinal diseases, cancer or allergies; no abnormal dietary habits; nonsmokers.

The study was carried out in accordance with the Helsinki Declaration and the Ethical Committee of the Universitary Hospital Virgen de la Arrixaca, Murcia, and Spain. Involvement was voluntary and all participants gave their informed consent to join the study.

Anthropometric measurements

After recording the clinical history and conducting the physical examination, we obtained the following anthropometric parameters measurements: weight, height, body mass index (BMI). Weight was measured while the subject was wearing underwear and was in a fasted state (after evacuation). A scale calibrated before each measurement, was used. Height was obtained with a cursor stadiometer graduated in millimeters. The subject was barefoot with the back and hands in contact with stadiometer in the Frankfurt horizontal plane. BMI was calculated by dividing weight (Kg) by height squared (m^2). Waist circumference (cm) was measured to the nearest 0.5 cm with a tape measure at the umbilical scar level.

Blood sampling

Blood samples were obtained from the median cubital vein and placed in EDTA-containing vials. Blood was centrifuged to obtain serum at 3.000 × g during 10 minutes at room temperature within 1 hour of collection and stored at 80°C until assays were performed.

Serum lipids

The concentrations of glucose, cholesterol total, LDLc, HDLc and TG were assayed using automated systems (Cobas 711, Roche Diagnostics).

Homocysteine

Homocysteine levels were measured by quantitative determination

by using an in t ensifying immunonephelometric particle test in a BN ProSpec® an a lyser (according to the protocol supplied in the kit for Siemens N Latex HCY OPAX 03). The reference interval for homocysteine concentration with the use of this method is from 4.9-14 μm/L.

Antioxidant enzymes

The determination of SOD and GPx was analyzed in total blood by a commercial kit (Randox Laboratories Ltd, UK). The concentration of GR was determined in serum by a commercial kit (Randox Laboratories Ltd, UK). These assays were carried out on a Hitachi 912 analyser (Roche Diagnostics Systems®). Values for SOD and GPx were normalized per gram of hemoglobin (Hb).

Oxidative stress biomarkers

• oxLDL (U/L): A competitive enzyme-linked immune-absorbent assay (ELISA; Mercodia, Uppsala, Sweden; with an intra-assay and interassay variation's coefficient of 4.8 and 4.5 respectively, for 82 U/L) was used to determine oxLDLc concentration in serum.

• F_2-isoprostanes (μg/g creatinine): (The urinary levels of 15-F_2-isoprostane were determined using a competitive enzyme-linked immunosorbent assay (Oxford Biomedical Research, Inc. Oxford, Michigan, USA). The results were normalized per milligram of creatinine measured in urine.

• 8-OHdG (ng/mL): The 8-hydroxiguanosine was measured with an ELISA kit (Japan Institute for the Control of Aging, Fukuroi, Shizuoka, Japan).

• PC (nmol/mg): The carbonylated proteins were measured by an ELISA kit (Biocell Corporation Ltd., New Zealand).

Statistical analysis

We performed a descriptive study in which we calculated the mean, standard deviation, minimum and maximum values for the quantitative measurements performed. The completion of this analyze was made with the entire sample and differentiated by study groups. We included the calculation of confidence intervals of 95%.

For the comparison of means with a dichotomous variable, we used the statistic test t-Student.

In cases where the qualitative variable had more than 2 categories, we used analysis of variance of one way (ANOVA) performing a posteriori the Tukey test with the correspondent corrections. All results were considered significant at a level of $p<0.05$. The analyses were performed using SPSS v18.0.

Results

Table 1 shows the anthropometric parameters and lipid profile of Control Group I compared to Control Group II; MetS patients compared to Control Group I and MetS patients compared to Control Group II (age, weight, BMI, glucose, total cholesterol, TG, LDLc, homocisteíne, HDLc, Apo A-I, Apo B, cholesterol/HDLc and TG/HDLc). The results are expressed as mean ± standard deviation.

According to lipid profile results, Control Group I presents levels (mean values) significantly higher ($p<0.05$) than those in Control Group II of total cholesterol (219.90 ± 40.46 mg/dL *vs* 172.25 ± 30.92 mg/dL) and LDLc (133.40 ± 29.99 mg/dL *vs* 92.60 ± 27.89 mg/dL).

The MetS patients compared to Control Group I presented significantly higher levels ($p<0.05$) of glucose (131.44 ± 26.05 mg/dL

Variable	Controls I: Adult Mean ± SD (n= 20)	Controls II: Young Mean ± SD (n= 20)	p-value (1)	MetS Patients Mean ± SD (n=32)	Controls I: Adult Mean ± SD (n= 20)	p-value (2)	MetS Patients Mean ± SD (n=32)	Controls II: Young Mean ± SD (n= 20)	p-value (3)
Age (years)	56.35 ± 4.58	24.70 ± 2.34	0.000*	58.03 ± 4.48	56.35 ± 4.58	0.261	58.03 ± 4.48	24.70 ± 2.34	0.000*
Weight (Kg)	73.36 ± 12.09	-	-	84.44 ± 16.08	73.36 ± 12.09	0.007*	84.44 ± 16.08	-	-
BMI (Kg/m^2)	27.43 ± 5.12	-	-	32.02 ± 4.98	27.43 ± 5.12	0.002*	32.02 ± 4.98	-	-
Glucose (mg/dL)	95.55 ± 13.45	89.95 ± 6.36	0.258	131.44 ± 26.05	95.55 ± 13.45	0.000*	131.44 ± 26.05	89.95 ± 6.36	0.000*
Total cholesterol (mg/dL)	219.90 ± 40.46	172.25 ± 30.92	0.001*	223.13 ± 41.72	219.90 ± 40.46	0.954	223.13 ± 41.72	172.25 ± 30.92	0.000*
TG (mg/dL)	108.70 ± 44.31	88.0 ± 51.79	0.450	155.69 ± 60.32	108.70 ± 44.31	0.009*	155.69 ± 60.32	88.0 ± 51.79	0.000*
LDLc (mg/dL)	133.40 ± 29.99	92.60 ± 27.89	0.000*	135.94 ± 32.72	133.40 ± 29.99	0.955	135.94 ± 32.72	92.60 ± 27.89	0.000*
Homocysteine (μmol/L)	11.575 ± 2.9088	11.511 ± 7.8024	0.999	11.672 ± 2.5840	11.575 ± 2.9088	0.997	11.672 ± 2.5840	11.511 ± 7.8024	0.992
HDLc (mg/dL)	62.55 ± 17.88	62.10 ± 13.75	0.996	53.72 ± 17.67	62.55 ± 17.88	0.161	53.72 ± 17.67	62.10 ± 13.75	0.192
Apo A-I (mg/dL)	175.0 ± 30.22	-	-	157.53 ± 31.22	175.0 ± 30.22	0.052	157.53 ± 31.22	-	-
Apo B (mg/dL)	99.10 ± 20.10	-	-	110.09 ± 18.31	99.10 ± 20.10	0.048*	110.09 ± 18.31	-	-
Cholesterol/HDLc	3.66 ± 0.80	2.91 ± 0.86	0.153	4.53 ± 1.66	3.66 ± 0.80	0.052	4.53 ± 1.66	2.91 ± 0.86	0.000*
TG/HDLc	19.2 ± 0.99	1.62 ± 1.40	0.787	3.31 ± 1.70	1.92 ± 0.99	0.003*	3.31 ± 1.70	1.62 ± 1.40	0.000*

SD: standard deviation, BMI: Body mass index, TG: Triglycerides, LDL-c: dense-low density lipoprotein, HDL-c: high-density lipoprotein. p-value (1): significance between Control I and Control II, p-value (2): significance between Control I and MetS patients, p-value (3): significance between Control II and MetS patients. Notes: Data are mean ± SD. * Statistically significant differences.

Table 1: Anthropometric parameters and Lipid profile by MetS status and age (n = 72).

Variable	Controls I: Adult Mean ± SD (n= 20)	Controls II: Young Mean ± SD (n= 20)	p-value (1)	MetS Patients Mean ± SD (n=32)	Controls I: Adult Mean ± SD (n= 20)	p-value (2)	MetS Patients Mean ± SD (n=32)	Controls II: Young Mean ± SD (n= 20)	p-value (3)
SOD (U/g Hb)	947.85 ± 272.04	904.55 ± 247.14	0.885	875.53 ± 323.03	947.85 ± 272.04	0.658	875.53 ± 323.03	904.55 ± 247.14	0.934
GPx (U/g Hb)	25.58 ± 15.91	29.12 ± 9.71	0.684	25.76 ± 13.14	25.58 ± 15.91	0.999	25.76 ± 13.14	29.12 ± 9.71	0.657
GR (U/L)	59.50 ± 9.98	51.19 ± 12.35	0.027*	50.31 ± 8.15	59.50 ± 9.98	0.005*	50.31 ± 8.15	51.19 ± 12.35	0.949
oxLDL (U/L)	86.25 ± 17.36	60.17 ± 16.28	0.000*	96.77 ± 23.05	86.25 ± 17.36	0.159	96.77 ± 23.05	60.17 ± 16.28	0.000*
8-OHdG (ng/mL)	18.76 ± 5.41	22.90 ± 7.55	0.310	21.41 ± 10.82	18.76 ± 5.41	0.552	21.41 ± 10.82	22.90 ± 7.55	0.823
F$_2$Isoprostanes (μg/g creatinine)	2.42 ± 1.14	2.04 ± 0.80	0.672	3.17 ± 1.78	2.42 ± 1.14	0.156	3.17 ± 1.78	2.04 ± 0.80	0.017*
PC (nmol/mg)	0.63 ± 0.19	0.29 ± 0.13	0.000*	0.56 ± 0.26	0.63 ± 0.19	0.425	0.56 ± 0.26	0.29 ± 0.13	0.000*

SOD: superoxide dismutase, GPx: glutathione peroxidase, GR: glutathione reductase, oxLDL: oxidized LDL; 8-0HdG: 8-hydroxy-2'-deoxyguanosine; PC: carbonyl protein. p-value (1): significance between Control I and Control II, p-value (2): significance between Control I and MetS patients, p-value (3): significance between Control II and MetS patients. Notes: Data are mean ± SD. * Statistically significant differences.

Table 2: Antioxidant status: enzymes and oxidative stress biomarkers by MetS status and age (N = 72).

vs 95.55 ± 13.45 mg/dL), TG (155.69 ± 60.32 mg/dL vs 108.70 ± 44.31 mg/dL), Apo B (110.09 ± 18.31 mg/dL vs 99.10 ± 20.10 mg/dL) and TG/HDLc (3.31 ± 1.70 vs 1.92 ± 0.99).

Moreover, the levels of glucose (131.44 ± 26.05 mg/dL vs 89.95 ± 6.36 mg/dL), total cholesterol (223.13 ± 41.72 mg/dL vs 172.25 ± 30.92 mg/dL), TG (155.69 ± 60.32 mg/dL vs 88.0 ± 51.79 mg/dL), LDLc (135.94 ± 32.72 mg/dL vs 92.60 ± 27.89 mg/dL), cholesterol/HDLc (4.53 ± 1.66 vs 2.91 ± 0.86) and TG/HDLc (3.31 ± 1.70 vs 1.62 ± 1.40) were significantly higher (p<0.05) in the MetS patients compared to Control Group II.

Table 2 presents the antioxidant status marked by: enzymes (SOD, GPx, GR) and certain biomarkers of oxidative damage as oxLDLc (endothelial damage), F$_2$-isoprostanes (lipid peroxidation) 8-OHdG (DNA damage), and PC (protein damage). We established the normal reference values for oxidative damage biomarkers in a previous article, as follows: SOD 931.97 ± 271.09 U/g Hb; GPx 27.58±6.89 U/g Hb; GR 46.56 ± 11.68 U/L; oxLDLc 63.23 ± 16.23 U/L; 8-OHdG 23.27 ± 10.58 ng/mL; F$_2$-isoprostanes 2.26 ± 0.9 μg/g creatinine; and PC 0.34 ± 0.15 nmol/mg.

Regarding the antioxidant status, we have observed statistically significant higher (p<0.05) levels in the Control Group I compared to Control Group II of GR (59.50 ± 9.98 U/L vs 51.19 ± 12.35 U/L), oxLDLc (86.25 ± 17.36 U/L vs 60.17 ± 16.28 U/L) and PC (0.63 ± 0.19 nmol/mg vs 0.29 ± 0.13 nmol/mg). In addition, only significant lower differences were observed in the values of GR between the MetS patients and Control Group I (50.31 ± 8.15 U/L vs 59.50 ± 9.98 U/L).

We found significantly higher levels in the MetS patients compared to Control Group II of oxLDL (96.77 ± 23.05 U/L vs 60.17 ± 16.28 U/L), F$_2$-isoprostanes (3.17 ± 1.78 μg/g creatinine vs 2.04 ± 0.80 μg/g creatinine) and PC (0.56 ± 0.26 nmol/mg vs 0.29 ± 0.13 nmol/mg) (Table 2).

Discussion

It was found significantly higher levels of glucose, TG and Apo B in the subjects with MetS compared with Control Group I according with our observational study recently published [19]. Several authors have also refered the elevation of TG values and glucose levels in MetS with respect to healthy population age-matched [20,21]. HDLc, LDLc and plasma cholesterol levels were not significantly higher in MetS patients with respect to Control Group I, previously reported fact [22]. This could be related to the inter-individual variability and also related to the age of the control Group I, so also could explain the lack of differences between the OxS biomarkers.

The Control Group I presented significantly higher (p<0.05) mean values than Control Group II of total cholesterol and LDLc, which could be related to the age difference between these groups (Table 1). Moreover, the levels of glucose, total cholesterol, TG and LDLc were significantly higher in the MetS patients compared to Control Group II.

Regarding the antioxidant status and its comparison between the two Control Groups, it was observed statistically significant higher (p<0.05) levels in the Control Group I compared to Control Group II of GR, oxLDLc and PC. These results suggest a superior OxS (endothelial and protein damage in the older subjects) due to aging, and a possible endogenous adaptation to an increase on the oxidative status of the organism (marked as the increase on GR). In addition, only significant differences were observed in the values of GR between Control Group I and the MetS patients, which may be due to a superior antioxidant capacity of the healthy individuals against those with MetS. However, Vávrová et al. [23] found higher activities of GR (p<0.001) for those subjects with MetS but altogether they found increased oxidative stress in MetS and a decreased antioxidative defense correlated with some laboratory (triglycerides, high-density lipoprotein cholesterol (HDL-C)) and clinical (waist circumference, blood pressure) components of MetS.

Significantly higher levels in MetS patients were also found compared to Control Group II of oxLDLc, F_2-isoprostanes and PC. These results indicate that the MetS patients have a superior endothelial, lipidic and protein damage than the younger controls. Furthermore, considering that MetS patients presented higher levels of oxLDLc compared to Control Group I and thath it had also shown significantly higher levels of oxLDLc than the Control Group II, it can be suggested that these results are probably due to aging. There were neither significant differences in the other antioxidant biomarkers nor the other enzymes between the MetS patients and the Control Groups.

Aging is a multifactorial complex process and its molecular mechanism remains unclear. It is now well established that biological aging correlates with the accumulation of oxidized biomolecules in most tissues [24]. In the present study of age-related increases in concentrations of oxidized biomolecules, disparities have been observed between intracellular and extracellular proteins. OxS induced peroxidation of membrane lipids is powerfull dangerous so it leads to a disfunction on the biological capacity of the cell membrane (such as the degree of fluidity). Moreover, it could lead to the inactivation of membrane-bound receptors or enzymes, which in turn may impair normal cellular function and increase tissue permeability. Moreover, lipid peroxidation may contribute to and strengthen cellular damage resulting from generation of oxidized products, some of which are chemically reactive and covalently modify critical macromolecules.

MetS is one of the major public health concerns as its prevalence increases worldwide with a subsequent predisposition to type II diabetes and CV disease [21]. Previous evidence supports the important role that OxS plays in MetS-related manifestations. The evidence for increased OxS is still a matter of debate. Fujita et al. [22] reported that systemic OxS increased in subjects with MetS, being closely related to the increase of visceral fat.

Moreover, Galle et al. [25] found that OxS promotes the formation of oxLDLc, which is involved in the initiation and progression of atherosclerosis [26]. Additionally, OxS has been suggested to be involved in the etiology of a host of chronic diseases and aging in general [23]. But there is controversy on the occurrence of OxS in patients with MetS. Some studies showed higher levels of markers

of oxidative damage (circulating oxidized LDL and plasma F_2-isoprostanes) between MetS patients and healthy individuals [27]. Meanwhile, others authors did not found found significant changes on the levels of these biomarkers [28,20,7]. In the present study OxS biomarkers and endogenous antioxidant enzymes (excepting GR) were found not to shown significant changes, comparing MetS patients and age-matched healthy individuals (Control Group I); according to Sjogren [28] Seet [20] and Shrestha [7]. That fact could be due to the similar plasmatic cholesterol level of MetS and Control I (223.13 ± 41.72 and 219.90 ± 40.46 mg/dL), col-LDL (135.94 ± 32.77 and 133.40 ± 29.99mg/dL) and BMI (32.02 ± 4.98 and 27.43 ± 5.12). Colas et al. [27] suggested an association between an excess of visceral fat and biochemical parameters associated with OxS in LDL. Obesity is quite associated with MetS, and may represent a major factor in the OxS evidenced in LDL from obese MetS patients. Sigurdardottir [21] established that circulating ox-LDL is associated with risk factors of MetS, but oxidation of LDL occurs in the arterial wall and not in the circulation. Comprehensive understanding of the molecular mechanism, underlying inflammation and OxS with implications for metabolic stress must be achieved to attenuate the impacts of obesity-induced insulin resistance and ensuing MetS.

Taking together, the present results do not show an increase on the OxS owing to the development of MetS disease. In fact, MetS patients compared to healthy younger subjects shown a superior endothelial, lipidic and protein oxidative damage (marked as oxLDL, 8-OHdG F_2-isoprostanes and PC).

Conclusion

The results of the study have shown that MetS patients don't present a superior OxS in comparison to age-related healthy individuals. Therefore, differences between MetS patients and Group I (same age) are quite minor that differences between MetS and Group II (younger). Consequently, aging is more relevant to OxS than the MetS *per se*. However; more research is needed to understand OxS induced damage and its relationship with the development of MetS and aging.

References

1. Farinha JB, Steckling FM, Stefanello ST, Cardoso MS, Nunes LS, et al (2015) Response of oxidative stress and inflammatory biomarkers to a 12-week aerobic exercise training in women with metabolic syndrome. Sports Med Open 2: 3.

2. Lorenzo C, Williams K, Hunt KJ, Haffner SM (2006) Trend in the prevalence of the metabolic syndrome and its impact on cardiovascular disease incidence: the San Antonio Heart Study. Diabetes Care 29: 625-630.

3. Syslová K, Böhmová A, Mikoška M, Kuzma M, Pelclová D, et al. (2014) Multimarker screening of oxidative stress in aging. Oxid Med Cell Longev 2014.

4. Dasuri K, Ebenezer P, Fernandez-Kim SO, Zhang L, Gao Z, et al. (2013) Role of physiological levels of 4-hydroxynonenal on adipocyte biology: implications for obesity and metabolic syndrome. Free Radic Res 47: 8-19.

5. Evans JL, Goldfine ID, Maddux BA, Grodsky GM (2002) Oxidative stress and stress-activated signaling pathways: a unifying hypothesis of type 2 diabetes. Endocr Rev 23: 599-622.

6. Ford ES (2006) Intake and circulating concentrations of antioxidants in metabolic syndrome. Curr Atheroscler Rep 8: 448-452.

7. Sjogren P, Basu S, Rosell M, Silveira A, de Faire U, et al. (2005) Measures of oxidized low-density lipoprotein and oxidative stress are not related and not elevated in otherwise healthy men with the metabolic syndrome. Arterioscler Thromb Vasc Biol 25: 2580-2586.

8. Holvoet P, Kritchevsky SB, Tracy RP, Mertens A, Rubin SM, et.al. (2004) The Metabolic Syndrome, Circulating Oxidized LDL, and Risk of Myocardial Infarction in Well-Functioning Elderly People in the Health, Aging, and Body Composition Cohort. Diabetes 53: 1068-1073.

9. Holvoet P, Lee DH, Steffes M, Gross M, Jacobs DR Jr (2008) Association between circulating oxidized low-density lipoprotein and incidence of the metabolic syndrome. JAMA 299: 2287-2293.

10. Holvoet P (2008) Relations between metabolic syndrome, oxidative stress and inflammation and cardiovascular disease. Verh K Acad Geneeskd Belg 70: 193-219.

11. Holvoet P, Mertens A, Verhamme P, Bogaerts K, Beyens G, et al. (2001) Circulating oxidized LDL is a useful marker for identifying patients with coronary artery disease. Arterioscler Thromb Vasc Biol 21: 844-848.

12. Hulthe J, Fagerberg B (2002) Circulating oxidized LDL is associated with subclinical atherosclerosis development and inflammatory cytokines (AIR Study). Arterioscler Thromb Vasc Biol 22: 1162-1167.

13. Tsimikas S, Bergmark C, Beyer RW, Patel R, Pattison J, et.al. (2003). Temporal increases in plasma markers of oxidized low-density lipoprotein strongly reflect the presence of acute coronary syndromes. J Am Coll Cardiol 41: 360-370.

14. Holvoet P, Theilmeier G, Shivalkar B, Flameng W, Collen D (1998) LDL hypercholesterolemia is associated with accumulation of oxidized LDL, atherosclerotic plaque growth, and compensatory vessel enlargement in coronary arteries of miniature pigs. Arterioscler Thromb Vasc Biol 18: 415-422.

15. Romano AD, Serviddio G, de Matthaeis A, Bellanti F, Vendemiale G (2010) Oxidative stress and aging. J Nephrol 23: 29-36.

16. Mendoza-Nunez VM, Ruiz-Ramos M, Sánchez-Rodríguez MA, Retana-Ugalde, R. Muñoz-Sánchez JL (2007) Aging-related oxidative stress in healthy humans. Tohoku J Exp Med 213: 261–268.

17. Jones DP, Mody VC, Carlson JL, Lynn MJ, Sternberg P Jr (2002) Redox analysis of human plasma allows separation of pro-oxidant events of aging form decline in antioxidant defenses. Free Radic Biol Med 33: 1290-1300.

18. Finkel T, Holbrook NJ (2000) Oxidants, oxidative stress and the biology of ageing. Nature 408: 239-247.

19. Sancho-Rodriguez N, Avilés-Plaza FV, Granero-Fernandez E, Hernández-Martinez A, Albaladejo-Oton MD, et al. (2011) Observational study of lipid profile and LDL particle size in patients with metabolic syndrome. Lipids Health Dis 10: 162.

20. Shrestha S, Chandra L, Aryal M, Das BK, Pandey S, et al. (2010) Evaluation of lipid peroxidation and antioxidants' status in metabolic syndrome. Kathmandu Univ Med J (KUMJ) 8: 382-386.

21. Sigurdardottir V, Fagerberg B, Hulthe J (2002) Circulating oxidized low-density lipoprotein (LDL) is associated with risk factors of the metabolic syndrome and LDL size in clinically healthy 58-year-old men (AIR study). J Intern Med 252: 440-447.

22. Fujita K, Nishizawa H, Funahashi T, Shimomura I, Shimabukuro M (2006) Systemic oxidative stress is associated with visceral fat accumulation and the metabolic syndrome. Circ J 70: 1437–1442.

23. Vávrová L, Kodydková J, Zeman M, Dušejovská M, Macášek J, et al. (2013) Alltered activities of antioxidant enzymes in patients with metabolic syndrome. Obes Facts 6: 39-47.

24. Linton S. Davies MJ, Dean RT (2001) Protein oxidation and ageing. Exp Gerontol 36: 1503-1518.

25. Galle J, Hansen-Hagge T, Wanner C, Seibold S (2006) Impact of oxidized low density lipoprotein on vascular cells. Atherosclerosis 185: 219-226.

26. Wallenfeldt K, Fagerberg B, Wikstrand J, Hulthe J (2004) Oxidized low-density lipoprotein in plasma is a prognostic marker of subclinical atherosclerosis development in clinically healthy men. J Intern Med 256: 413-420.

27. Colas R, Sassolas A, Guichardant M, Cugnet-Anceau C, Moret M, et al. (2011) LDL from obese patients with the metabolic syndrome show increased lipid peroxidation and activate platelets. Diabetologia 54: 2931-2940.

28. Seet RC, Lee CY, Lim EC, Quek AM, Huang SH, et al. (2010) Markers of oxidative damage are not elevated in otherwise healthy individuals with the metabolic syndrome. Diabetes Care 33: 1140-1142.

14

Assessment of Diabetic Patient Perception on Diabetic Disease and Self-Care Practice in Dilla University Referral Hospital

Yohannes Addisu[1], Akine Eshete[1] and Endalew Hailu[2]*

[1]*College of Health and Medical Sciences, Dilla University, Ethiopia*
[2]*Department of Nursing, College of Public Health and Medical Sciences, Jimma University, Ethiopia*

Abstract

Background: Diabetes is a chronic and irreversible disease that lasts, lifelong, directly concerns any individual of all ages and their relatives, and brings heavy economic burden, affects self-care activities and shortens life expectancy due to the chronic damages it causes, Thus, before considering any possible intervention it was imperative to assess present knowledge, perception, and self-care practices of patients towards the management of diabetes.

Methods: A facility based cross-sectional study supplemented by using both quantitative and qualitative methods was conducted from April – June 2013 in Dilla referral hospital. A total of 310 participants with Diabetes Mellitus were interviewed. Face-to-face interviews were used for quantitative data; and qualitative data were collected by in-depth interview. SPSS version 20 was used to perform descriptive and logistic regression analyses. Statistical significance was set at P-value <0.05 to judge the association.

Result: Two third, 238 (76.8) of them had good practiced on the recommended self-care practices. Among the recommended self-care behaviors, drug adherence 289 (93.2%), dietary intake 154 (49.7%) and regular exercise 138 (44.5%) were the most practiced self-care. Self-blood glucose monitoring was the least practiced which accounted 62 (20%). Approximately 78 % of diabetic patients were developed positive perception towards DM and has a significant effect for patients with diabetes to provide own self-care practice [OR-2.74, 95% CI (1.27, 5.91)]. Majority 79.4% of the respondents were knowledgeable about diabetes, but those diabetic patients who were knowledgeable on DM were less likely performed recommended self-care to manage the disease [OR-0.29, 95% CI (0.10, 0.80)]. On other hand those diabetic patients who were knowledgeable on DM self-care were more likely performed recommended self-care [OR-6.52, 95% CI (2.88, 14.78)]. Education also has a significant effect for patients with diabetes in their own self-care practice. A major point to address therefore is regular access to/contact with diabetic educators which currently is severely substandard.

Conclusions: Management of diabetes may be enhanced by reinforcing patients' knowledge, developing positive perception and encouraging behavior change whilst taking into consideration patients' backgrounds. To increase the self-care behavior, the health care team should be utilizing a patient-centered approach in order to deliver diabetes messages on specific issues of management practice.

Keywords: Diabetes; Insulin; Blood glucose; Alcohol; Smoking

Introduction

Background

Diabetes mellitus (DM) is "a group of metabolic diseases characterized by hyperglycemia resulting from defects in insulin secretion, insulin action or both" (American diabetes association, 2005), manifested by carbohydrates, fat, protein metabolism abnormality. It is a chronic disease, which has no cure and associated with high rate of morbidity and mortality in both developing and developed countries and also becoming a pandemic in the world, with increased need for health care [1,2]. DM is increasingly prevalent and one of the top public health concerns all over the world. The International Diabetes Federation (IDF) estimates that 23 million years of life are lost due to disability and reduced quality of life as a result of complications associated with diabetes. Evidence has shown that $232 billion U.S. dollars were spent worldwide in 2007 to treat and prevent diabetes. This figure is expected to climb to a minimum of over $ 300 billion in 2025 [3]. The Diabetic Prevention Programs (DPP) found conclusively that with moderate exercise and change in diet people can reduce the risk of developing type 2 diabetes by 58%. Sub-Saharan Africa, like the rest of the world, is experiencing an increasing prevalence of diabetes alongside other non-communicable diseases [2].

Even though the actual number was not known, World health organization has estimated the number of diabetic cases in Ethiopia to be 800,000 by the year 2000, and the number is expected to increase to 1.8 million by 2030 [4]. To prevent serious morbidity and mortality, diabetes treatment requires dedication to demanding self-care behaviors in multiple domains, including food choices, physical activity, proper medications intake and blood glucose monitoring [5]. Self-care in diabetes is a process where the person attempts a variety of self-care strategies, according to her/his unique body's cues, until discovering what is effective for her/his lifestyle and contextual situation and is individuals' taking the necessary action to protect their lives, health and well-being [6-8]. In order to control their disease, patients with diabetes need to adopt self-care activities such as exercising, an appropriate diet, regular exercises, control of blood glucose, appropriate use of oral antidiabetics, awareness of the effects and side effects of insulin treatment, avoiding alcohol use and smoking, preventing complications of diabetes, and compliance to life-long medication [9,10].

In addition there are no studies that have addressed the assessment

*Corresponding author: Endalew Hailu, Department of Nursing, College of Public Health and Medical Sciences, Jimma University, Ethiopia,
E-mail: endale.10@gmail.com

of diabetic patient perception on diabetic disease and self-care practice in Dilla university referral hospital, South Ethiopia

Hence this study is designed to address this gap. So, the purpose of this study is assess the perception of diabetic patients about diabetic related education and self-care practice in in Dilla university, referral hospital, Southwest Ethiopia.

Significance of the Study

Diabetes is a chronic disease that requires lifelong self-care behavior, today, successful treatment of diabetes mellitus is closely associated with the education of both Patients and their relatives and patient education is one of the most important responsibilities of health professions. Educators emphasize that learning depends on the individual's level of development, and patients should have awareness in diabetes education. In the management of diabetes, helping patients improve their health and quality of life is considered an important aspect of diabetes self-care education. Local evidences are limited on the assessment of diabetic patient perception on diabetic disease and self-care practice in Dilla university referral hospital, South Ethiopia, Factors influence self-care practices and Studies conducted elsewhere could not be used to infer about diabetic patients in the study area, as these differences in cultures and life style.

Therefore, the finding of the current study will be helpful to design self-care practice and to assess their perception on disease process and also it helps every staff in diabetic clinic to improve or maintain the health information about self-care practice. Thus, this study will be designed, the assessment of diabetic patient perception on diabetic disease and self-care practice in Dilla university referral hospital, South Ethiopia.

Methods and Materials

Study setting

Cross sectional study was conducted in Dilla university referral hospital, which is located about 365 Kms to the south of Addis Ababa, the capital city of Ethiopia, and 85 Kms to Awassa the regional capital city of SNNPR. DURH is one of the teaching hospital in Ethiopia and currently the only referral hospital in the Gedeo Zone of south part. The hospital is rapidly expanding in terms of services and provides multi-dimensional aspects of care to clients who need health service. There are five units (internal medicine, surgery, gynecology/ obstetrics, pediatrics, and psychiatry) run by the hospital. Diabetic patients get service from Diabetic clinic and admitted service also get medical wards. The service is rendered by internists, medical residents, medical interns and nurses. The study was conducted over two month from April – June, 2013.

Populations

A patients is included in the study if he/she was 18 years and older and must on follow up for a least Diabetic patients who have at least three visit on diabetic follow up units and had an appointment during the study period, patient Patients with hearing impartment or any other serious health problem who were unable to provide appropriate information were excluded.

Sample size

Sample size is calculated by using single population proportion formula by considering the following assumptions; 50% prevalence assumption, 95% confidence level of significance alpha 0.05 = 1.96, and 5% margin of error, which results in the sample size of 384. Since the source population is less than 10,000 the sample size is adjusted with correction formula and the final sample size was became 310.

For the qualitative study part of the study using in-depth interview; ten patients with diabetes were included. The in-depth interview was conducted separately for males and females patients. The selected patients were not included in the quantitative part of the study.

Sampling methods

Health institutions available in Gedeo zone were grouped by ownership into Government and Privates. Of these, only one government hospital of Dilla university referral hospital is render diabetic follow up clinic. The lists of respondents were prepared based on their updated registration log book. After establishing the sampling frames of respondents, we would use random sampling technique to identify the study unit to be included to the survey. The eligible attending respondents were recruited in order of their appointments. Therefore, every other patients coming to the follow up clinic was interviewed until reach 310 samples. The first diabetic patient was selected by lottery method using their card number. In cases where the patients have two follow up appointments within a month, the patient's appointment date was checked and he/she was excluded from the interview.

For the qualitative part of the study participants were selected using purposive sampling technique till reached to a point of redundancy of information. The participants were interviewed after informed by principal investigator about the purpose of the study.

Measurements

Structured questionnaire is originally developed in English and this be translated to Amharic and then back translated into English by another person to ensure validity. For the validity of the questioners, it was adapted the tool from similar study done in Malaysian and also uses questioner that was prepared by Spain diabetic association and North western university of Chicago [8,11]. The questionnaire is slightly modified in order to fit, the purpose of this study. Each question was checked for the relationships with variables and study objectives. Pretest was carried out in Hawassa hospital. Pretest was conducted in 5% of the sample from the same source population to check clarity and consistency of the questionnaires prior to the actual data collection. Area of pretest were determine the acceptability of the questions to be asked and the methods used, reaction and willingness of the respondents, time required, performance and adequacy of data collectors and either to modify or change ambiguous and clear ideas. Far qualitative part of the study, in-depth interview was performed to get insight knowledge, perception and self-care practice.

Measurement of variables

a) **Knowledge about diabetic disease:** Is measured by seven items in true-false format. Correct answer will be given "1" and "0" is given for incorrect and don't know. Then a total score is computed out of seven marks (with the range of 0-7) the median score and those who Score above50% have a good knowledge where as those score below 50% low knowledge.

b) **Knowledge about diabetic self-care practice:** Is measured by four items in true-false format. Correct answer will be given "1" and "0" is given for incorrect and don't know. Then a total score is computed out of four marks (with the range of 0-7) the median score and those who Score above 50% have a good knowledge self-care practice where as those score below 50% low knowledge self-care practice.

c) Perception is measured by three item (with the range of 0-3) the median score is 2 and those who Score above 50% have a good Perception where as those score below 50% poor Perception.

d) Diabetes self-care practice was measured by using items on physical exercise, diet, medication, and blood glucose measurement. Then classified the self-care as 'good self-care practice' and 'not have good self-care practice'; respondents were labeled to have "good self-care" if they scored above 50% of the total self-care practices in the last three days.

Data collection methods

A total of four data collectors were participated in the actual data collection; they are diploma Nurses who were not working in the Diabetic follow up clinic and three supervisors who are residents in the department of internal medicine. Trained data collectors were collect the data by using a pretested and structured questioner. The investigators were give one day training to data collectors and supervisors before data collection, the training was include briefing on the general objectives of the study, discussing the contents of the questionnaires one by one and the type of information needed to handle any questions arising during data collection time; and discussions on how to maintain confidentiality and privacy. And both the principal investigator and the supervisors regularly supervise them on daily basis; there by formats was checked for its completeness, accuracy and consistency.

Data quality control

Trained data collectors who collect the data and pretesting of the instruments were made before the actual data collection. So that corrections was made accordingly. More over the principal investigator was supervise the data collection on daily basis for completeness and consistence, of the filled questionnaires. In addition to this, we were thoroughly clean and carefully enter the data to computer for commencement of analysis.

Data processing and analysis

The data was cleaned, edited, entered in to computer and analyzed using SPSS for windows program version 20. Descriptive statistics of different variables was computed to see the overall distribution of the study variable. Binary logistic regression was used for bivariate analysis and finally multiple logistic regressions were used to identify factors associated with self-care practice. To avoid many variables and unstable estimates in the subsequent model, only variables that reached a p-value less than 0.05 at bivariate analysis was kept in the subsequent model analysis. 95% confidence interval (CI) for OR are used in judging the significance of the associations. The recorded interview were transcribed first to the language of the interview and fully translated into English. Responses and comments were grouped according to the theme and finally triangulation was performed by relating thematic areas and explaining with related to the study questions.

Ethical consideration

Dilla University, research and publication of college of Health and Medical Sciences approved this study. An official letter was written to the DURH then to Diabetic follow up clinic by DURH. Verbal consent was obtained from each respondent and the research and publication committee approved the procedure since the study was a survey and with no any harm to the respondents.

Results

Socio-demographic characteristics of the study participants

A total of 310 respondents were included in the study and giving 100% response rate. From the total participate, 200 (64.5%) were males and 110 (35.5%) were females. The mean ages of the respondent was 41.9 (SD ± 1.4) with a range age of 18 to70 (Table1).

S.No	Variable	Frequency	Percentage
1	**Sex of respondents**		
	1.Male	200	64.5
	2.Female	110	35.5
	Total	310	100
2	**Age of respondents**		
	1. <39	112	36.1
	2.40-44	43	13.9
	3.45-49	39	12.6
	4.>50	116	37.4
	Total	310	100
3	**Religion of respondents**		
	1.Orthdox	115	37.1
	2.Catholic	5	1.6
	3.Protestant	159	51.3
	4.Muslim	24	7.7
	5.Other (Tradional)	7 (3 Joba and 4 traditional)	2.3
	Total	310	100
4	**Ethnicity of respondents**		
	1.Gedeo	123	39.7
	2.Sidama	6	1.9
	3.Gurage	22	7.1
	4.Walyeta	11	3.5
	5.Amhara	81	26.1
	6.Oromo	51	16.5
	7.Other	16 (3 Gamo, 5 hadiya and 8 cafa)	5.2
	Total	310	100
5.	**Marital status of respondents**		
	1.Single	77	24.8
	2.Married & live together	206	66.5
	3.Married but not live	12	3.9
	Together		
	4.Divorced	0	
	5.Widowed	15	4.8
	6.Other		
	Total	310	100
6	**Living with**		
	1. My Spouse	213	68.7
	2.Alone	50	16.1
	3.Family	19	6.1
	4.Father	8	2.6
	5.Mother	5	1.6
	6.Childeren	15	4.8
	Total	310	100
7	**Educational status**		
	1.Illiterate	39	12.6
	2.Grade 1-8	76	24.5
	3. Grade 9-10	28	9
	4. preparatory	41	13.2
	5.Higher Education	126	40.6
	Total	310	100

	Occupation status		
8	1.goverment Employ	117	37.7
	2.Private Employ	7	2.3
	3.Merchant	29	9.4
	4.Farmer	53	17.1
	5.Driver		
	6.Daily laborer	8	2.6
	7.Unemployed	26	8.4
	8.Other	70 (8 house wife,13 pension, 49 student)	22.6
	Total	310	100
9	Residence of subjects		
	1.Urban	93	30
	2.Rural	217	70
10	Income level		
	1.low level	125	40.3
	2.medium level	101	32.6
	3.High level	84	27.1
	Total	310	100

Table 1: Socio-demographic characteristics of patients with diabetes in Dilla referral hospital, 2014.

S.No	Variable	Frequency	Percentage
1.	**Type of DM**		
	1.Type I	123	39.7
	2.Type II	187	60.3
	Total	310	100%
2.	**Duration of DM**		
	1.<1Yr	84	27.1
	2.1-2 Yr	47	15.2
	3.3-5 Yr	74	23.9
	4.>5 Yr	105	33.9
	Total	310	100
3.	**Follow Up of DM**		
	1.Always	115	37.1
	2.Sometimes	195	62.9
	Total	310	100
9.	**Average of three consecutive blood glucose level**		
	1.Normal (<FBG127)	44	14.2
	2.Abnormal (>FBG127)	266	85.8
	3.Total	310	100

Table 2: Clinical Characteristics and related history of patients with diabetes in Dilla university referral hospital, 2014.

DM related history of study participants

Among the total respondents, 187 (60.3%) of them were medically diagnosed with type-2 diabetes. The mean duration since medically diagnosed for diabetes was 2.5 (SD ± 1.40) years. The majority 195 (62.9%) of the study participant did not have follow up for their health impairment. As result a substantial proportion 266 (85.5%) patients had abnormal blood glucose level or glycemic control (Table 2).

Perception of patients towards diabetes mellitus

Among the total participants, the majority 242 (78.1%) of patients had positive Perception towards DM and diabetes complications. More than half of the respondent 174 (56.1%) perceives or agree that DM never get break and the remaining 105 (35.2%) were not agree. Regarding severity of diabetes and its related complications, a total of

215 (65.4%) respondents were agreed on DM is very serious disease. about half, 162 (52.3%) participants were disagreed on DM changes personal outlook in life and the remaining 128 (41.3%) were agreed (Table 3).

Patient diabetic self-care practice among study participants

We measured diabetes self-care practice using the following recommended self-care items like physical exercise, diet, medication and blood glucose measurement. We classified the self-care as 'good self-care practice' and 'not good self-care practice'; respondents were labeled to have "good self-care" if they scored above 50% of the total self-care practices.

Among the total respondents, majority 238 (76.8%) of them had good practiced on the recommended self-care practices. Almost half of the respondents 154 (49.7%) followed the recommended dietary intake for controlling DM. Only 138 (44.5%) had exercise for average of 30 minutes per day. Regarding blood glucose monitoring only 62 (20%) of patients measured their blood glucose by themselves one per day. Almost all of the respondents 289 (93.2%) had taken the prescribed drugs appropriately whereas 21 (6.8%) did not take the prescribed drugs as prescribed (Table 4).

Self-care practice on blood glucose monitoring and it's predictors among study participants

Among the total respondents, 62 (20%) of patients reported that they performed self-measuring for blood glucose. Almost 35 (55.5%) of the patients did not control their blood glucose regularly ,According to the result of the multivariate analysis, individuals' with high income levels were 5.8 times more likely to perform self-blood glucose monitoring than less income levels [OR-5.83, 95% CI (2.41, 14.12)]. On the other side, diabetic patients with medium income level were 2.99 times more likely to perform self-blood glucose monitoring than less income level [OR-2.99, 95% CI (1.32, 6.78)]. Diabetic patients who were type one were 4.2 times more likely performed self-blood glucose monitoring than type two patients (AOR: 4.17, 95% CI: 2.06-8.45).

S.No	Variable	Frequency	Percent
1	General Perception score towards DM		
	1. positive perception	242	78.1
	2. negative perception	68	21.9
	Total	310	100
2	You never get a break from DM		
	1.Agree	174	56.1
	2.Disagree	109	35.2
	3.Neutral	27	8.2
	Total	310	100
3	DM changes personal outlook in life		
	1.Agree	128	41.3
	2.Disagree	162	52.3
	3.Neutral	20	6.5
	Total	310	100
4	DM is very serious disease		
	1.Agree	215	69.4
	2.Disagree	74	23.9
	3.Neutral	21	6.8
	Total	310	100
5	Perceived Health Status of the respondent		
	1.Exellent	11	3.5
	2.V.good	53	17.1
	3.good	178	57.4
	4. Medium	57	18.4
	5.Dangerous	11	3.5
	Total	310	100

Table 3: Perception of Patients with diabetes on Self-care practice in Dilla university referral hospital, 2014.

S. No	Variable	N (%)
1	DM self- care practice scores levels: (n=310) 1. Having self-care practice 2. Not have self- care practice	238 (76.8%) 72 (23.2%)
2	Patients self-blood glucose monitoring practice: (n= 310) 1.Yes 2.No	62 (20%) 248 (80 %)
3	Patients Self-care practice of insulin intake to control DM: (n=310) 1.Yes2.No	90 (29%) 220 (71%)
4	Patients' physical exercise to control DM: (n=310) 1.Yes 2.No	138 (44.5) 172(55.5)
5	Patients' Regular Dietary Adjustment to control DM: (n=310) 1. Yes 2. No	154 (49.7%) 156 (50.5%)
6	Patients Self-care practice on taking medication adherence 1. Taken as prescribed by physician 2. not follow as prescribed by physician	289 (93.2) 21(6.8)

Table 4: Patient self-care practice among patients with diabetes in Dilla university referral hospital, 2014.

S.No	Variable	Patients self-blood glucose monitoring practice: N (%)		COR (CI)
		yes	No	
1	Income level of the respondents 1. Low level 2. Medium level 3. Highest level	14 (4.5) 26 (8.4) 22 (7.1)	111 (35.8) 75 (24.2) 62 (20.2)	1 2.99 (1.32-6.78) 5.83 (2.41-14.12)
2	Type of DM 1. Type 1 2. Type 2	39 (12.6) 23 (7.1)	84 (27.1) 164 (52.9)	4.17 (2.06-8.45) 1
3	Perception of DM 1. Correct perception 2. Incorrectperception	59 (19) 3 (1.0)	183 (59) 65 (21)	4.86 (1.40-16.90) 1
4	General knowledge of DM 1. Low knowledge of DM 2. Good knowledge of DM	6 (1.9) 56 (18.1)	58 (18.7) 190 (61.3)	1 1.33 (0.31-5.74)
5	Knowledge about diabetes self-care 1. Low Knowledge about diabetes self-care 2. Good Knowledge about diabetes self-care	7 (2.4) 53 (17.8)	84 (28.3) 153 (51.5)	1 2.74 (0.86-8.72)
6	Information received about DM 1. Yes 2. No	24 (7.7) 38 (12.3)	59 (19.0) 189 (61)	2.27 (1.13-4.58) 1

Table 5: Multivariate analysis for Predictors of Self-care Practice on Blood Glucose Monitoring among patients with diabetes in Dilla university referral hospital, 2014.

Individuals who had positive perception towards diabetes disease were 4.9 times more likely to perform self-blood glucose monitoring than negative perception [OR-4.86, 95% CI (1.40, 16.90)]. In addition, patients with frequently received information on DM were two times more likely to perform self-blood glucose monitoring [OR- 2.27, 95% CI (1.13, 4.58)] than patients who did not received information about the disease. However, in multivariate analysis knowledgeable on DM and knowledgeable on self-care did not show significant relation with self-blood glucose monitoring practice (Table 5).

Self-care practice on physical exercise and it's predictors among study participants

Among the total respondents, 138 (44.5%) patients had different type of physical exercise to control DM. Of which 122 (79.2%) of patients exercised walking and followed by 27 (17%) gymnastic. Among those who had walking, 90 (73.8%) of patients had been walking on foot with in an average of forty minutes interval.

In multivariate analysis, male diabetic patients were two times more likely to have physical exercise than females, (AOR: 2.32, 95% CI: 1.32-4.06). Individuals who had less than one and 3-5 years duration

of DM were around 2.26and 2.4 times more likely to perform exercise than those who had greater than five years duration of DM [OR2.26, 95% CI (1.14-4.49)] and [OR2.40, 95% CI (1.18-4.87)] respectively. On the other hand, diabetic patients who were good knowledgeable on DM were two times more likely to perform exercise than with low knowledgeable on DM [OR 2.12, 95% CI (1.02, 4.38)]. Lastly occupational statuses of respondents showed significant relation with performing exercise (Table 6).

Patients' dietary adjustment for recommended foods intake and its predictors

regarding regular dietary adjustment of recommended food intake, almost half 154 (49.7%) of them had regular dietary adjustment intake. The recommended dietary adjustment intake time for patients with diabetes were (breakfast, lunch, snack and dinner) and different types of food which was recommended for patients with diabetes (vegetables, cereals, rice, wheat and its products, potatoes and sweet potatoes, and fruits). Among those who had regular dietary intake time, 139 (27.2%) of them had regular time adjustment for breakfast followed by dinner 131(25.6%). Less proportion 51(16.5%) of them answered that taken special diet when blood glucose level was high such as Besso 18 followed by Shiferraw.

In multivariate analysis, male diabetic patients were two times more likely to have diet adjustment than females, (AOR: 2.17, 95% CI: 1.25, 3.76). On the other hand, diabetic patients with very high income were 2.5 times more likely to have diet adjustment than with less income [OR-2.49, 95% CI (1.25, 4.94)]. In addition, patients with frequent received information on DM were nearly three times more likely to have diet adjustment [OR- 2.94, 95% CI (1.59, 5.42)] than patients with no received information about DM disease. Individuals who had 3-5 years of duration of DM were 0.5 times less likely to have diet adjustment than those who had less than one year's duration of DM [OR 0.47, 95% CI (0.23 -0.95)]. Age of respondents showed significant relation with diet adjustment (Table 7).

Patients' received health information about DM

Less than half 83 (26.8%) of the surveyed patients had been received information about DM since their diagnosis. Surveyed patients cited that doctors and nurses are the primary source of information for DM, but majority of surveyed patients mentioned that there was no

S.No	Variable	Frequency	Percentage
1	**Having Physical exercise**		
	1.Yes	138	44.5
	2.No	172	55.5
	Total	310	100
2	**Type of physical Exercise**		
	1.Waking	122	79.2
	2.Swming	5	3.2
	4.Gymnastic	27	17.5
	5.Total	154	100
3	**How long do u wake**		
	1.<40 min	90	73.8
	2.40-60 min	26	21.3
	3.> 60 min	6	4.9
	Total	122	100

Table 6: Patients' physical exercise to control DM among patients with diabetes in Dilla university referral hospital, 2014.

S.No	Variable	Frequency	Percentage
1	Do You have diet adjustment		
	1.Yes	154	49.7
	2.No	156	50.3
	Total	310	100
2	Which meals		
	1.Breakfast	139	27.2
	2.Lunch	125	24.5
	3.Snak	116	22.7
	4.Dinner	131	25.6
	Total	511	100
3	Special diet when Blood Glucose level is high		
	1.Yes	51	16.5
	2.No	259	83.5
	Total	310	100
4	Which type of diet?		
	1.Beso	18	35.3
	2.kollo	8	15.7
	3.shiferaw	10	19.6
	4.Sugar	15	29.4
	Total	51	100

Table 7: Patients' Dietary Adjustment for recommended foods to control DM among patients with diabetes in Dilla university referral hospital, 2014.

S.No	Variable	Frequency	%
1	Do You receive information about DM		
	1.Yes	83	26.8
	2.No	224	72.3
	3.Not sure	3	1
	Total	310	100
2	If yes, what is the Topic		
	1.About Foot Care	58	28.7
	2.About diet	78	38.6
	3.About Physical exercise	66	32.7
	4.Total	202	100
3	Reason for not received information on DM		
	1. No HE about DM	161	64.1
	2. Busy schedule of health care provider	57	22.7
	1. un readiness of health care provider to provide information	33	13.4
	Total	251	100
4	Which Topic is more clear for You		
	1.About foot care	54	22
	2.About diet	72	29.4
	3.About Exercise	58	23.7
	4.About drug intake	61	24.9
	Total	245	100

Table 8: Patients' received Health information about DM among patients with diabetes in Dilla university referral hospital, 2014.

formal health education on DM. The available scientific knowledge concerning diabetes mellitus is an important resource to guide and educate diabetes patients concerning self-care. Self-care concepts that can benefit patients include adherence to diet, physical activity, blood glucose monitoring, and taking oral medication and insulin. For those among Surveyed patients, 78 (38.8%) had been received information about diet followed by exercise 66 (32.7%) during their diagnosis. Among those who had not received information concerning self-care and information about DM, the most commonly mentioned reasons were unavailability of health education which accounted 161 (64.1%) followed by busy Schedule of health care provider which accounted 57(22.7%) (Table 8).

Discussion

This study has tried to assess diabetic patient perception on diabetic disease and self-care practice in Dilla university referral hospital, South Ethiopia. This study revealed that 79.4% of them were knowledgeable about diabetes this finding is consistent with a study done in Bangladesh (75 %) (38). whereas the finding from Harer is incomparable to our study where (93.7%) is knowledgeable about DM this might be because of health education/information given in our study area is only 59 (19%) (39). Contrary to this Scenario study from Egypt finding show that (90%) were poor knowledgeable about diabetes. With regard to knowledge on DM symptoms and diabetes self-care practices, 52.1% and 69.1% of them were knowledgeable on DM symptoms and diabetes self-care practices respectively but this finding was incongruent with a study done in Harer (88.3% and 93.2%) regarding knowledgeable on DM symptoms and diabetes self-care practices respectively. The cause for the discrepancy may be the same with knowledge gap created between Harer and our study area with similar pattern self-care result is lower in our study area than the studies done in Sewden 56%.

This means that health care setting, communities, service providers and patients with diabetes should work together to manage the disease. This finding is consistent to qualitative finds according to one in-depth interview respondents said that "We need to be work holistically and work hand in hand with one another as a health team". This approach helps to explores patients' understanding of the disease, treatment options and self-care practice. Successful chronic disease management is dependent on effective, systematic and interactive communication between patients and service providers as well as the health system with which they make contact.

In this study patient showed understanding of the causes and complications of the disease and most of (78.1%) them developed positive perception towards DM. However this finding differs where a study conducted in United Arab Emirates (72%) had a negative attitude towards having diabetes [12]. Finding from United Arab Emirates is supported by our qualitative study according to respondent from in-depth result one female participant said that "DM patient always ask themselves the following questions after the diagnosis: Why me? What am I going to eat? What are the people going to say about me? Where will I get money to buy food?" This question that comes to the mind of patient may make a patent to perceive negatively. It is therefore that patients should be encouraged to understand the meaning of chronic disease and its management. This means that Patients with positive beliefs will have positive attitudes towards behavioral change and will be motivated to comply, and those with negative will be less motivated and will resist behavior change. In this study individuals who were positive perception towards diabetes disease were 2.7 times more likely to perform recommended self-care than negative perception (OR-2.74, 95% CI (1.27, 5.91). Similarly a study conducted in Jimma university hospital Patients with high perceived severity of the disease was more likely to adhere to self-care practice [13].

The available scientific knowledge and perception concerning diabetes mellitus is an important resource to guide and educate diabetes patients concerning self-care. Self-care concepts that can benefit patients include adherence to diet, physical activity, blood glucose monitoring and taking oral medication and insulin [6,7]. In the current study, 238 (76.8%) of them had good practiced on the recommended self-care practices. Among the recommended self-care behaviors, drug adherence 289 (93.2%), dietary intake 154 (49.7%) and regular exercise 138 (44.5%) were the most practiced recommended self-care. On the other hand, self-blood glucose monitoring was the least practiced which accounted 62 (20%). In this study, the recommended self-care practice was higher (76.8%) where compare to a study conducted in Harer (39.2%) and in United Arab Emirates (37.7%). With regarded to specific recommended self-care practices, dietary intake 154 (49.7%) and regular exercise 138 (44.5%) were less likely practiced with compare to a study conducted in Harer [12,14]. In this study there was a consistence finding from in-depth interview according to one female DM patient she said that "some patients knew about the recommended food practices, but because of socio-economic barriers (lack of finances) were unable to acquire the right kind of food. Some of the challenges to dietary adherence involve avoiding favorite foods, selecting healthful alternatives, time management (patients find it difficult to plan food with insulin or oral medication) and social support (as most women prepare food for their families).

For successful diabetes management individuals should pay more attention for knowledge on the recommended self-care practices. The gain of knowledge on management of diabetes is to help patients to make life skill changes and offer the support needed to achieve optimal health [15]. In line with in the current study patients who were knowledgeable on DM self-care 6.52 were times more likely performed recommended self-care (OR-6.52, 95% CI (2.88, 14.78) than patients who were low knowledgeable on DM self-care. This finding was supported the studies conducted in Bangladesh and United Arab Emirates knowledge was significant independent predictors of good practice (OR- 1.28 (95% CI: 1.03 to 1.60) and (r = 0.320, p, 0.001) respectively (38, 55). However, in this study diabetic patients who were knowledgeable on DM were 0.3 times less likely performed recommended self-care to manage the disease (OR-0.29, 95% CI (0.10, 0.80).

On the other hand, individuals with educational level of grade 9-12 and higher educational status were more likely to adhere on self-care practice than patients who were illiterate (OR-3.96, 95% CI (1.25, 12.55)) and[OR-3.45, 95% CI (1.16, 10.29)] respectively. Similar results were found in other studies in Harer, and Egypt [14,16] educational statuses were more likely to adhere on self-care practice.

However in the current study patients with less frequent information received on DM did not show significant relation with self-care practice to control DM, but a study conducted in Harer, patients with less frequent information received were less likely performed self-care (OR-0.3, 95% CI (0.09, 0.79). This finding was strongly support in-depth interview he said that "There was the problem of limited time for consultation with the health profession was seen as one of the possible problems that could contribute to patients being non-adherent in their management. Another participants expressed the view that 'we need a patient-centered approach health care providers can give care that is more effective over time".

In this study, several explanations were possible for the fact that respondents had knowledge of DM but inappropriate self-care practices. The results of this study encourage a positive outlook for requiring a diabetes education during every visit and counseling that have an impact in improving the perception about disease, knowledge on DM, Self-care practice that include adherence to diet, physical activity, blood glucose monitoring and taking medication. This is supported with in-depth findings; "one participant said that Patients need to be encouraged always to 'think out of the box' in order to discourage them from negative thoughts. 'Patients need to cut down their food portions, they also need to exercise; but they need to know what is regarded as sufficient exercise or physical activity and how much is sufficient".

Limitations

The finding of this study may be interpreted with caution as it is facility –based which may produce more. Self-reported about self-care practice, self-reported dietary habits.

Conclusion

In this study (78.1%) diabetic patients were developed positive perception towards DM and has a significant effect for patients with diabetes to provide own self-care practice. Two third, 238 (76.8%) of them had good practiced on the recommended self-care practices. Among the recommended self-care behaviors, drug adherence 289 (93.2%), dietary intake 154 (49.7%) and regular exercise 138 (44.5%) were the most practiced recommended self-care. Self-blood glucose monitoring was the least practiced which accounted 62 (20%). Majority 79.4% of the respondents were knowledgeable about diabetes, but those diabetic patients who were knowledgeable on DM were less likely performed recommended self-care to manage the disease. On other hand those diabetic patients who were knowledgeable on DM self-care were more likely performed recommended self-care. Education also has a significant effect for patients with diabetes in order to provide own self-care practice. From this study we can also conclude that income level, perception towards DM and patients who received information were more likely to adhere to self-care practice of SMBG. This finding also showed that duration of DM and knowledgeable about diabetes has significant statistical effect on self-care behavior of physical exercise. Patient's income also another determining factor for diabetes self-care practices of diet adjustment. Patients with regularly received information and duration of DM were more likely to adhere to self-care practice of diet adjustment. Lastly A major point to address therefore is regular access to/contact with diabetic educators which currently is severely substandard.

References

1. Lawal M (2008) Management of diabetes mellitus in clinical practice. Br J Nurs 17: 1106-1113.

2. American Diabetic Association (2008) Standard of medical care in diabetes. Diabetes care 31:43.

3. Mensing C, Boucher J, Cypress M, Weinger K, Mulcahy K, et al. (2005) National standards for diabetes self-management education. Diabetes Care 28 Suppl 1: S72-79.

4. Lin C, Anderson R, Hagerty B, Lee B (2007) Diabetes self management experience among Taiwanese patients with type two diabetes mellitus. J Clin Nurs 9: 1-3.

5. Tan MY, Magarey J (2008) Self-care practices of Malaysian adults with diabetes and sub-optimal glycaemic control. Patient Educ Couns 72: 252-267.

6. WHO (2003) Diabetes estimates and projection. Geneva.

7. WHO (2005) World Health Organization Health Action in Crises, Ethiopia Strategy Paper.

8. Lester FT (1991) Clinical status of Ethiopian diabetic patients after 20 years of diabetes. Diabet Med 8: 272-276.

9. Feleke Y, Enquselassie F (2005) An assessment of the health care system for diabetes in Addis Ababa. Ethiop J Health dev 19: 203-210.

10. Peyrot M, Rubin RR, Lauritzen T, Snoek FJ, Matthews DR, et al. (2005) Psychosocial problems and barriers to improved diabetes management: results of the Cross-National Diabetes Attitudes, Wishes and Needs (DAWN) Study. Diabet Med 22: 1379-1385.

11. Harris MI, Klein R, Welborn TA, Knuiman MW (1992) Onset of NIDDM occurs at least 4-7 yr before clinical diagnosis. Diabetes Care 15: 815-819.

12. Mshunqane N, Stewart AV, Rothberg AD (2012) Type 2 diabetes management: Patient knowledge and health care team perceptions, South Africa. Afr J Prm Health Care Fam Med. 4: 7.

13. Lawal M (2008) Management of diabetes mellitus in clinical practice. Br J Nurs 17: 1106-1113.

14. Gillibrand R, Stevenson J (2006) The extended health belief model applied to the experience of diabetes in young people. Br J Health Psychol 11: 155-169.

15

Correlation between CMV Infection and NODAT

Dedinská I[1], Stančík M[2]*, Laca L[1], Miklušica J[1], Kantárová D[2], Ulinako J[3], Janek J[4], Galajda P[2] and Mokáň M[2]

[1]Surgery Clinic and Transplant Center, University Hospital Martin and Jessenius Faculty of Medicine, Comenius University, Slovak Republic
[2]Clinic of Internal Medicine I, University Hospital Martin and Jessenius Faculty of Medicine, Comenius University, Slovak Republic
[3]Department of Plastic Surgery, F.D.Roosevelt's Faculty Hospital in Banská Bystrica, Slovak Republic
[4]Department of Vascular Surgery, F.D.Roosevelt's Faculty Hospital in Banská Bystrica, Slovak Republic

Abstract

Purpose: New-onset diabetes mellitus after transplantation (NODAT) is a well-known complication of transplantation.

Materials and methods: Retrospectively, we detected CMV replication (PCR) in every month after transplantation of kidney in the first 12 months after transplantation in patients in a homogenous group from the aspect of immunosuppresion.

Results: In the group of 167 patients (control group: n = 103, NODAT group: n = 64), the average value of CMV viremia was without any significant difference between the NODAT group and the control group (P = 0.9285). In the 10th month after kidney transplantation, we recorded significantly higher CMV viremia in the NODAT group (p < 0.0001), however, in the multi variant analysis, that difference was not confirmed. Thus, in our group, CMV is of no relevance with the development of NODAT in the monitored period. The survival of patients and graft was 12 months after kidney transplantation without any statistically significant difference between the monitored groups (P = 0.6113 - survival of the patient; P = 0.5381 – survival of the graft).

Conclusion: Our analysis shows that in regular monitoring of CMV viremia and applying chemoprophylaxison the risk recipeints, CMV is not the risk factor for NODAT.

Keywords: Cytomegalovirus; New-onset diabetes after transplantation; Kidney transplantation; Chemoprophylaxis; Immunosuppressive drugs

Introduction

New-onset diabetes mellitus after transplantation (NODAT) is a well-known complication of transplantation and its development is associated with lower graft function and survival and reduced long-term patient survival mainly because of cardiovascular events [1-3]. Kidney transplant recipients who develop NODAT have variably been reported to be at increased risk of fatal and nonfatal cardiovascular events and other adverse outcomes including infection, reduced patient survival, graft rejection, and accelerated graft loss compared with those who do not develop diabetes. Identification of high-risk patients and implementation of measures to reduce the development of NODAT may improve the long-term patient and graft outcome [4]. In 2003, the International Expert Panel consisting of experts from both the transplant and diabetes fields set forth the International Consensus Guidelines for the diagnosis and management of NODAT [5,6]. It was recommended that the definition and diagnosis of NODAT should be based on the definition of diabetes mellitus and impaired glucose tolerance (IGT) described by the World Health Organization (WHO) [6,7]. The American Diabetes Association (ADA) guidelines for the diagnosis diabetes mellitus are provided in Table 1 [4].

Cytomegalovirus (CMV) is one of the most important infections in renal transplant recipients [8-12]. Exposure to the virus, as indicated by presence of detectable immunoglobulin G (IgG) anti-CMV antibodies in the plasma, increases with age in the general population and is present in more than two-thirds of donors and recipients prior to transplantation [8]. It is therefore common for the donor and/or recipient to be CMV-positive at the time of transplantation.

CMV can be transmitted from the donor either by blood transfusion or by the transplanted kidney; the concurrent administration of immunosuppressive drugs to prevent rejection further increases the risk of clinically relevant CMV disease, with induction therapy principally

being associated with an increased risk of disease [13,14]. Thus, both the recipient and the donor are routinely tested for anti-CMV antibodies prior to transplantation. CMV disease may manifest as a nonspecific febrile syndrome (e.g. fever, leukopenia, and atypical lymphocytosis) or tissue-invasive infections (e.g. hepatitis, pneumonitis, and enteritis). Tissue-invasive CMV disease is defined as CMV disease and CMV detected in tissue with histology, NAT or culture [15].

The link between cytomegalovirus (CMV) infection and the development of NODAT was first reported in 1985 in a renal transplant recipient [16]. Limited studies suggested that both asymptomatic CMV infection and CMV disease are independent risk factors for the development of NODAT. In a study consisting of 160 consecutive non-diabetic renal transplant recipients who were prospectively monitored for CMV infection during the first three months after transplantation, Hjelmesaeth and colleagues found that asymptomatic CMV infection was associated with a four-fold increased risk of new-onset diabetes (adjusted RR = 4.00; p = 0.025) [17]. Patients with active CMV infection had significantly lower median insulin release compared to their CMV negative counterparts, suggesting that the impaired pancreatic β

Diagnostic criteria for diabetes mellitus
symptoms of diabetes mellitus: polyuria, polydipsia, unexplained weight loss
or
fasting blood glucose ≥ 7 mmol/l
or
glycemia in the 2nd hour of oGTT ≥ 11.1 mmol/l

Table 1: ADA diagnostic criteria for diabetes mellitus.

*Corresponding author: Dr. Matej Stančík, Clinic of Internal Medicine I, University Hospital Martin and Jessenius Faculty of Medicine, Comenius University, Slovak Republic. E-mail: matej_stancik@hotmail.com

cell insulin release may be involved in the pathogenic mechanism of CMV-associated NODAT. It is speculated that CMV-induced release of proinflammatory cytokines may lead to apoptosis and functional disturbances of pancreatic β-cells [18]. Randomized controlled trials have demonstrated that the incidence of CMV disease can be reduced by prophylaxis and preemptive therapies in solid-organ transplant recipients [19-21].

According to the recommendations of KDIGO, CMV chemoprophylaxis is indicated (except when donor and recipientboth have negative CMV serologies) by applying the oral ganciclovir or valganciclovir for the period of minimum 3 month after kidney transplantation and for the period of 6 weeks after the kidney transplantationin case of T-cell-depleting antibody therapy [15].

In our department, we apply chemoprophylaxis (valganciclovir) in case of seronegative recipient or seropositive donor (R+/D-) 100 days after transplantation. In case of applying antithymocyte globulin, we apply the prophylaxis for the period of 6 weeks. However, CMV viremia (by using the polymerase chain reaction – PCR) is monitored regularly in all recipients, except for R+/D-, as follows: the first 6 months after transplantation every 2 weeks, and from the 6th – 12th month after transplantation 1x per month.

Materials and Methods

In the retrospective analysis, we monitored CMV viremia as the risk factor for NODAT in the group of patients who underwent primary transplantation of kidney from a deceased donor in the Transplantation Center in Martin in the years 2009-2013. The patients with diabetes mellitus type 1 and 2 and the patients who had not finished 12 months from kidney transplantation were excluded from monitoring. The patients who had the mTOR inhibitor or cyclosporin A in their immunosuppresive regime were also excluded from monitoring because of prevent of results distortion by immunosuppression. In each patient, we recorded the age at the time of transplantation, sex, we identified recipients with risky HLA for NODAT and with polycystic kidney diseases, we recorded the number of HLA mismatches and the type of donor (ECD). In each patient, we identified CMV viremia (by PCR) as customary in our department: 2x per month during the first 6 months from kidney transplantation and 1x per month from the 6th- 12th month after kidney transplantation. Retrospectively, we identified the patients who had a symptomatic CMV disease in the monitored period. The patients were divided into two sub-groups according to the development of NODAT in the monitored period – the control group and the NODAT group. NODAT was diagnosed in a standard way according to the ADA criteria. The groups were compared from the aspect of development of NODAT and CMV viremia during the entire monitored period, during the first 6 months after transplantation and the next following 6 months after transplantation, and we also compared CMV viremia in every month after kidney transplantation. In the end, we compared the function of the graft 1 year after kidney transplantation (by the estimate of glomerular filtration - eGFR by applying the CKD-EPI creat 2009 formula) and we compared the 12-month survival of the graft (censored for death) and the patients. By the correlation coefficient, we identified whether CMV viremia affects the function of the graft 12 months after kidney transplantation. All risk patients in the monitored group, i.e. the seronegative recipients who received the organ from a seropositive donor and the recipients who received the T-cell-depleting antibody were administered chemoprohylaxis. In case of a seronegative recipient, it was 100 days from kidney transplantation and in case of the T-cell-depleting antibody, it was 6 weeks from administration.

We used a certified statistical program MedCalc version 13. 1. 2. for statistical evaluation and we used the following statistical analyses: Student's t-test, chi-square test, correlation coefficient, Logistic regression, Cox proportional hazard model, Kaplan-Meier curves of survival. We consider the value p < 0.05 to be statistically significant.

Results

The group was composed of 167 patients, including 103 (61.7%) patients who were included in the control group and 64 (38.3%) patients in the group with development of NODAT in the monitored period. The average level of tacrolimus (during the monitored 12 months from kidney transplantation) was in both groups without any statistically significant difference (P = 0.5592), and similarly was the average dose of prednisone/day (P = 0.0877). The average dose of mycophenolate mofetil/dayor mycophenolate sodium was also without any statistically significant difference between the monitored groups (P = 0.0919 – mycophenolate mofetil and P = 0.1734 – mycophenolate sodium). In view of that, both groups were homogenous from the aspect of the applied immunosuppression, and the individual monitored parameters were not distorted by the applied immunosuppresion (Table 2). The characteristics of the group are given in Table 3. The patients in the NODAT group were significantly older than the patients in the control group, and during the monitored 12 months, the patients in the NODAT group received a statistically significant higher dose of methylprednisolone. However, in the multivariant analysis, the dose of methylprednisolone as an independent risk factor for NODAT was not identified (Table 4). Average methylprednisolone dose correlated with the incidence of acute rejection [r = 0.2614; 95 % CI for r = 0.06098-0.4416 (P = 0.0114)], but CMV replication was not linked to the average

	Control group n = 103	NODAT group n = 64	p value
Average level of TAC (ng/ml)	4.7 ± 0.9	4.8 ± 1.2	0.5592
Average dose of prednisone/day (mg)	8.2 ± 2.3	8.8 ± 2.0	0.0877
Average dose of MMF/day (mg)	849.4 ± 264.2	911.7 ± 175.4	0.0919
Average dose of mycophenolate sodium/day (mg)	670.7 ± 292	721.9 ±113	0.1734

TAC – Tacrolimus; MMF – Mycophenolate Mofetil

Table 2: Comparison of the control group versus NODAT from the aspect of immunosuppression.

	Control group n = 103	NODAT group n = 64	p value
Age at the time of transplantation (years)	**43 ± 12.1**	**50.5 ± 9.6**	**<0.0001**
Males (%)	62.1	59.4	0.8627
HLA A30 (%)	2.9	0	0.4375
HLA B27 (%)	9.6	10.9	0.9937
HLA B42 (%)	1	0	0.8335
Average number of HLA mismatches	3.5 ± 1.2	3.7 ± 1.4	0.3266
APKD (%)	10.4	17.2	0.2839
ECD donor (%)	17.3	21.9	0.5926
Pulse therapy by methylprednisolone (%) except for induction	36.4	34.9	0.9792
average dose of (g) except for induction	**2.0 ± 0.7**	**2.3 ± 0.7**	**0.0086**
CMV replication (%)	45.8	45.2	0.9286
Average number of copies (cop/ml)	3500	3800	0.9763

DM2 – Diabetes Mellitus Type 2; APKD – Polycystic Kidney Disease; ECD – Extended Criteria Donor; CMV – Cytomegalovirus

Table 3: Characteristics of the group – univariant analysis.

	Hazard ratio	CI 95 %	p value
Age at the time of transplantation < 30 years	0.3065	0.08262-1.1363	0.0769
Age at the time of transplantation 30-39 years	0.5000	0.0526-4.7518	0.5714
Age at the time of transplantation 40-49 years	0.7000	0.4292-1.1416	0.1529
Age at the time of transplantation 50-59 years	1.1376	1.0437-1.2399	0.0034
Age at the time of transplantation ≥ 60 years	2.5038	1.7179-3.6492	<0.0001
Pulse therapy by methylprednisolone (yes/no)	2.6024	0.7415-9.1334	0.1354
Average dose of (g) except for induction	1.1026	0.7115-1.7086	0.6622
DM2 – Diabetes Mellitus Type 2			

Table 4: Characteristics of the group– multivariant analysis.

methylprednisolone dose [r = 0.1633; 95 % CI for r = -0.0462-0.3542 (P = 0.1157)].

The average value of the CMV viremia (cop/ml) in the NODAT group and in the control group was without any statistically significant difference. We compared replication of CMV in the first 6 months after kidney transplantation with replication during the second half-year after transplantation, and we recorded in both groups significantly higher replication of CMV infection in the first half-year after transplantation. However, upon comparing the control group versus the NODAT group, no difference in replication in the first and in the second half-year after kidney transplantation was recorded (Figures 1-4).

CMV viremia in individual months after kidney transplantation is presented in Table 5. In the 10th month after kidney transplantation, we recorded significantly higher CMV viremia in the NODAT group, however, such difference was not confirmed in the multivariant analysis (Tables 5 and 6). In view of the foregoing, in our group, CMV is of no relevance to development of NODAT in the monitored periodin

the first 12 months from kidney transplantation. We discovered that significantly more patients (70%) had diagnosed NODAT in the first 6 months after transplantation (P < 0.001) (Figure 5).

In the whole group, we identified the patients who developed the symptomatic form of CMV infection. In the whole group, it was only 6% patients. In the NODAT group, 10.9% patients had the symptomatic CMV infection, and in the control group it was 2.9% (0.0741).

The value of creatinine 12 months after transplantation was comparable in both groups, and also the eGFR (the limit of statistical significance) (Table 7). By the correlation coefficient we discovered that the higher number of copies CMV/ml worsens the function of the graft (characterized eGFR) 12 months after kidney transplantation (Figures 6 and 7).

Discussion

Many risk factors have been found to have influence on the development of NODAT. In 1985 Lehr et al. reported a case of cytomegalovirus (CMV) induced NODAT in a kidney recipient patient, after that the role of CMV infection in NODAT has been an area of interest to researchers [16]. Since then, other studies have supported [17,22] the relationship between them whilst other studies [23,24] have failed to prove this association. However, the influence of CMV infection on developing NODAT still remains a question. If the impact of CMV infection on higher incidence of NODAT is proven, initiating prophylaxis against CMV infection after transplantation will be strongly suggested [25]. In meta-analysis of authors Einollahi et al., it was discovered that the risk of NODAT in kidney transplants with CMV infection was 1.94 fold more as compared to individuals without CMV infection using adj ORs from the studies [26]. This significant relationship was proved by overall pooled OR using un-adj ORs. There was a difference in the result of evaluated studies in term of CMV induced NODAT. Though, three studies [27,28] reported no significant relationship between CMV infection and NODAT; other studies [17,23,29] detected CMV infection as the risk factor for NODAT. In

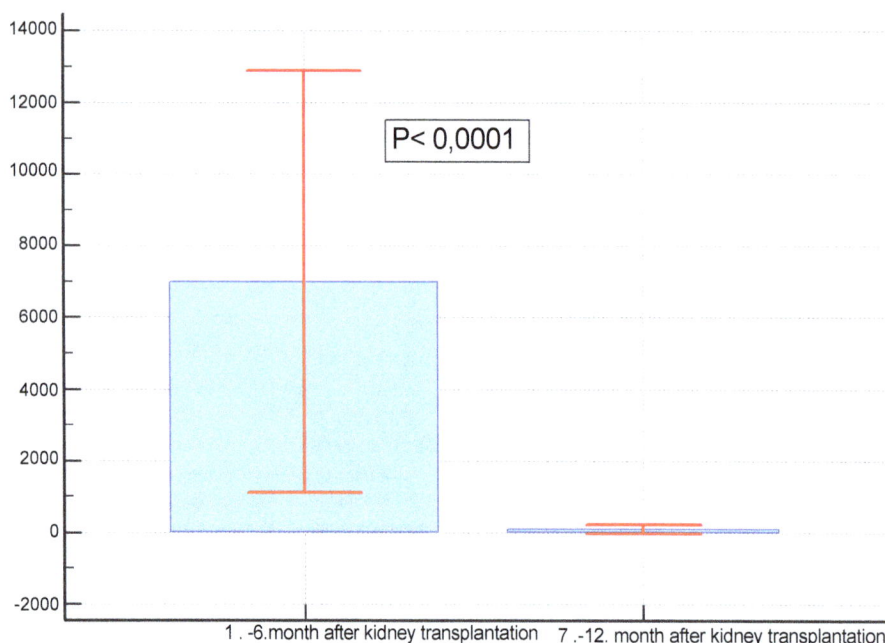

Figure 1: Replication of CMV 1st – 6th month versus 7th – 12th month after kidney transplantation – control group.

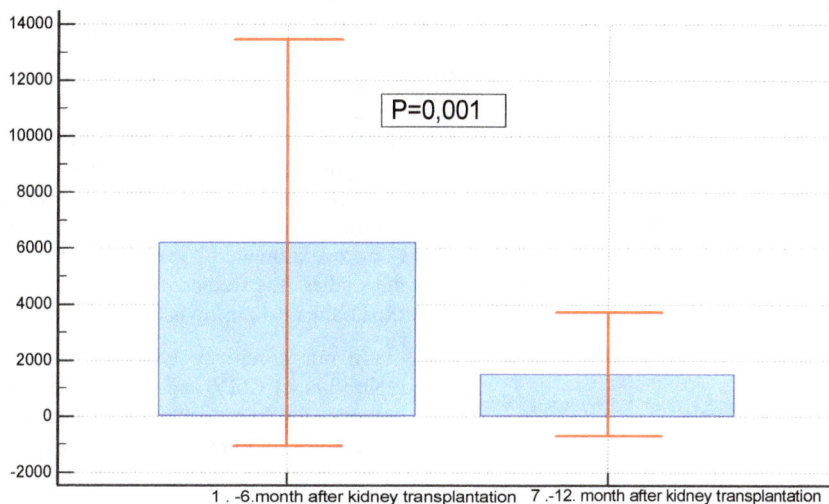

Figure 2: Replication of CMV 1st – 6th month versus 7th – 12th month after kidney transplantation – NODAT group.

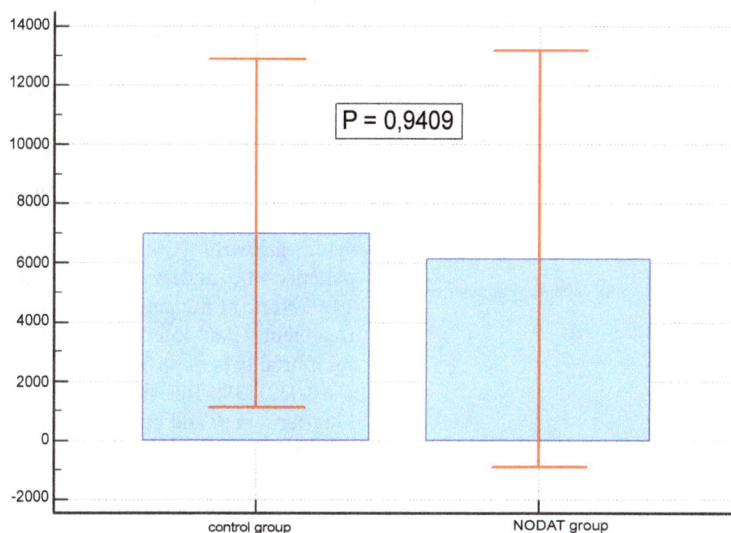

Figure 3: Replication of CMV 1st – 6th month after kidney transplantation: control group versus NODAT group.

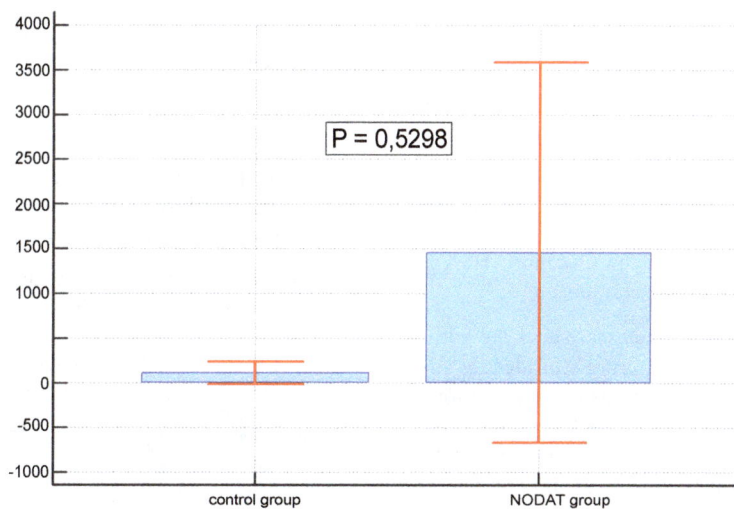

Figure 4: Replication of CMV 7th – 12th month after kidney transplantation: control group versus NODAT group.

Months after transplantation	control group (n=103) CMV PCR (cop/ml)	NODAT group (n=64) CMV PCR (cop/ml)	p value
1	1177.1	0	0.3568
2	6489.6	24241.9	0.3281
3	26346	4975.8	0.3080
4	4578.9	6770.9	0.6551
5	659.4	601.6	0.9007
6	2729.2	270.9	0.2195
7	52.1	2233.9	0.2138
8	338.5	250	0.8397
9	0	41.9	0.0858
10	**104.2**	**48256.6**	**<0.0001**
11	177.1	16.1	0.4674
12	0	48.4	0.4382

Table 5: CMV replication – individual months after kidney transplantation (univariant analysis).

Months after transplantation	Odds ratio	95% CI	p value
1	0.9990	0.6843-1.4582	0.9957
2	1.0000	1.0000-1.0000	0.5884
3	1.0000	1.0000-1.0000	0.1969
4	1.0000	1.0000-1.0000	0.8043
5	1.0001	0.9999-1.0003	0.3769
6	0.9999	0.9998-1.0001	0.3515
7	1.0000	0.9999-1.0001	0.5512
8	0.9999	0.9994-1.0003	0.6266
9	1.0210	0.0000-24969.8938	0.9968
10	1.0000	1.0000-1.0001	0.6025
11	0.9989	0.3234-3.0852	0.9985
12	1.0066	0.0031-328.3802	0.9982

Table 6: CMV replication – individual months after kidney transplantation (multivariant analysis).

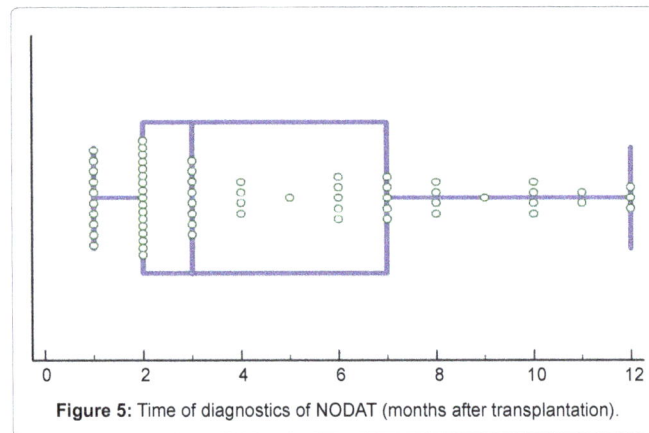

Figure 5: Time of diagnostics of NODAT (months after transplantation).

addition, Valderhaug et al. [30] only found the relationship between CMV infection and NODAT in univariate analysis whilst a multivariate analysis, adjusted for age, prednisolone, type of cohort, HLA-B27 phenotype and BMI did not support this association.

According to the above mentioned metaanalysis of the authors Einollahi et al., the studies used different criteria to identify CMV infection. Isolation of the CMV virus and detection of viral proteins or nucleic acid are different ways to recognize CMV infection [27]. In addition, active systemic CMV infection can be diagnosed as CMV-DNA in plasma by polymerase chain reaction methods or by detection of CMV-antigenemia in leucocytes (i.e., CMVpp65) (18). Four from seven works in analysis did not report a criterion for identifying CMV

infection [22,27-29]. Three remaining studies used different criterion to recognize CMV infection; Hjelmesaeth et al. [17] defined CMV infection as one or more CMV pp65 antigen-positive cells per 100.000 leucocytes, Marin et al. [24] defined it as more than 50 infected cells per 200,000 leucocytes using the pp65 assay or isolation of CMV antigenemia or fourfold increase in the baseline IgG and Valderhaug et al. [30] diagnosed it by CMV-pp65 antigen in leucocytes or CMV-DNA in plasma, but they did not report any details. Thus using various criteria and methods with different sensitivity and specificity can lead to an overestimate or may in fact underestimate CMV infection in the studies. The studies which determine CMV viremia by PCR may expain the relationship between CMV and NODAT.

In our group, we had not detected any relationship between replication of CMV and development of NODAT. The group was homogenous from the aspect of immunosuppresion. The results of our analysis and the low occurrence of symptomatic CMV infection is, in our opinion, related to the intensive monitoring of CMV viremia (PCR) after transplantation (the first 6 months, CMV viremiais determined every 1 month, in the second half-year every 6 weeks). In the risk patients (seronegative donor and seropositive recipient), we monitor CMV viremia also in the second year after transplantation, every 2 months. The patients who were treated by T-cell-depleting antibody, have in our center monitored CMV viremia every 1 month for 3 months after the end of therapy. All recipients with the increased risk of CMV infection were administered chemoprophylaxis according to the KDIGO recommendations of 2009 [15].

Prospective observational cohort study of authors Smedbråten et al. is an extension of the previous study reporting effects of cytomegalovirus (CMV) on the graft and patient survival in 471 patients who underwent kidney transplantation between 1994 and 1997. None of the patients received CMV prophylaxis or preemptive treatment. CMV infection was an independent significant risk factor for mortality in multivariate analysis (HR = 1.453, 95% CI 1.033–2.045, p = 0.032) [31]. This observed association between CMV infection and long-term graft and patient outcome may be altered by prophylaxis or preemptive CMV therapy. In a study by Kliem et al., oral ganciclovir prophylaxis was compared to intravenous preemptive CMV therapy [32]. Compared to preemptive therapy, prophylaxis was found to be significantly associated with improved long-term (4 yr) uncensored graft survival, with the greatest benefit observed in the donor +/recipient + CMV serostatus group. Moreover, when analyzing the death-censored graft survival, prophylaxis significantly improved graft survival in the donor +/recipient + CMV serostatus group. Opelz et al. reported from analyses of register data that CMV prophylaxis was significantly associated with improved graft survival both censored and uncensored for death; but in both cases only in the donor +/recipient – CMV serostatus group [33]. In our group, we identified relationship between CMV viremia and function of the graft 12 months after kidney transplantation. With the increasing number of CMV copies/ml, eGFR is worsened one year after kidney transplantation.

CMV replication after transplantation may contribute to reduced graft function and survival through the associated inflammation and

	Control group n = 103	NODAT group n = 64	p value
Creatinine 12 months after transplantation (μmol/l)	139.4 ± 38.1	140.1 ± 43.6	0.9144
eGFR 12 months after transplantation (ml/min)	51 ± 14.4	46.8 ± 13.2	0.0635

Table 7: Comparison of function of the graft (creatinine and eGFR) 12 months after transplantation.

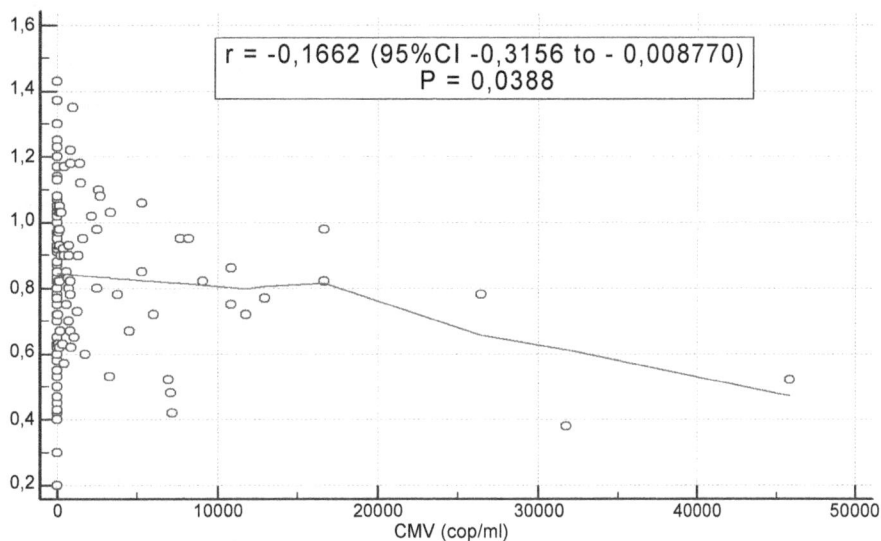

Figure 6: Correlation between CMV and eGFR (CKD-EPI) 12 months after kidney transplantation.

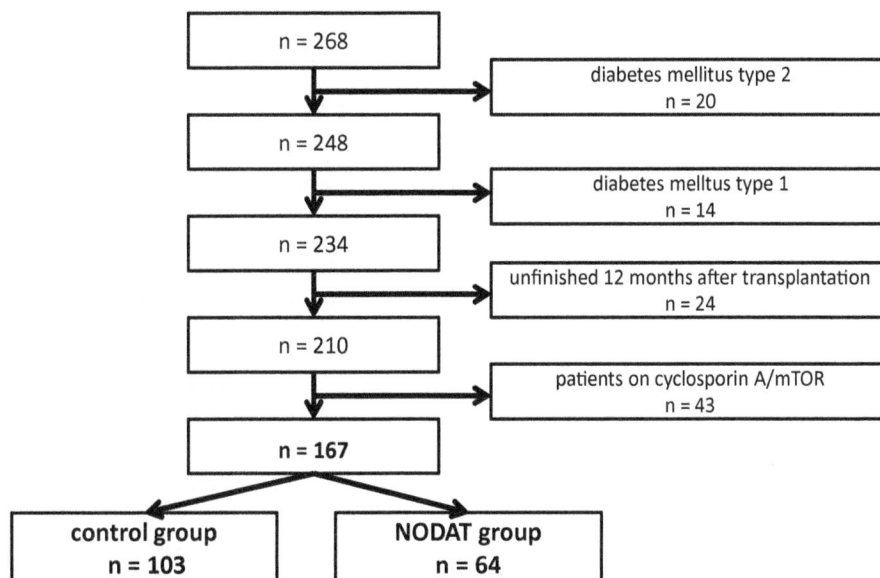

Figure 7: Selection of patients for the analysis.

cytokine release [34]. Uncontrolled replication of CMV triggers direct and/or indirect effect in transplant recipients [35]. When CMV is reactivated under immunosuppressive conditions, it has both direct effects, such as development of CMV disease, and indirect effects on transplantation, including increased incidence of allograft rejection [36].

In our study, survival of the patients (censored for death) as well as survival of the graft is numerically worse in the NODAT group, no statistically significant difference was confirmed. We assume that the survival of patients with NODAT is significantly worse from the long-term aspect (10 and more years). Intensive monitoring of glycaemia and early diagnostics and treatment of NODAT, as well as check-up of the other affectable risk factors for NODAT are able to significantly improve survival of both the patients and the graft and to decrease the cardiovascular mortality and morbidity.

Conclusion

Our analysis suggests that by regular monitoring of CMV viremia and applying chemoprophylaxis for risk recipients (in our case, seropositive donor/seronegative recipient or recipient after T-cell-depleting antibody therapy) is not the CMV risk factor for NODAT. The results of the analysis (or CMV viremia or development of NODAT) are not distorted by the administered immunosuppressive treatment – from the aspect of immunosuppression, the group was homogenous. Regular monitoring of CMV viremia and chemoprophylaxis may affect not only development of NODAT, but it is possible (as in our group) to eliminate the number of patients with symptomatic CMV infection. Frequent monitoring of CMV viremia may increase the costs on care about the recipient after kidney transplantation, however, we eventually decrease the costs on treatment of later complications arising from CMV infection. In the patients after kidney transplantation, the most important risk factor for NODAT is the age at the time of transplantation (more than 50 years of age), prediabetes before transplantation, positive family history of diabetes mellitus type 2, and the body mass index of more than 30 kg/sqm at the time of transplantation. Regular weight and waist circumference control in patients after kidney transplantation leads to identification of risk patients for NODAT. Screening of risk factors for diabetes mellitus should be done even before placing the patient on the waiting list and it is advisable to carry out the oral glucose tolerance test (oGTT) also in patients with physiological levels of fasting glycemia [37,38].

Funding

This paper was supported by VEGA grant 1/0160/16 Diagnostic - prognostic relevance of adipocytokine network and glucose homeostasis assessment in cachexia.

References

1. Hjelmesaeth J, Hartmann A, Leivestad T, Holdaas H, Sagedal S, et al. (2006) The impact of early-diagnosed new-onset post-transplantation diabetes mellitus on survival and major cardiac events. Kidney Int 69: 588-595.

2. Bee YM, Tan HC, Tay TL, Kee TY, Goh SY, et al. (2011) Incidence and risk factors for development of new-onset diabetes after kidney transplantation. Ann Acad Med Singapore 40: 160-167.

3. Cosio FG, Pesavento TE, Kim S, Osei K, Henry M, et al. (2002) Patient survival after renal transplantation: IV. Impact of post-transplant diabetes. Kidney Int 62: 1440-1446.

4. Pham PT, Pham PM, Pham SV, Pham PA, Pham PC (2011) New onset diabetes after transplantation (NODAT): an overview. Diabetes Metab Syndr Obes 4: 175-186.

5. Davidson J, Wilkinson A, Dantal J, Dotta F, Haller H, et al. (2003) New-onset diabetes after transplantation: 2003 International consensus guidelines. Proceedings of an international expert panel meeting. Barcelona, Spain, 19 February 2003. Transplantation 75: SS3-24.

6. Wilkinson A, Davidson J, Dotta F, Home PD, Keown P, et al. (2005) Guidelines for the treatment and management of new-onset diabetes after transplantation. Clin Transplant 19: 291-298.

7. Montori VM, Basu A, Erwin PJ, Velosa JA, Gabriel SE, et al. (2002) Posttransplantation diabetes: a systematic review of the literature. Diabetes Care 25: 583-592.

8. Rubin RH (1993) Infectious disease complications of renal transplantation. Kidney Int 44: 221-236.

9. Farrugia E, Schwab TR (1992) Management and prevention of cytomegalovirus infection after renal transplantation. Mayo Clin Proc 67: 879-890.

10. Brennan DC (2001) Cytomegalovirus in renal transplantation. J Am Soc Nephrol 12: 848-855.

11. Smith SR, Butterly DW, Alexander BD, Greenberg A (2001) Viral infections after renal transplantation. Am J Kidney Dis 37: 659-676.

12. Kotton CN, Fishman JA (2005) Viral infection in the renal transplant recipient. J Am Soc Nephrol 16: 1758-1774.

13. Büchler M, Hurault de Ligny B, Madec C, Lebranchu Y (2003) Induction therapy by anti-thymocyte globulin (rabbit) in renal transplantation: a 1-yr follow-up of safety and efficacy. Clin Transplant 17: 539-545.

14. Burke GW 3rd, Kaufman DB, Millis JM, Gaber AO, Johnson CP, et al. (2004) Prospective, randomized trial of the effect of antibody induction in simultaneous pancreas and kidney transplantation: three-year results. Transplantation 77: 1269-1275.

15. Kidney Disease: Improving Global Outcomes (KDIGO) Transplant Work Group (2009) KDIGO clinical practice guideline for the care of kidney transplant recipients. Am J Transplant 9: S1-155.

16. Lehr H, Jao S, Waltzer WC, Anaise D, Rapaport FT (1985) Cytomegalovirus-induced diabetes mellitus in a renal allograft recipient. Transplant Proc 17: 2152-2154.

17. Hjelmesaeth J, Sagedal S, Hartmann A, Rollag H, Egeland T, et al. (2004) Asymptomatic cytomegalovirus infection is associated with increased risk for new-onset diabetes and impaired insulin release after renal transplantation. Diabetologia 47: 1550-1556.

18. Hjelmesaeth J, Muller F, Jenssen T, Rollag H, Sagedal S, et al. (2005) Is there a link between cytomegalovirus infection and new-onset posttransplantation diabetes mellitus? Potential mechanisms of virus induced β-cell damage. Nephrol Dial Transplant 20: 2311-2315.

19. Hodson EM, Craig JC, Strippoli GF, Webster AC (2008) Antiviral medications for preventing cytomegalovirus disease in solid organ transplant recipients. Cochrane Database Syst Rev.

20. Hodson EM, Jones CA, Strippoli GF, Webster AC, Craig JC (2007) Immunoglobulins, vaccines or interferon for preventing cytomegalovirus disease in solid organ transplant recipients. Cochrane Database Syst Rev: CD005129.

21. Strippoli GF, Hodson EM, Jones C, Craig JC (2006) Preemptive treatment for cytomegalovirus viremia to prevent cytomegalovirus disease in solid organ transplant recipients. Transplantation 81: 139-145.

22. Hjelmesaeth J, Hartmann A, Kofstad J, Stenstrøm J, Leivestad T, et al. (1997) Glucose intolerance after renal transplantation depends upon prednisolone dose and recipient age. Transplantation 64: 979-983.

23. Sulanc E, Lane JT, Puumala SE, Groggel GC, Wrenshall LE, et al. (2005) New-onset diabetes after kidney transplantation: an application of 2003 International Guidelines. Transplantation 80: 945-952.

24. Marin M, Renoult E, Bondor CI, Kessler M (2005) Factors influencing the onset of diabetes mellitus after kidney transplantation: a single French center experience. Transplant Proc 37: 1851-1856.

25. Nemati E, Taheri S, Pourfarziani V, Einollahi B (2008) Cytomegalovirus disease in renal transplant recipients: an Iranian experience. Exp Clin Transplant 6: 132-136.

26. Einollahi B, Motalebi M, Salesi M, Ebrahimi M, Taghipour M (2014) The impact of cytomegalovirus infection on new-onset diabetes mellitus after kidney transplantation: a review on current findings. J Nephropathol 3: 139-148.

27. Madziarska K, Weyde W, Krajewska M, Patrzalek D, Janczak D, et al. (2011) The increased risk of post-transplant diabetes mellitus in peritoneal dialysis-treated kidney allograft recipients. Nephrol Dial Transplant 26: 1396-1401.

28. Numakura K, Satoh S, Tsuchiya N, Horikawa Y, Inoue T, et al. (2005) Clinical and genetic risk factors for posttransplant diabetes mellitus in adult renal transplant recipients treated with tacrolimus. Transplantation 80: 1419-1424.

29. Yang WC, Chen YS, Hsieh WC, Shih MH, Lee MC (2006) Post-transplant Diabetes Mellitus in Renal Transplant Recipients-Experience in Buddhist Tzu Chi General Hospital. Tzu Chi Med J 18: 185-191.

30. Valderhaug TG, Hjelmesaeth J, Rollag H, Leivestad T, Røislien J, et al. (2007) Reduced incidence of new-onset posttransplantation diabetes mellitus during the last decade. Transplantation 84: 1125-1130.

31. Smedbråten YV, Sagedal S, Leivestad T, Mjøen G, Osnes K, et al. (2014) The impact of early cytomegalovirus infection after kidney transplantation on long-term graft and patient survival. Clin Transplant 28: 120-126.

32. Kliem V, Fricke L, Wollbrink T, Burg M, Radermacher J, et al. (2008) Improvement in long-term renal graft survival due to CMV prophylaxis with oral ganciclovir: results of a randomized clinical trial. Am J Transplant 8: 975-983.

33. Opelz G, Döhler B, Ruhenstroth A (2004) Cytomegalovirus prophylaxis and graft outcome in solid organ transplantation: a collaborative transplant study report. Am J Transplant 4: 928-936.

34. Helanterä I, Loginov R, Koskinen P, Törnroth T, Grönhagen-Riska C, et al. (2005) Persistent cytomegalovirus infection is associated with increased expression of TGF-beta1. PDGF-AA and ICAM-1 and arterial intimal thickening in kidney allografts. Nephrol Dial Transplant 20: 790-796.

35. Helanterä I, Egli A, Koskinen P, Lautenschlager I, Hirsch HH (2010) Viral impact on long-term kidney graft function. Infect Dis Clin North Am 24: 339-371.

36. Ishibashi K, Tokumoto T, Shirakawa H, Oguro T, Yanagida T, et al. (2014) The presence of antibodies against the AD2 epitope of cytomegalovirus glycoprotein B is associated with acute rejection after renal transplantation. Microbiol Immunol 58: 72-75.

37. Zilinska Z, Chrastina M, Trebaticky B, Breza J Jr, Slobodnik L, et al. (2010) Vascular complications after renal transplantation. Bratisl Lek Listy 111: 586-589.

38. Dedinská I, Laca Ľ, Miklušica J, Rosenberger J, Žilinská Z, et al. (2015) Waist circumference as an independent risk factor for NODAT. Ann Transplant 20: 154-159.

16

Association of Deoxyribonuclease I Gene Polymorphisms with Graves' Disease

Jingyan Chen[1], Hua Zeng[2], Zhixian Zhang[2], Tingting Li[1], Lei Bi[2], Helin Ding[1#] and Jin Zhang[1*#]

[1]Department of Endocrinology, Sun Yat-Sen Memorial Hospital of Sun Yat-Sen University, Guangzhou, PR China
[2]Department of Clinical Laboratory, Sun Yat-Sen Memorial Hospital of Sun Yat-Sen University, Guangzhou, PR China
#Contributed equally to this work

Abstract

Background: This study aimed to investigate the association between the single nucleotide polymorphism (SNP) rs1053874 in the deoxyribonuclease I (DNASE1) gene and Graves' disease (GD) in the Han Chinese population.

Methods: Polymerase chain reaction-restriction fragment length polymorphism analysis and direct sequencing were used to identify the distribution of the SNP rs1053874 in the DNASE1 genes from 284 GD patients and 203 healthy controls, and associations between clinical manifestations of GD and the observed genotype and allele frequencies at the DNASE1 gene were analyzed.

Results: In the Han Chinese population, there were significant differences between the GD groups and the controls with respect to genotype and allele frequencies associated with theSNPrs1053874. The risk of GD was greater among carriers of the G allele than non-carriers (OR=0.65, 95% CI: 0.49- 0.86). There were significant differences in genotype and allele frequencies between the GD patients with a history of relapse and the GD patients without history of relapse; furthermore, the G allele of the SNP rs1053874 was associated with relapse in GD patients.

Conclusion: This study confirmed that the DNASE1 gene may be a GD susceptibility gene in the in the Southern Chinese Han population. The G allele at the rs1053874 SNP would be a direct genetic risk factor for GD in this population. Furthermore, this allele may be associated with disease relapse.

Keywords: Deoxyribonuclease I (DNASE1); Single nucleotide polymorphisms (SNPs); Graves' disease

Abbreviations: MAF: Minor Allele Frequency; RFLP: Restriction Fragment length polymorphism; SRED: Single Radial Enzyme Diffusion; cAMP: Cyclic Adenosine Monophosphate; CV: Coefficient of Variation; ELISA: Enzyme-Linked Immunosorbent Assay; GD: Graves' disease; Ig: immunoglobulin mRNA: Messenger Ribonucleic acid; OD: Optical Density; PCR: Polymerase Chain Reaction; qRT-PCR: Quality Real Time-Polymerase Chain Reaction; RA: Rheumatoid arthritis: SD: Standard Deviation; SLE: Systemic Lupus Erythematousdeviation; TSH: Thyrotropin; TGAb: Thyroglobulin Antibody; TPOAb: Thyroperoxidase Antibody; TRAb: TSH Receptor Antibody; TSH: thyroid-stimulating hormone; TSHR: Thyrotropin Teceptor; TSAb: Thyroid Stimulatory Antibodies; SNP: Single Nucleotide Polymorphism

Introduction

Graves' disease (GD), which is an autoimmune disease associated with the increased secretion of thyroid hormone, is the major cause of hyperthyroidism. Although the pathogenesis of GD has not been fully elucidated, it is known that genetic factors play an important role in the development of this disease [1]. The incidence of GD exhibits a clear pattern of familial aggregation; however, as a polygenic disease, GD does not follow a Mendelian pattern of inheritance. Genetic susceptibility to GD may be determined by the penetrance of a number of different genes; but the pathogenesis of GD may be affected by environmental factors [1].

Deoxyribonuclease I (DNase I; Enzyme Commission (EC) number 3.1.21.1) is the earliest discovered DNA hydrolase. Recent studies have found that DNase I is a multifunctional enzyme involved in cellular apoptosis, necrosis, and other relevant processes; this enzyme can also participate in the degradation of chromatin from ne- crotic cells [2].

DNase I is encoded by the DNASE1 gene, which is located on chromosome 16p13. 3. Many studies have demonstrated that polymorphisms in DNase I, which exist at both the gene and protein levels, are regulated by autosomal genes and are unrelated to sex chromosomes. To date, six alleles of DNASE1 (DNASE1*1–6) associated with enzyme polymorphisms have been identified; these alleles differ only by point mutations in single nucleotides in the coding region of the gene [3-5].

Among these polymorphisms, DNASE1*1 and DNASE1*2 are the two alleles that are most widely distributed in populations. The only difference between DNASE1*1 and DNASE1*2 is the single nucleotide polymorphism (SNP) rs10538746 in exon 8 of the DNASE1 gene [4]. Prior research [6] has not only revealed that DNase I exhibits reduced enzymatic activity and thermal stability in auto- immune thyroid disease (AITD) patients and their families but also that several SNPs may be associated with AITD pathogenesis. However, so far there is no other related research on the associations between DNASE1 polymorphisms and GD in Han Chinese populations. In this study, a case-control association study of the patients with GD and healthy controls was performed to analyze the distribution of a polymorphism in the DNASE1 gene in the Han Chinese population and the associations between this polymorphism and GD.

*Corresponding authors: Jin Zhang, Department of Endocrinology, Sun Yat-Sen Memorial Hospital of Sun Yat-Sen University, Guangzhou, PR China, E-mail: zhangjinchina@163.com

Helin Ding, Department of Clinical Laboratory, Sun Yat-Sen Memorial Hospital of Sun Yat-Sen University, Guangzhou, PR China, E-mail: dinghelin@aliyun.com

Materials and Methods

Study subjects

284 unrelated Han Chinese patients with GD were enrolled in this study. The study was conducted at the Department of Endocrinology in the Sun Yat-Sen Memorial Hospital of Sun Yat-Sen University. All GD patients were diagnosed on the basis of the clinical criteria and confirmed by thyroid function testing and thyroid antibody measurements. The clinical evaluation included the patient's history as well as the presence of typical symptoms and signs of hyperthyroidism. The laboratory diagnosis included elevated serum free triiodothyronine (FT3) and free thyroxine (FT4) concentrations, low or undetectable serum sensitive TSH (sTSH), and positive thyrotropin (TSH) receptor antibodies (TRAb). Meanwhile, goiter was assessed by experienced endocrinologists and confirmed by thyroid ultrasonography; Graves' ophthalmopathy (GO) was diagnosed by complete eye examination performed by experienced oph- thalmologists. The exclusion criteria were as follows: patients with other coexisting autoimmune diseases or other thyroid disease. There were 209 females (73.59%) and 75 males (26.41%), who ranged from 13–80 years of age, with a mean age of 39 years (29–50 years). The median disease duration was 1.5 years (1 month–40 years). Simultaneously, 203 healthy volunteers were recruited as the control subjects, which included 133 females (65.52%) and 70 males (34.48%). The exclusion criteria for the healthy controls were as follows: normal subjects with a history of thyroid or other autoimmune diseases and with abnormal thyroid function and autoantibodies [FT3, FT4, sTSH, thyroperoxidase antibodies (TPOAb), thyroglobulin antibodies (TGAb), or TRAb]. All study participants were unrelated Han Chinese individuals who resided in Guangdong Province in the southern region of China. Informed consent was obtained from all participants before the study samples were collected; the study protocol was approved by the Ethics Committee of Sun Yat-Sen Memorial Hospital of Sun Yat-Sen University and registered in the Chinese Clinical Trial Registry.

Clinical data collection and laboratory examinations

Baseline clinical and lab data for all subjects were collected. The medical histories of the GD patients were obtained, including gender, age, disease duration, family history, and history of GD relapse. Medical examinations were conducted to record patients' physical conditions conditions, including extent of goiter and ophthalmological parameters. In addition, peripheral blood samples from all subjects were collected by venipuncture in the fasting state in the morning for DNA extraction and biochemical markers. The serum FT3, FT4, sTSH, TGAb, and TPOAb were assayed by automated chemiluminescent immunoassays (Siemens ADVIA Centaur CP, MA, USA), and the serum TRAb was measured using a commercially available enzyme-linked immunosorbent assay (ELISA) kit (RSR Ltd., Cardiff, UK).

Detection of the rs1053874 SNP

A whole blood genomic DNA extraction kit (Omega Bio-Tek, GA, US) was used to extract genomic DNA from 0.25 ml samples of peripheral venous blood containing an anticoagulant. Polymerase chain reaction (PCR) was used to amplify target fragments. PCR primers for rs1053874 were designed by PRIMER 5.0 software (Microsoft Corp, PREMIER Biosoft International) and were synthesized by Sangon Biotech (Sangon Biotech CO. LTD, Shanghai, China) [8]. The upstream primer was 5'-ATCGTGGTTGCAGGGATGCTGCCTC-3', and the downstream primer was 5'-AGTTCAACAGGTGTGGGGAG-3'.

For each PCR amplification, the reaction system, which consisted of a total volume of 25 μl, contained 150 ng of DNA template, 2.5 pmol of each upstream and downstream primer, 500 μM of deoxyribonucleotide triphosphate (dNTP) mix, 12.5 μl of 2 ×GC Buffer I (including $MgCl_2$), and 1 U of Taq Hot Start enzyme. The following PCR conditions were utilized: an initial denaturation at 94°C for 5 minutes; 32 cycles of denaturation at 94°C for 30 seconds, annealing at 61°C for 45 seconds, and 9 extension at 72°C for 1 minute; and a final extension at 72°C for 5 minutes. Restriction fragment length polymorphism (RFLP) was used to identify the A2317G genotype. More specifically, 10 μl of PCR product was uniformly mixed with 1 μl of endonuclease and 2 μl of 10 × Buffer R, and the resulting solution was incubated in a 37°C water bath for 4 hours. Then, to identify the genotypes, the products of this endonuclease digestion were analyzed by electrophoresis on a 3% agarose gel run at 70 V for 45 minutes. Samples of each genotype were sent for sequencing.

The substitution of G for A at the rs1053874 site can produce a restriction site recognized by the restriction endonuclease XhoI. Thus, the amplification products were digested by XhoI. The three genotypes of the rs1053874 SNP in the DNASE1 gene could then be identified based on the lengths of the digested fragments. In particular, agarose gel electrophoresis of the digested fragments should result in a single band at 261bp for the AA genotype; three bands at 261bp, 239bp, and 22bp for the heterozygous AG genotype; and two bands at 239bp and 22bp for the GG genotype.

Statistical Analysis

All data were analyzed using the SPSS17.0 software package. Hardy-Weinberg equilibrium testing was used to examine whether each groups of the studied population could be representative of the overall population with respect to genotype frequencies. All data were tested for normality. Normally distributed data were expressed as the means ± standard deviation (x ± s), whereas non-normally distributed data were expressed as median (interquartile range). Two independent sample t-tests were used for between-group comparisons of normally distributed data. Non-normally distributed data were analyzed using rank-based nonparametric tests. χ^2 tests were used for between-groups comparisons of genotype frequencies, allele frequencies, and complication rates. Two-sided probabilities were computed for all statistical analyses, and $P < 0.05$ was regarded as significant.

Results

Comparisons of general characteristics of the study subjects

The clinical characteristics of the patients with GD and healthy volunteers are shown in Table 1. According to the Pearson Chi-Square test, no significant difference in gender or age was exhibited between the control and GD groups ($P > 0.05$); furthermore, there was no significantly differ with respect to either age or gender in the GD patients with or without a family history (all $P > 0.05$). The patients with GO or without GO did not significantly differ with respect to either age ($P = 0.09$) or gender ($P = 0.36$). The patients with or without a history of relapse also did not significantly differ with respect to age ($P = 0.18$) or gender ($P = 0.18$).

Association of rs10583874 polymorphism between GD and control subjects

To examine the reliability of the observed data, the genotype frequencies in the control subjects for the rs1053874 SNP in DNASE1 were tested for Hardy-Weinberg equilibrium. The results demonstrated that the observed genotype frequencies did not significantly differ from the expected genotype frequencies associated with Hardy-Weinberg

(X ± SD)									
GD-total		**GD-family history**		**GO**		**GD-recurrence**		**Controls Normal range**	
		(+)	(-)	(+)	(-)	(+)	(-)		
n	284	81	203	22	262	35	249	203	
Gender (M/F)	75/209	24/57	51/152	4/18	71/191	6/29	69/180	70/133	
Age (year)	38.0 ± 14.3	36.0 ± 14.5	38.8 ± 14.1	33.2 ± 12.3	38.4 ± 14.4	40.7 ± 13.6	38.0 ± 14.3	42.8 ± 13.2	
FT$_3$ (pmol/L)	33.0 ± 23.5	40.4 ± 24.5	36.7 ± 21.1	19.6 ± 12.7	17.8 ± 8.9	15.3 ± 7.5	19.7 ± 5.4	5.2 ± 1.3	3.5~6.5
FT$_4$ (pmol/L)	29.5 ± 10.9	27.1 ± 13.4	26.5 ± 14.1	23.7 ± 13.6	26.4 ± 18.2	25.6 ± 15.3	26.6 ± 18.3	14.5 ± 6.6	11.5~22.7
TSH(mU/L)	0.4 ± 1.1	0.2 ± 0.7	0.3 ± 0.6	0.3 ± 0.5	0.4 ± 0.6	0.6 ± 1.4	0.5 ± 1.0	3.50 ± 1.3	0.5~4.9

Note: GD: Graves' disease; GO: Graves' Ophthalmopathy; M: Male; F: Female; FT3: Free Triiodothyronine; FT4: Free Thyroxine; TSH: Thyrotropin

Table 1: Baseline clinical characteristics of GD patients and healthy controls.

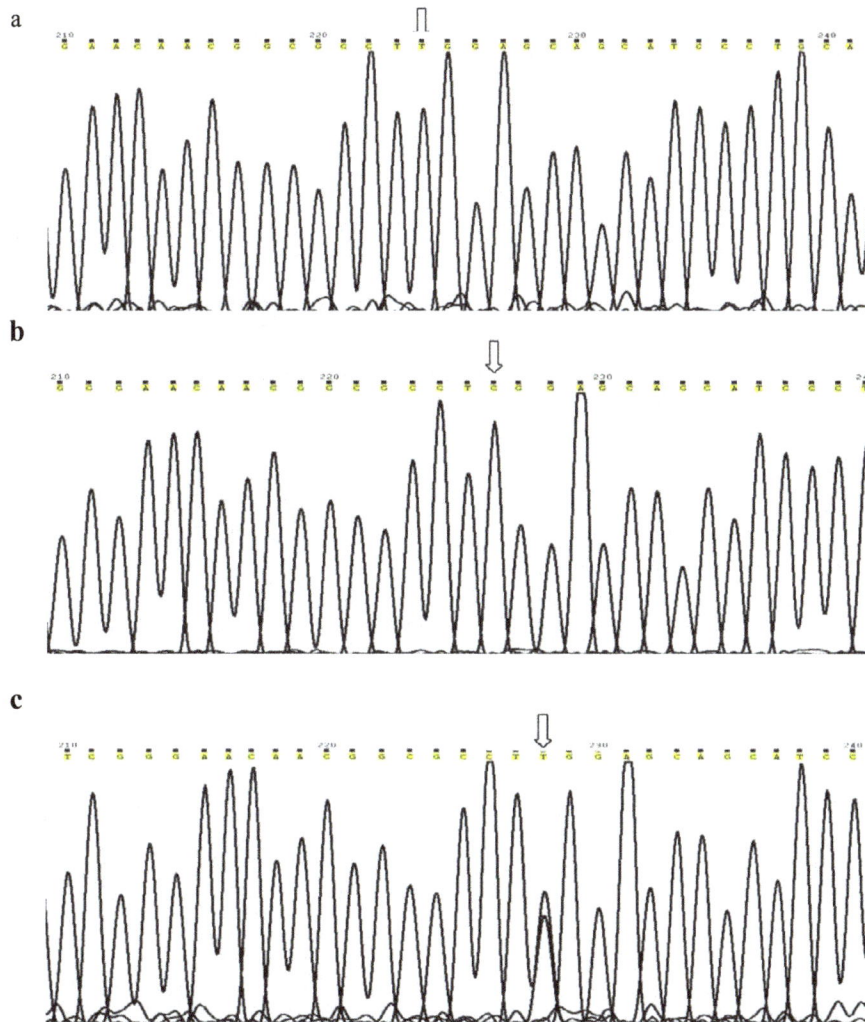

Figure 1: Sequencing results of rs1053874 in the in the Southern Chinese Han population. The three genotypes of the rs1053874 Single-nucleotide polymorphism (SNP) in the DNASE1 gene were performed by PCR-RFLP method in the in the Southern Chinese Han population.
a) The sequence from the patient with AA genotype of rs1053874;
b) The sequence from the patient with GG genotype of rs1053874;
c) The sequence from the patient with AG genotype of rs1053874.

equilibrium ($\chi^2 = 1.35$, P = 0.25), suggesting that the subjects were representative of the overall population of interest. The frequencies of the A/A, A/G, and G/G genotypes in the control groups were 29.56%, 45.81%, and 24.63%, respectively; while 23.94%, 38.03%, and 38.03% in the GD group, respectively (Figure 1). The differences in the genotype frequencies of the controls and GD groups were significant ($\chi^2 = 9.71$, P = 0.00). In the controls groups, the major allele was A (52.46%), whereas in the GD groups, the major allele was G (57.04%). The differences in the allele frequencies of the controls and GD groups were significant ($\chi^2 = 8.59$, P = 0.00). The number of instances and proportion of each genotype and allele in the two groups are presented in Table 2A.

Among the GD patients, the median ages of GD onset for the three

Genotype frequencies	Control (%)	GD (%) OR (95%CI)	χ2	P
A/A	60 (29.56)	68 (23.94)		
A/G	93 (45.81)	108 (38.03)	9.71	0.01
G/G	50 (24.63)	108 (38.03)		
Allele frequencies				
A	213 (52.46)	244 (42.96) 0.68ᵃ (0.53-0.88)	8.59	0
G	193 (47.54)	324 (57.04)		

GD: Graves' Disease; M: Male; F: Female

Table 2a: Genotype distribution and allele frequencies of rs1053874 In GD patients and healthy controls.

genotypes of A/A, A/G, and G/G were 30 years (24–44 years), 34 years (25–42 years), and 32 years (25–43 years), respectively. There were no significant differences in the ages of onset associated with these three genotypes ($\chi^2 = 0.34$, P = 0.84).

Comparisons of genotype and allele frequencies for rs1053874 after stratification

Stratification by gender: The data revealed that A/G was the most common genotype among males of the control groups (5.71%) but that G/G was the most common genotype among males of the GD groups (38.66%). Male subjects from the controls and GD groups exhibited no significant differences in genotype distribution ($\chi^2 = 4.09$, P = 0.13). While for female subjects, the major genotype was A/G in both the control and GD groups (45.86% and 40.67%, respectively), and the two groups exhibited a significant difference in genotype distribution ($\chi^2 = 7.63$, P = 0.02) (Table 2B).

In addition, among males from the control and GD groups, the frequencies of the A allele were 51.43% and 46.00%, respectively, whereas the frequencies of the G allele were 48.57% and 54.00%, respectively. There was no significant difference in allele frequency between male subjects from the control and GD groups ($\chi^2 = 0.85$, P = 0.36). Furthermore, among females from the control and GD groups, the frequencies of the A allele were 53.01% and 41.87%, respectively, whereas the frequencies of the G allele were 46.99% and 58.13%, respectively. Female subjects from the control and GD groups significantly differed with respect to allele frequency ($\chi^2 = 8.12$, P = 0.00) (Table 2C). Moreover, between male and female subjects from the GD groups, there was no significant difference in genotype distribution ($\chi^2 = 3.39$, P = 0.18), also in allele frequencies ($\chi^2 = 0.77$, P = 0.38) (Table 2D).

Stratification by ophthalmopathy: The frequencies of the A/A, A/G, and G/G genotypes were 36.36%, 13.64%, and 50.00%, respectively, in the GO patients and 29.56%, 51.72%, and 47.78%, respectively, in the No-GO patients. There were significant differences in the overall distribution of genotypes among the controls, the GO patients, and the No-GO patients ($\chi^2 = 15.60$, P = 0.00). Compared with the controls, the GO patients and the No-GO patients exhibited significantly different genotype distributions ($\chi^2 = 9.83$ and 8.40, respectively; P = 0.00 and 0.02, respectively). In addition, there was a significant difference between the genotype distributions of the GO patients and the No-GO patients ($\chi^2 = 6.17$, P = 0.046). The three aforementioned groups exhibited significantly different frequencies of the A and G alleles ($\chi^2 = 8.59$, P = 0.01). In the groups of GO patients and the groups of No-GO patients, the major allele was the G allele, which was found at frequencies of 56.82% and 57.06%, respectively; these frequencies were higher than the frequency of the G allele in the control groups (47.54%). Comparisons revealed a significant difference in allele frequency between the No-GO patients and the controls ($\chi^2 = $

8.33, P = 0.00) but no significant differences in allele frequency between the GO patients and either the con- trols ($\chi^2 = 1.37$, P = 0.24) or the No-GO patients ($\chi^2 = 0.00$, P = 0.98) (for detailed information, Table 2E).

Stratification by family history: The frequencies of the A/A, A/G, and G/G genotypes were 29.56%, 45.81%, and 24.63%, respectively, in the control groups; 20.99%, 45.68%, and 33.33%, respectively, in the groups of GD patients with a family history; and 25.12%, 34.98%, and 39.90%, respectively, in the GD patients without family history. There were significant differences among these three groups with respect to the overall distribution of genotypes ($\chi^2 = 12.46$, P = 0.01). The genotype distributions of the control and the GD patients with no family history significantly differed ($\chi^2 = 11.02$, P = 0.00). When the groups of GD patients with a family history was compared first with the control groups and subsequently with the groups of GD patients with no family history of the disease, no significant differences in genotype

Gender	Controls between male and female				
	Genotype frequencies	Control (%)	GD (%)	χ²	P
Male	A/A	20 (28.57)	23 (30.67)		
	A/G	32 (45.71)	23 (30.67)	4.09	0.13
	G/G	18 (25.72)	29 (38.66)		
Female	A/A	40 (30.08)	45 (21.53)		
	A/G	61 (45.86)	85 (40.67)	7.63	0.02
	G/G	32 (24.06)	79 (37.80)		

Table 2b: rs1053874 gene polymorphisms in GD patients and healthy controls between male and female.

Gender	Allele	Control (%)	GD (%)	OR (95%CI)	χ²	P
Male	A	72 (51.43)	69 (46.00)	0.81		
	G	68 (48.57)	81 (54.00)	(0.51-1.28)	0.85	0.36
Female	A	141 (53.01)	175 (41.87)	0.64		
	G	125 (46.99)	243 (58.13)	(0.47-0.87)	8.12	0

Table 2c: Genotype distribution rs1053874 in GD patients and healthy controls between male and female.

Genotype frequencies	Male (%)	Female (%)	χ²	P
A/A	23 (30.67)	45 (21.53)		
A/G	23 (30.67)	85 (40.67)	3.39	0.18
G/G	29 (38.66)	79 (37.80)		
Allele frequencies				
A	57 (46.00)	175 (41.87)	0.77	0.38
G	71 (54.00)	243 (58.13)		

Table 2d: Genotype distribution and allele frequencies ofrs1053874in GD patients between male and female.

		Control (%)	GO (%)	NO-GO (%)	χ²	P
Genotype frequencies	A/A	60 (29.56)	8 (36.36)	60 (29.56)	ᵃ9.83	ᵃ 0.00
	A/G	93 (45.81)	3 (13.64)	105 (51.72)	ᵇ6.17	ᵇ0.046
	G/G	50 (24.63)	11 (50.00)	97 (47.78)	ᶜ8.40	ᶜ0.02
Allele frequencies	A	213 (52.46)	19 (43.18)	225 (42.94)	8.59	0.01
	G	193 (47.54)	25 (56.82)	299 (57.06)	ᶜ8.33	ᶜ0.00

Note: There were significant differences in the genotype among the three groups. χ 2 =15.60, P=0.00)
ᵃGO patients compared with controls;
ᵇNO-GD patients compared with GO patients;
ᶜNO-GD patients compared with controls; GO: GD patients with ophthalmopathy.

Table 2e: Genotype distribution and allele frequencies of rs1053874 in GD patients with or without ophthalmopathy and healthy controls.

distributions were observed (χ^2 = 3.19 and 2.82, respectively; P = 0.20 and 0.25, respectively). There were significant differences among these three groups with respect to the overall frequencies of the A and G alleles (χ^2 = 8.66, P = 0.01). In the GD groups with a family history and the GD groups of without family history ,the major allele was the G allele, which was found at frequencies of 56.71% and 57.39%, respectively; these frequencies were higher than the frequency of the G allele in the control groups (47.54%) (in comparisons with the control groups, χ^2= 3.45 and 7.90, respectively; P = 0.06 and 0.00, respectively). There was not significantly differ with respect to allele frequency in the GD groups with or without a family history (χ^2 = 0.07, P = 0.79) (Table 2F).

Stratification by history of relapse: The frequencies of the A/A, A/G, and G/G genotypes were 17.14%, 14.29%, and 68.57%, respectively, in the relapsed GD patients and 24.90%, 41.37%, and 33.73%, respectively, in the newly diagnosed GD patients (with no history of relapse). There were significant differences in the overall distribution of genotypes between the control groups, the relapsed-GD groups, and the newly diagnosed GD groups (χ^2 = 27.34, P = 0.00). With respect to genotype distribution, the control groups significantly differed from the relapsed-GD groups (χ^2 = 27.40, P = 0.00) but did not significantly differ from the newly diagnosed GD groups (χ^2 = 4.54, P = 0.10). There was a significant difference in genotype distribution between the groups of GD patients with a history of relapse and the newly diagnosed GD groups (χ^2 = 16.48, P = 0.00). The three aforementioned groups exhibited significantly different frequencies of the A and G alleles (χ^2 = 19.77, P = 0.00). In the relapsed-GD patients and the newly diagnosed patients, the major allele was the G allele, which was found at frequencies of 75.71% and 54.42%, respectively; these frequencies were higher than the frequency of the G allele in the control groups (47.54%). Compared with the control groups, both the relapsed GD patients and the relapsed-GD patients GD patients exhibited significant differences in allele frequency (χ^2 = 18.98 and 4.24, respectively, P = 0.00 and 0.04, respectively). There was also a significant difference in allele frequency between the relapsed-GD patients and the newly-diagnosed patients (χ^2 = 11.36, P = 0.00) (Table 2G).

Discussion

GD is an organ-specific autoimmune disease that is influenced by interactions among genetic and environmental factors. No prior research has examined the associations between a polymorphism in the DNASE1 gene and GD in the Han Chinese population. This study utilized a case control approach. PCR-RFLP and direct sequencing techniques were used to comprehensively analyze the association

Genotype frequencies	Control(%)	Relapsed GD (%)	GD-newly diagnosed (%)	χ^2	P
A/A	60 (29.56)	6 (17.14)	62 (24.90)	[a]27.40	[a]0.00
A/G	93 (45.81)	5 (14.29)	103 (41.37)	[b]4.54	[b]0.10
G/G	50 (24.63)	24 (68.57)	84 (33.73)	[c]16.48	[c]0.00
Allele frequencies					
A	213 (52.46)	17 (24.29)	227 (45.58)	19.77	0
G	193 (47.51)	53 (75.71)	271 (54.42)	[a]18.98	[a]0.00
				[b]4.24	[b]0.04
				[c]11.36	[b]0.00

Note: *There were significant differences in the genotype among the three groups.
(χ^2 =37.34 P=0.00)
[a]GD patients with history of relapse compared to healthy controls;
[b]Newly diagnosed GD patients compared to controls;
[c]GD patients with history of relapse compared to newly diagnosed GD patients.

Table 2g: Genotype distribution and allele frequencies of rs1053874 in GD patients with or without history of relapse and healthy controls.

between the rs1053874 polymorphism in the DNASE1 gene and GD in Han Chinese populations.

The study results revealed that the DNASE1 gene may be a GD susceptibility gene in the Han Chinese population of Guangdong Province. The G allele at the rs1053874 SNP is a predisposing factor for GD in this population. This allele did not appear to be correlated with gender, family history of GD, or the presence of ophthalmopathy, although it may be associated with disease relapse. The allele frequencies determined for the rs1053874 polymorphism did not significantly differ from those reported in a previous investigation of a Han Chinese population (9)(P > 0.05). In the examined Han Chinese population, the frequencies of the A allele (the major allele) and the G allele of the rs1053874 polymorphism were 0.52 and 0.48, respectively; comparisons of these results with the corresponding findings for other populations reveal that the allele frequencies determined in this study are similar to the allele frequencies for other Asian populations, such as Japanese, Mongolian, and Korean populations (P > 0.05), but significantly different from the allele frequencies in Turkish, Namibian, and German populations (P < 0.05) [9,10].

We selected only one SNP locus in DNASE1 (rs1053874, which is associated with DNASE1*1 and DNASE1*2) for examination in this study. This approach was utilized for the following reasons. First, after the data for DNASE1 in the Han Chinese population were downloaded from HapMap (http://snp.cshl.org/) and introduced into Haploview for computational analysis, it was found that the minor allele frequency (MAF) was significantly lower for other SNPs than for rs1053874. Moreover, the alleles associated with these other DNASE1 SNPs occur at extremely low frequencies. Takeshita et al. [11] reported that in the Japanese population, the frequencies of the four other alleles were 0.0074 for DNASE1*3, 0.0009 for DNASE1*4, 0.0002 for DNASE1*5, and 0.0002 for DNASE1*6. Furthermore, these four alleles have not been detected in German, Turkish, or Namibian populations [12]. Moreover, the sys- tematic selection of SNP loci should account for mutations in the conserved regions of genes. Yasuda et al. [3] considered the DNASE1*1 allele to be the original allele for DNase I in mammalian species, and the DNASE1*2 allele can arise from the DNASE1*1 allele via a point mutation in exon 8 of the DNASE1 gene. Based on the two major reasons above, we selected the rs1053874 polymorphism as our target site, ignoring the distributions of other alleles, thereby avoiding complicated examination procedures and greatly improving screening efficiency for large populations.

Genotype Frequencies	Control(%)	GD-Family History (%)	GD- No-Family History (%)	χ^2	P
A/A	60 (29.56)	17 (20.99)	51 (25.12)	[a]3.19	[a] 0.20
A/G	93 (45.81)	37 (45.68)	71 (34.98)	[b]2.82	[b]0.25
G/G	50 (24.63)	27 (33.33)	81 (39.9)	[c]11.02	[c]0.00
Allele frequencies					
A	213 (52.46)	71 (43.18)	173 (42.61)	8.66	0.01
G	193 (47.54)	91 (56.17)	233 (57.39)	[c]7.90	[c]0.00

Note: There were significant differences in the genotype among the three groups.
(χ^2 =12.46, P=0.01).
[a]GD with family history compared with controls;
[b]GD with family history compared with GD with-out family history;
[c]GD without family history compared with controls.

Table 2f: Genotype distribution and allele frequencies of rs1053874 in GD patients with or without family history and healthy controls.

The results of this study demonstrated that in the Han Chinese population, the rs1053874 SNP of the DNASE1 gene is associated with GD. Carriers of the G allele of this polymorphism had a higher risk of GD than non-carriers of this allele (odds ratio (OR) = 0.65, 95% confidence interval (CI): 0.49–0.86). There were no significant differences among the three examined genotypes with respect to the age of GD onset. Analyses after stratifying by gender indicated that the G/G genotype and the G allele were significantly more frequent in the male GD patients and the female GD patients than in the controls. However, there were no significant differences in genotype and allele frequencies between the male and female GD patients (P > 0.05). Analyses after stratifying by family history revealed no significant differences in allele frequency between the GD patients with a family history and the GD patients without family history. Analyses after stratifying by ophthalmopathy found no significant differences between the patients with GO and the patients without GO. However, we found differences in G allele frequencies between the No-GO group and control group are significant, and differences of the same allele frequencies between the GO group and control group are not significant. For this result, we think there are two reasons. Firstly, maybe not the SNP rs1053874 its own polymorphism associated with GD, but with a chain polymorphism loci in the coding and show the relevance to GD. Secondly, individual differences exist from patient to patient, and the number of GO patients is low; we need sufficient number of patients to achieve a sufficient effect to find a better results in the further. Analyses after stratifying by a history of relapse demonstrated that the relapsed-patients and the newly diagnosed patients significantly differed with respect to genotype distributions and allele frequencies. These results suggest that the DNASE1 gene is unrelated to the age of onset, gender, family history, or presence of ophthalmopathy in GD patients but could be associated with the relapse of GD. The stratified analyses of this study demonstrated that although the G/G genotype frequencies in the subgroups of male GD patients and the subgroups of GD patients with a family history did not significantly differ from the G/G genotype frequency of the control groups, the other subgroups of GD patients exhibited higher G/G genotype frequencies than the control groups. These results suggested that the G/G genotype and the G allele may be associated with the pathogenesis of GD. The two aforementioned subgroups and the control groups exhibited no significant differences with respect to G/G genotype frequency. It may be related to the reduction of the sample size after the stratification. After stratificated by gender, the number of GD male groups is much less than the female groups, so only the female's differences were significant in our study. Additionally, possible reason is that GD is not a monogenic disease; it is an autoimmune disease in which multiple genetic factors are suspected to play an important role. Though only a few risk factors for these diseases have been identified. Susceptibility seems to be stronger in women, pointing toward a possible role for genes related to sex steroid action or mechanisms related to genes on the X-chromosome [13].

So in the further more research is required to explore the complex interactions that relate to the development of GD, which include interactions between genes, between genetic and environmental factors, and between genes and organs. Dittmar et al. [14] demonstrated that the enzymatic activity of DNase I was significantly lower in patients with monoglandular or polyglandular autoimmune syndromes than in normal individuals. In particular, DNase activity was reduced by 54%, 31%, and 24% in patients with a monoglandular autoimmune disease, patients with a polyglandular autoimmune disease, and the healthy relatives of individuals with autoimmune diseases, respectively. In addition, AITD patients exhibited reduced mRNA expression of the DNASE1 gene [15]. Fujihara et al. [16] found that DNASE1 genotype

affected the serum activity of this enzyme; in particular, relative to the A/A genotype, the G/G and A/G genotypes were associated with higher serum activity but decreased thermal stability of DNase I. In vitro experiments by Kumamoto et al. [17] revealed that an A to G substitution at the rs1053874 locus leads to the replacement of a glutamine (Gln) with an arginine (Arg) in the resulting protein, which appeared to significantly reduce the enzymatic activity of DNase I. This result was inconsistent with Fujihara's findings. Dittmar et al. [6] found that a G to A substitution at position 1218 in exon 5 of the DNASE1 gene could reduce DNase I activity. However, this reduction was only observed for DNASE1*1 that is, the effect was only observed for the A allele of the rs1053874 locus. The aforementioned substitution caused no change in DNase I activity for the G allele of the rs1053874 locus, suggesting that DNase I activity is not only associated with the genotype of the rs1053874 locus but may also be affected by other SNP genotypes. The mechanisms involved in the associations between DNase I and susceptibility to GD require additional study. A possible mechanism is that a reduction in DNase I activity leads to cellular apoptosis and secondary necrosis, causing the exposure of chromatin fragments; the recognition of these fragments by Toll-like receptor 9 (TLR9) could trigger autoimmune diseases [18]. Leadbetter et al. [19] found that after anti-DNA B cell antigen receptors (BCRs) bind hypomethylated CpG DNA, this DNA can be internalized or endocytosed into B cells. At a later stage, TLR9 combines with CpG DNA to form complexes in lysosomes and endosomes, eventually activating B cells. Although unmethylated CpG DNA is rarely found in the body under normal conditions, self DNA from apoptotic cells or necrotic tissues may combine with antibodies and TLR9 to form immune complexes that disrupt the tolerance status of autoreactive B cells and can thereby act as potential predisposing factors of autoimmune diseases. In addition, under certain circumstances, immune complexes containing self DNA from apoptotic cells or necrotic tissues have the potential to self activate. Anti-DNA B cells can bind DNA through BCRs and TLR9 to directly activate hypomethylated CpG DNA without involving the immune complexes described above. Thus, irrespective of whether this DNA is in these immune complexes, it can facilitate the disruption of the tolerance status of autoreactive B-cells, thereby initiating or promoting the development and progression of autoimmune diseases [19-21].

Conclusion

This study confirmed that the DNASE1 gene may be a GD susceptibility gene in thein the Southern Chinese Han population. The G allele at the rs1053874 SNP would be a direct genetic risk for GD in this population. This allele did not appear to be correlated with gender, family history of GD, or the presence of ophthalmopathy among GD patients, although it may be associated with disease relapse. The results contribute to the accumulation of data for population genetics and anthropological research and helping to establish a genetic database for the Han population.

Funding

This work supported by Guangdong Provinces Science and Technology Project (grant number: 2011B031800162); Guangdong Medical Science and Technology research foundation (grant number:A2010166), and key Project of Guangzhou Science and Technology Project (grant numbers: 2011J4100114).

Acknowledgements

We would like to thank the participation of the patients and healthy volunteers. We also thank to Tingting Li, Feng Li and Xiaoyi Wang (Department of Endocrinology) for excellent technical assistance, valuable suggestions and/or critical comments.

References

1. Weetman AP (2000) Graves' disease. N Engl J Med 343: 1236-1248.

2. Yasuda T, Nadano D, Sawazaki K, Kishi K (1992) Genetic polymorphism of human deoxyribo-nuclease II (DNase II): low activity levels in urine and leukocytes are due to an autosomal recessive allele. Ann Hum Genet 56: 1-10.

3. Yasuda T, Takeshita H, Iida R, Kogure S, Kishi K (1999) A new allele, DNASE1*6, of human deoxyribonuclease I polymorphism encodes an Arg to Cys substitution responsible for its instability. Biochem Biophys Res Commun 260: 280-283.

4. Yasuda T, Kishi K, Yanagawa Y and Yoshida (1995) A Structure of the human deoxyribonuclease I (DNase I) gene: identification of the nucleotide substitution that generates its classical genetic poly-morphism. Ann Hum Genet 59: 1-15.

5. Iida R, Yasuda T, Aoyama M, Tsubota E, Kobayashi M, et al. (1997) The fifth allele of the human deoxyribonuclease I (DNase I) polymorphism. Electrophoresis 18: 1936-1939.

6. Dittmar M, Bischofs C, Matheis N, Poppe R, Kahaly GJ (2009) A novel mutation in the DNASE1 gene is related with protein instability and decreased enzyme activity in thyroid autoimmunity. J Autoimmun 32: 7-13.

7. Yasuda T, Iida R, Ueki M, Tsukahara T, Nakajima T, et al. (2004) A novel 56-bp variable tandem repeat polymorphism in the human deoxyribonuclease I gene and its population data. Leg Med (Tokyo) 6: 242-245.

8. Takeshita H, Soejima M, Koda Y, Yasuda T, Takatsuka H, et al. (2009) Gln222Arg (A2317G) polymorphism in the deoxyribonuclease I gene exhibits ethnic and functional differences. Clin Chem Lab Med 47: 51-55.

9. Ni Y, Zhang J, Sun B (2008) Deoxyribonuclease I gene polymorphism in Han Chinese population: frequency and effect on glucose and lipid parameters. Mol Biol Rep 35: 479-484.

10. Takeshita H, Yasuda T,Nakashima Y, Mogi K, Kishi K, et al. (2001) Geographical north-south decline in DNASE1*2 in Japanese populations. Hum Biol 73: 129-134.

11. Fujihara J, Hieda Y, Takayama K, Xue Y, Nakagami N, et al. (2005) Analysis of genetic polymorphism of deoxyribonuclease I in Ovambo and Turk populations using a genotyping method. Biochem Genet 43: 629-635.

12. Barbesino G, Tomer Y, Concepcion ES, Davies TF, Greenberg DA (1998) Linkage analysis of candidate genes in autoimmune thyroid disease. II. Selected gender-related genes and the X-chromosome. International Consortium for the Genetics of Autoimmune Thyroid Disease. J Clin Endo-crinol Metab 83: 3290-3295.

13. Dittmar M, Poppe R, Bischofs C, Fredenhagen G, Kanitz M, et al. (2007) Impaired deoxyribonuclease activity in monoglandular and polyglandular autoimmunity. Exp Clin Endocrinol Diabetes 115: 387-391.

14. Dittmar M, Woletz K, Kahaly GJ (2013) Reduced DNASE1 gene expression in thyroid autoim-munity. Horm Metab Res 45: 257-260.

15. Fujihara J, Takatsuka H, Kataoka K, Xue Y, Takeshita H (2007) Two deoxyribonuclease I gene polymorphisms and correlation between genotype and its activity in Japanese population. Leg Med (Tokyo) 9: 233-236.

16. Kumamoto T, Kawai Y, Arakawa K, Morikawa N, Kuribara J, et al. (2006) Association of Gln222Arg polymorphism in the deoxyribonuclease I (DNase I) gene with myocardial infarction in Japanese patients. Eur Heart J 27: 2081-2087.

17. Ueki M, Kimura-Kataoka K, Fujihara J, Takeshita H, Iida R (2014) Evaluation of all nonsynonymous single-nucleotide polymorphisms in the gene encoding human deoxyribonuclease I-like 1, possibly implicated in the blocking of endocytosis-mediated foreign gene transfer. Dna Cell Biol 33: 79-87.

18. Leadbetter EA, Rifkin IR, Hohlbaum AM, Beaudette BC, Shlomchik MJ, et al. (2002) Chromatin-IgG complexes activate B cells by dual engagement of IgM and Toll-like re-ceptors. Nature 416: 603-607.

19. Viglianti GA, Lau CM, Hanley TM, Miko BA, Shlomchik MJ, et al. (2003) Activation of autoreactive B cells by CpG dsDNA. Immunity 19: 837-847.

20. Peng SL (2005) Signaling in B cells via Toll-like receptors. Curr Opin Immunol 17: 230-236.

17

Effects of Combined Resveratrol Plus Metformin Therapy in *db/db* Diabetic Mice

Duarte-Vázquez Miguel Ángel[1,3], **Gómez-Solís María Antonieta**[2], **Gómez-Cansino Rocio**[2], **Reyes-Esparza Jorge**[2], **Jorge Luis Rosado**[1,3] and **Rodríguez-Fragoso Lourdes**[2]*

[1]*CINDETEC A.C. Avenida Jurica, Industrial Park Querétaro, Querétaro, México*
[2]*Faculty of Pharmacy, Autonomous University of the State of Morelos, Cuernavaca, Morelos, México*
[3]*Nucitec, S. A. de C. V. Avenida Jurica, Industrial Park Querétaro, Querétaro, México*

Abstract

Background: The worldwide prevalence of Type 2 diabetes mellitus is associated with other conditions that trigger metabolic syndrome. Although several studies on the benefits of resveratrol have been carried out, few have assessed this drug in combination with metformin.

Objectives: This study looks at the effects that combined metformin/resveratrol therapy has on body weight gain and liver and renal damage of *db/db* diabetic mice. It also addresses biochemical findings.

Method: Diabetic mice were treated with resveratrol (20 mg/kg/day), metformin (150 mg/kg/day) and combined metformin/resveratrol therapy for 5 weeks. Histopathological tissue analyses and biochemical parameters (glucose, insulin, triglycerides and cholesterol), functional liver enzymes (AP, AST and GGT) and renal parameters (urea and uric acid) were examined.

Results: Our data clearly showed that combined metformin/resveratrol treatment reduced obesity, glucose and triglyceride levels, as well as improving renal function and partially improving liver function in diabetic mice.

Conclusion: The combined therapy may enhance remedial effects in diabetic patients as well as in other metabolic disorders, such as metabolic syndrome.

Keywords: Type 2 diabetes mellitus; Metabolic syndrome; Metformin; Resveratrol; Glucose; Triglycerides; Steatosis

Introduction

Type 2 Diabetes mellitus (T2DM) is a globally prevalent chronic illness associated with high morbidity, disability, and mortality rates, especially in developing countries [1]. T2DM is a multifactorial disease that combines hereditary and environmental factors. Diabetes mellitus is characterized by two major metabolic dysfunctions: decreased insulin secretion by pancreatic beta cells, and peripheral resistance to insulin action [2]. T2DM in combination with other metabolic alterations is known as metabolic syndrome. This is a common disorder characterized by increases in waist circumference, blood pressure and triglyceride levels, as well as a reduction in high-density lipoprotein cholesterol (HDL-C) levels and evidence of glucose intolerance [3].

Metformin is unanimously considered a first-line glucose-lowering agent in the pharmacological management of type 2 diabetes, used either alone or in combination with other antihyperglycaemics [4]. There are no clinically relevant pharmacological interactions with metformin because this compound is not metabolized and does not inhibit the metabolism of other drugs [5]. The antihyperglycaemic properties of metformin are mainly attributed to its suppression of hepatic glucose production, especially hepatic gluconeogenesis, and slightly increased peripheral tissue insulin sensitivity. This drug has hypoglycemic effects by reducing basal and postprandial blood glucose [4].

Resveratrol is an antioxidant found in several plants, especially in the skin of red grapes, and has numerous health-promoting effects in both animals and humans. It has been recently found to have beneficial effects in animals with experimental insulin-deficient diabetes, including antihyperglycemic action and protection of pancreatic β-cells, and could potentially support the conventional treatment of type 1 diabetes [6-8]. Resveratrol regulates numerous intracellular signaling pathways in both humans and other animals, resulting in disparate cellular functional alterations with distinct clinical implications. Although resveratrol is still not an approved drug for use in humans, it has yielded beneficial effects in patients suffering from a wide variety of diseases, including diabetes, arthritis, cancer, epilepsy, proliferative retinopathy and renal failure [9-13].

Metformin appears to be more effective at treating insulin resistance than resveratrol. However, the potential beneficial effects of combined metformin/resveratrol therapy on glucose homeostasis has been previously reported given it increases insulin signaling in adipose tissues and muscle [7]. Our aim was to evaluate the pharmacological effects of resveratrol and metformin, alone and in combination, in obese *db/db* diabetic mice.

Material and Methods

Animal maintenance

Six-week-old male *db/db* diabetic mice (BKS.Cg-+ Lepr[db]/+Lepr[db]/OlaHsd) were obtained from Envigo Laboratories Inc. Mexico (Cat. No. T.2018S.15). The animals were housed in a temperature and humidity controlled environment and allowed food (Standard Purina Chow Diet, Mexico) and water *ad libitum*. The experiments were conducted in accordance with the Guide for the Care and Use of Laboratory Animals [14].

*Corresponding author: Lourdes Rodríguez Fragoso, M.D, Ph.D, Faculty of Pharmacy, Autonomous University of the State of Morelos, Cuernavaca, Morelos, CP 62209, Mexico, E-mail: mrodriguezf@uaem.mx

Pharmacological treatments and sample collection

After acclimatization, the animals were divided into the following groups, each one consisting of 5 animals. Non-diabetic lean mice comprised the control group. The diabetic mice were randomly assigned to four groups: group 1 received 500 μL of water orally; group 2 received metformin at a daily dose of 150 mg/kg body weight p.o. in 500 μL of water; group 3 received resveratrol in doses of 20 mg/kg body weight/day p.o. in 500 μL of water, and group 4 received a combined metformin/resveratrol treatment (150/20 mg/kg). During treatment, all groups were under a controlled diet and received water *ad libitum*. All treatments were administered for 5 weeks. Metformin hydrochloride was purchased from Wanbury Limited (Maharashtra, India), and resveratrol (resVida®) was supplied by DSM Nutritional Products (Mexico, Mexico). Both were dissolved in sterile deionized water prior to experimental use. Mice body weight was monitored throughout the study. After treatment, animals were starved overnight and sacrificed under light chloroform anesthesia. Blood and tissue samples (pancreas, kidney, liver and fat) were collected from each animal and kept at -4°C until further study.

Biochemical analysis

Serum from blood samples was collected by centrifugation, and triglycerides, cholesterol, glucose and insulin levels were quantified using colorimetric methods (Triglycerides SL, Cholesterol PAP SL, Glucose PAP SL, ELITech, Mexico and rat/mouse insulin ELISA kit from Millipore, USA). Liver enzymes, aspartate amino transferase (AST), gamma glutamyl transpeptidase (GGT) and alkaline phosphatase (AP) were also quantified using a colorimetric method (AST, GGT and AP SL, ELITech, Mexico). Renal function was analyzed by measuring urea and uric acid levels in blood using commercial kits (Urea SL and Uric Acid Mono SL, ELITech, Mexico) and in accordance with manufacturer protocol.

Histopathological analysis

Tissue fragments of pancreas, kidney, liver and fat were fixed in 10% formaldehyde solution, dissolved in phosphate-saline buffer (pH 7.4), dehydrated in alcohol and embedded in paraffin. Four-micrometer paraffin sections were stained with hematoxilin and eosin (H&E) and subjected to histopathological examination.

Data Analysis

Weight control values from mice in each treatment group were analyzed and compared; we employed descriptive statistical parameters as means ± standard error of the mean (SEM). The biochemical data (hepatic enzymes, renal parameters, triglycerides, cholesterol, glucose and insulin) were analyzed with SPSS 10.0 software (SPSS Inc., Chicago, Ill, USA) using ANOVA, as well as Dennett's test for multiple comparatives. Differences were considered significant if the p value was less than 0.05.

Results

Body weight gain of *db/db* diabetic mice

Figure 1 shows body weight gain for all groups. This was significant in diabetic mice when compared to the control group (p<0.05). Diabetic mice treated with metformin showed a weight gain similar to that of untreated diabetic mice. Animals treated with resveratrol alone showed a significant body weight reduction when compared with diabetic mice, as well as those mice treated with metformin alone (p<0.05). However, animals treated with metformin and resveratrol showed a significant reduction in weight gain, mainly during the first three weeks (p<0.05). During the last two weeks of treatment, their weight gain was similar to that of animals treated only with resveratrol. All animals had a gradual increase in body weight, but weight-gain reduction was better among those groups treated with resveratrol, either alone or combined.

Biochemical findings in *db/db* diabetic mice

Table 1 shows the biochemical parameter analysis of all groups at the end of treatment. All diabetic animals had high levels of glucose as compared with non-diabetic lean mice (p<0.05). However, a significant decrease in glucose levels was observed in groups treated with metformin, resveratrol, and both drugs combined when compared with untreated diabetic mice (p<0.05). The lowest observed value (308 ± 37 mg/dL) belonged to those animals treated with the metformin/resveratrol combination (p<0.05).

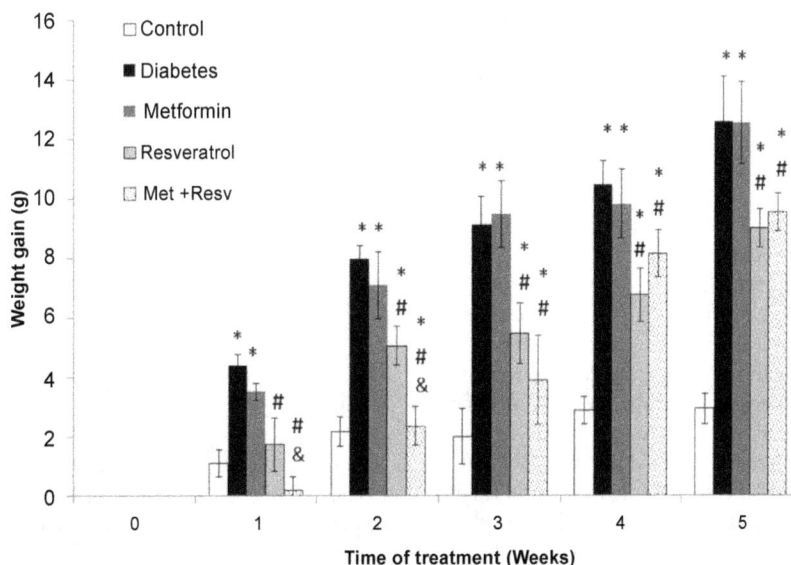

Note: Data are means ± S.D. n=5, *p<0.05 compared with control group, #p<0.05 compared with diabetic group and p<0.05 compared with single treatment group.

Figure 1: Body weight gain of *db/db* diabetic mice.

Group	Glucose mg/dL	Triglycerides mg/dL	Cholesterol mg/dL	Insulin ng/mL
Control	189.0 ± 4.3	148.0 ± 13	101.0 ± 5.5	1.8 ± 0.6
Diabetes (D)	486.0 ± 32*	505.0 ± 89*	167.0 ± 20*	10.0 ± 2.1*
D + Metformin	362.0 ± 31*#	325.0 ± 63*#	142.0 ± 21*	7.1 ± 3.2
D + Resveratrol	387.0 ± 20 *#	312.0 ± 95*#	90.0 ± 25*#	8.1 ± 1.6*
D + Metformin + Resveratrol	308.0 ± 37 *#	288.0 ± 86*#	136.0 ± 8.34*	10.6 ± 3.5*
Data are means ± S.D. n=5, *p<0.05 compared with control group, #p<0.05 compared with diabetic group.				

Table 1: Biochemical parameters analyzed in diabetic mice.

All diabetic animals had high triglyceride levels when compared with non-diabetic lean mice ($p<0.05$). However, all treatments significantly decreased serum triglyceride levels ($p<0.05$). The combined metformin/resveratrol treatment reduced 57% of these values when compared with diabetic mice ($p<0.05$). The resveratrol treatment lowered cholesterol the most effectively ($p<0.05$). Although animals treated with metformin and combined therapy also showed a reduction in cholesterol levels, there were no significant differences with diabetic mice (Table 1).

On the other hand, diabetic mice showed increased insulin levels when compared with the control group ($p<0.05$). However, no significant changes were observed in the insulin levels of animals treated with metformin, resveratrol and combined therapy as compared with those of diabetic mice.

Hepatocellular damage and cholestasis analysis in *db/db* diabetic mice

Table 2 shows the analysis of liver enzymes in animals treated with metformin, resveratrol and combined metformin and resveratrol. As we can see, the *db/db* diabetic mice showed a significant increase in AP (1.95-fold), GGT (2.12-fold) and AST (1.65-fold) levels when compared with the control group ($p<0.05$). Diabetic mice treated with resveratrol, metformin and combined therapy showed a significant reduction in AP levels ($p<0.05$) when compared with diabetic mice. Only the resveratrol treatment reduced AST levels in diabetic mice ($p<0.05$).

Renal function analysis in *db/db* diabetic mice

Renal function analysis of *db/db* diabetic mice showed a significant increase in urea and uric acid levels ($p<0.05$) (Table 2). Diabetic animals treated with metformin, resveratrol or combined therapy showed a significant reduction in urea and uric acid when compared with untreated diabetic mice ($p<0.05$), though this decrease did not compare to that of the control group.

Histopathological findings

Figure 2 shows the representative histological changes observed in the livers of the different treatment groups. By week 5, diabetic mice showed hepatocellular injuries characterized by centrilobular, micro and macrovesicular fatty infiltration, necrosis, ballooning degeneration and pleomorphic nuclei; the same liver architecture was observed in those mice treated with metformin. Resveratrol treatment showed a significant improvement in liver architecture, non-fatty infiltration and hepatocellular degeneration. Although the combined metformin/resveratrol therapy likewise showed an improvement in liver architecture, we also observed areas with fatty infiltration (Figure 2). These results correlated with improvements in hepatocellular damage and cholestasis (Table 2). Figure 3 shows a representative microphotography of the pancreas. As we can see, the size of the islets of Langerhans in the pancreatic tissues of diabetic mice was large and more abundant in the lobule when compared to normal mice tissues;

the acini (exocrine pancreas) did not show significant changes. Diabetic mice treated with metformin showed reduced islets of Langerhans and more abundant acini when compared with diabetic mice, the size of their islets and acini were quite similar to those found in control mice. Animals treated with resveratrol showed large and small islets and a reduction of the exocrine pancreas; pancreas characteristics were similar to those of diabetic mice.

Combined therapy yielded similar results. However, the size of the islets was smaller than in diabetic mice and those animals treated with resveratrol alone. The exocrine pancreas did not show significant changes. All treatments showed an absence of necrosis and fibrotic changes. Figure 4 shows the morphological aspect of the kidneys of diabetic mice. There was an absence of Bowman's capsule, glomerular atrophy, while tubular necrosis and inflammatory infiltration were present. Animals treated with either metformin or resveratrol showed normal kidney tissue architecture when compared with the control group (normal renal tubules and glomerulus). The combined therapy yielded similar results.

Finally, Figure 5 shows the difference in adipocyte size under each of the treatments. Diabetic mice showed a significant increase in the size of all fat cells. Metformin, resveratrol and combined therapy greatly decreased the size of adipocytes when compared with untreated diabetic mice.

Discussion

This study examined the benefits of metformin, resveratrol and metformin/resveratrol combined treatment in *db/db* diabetic mice. These treatments were administered for 5 weeks, at the end of which we evaluated different parameters such as glucose, triglycerides, cholesterol, insulin, liver and kidney function, as well as ultrastructural changes in tissues (pancreas, kidney, liver and fatty tissue) to determine the benefits of resveratrol alone and in combination with a reference drug (metformin).

The diabetic mice model was employed given its usefulness in the study of diabetes and other co-morbidities. *db/db* diabetic mice have an autosomal recessive mutation in the Leprdb gene in chromosome 4 plus a Leptin receptor deficiency. They are obese and exhibit several metabolic characteristics such as hyperinsulinemia, depletion of insulin-producing islets, hyperglycemia, hyperlipidemia, hypertriglyceridemia, insulin resistance, and hyperglucagonaemia. They also show non-alcoholic steatohepatitis, nephropathy and pancreatitis [15,16].

The effects of resveratrol on metabolic health have been well-studied during the past decade. Preclinical studies have established this compound has beneficial effects in animals with experimental insulin-deficient diabetes, including antihyperglycemic action and protection of pancreatic β-cells. It has the potential to support the conventional treatment of type 1 diabetes, though its beneficial effects are not exclusive to glucose metabolism. Previous research demonstrates that resveratrol can reduce glucose, triglyceride and cholesterol blood levels, as well as ameliorate renal and hepatic function in obese Zucker

Group	Alkaline phosphatase (U/L)	Glutamyl transpeptidase (U/L)	Aspartate amino transpherase (U/L)	Urea (mg/dL)	Uric acid (mg/dL)
Control	122.0 ± 16.0	6.2 ± 0.09	230.0 ± 15.0	78.0 ± 4.0	4.2 ± 0.75
Diabetes (D)	239.0 ±13.1*	13.2 ± 2.19*	380.0 ± 110.0*	105.0 ± 6.0*	18.0 ± 0.5*
D + Metformin	171.2 ± 14.3*#	12.0 ± 3.84*	260.0 ± 10.0*	66.0 ± 2.0 #	8.7 ± 0.6*#
D + Resveratrol	152.5 ± 4.7*#	10.8 ± 1.09*	252.0 ± 30.0*#	51.6 ± 0.5 #	7.5 ± 1.2 *#
D +Metformin + Resveratrol	178.0 ± 16.0*#	17.0 ± 0.08*	340.0 ± 98.0*	54.0 ± 6.0 #	10.6 ± 0.4 *#

Data are means ± S.D. n=5, *$p<0.05$ compared with control group, #$p<0.05$ compared with diabetic group.

Table 2: Renal and hepatical parameters analyzed in diabetic mice.

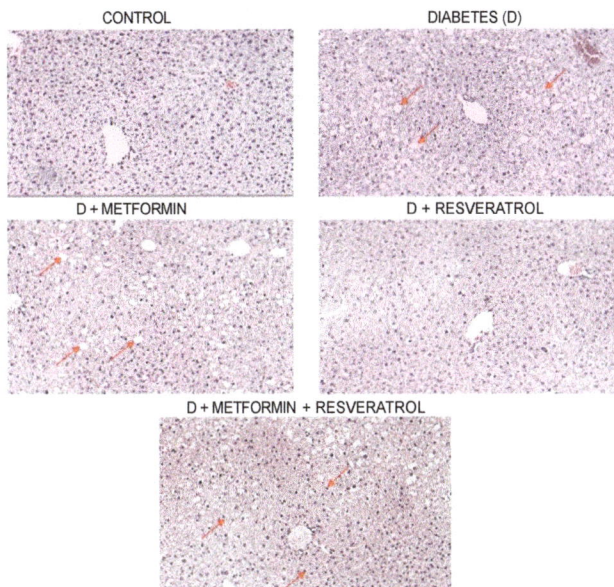

Note: Our analysis does not exhibit signs of toxicity. The arrows point to fat accumulation. The integrity of tissues was analyzed after staining with hematoxylin and eosin (magnification 20X).

Figure 2: Representative light microscopy of liver tissues from male *db/db* mice groups for control, diabetic, metformin, resveratrol and metformin+resveratrol treatments.

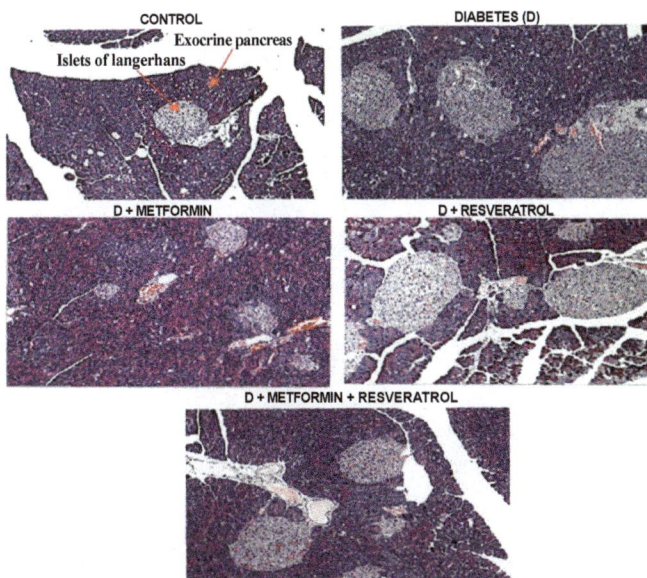

Note: The integrity of tissues was analyzed after staining with hematoxylin and eosin (Magnification 20X).

Figure 3: Representative light microscopy of pancreas tissues from male *db/db* mice groups for treatments control, diabetic, metformin, resveratrol and metformin+resveratrol treatments.

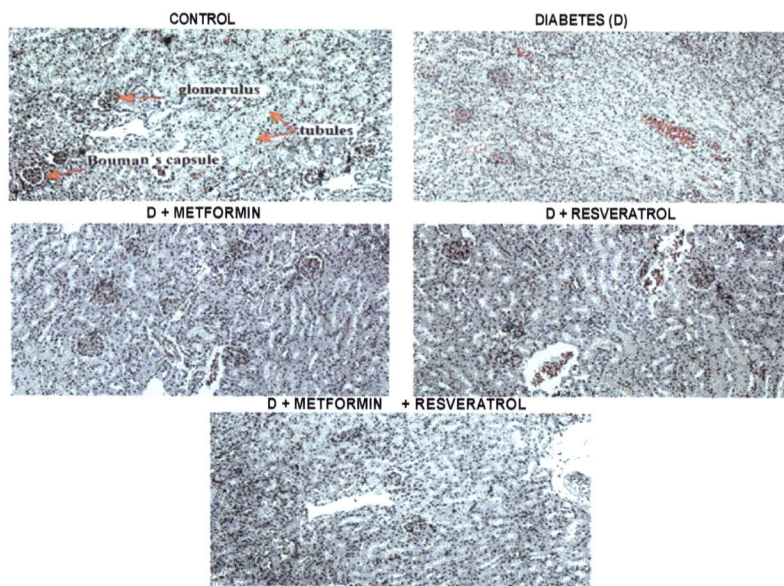

Note: The integrity of tissues was analyzed after staining with hematoxylin and eosin (magnification 20X).

Figure 4: Representative light microscopy of kidney tissues from male *db/db* mice groups for control, diabetic, metformin, resveratrol and metformin+resveratrol trreatments.

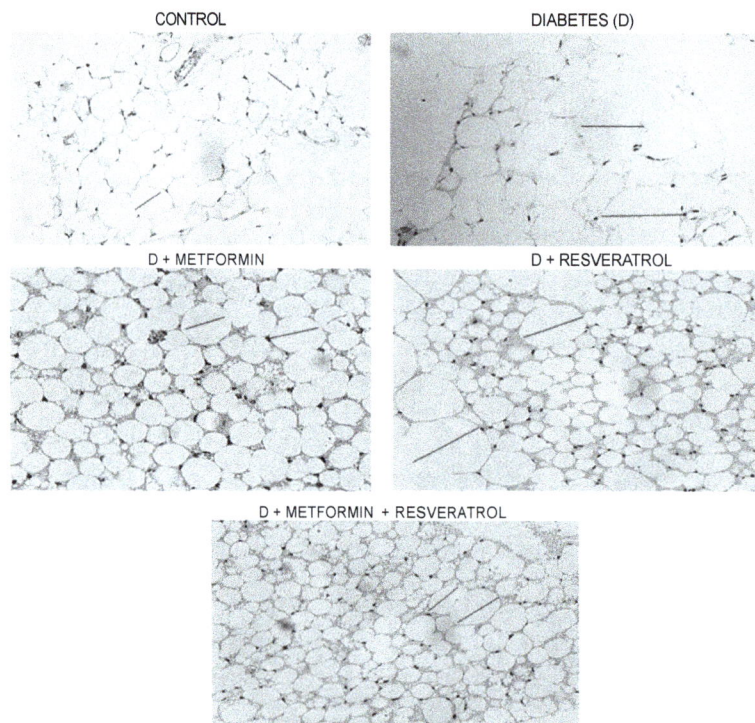

Note: The integrity of tissues was analyzed after staining with hematoxylin and eosin (magnification 20X).

Figure 5: Representative light microscopy of fat tissues from male *db/db* mice groups for control, diabetic, metformin, resveratrol and metformin+resveratrol treatments.

rats when administered 5 mg/kg/day for 30 days [17]. Thus, we decided to evaluate the combination of this compound with a reference drug, metformin, in diabetic mice with additional metabolic disorders.

Animal models of obesity have demonstrated resveratrol can have beneficial effects on glucose homeostasis, diabetes and metabolic dysfunction [18]. Different researchers have shown that resveratrol decreases blood glucose and increases insulin secretion [8,19]. Rivera et al. found that 10 mg/kg/day of resveratrol doses over 30 days improved insulin sensitivity and decreased hyperglycemia in Zucker fat rats [20]. Administration of resveratrol to streptozotocin/nicotinamide-induced diabetic rats significantly decreased insulin resistance [21]. Our results agree with previous reports and demonstrate a significant decrease in glucose levels in *db/db* diabetic mice treated with metformin, resveratrol and combined therapy. However, although all three therapies reduced glucose levels, the pharmacological treatment produced different effects on the pancreas. The histological findings showed reduced islets of Langerhans in animals treated with metformin, while resveratrol and metformin/resveratrol treatments yielded large and numerous islets and a reduction of exocrine acini. In type 2 diabetic human disease, insulin resistance leads to an increased demand for insulin, β-cells secrete more hormone and blood insulin levels are initially elevated. Although the histological findings showed large islets of Langerhans in diabetic mice, as well as in those animals treated with resveratrol alone and combination therapy, these results were not functional because the insulin serum levels did not show a significant reduction. Animals treated with metformin showed a significant reduction in the size and number of islets, but these findings did not correlate with insulin levels.

Excessive body weight and obesity can exert negative metabolic health effects, partly via accumulation of fat in the liver [22]. Such accumulation, when unrelated to alcohol intake, is a strong independent marker of dyslipidaemia and insulin resistance [22]. Pre-clinical studies have revealed promising results regarding the beneficial effects of resveratrol in preventing and reversing obesity-induced metabolic disturbances [23]. Specifically, rodents supplemented with resveratrol have shown improved mitochondrial function, insulin sensitivity and liver fat accumulation [18]. Here we used obese diabetic mice with liver steatosis and demonstrated that resveratrol administration (20 mg/kg/day) and combined treatment (resveratrol/metformin) produced a significant reduction in weight-gain, mainly during the first three weeks, which metformin did not do. The weight-gain reduction induced by resveratrol alone and metformin/resveratrol was associated with a significant reduction in the size of adipocytes at the end of treatment; we believe that the decrease in weight-gain was directly related to the reduction in the size of fat cells.

Hepatic fat accumulation is a well-known complication of type 2 diabetes. Fat is stored in the form of triglycerides and may be a manifestation of increased fat transport to the liver, enhanced hepatic fat synthesis, and decreased oxidation or removal of fat from the liver. Obesity entails excessive fat accumulation accompanied by lobular inflammation and steatonecrosis. Our study showed diabetic mice with high levels of triglycerides and cholesterol, fatty infiltration and necrosis in the liver, and alterations in hepatic enzymes. Previous studies report that metformin and resveratrol diminished the activity of pathophysiological enzymes such as aspartate transaminase (AST), alanine transaminase (ALT) and alkaline phosphatase (AP) [24,25]. Our results are consistent with previous reports, although our study only showed a reduction in AP levels under all treatments (p<0.05). Only resveratrol treatment reduced AST levels in diabetic mice, and those animals showed amelioration of hepatic steatosis. Animals treated with combined therapy showed a reduction in liver hepatic steatosis. There were no observable changes in liver transaminase levels.

It has been reported that resveratrol ameliorates hyperglycemia-mediated renal dysfunction or diabetic nephropathy by reducing urinary levels of urea, creatinine, albumin and albumin to creatinine ratio, as well as by increasing levels of proinflammatory proteins [26]. Previous studies show diabetic rats treated with resveratrol (5 mg/kg) for 30 days had a significant decrease in urea, uric acid and creatinine levels [17]. Our results showed that all treatments decreased urea and uric acid levels, and those findings correlated with the histological changes in kidney tissue.

This study demonstrated that metformin/resveratrol combination therapy reduces obesity, glucose and triglyceride levels, as well as improving renal function and partial liver damage in diabetic mice. These data suggest said combined therapy may enhance remedial effects in diabetic patients as well as those suffering other metabolic disorders, such as metabolic syndrome. Because of we used a mouse model the sample amount obtained was small and was not enough for performing others experimental analyzes contemplated by the authors.

Acknowledgements

Rocio Gómez wants to thank CONACYT (CVU: 363314) and the Pharmacy School at the University of Morelos State for supporting her postdoctoral studies.

References

1. Rosas-Guzmán J, Rosas-Saucedo J, Romero-García AR (2016) SGLT2 inhibitors in diabetes mellitus treatment. Rev Recent Clin Trials.

2. Berry C, Tardif JC, Bourassa MG (2007) Coronary heart disease in patients with diabetes: part I: recent advances in prevention and noninvasive management. J Am Coll Cardiol 49: 631-642.

3. Alberti KGMM, Eckel RH, Grundy SM, Zimmet PZ, Cleeman JI, et al. (2009) Harmonizing the metabolic syndrome: A joint interim statement of the international diabetes federation task force on epidemiology and prevention, national heart, lung, and blood institute, American heart association, world heart federation, international atherosclerosis society and international association for the study of obesity. Circulation 120: 1640-1645.

4. Scheen AJ, Paquot N (2013) Metformin revisited: a critical review of the benefit-risk balance in at-risk patients with type 2 diabetes. Diabetes Metab 39: 179-190.

5. Scheen AJ (2005) Drug interactions of clinical importance with antihyperglycaemic agents: an update. Drug Saf 28: 601-631.

6. Beaudoin MS, Snook LA, Arkell AM, Simpson JA, Holloway GP, et al. (2013) Resveratrol supplementation improves white adipose tissue function in a depot-specific manner in Zucker diabetic fatty rats. Am J Physiol Regul Integr Comp Physiol 305: 542-551.

7. Frendo-Cumbo S, MacPherson RE, Wright DC (2016) Beneficial effects of combined resveratrol and metformin therapy in treating diet-induced insulin resistance. Physiol Rep 4: 1-12.

8. Szkudelski T, Szkudelska K (2015) Resveratrol and diabetes: from animal to human studies. Biochim Biophys Acta 1852: 1145-1154.

9. Bagul PK, Banerjee SK (2015) Application of resveratrol in diabetes: rationale, strategies and challenges. Curr Mol Med 15: 312-330.

10. Bagul PK, Dinda AK, Banerjee SK (2015) Effect of resveratrol on sirtuins expression and cardiac complications in diabetes. Biochem Biophys Res Commun 468: 221-227.

11. Lin CT, Sun XY, Lin AX (2016) Supplementation with high-dose trans-resveratrol improves ultrafiltration in peritoneal dialysis patients: a prospective, randomized, double-blind study. Ren Fail 38: 214-221.

12. Liu K, Zhou R, Wang B, Mi MT (2014) Effect of resveratrol on glucose control and insulin sensitivity: a meta-analysis of 11 randomized controlled trials. Am J Clin Nutr 99: 1510-1519.

13. Łukawski K, Gryta P, Luszczki J, Czuczwar SJ (2016) Exploring the latest avenues for antiepileptic drug discovery and development. Expert Opin Drug Discov 11: 369-382.

14. National Research Council (US), Committee for the Update of the Guide for the Care and Use of Laboratory Animals (2011) Guide for the Care and Use of Laboratory Animals (8th edn.). National Academies Press, Washington (DC).

15. Laskewitz AJ, van Dijk TH, Grefhorst A, van Lierop MJ, Schreurs M, et al. (2012) Chronic prednisolone treatment aggravates hyperglycemia in mice fed a high-fat diet but does not worsen dietary fat-induced insulin resistance. Endocrinology 153: 3713-3723.

16. Soto-Urquieta MG, Lopez-Briones S, Perez-Vazquez V, Saavedra-Molina A, Gonzalez-Hernandez GA, et al. (2014) Curcumin restores mitochondrial functions and decreases lipid peroxidation in liver and kidneys of diabetic db/db mice. Biol Res 47: 2-8.

17. Palsamy P, Subramanian S (2008) Resveratrol, a natural phytoalexin,

normalizes hyperglycemia in streptozotocin-nicotinamide induced experimental diabetic rats. Biomed Pharmacother 62: 598-605.

18. de Ligt M, Timmers S, Schrauwen P (2015) Resveratrol and obesity: Can resveratrol relieve metabolic disturbances? Biochim Biophys Acta 1852: 1137-1144.

19. Gambini J, Ingles M, Olaso G, Lopez-Grueso R, Bonet-Costa V, et al. (2015) Properties of resveratrol: In vitro and in vivo studies about metabolism, bioavailability, and biological effects in animal models and humans. Oxid Med Cell Longev 2015: 1-13.

20. Rivera L, Moron R, Zarzuelo A, Galisteo M (2009) Long-term resveratrol administration reduces metabolic disturbances and lowers blood pressure in obese Zucker rats. Biochem Pharmacol 77: 1053-1063.

21. Asadi S, Goodarzi MT, Saidijam M, Karimi J, Azari RY, et al. (2015) Resveratrol attenuates visfatin and vaspin genes expression in adipose tissue of rats with type 2 diabetes. Iran J Basic Med Sci 18: 537-543.

22. van Herpen NA, Schrauwen-Hinderling VB, Schaart G, Mensink RP, Schrauwen P (2011) Three weeks on a high-fat diet increases intrahepatic lipid accumulation and decreases metabolic flexibility in healthy overweight men. J Clin Endocrinol Metab 96: E691-E695.

23. Lasa A, Schweiger M, Kotzbeck P, Churruca I, Simon E, et al. (2012) Resveratrol regulates lipolysis via adipose triglyceride lipase. J Nutr Biochem 23: 379-384.

24. Linden MA, Lopez KT, Fletcher JA, Morris EM, Meers GM, et al. (2015) Combining metformin therapy with caloric restriction for the management of type 2 diabetes and nonalcoholic fatty liver disease in obese rats. Appl Physiol Nutr Metab 40: 1038-1047.

25. Loomba R, Lutchman G, Kleiner DE, Ricks M, Feld JJ, et al. (2009) Clinical trial: pilot study of metformin for the treatment of non-alcoholic steatohepatitis. Aliment Pharmacol Ther 29: 172-182.

26. Park EJ, Pezzuto JM (2015) The pharmacology of resveratrol in animals and humans. Biochim Biophys Acta 1852: 1071-1113.

18

Metabolic Syndrome in First Manic Episode: A Comparison between Patients with or without Previous Depressive Episode

Sermin Kesebir*, Merih Altıntaş, Elif Tatlıdil Yaylacı, Boray Erdinç and Nevzat Tarhan

Uskudar University, Turkey

Abstract

Objective: The purpose of this study was to investigate, whether an association between metabolic syndrome (MetS) and clinical features and affective temperaments exists or not in first manic episode of bipolar disorder (BD) with or without previous depressive episode.

Methods: Diagnosed with dipolar disorder type I according to DSM-IV criteria fifty four patients who were had a least one previous depressive episode (PDE) and 87 patients who were experiencing their first manic episode (FME) evaluated consecutively for inclusion. Comorbid axis I disorders and alcohol or substance use were excluded. NCEP ATP III formulated an operational definition of MetS based on the presence of three or more of the following characteristics: abdominal obesity (waist circumference), hypertriglyceridemia, low HDL or being on an antilipidemic agent, high blood pressure or being on an antihypertensive agent, and fasting hyperglycemia or being on antiglycemic agent. The patients who had been in remission period for at least 8 weeks were evaluated with SCIP-TURK and TEMPS-A. Remission was defined as YMRS score<5.

Results: MetS was found to be more frequent in these patients than the patients who didn't have a PDE. PDE, negative family history, childhood trauma and seasonality are determined as the predictors of MetS. Anxious temperament scores were higher in MetS (+) FME patients of both groups. Irritable temperament scores were higher only in MetS (+) FME patients without PDE group.

Conclusion: The presence of MetS seems to be correlated with the onset and progression of BD. This may also contribute to the discovery of biological markers, increase in our diagnostic tools, development of protective and individual-spesific treatment options.

Keywords: Metabolic syndrome; First episode mania; Previous depressive episode

Introduction

Bipolar disorder (BD) is known to be associated with premature mortality [1]. Excess mortality rates due to medical disorders are between 1.5-3 times higher in adults with BD compared to general population. There is increasing evidence that indicates an inter-relationship between mood disorders and some physical diseases [2]. Glucocorticoid/insulin signalling mechanisms and inflammatory effector systems are intersections pointing to pathophysiological relationships between bipolar disorder and general medical conditions that are susceptible to stress as metabolic syndrome (MetS).

MetS is more prevalent in those with bipolar disorder than in the general population [3]. A subgroup of patients with bipolar disorder have a higher risk of developing MetS based on their habits, lifestyles, genetic susceptibility, and choices of treatment. A 35-40% prevalence of MetS has been reported in patients with bipolar disorder, and the MetS includes obesity, diabetes, hypertension, and dysplipidemia. Although they are not among the diagnostic criteria of MetS, the proinflammatory and prothrombotic states and purinerjic dysfunction are considered to be in the framework of metabolic syndrome [4,5].

Bipolar patients with a MetS have an adverse course and outcome, less favorable response to treatment, a greater risk for suicidality, higher rates of unemployment and thus higher cost [6]. On the other hand, having a medical condition was associated with longer duration of untreated illness and female gender [7]. In Perugi et al. study, length of pharmacological treatment and age at onset of first major episode were associated with the presence of comorbid MetS [8].

There aren't any studies that investigate MetS and their clinical and temperamental correlates in the first episode mania with drug naive patients and at the onset of the illness. In the present study we aimed to investigate, whether an association between MetS and clinical features and affective temperaments exists or not in first manic episode of BD with or without previous depressive episode, and to clarify the prevalence and predictors of MetS in patients which were robustly defined.

Methods

Sample

A total of 200 patients who were admitted to the Erenköy Mental and Neurological Diseases Training and Research Hospital (Istanbul, Turkey) outpatient clinics or emergency services between 1 April 2011 and 1 April 2014 and received a diagnosis of bipolar disorder type I according to DSM-IV criteria and who were experiencing their first episode were screened consecutively for inclusion. Comorbid axis I disorders were excluded (n=41). Additional exclusion criteria were: (i) being outside the 18-45 age range (n=4), (ii) alcohol or substance use (n=6, and (iii) use of any psychotropic drugs within the last 24 hours for current manic episode (n=8).

*Corresponding author: Sermin Kesebir, Uskudar University, Turkey,
E-mail: serminkesebir@hotmail.com

Assesment tools

Structured Clinical Interview for DSM-Axis I Disorders-SCID-I Turkish version [9]. Mood Disorders Diagnosis and Following Form (SKIP-TURK) [10]. The SKIP-TURK was used to record age at disorder onset, duration of the disorder, age at treatment initiation, physical and sexual abuse in the history, family history, academic and social functioning, age at menarche, premenstrual syndrome, stressor prior to first episode, the type of first episode, severity of the episode (Global Assessment of Functionality –GAF- score), postpartum onset, seasonality, depression subtype, psychotic episode, suicide, hospitalization, duration of the episode, the number of the episodes, dominant course pattern, acute onset and remission, chronicity and rapid cycling, switch, cigarette smoking, and alcohol and other substance use.

Young Mania Rating Scale (YMRS) [11] was used to measure the severity of manic symptoms before treatment in manic cases and to confirm the state of remission in the recovery episode. We used the Turkish version, developed by Karadağ et al., which provides equivalent reliability to the original version [12].

Temperament Evaluation of Memphis, Pisa, Paris and San Diego Autoquestionnaire (TEMPS-A) [13]. It wasdeveloped by Akiskal et al. to evaluate depressive, cyclothymic, hyperthymic, irritable and anxious temperaments.The reliability and validity study for the Turkish form was done by Vahip et al. [14].

Procedures

Ethical permission for the study was obtained from the Local Ethical Committee of Erenköy Mental and Neurological Disease Training and Research Hospital (Istanbul, Turkey). The cost for blood level measurements was met by our hospital's Investigation Budget Fund. An informed consent form was signed by a first-degree relative of patients experiencing a manic episode, than confirmed by the patient in remission period. Information for the SKIP-TURK was collected during the remission period with the patient and at least one first-degree relative. When a clear evaluation could not be performed, information about the illness was obtained from other relatives of the patient.

Blood samples necessary for the measurement were drawn from the brachial vein after at least eight hours of fasting within the first 24 hours. Use of a benzodiazepine was allowed for reasons of agitation. Simultaneous fasting blood glucose (FBG), C-reactive protein (CRP), uric acid and lipid levels (cholesterol, high and low density lipoprotein and trygliceride) were measured in the biochemistry laboratory of our hospital, using standard enzymatic procedures. Abdominal obesity was evaluated by measure of waist circumference.

The National Cholesterol Education Program Expert Panel on Detection, Evaluation, and Treatment of High Blood Cholesterol in Adults (NCEP ATP III) formulated an operational definition of MetS based on the presence of three or more of the following characteristics: abdominal obesity (waist circumference), hypertriglyceridemia, low HDL or being on an antilipidemic agent, high blood pressure or being on an antihypertensive agent, and fasting hyperglycemia or being on antiglycemic agent [15].

The patients who had been in remission period for at least 8 weeks were evaluated with TEMPS-A. Remission for the patients was defined as YMRS score<5.

Statistical analysis

The comparison of numerical variables was carried out using t-tests, and Pearson's correlation test was used for correlation analysis. The comparison of categorical variables was carried out using chi-square test. Logistic regression was performed for obtain the predictive variables. Two-tailed tests were used on all findings and a p-value of <0.05 was considered statistically significant.

Results

Sample

75 female and 66 male first manic episode (FME) patients means of age was 28.3 ± 5.1. 54 patients had a at least one previous depressive episode (PDE) and 44 of them had a psychopharmacological treatment for concurrent depressive episode (81.5%). MetS was found to be more frequent in these patients than the patients who didn't have a PDE (Table 1). Female gender was more frequent in FME with PDE group, while FME without PDE group was older.

The predictors of MetS in first manic episode

Presence of PDE, negative family history of BD, presence of childhood trauma and seasonality are determined as the predictors of MetS (OR=9.3, CI 95% 2.5-10.2, p<0.001; OR=7.8, CI 95% 4.5-11.8, p<0.001; OR=5.6, CI 95% 1.3-7.8, p=0.005; OR=2.1, CI 95% 2.1-4.2, p=0.030).

Comparing of MetS (+) and (–) patients

Mean of age of MetS (+) patients was lower in FME with PDE group while mean of age of MetS (+) patients was higher in FME without PDE group (Table 2).

Family history of BD was less frequent in MetS (+) FME patients with or without PDE while childhood trauma was more frequent (Table 2). Frequency of psychotic symptoms were similar between MetS (+) and (-) patients in two group. Premenstrual syndrome (PMS) was found to be more frequent only in MetS (+) patients who were FME with PDE.

Anxious temperament scores were higher in MetS (+) FME patients of both groups. Irritable temperament scores were higher only in MetS (+) FME patients without PDE group (Table 2).

Discussion

This is the first study that investigates MetS in patients with first manic episode which take into consideration of the presence of a previous depressive episode. MetS was found to be more frequent in FME with PDE group than FME without PDE. Moreover, presence of previous depressive episode was found to be the strongest predictor of MetS in regression analysis. Obviously, individuals with depression have an elevated risk of MetS [16]. At the same time according to our results, four-fifths of the patients with previous depressive episode, had used a psychopharmacological treatment for their mentioned depressive disorders. As a result it is worth to ask whether depressive episode itself or the psychopharmacological agents used to treat it was the cause of the higher MetS in these FEM patients with PDE.

According to Vancampfort et al. meta-analysis, antipsychotic use significantly explained higher MetS prevalence estimates in major

	FME with PDE n= 54	FME without PDE n= 87	Analysis p
MetS (%)	44.8	28.7	0.012
Age (mean ± SD)	26.1 ± 4.7	30.2 ± 5.3	0.027
Gender (female/male)	19/8	42/45	< 0.001

Table 1: Sample.

	FME with PDE n= 54			FME without PDE n= 87		
	MetS (+) n= 24	MetS (-) n= 30	Analysis P	MetS (+) n= 25	MetS (-) n= 62	Analysis p
Age (mean ± SD)	23.7 ± 3.5	31.1 ± 4.2	**0.005**	34.5 ± 4.1	26.3 ± 2.9	**0.001**
Gender (female/male)	8/4	11/4	0.055	12/13	30/32	0.722
Family history (%)	16.6	66.6	<0.001	28	50	0.001
Childhood trauma (%)	41.6	26.6	0.018	64	35.5	0.015
YMRS (Mean ± SD)	27.5 ± 2.9	30.1 ± 3.2	0.422	34.3 ± 4.1	32.6 ± 2.7	0.375
Psychotic symptom (%)	25	33.3	0.279	32	33.9	0.831
Seasonality (%)	66.6	13.3	<0.001	-	-	-
PMS (%)	50	20	0.010	44	32.2	0.467
Depressive temperament (mean ± SD)	15.6 ± 2.5	14.7 ± 1.8	0.462	16.5 ± 2.3	17.7 ± 2.8	0.423
Cyclothymic temperament (mean ± SD)	13.4 ± 2.8	12.6 ± 1.5	0.567	14.3 ± 2.5	12.9 ± 1.7	0.267
Hyperthymic temperament (mean ± SD)	11.6 ± 3.4	12.1 ± 2.3	0.755	13.6 ± 3.4	15.1 ± 2.3	0.155
İrritable temperament (mean ± SD)	17.8 ± 2.3	16.3 ± 1.9	0.232	20.8 ± 2.1	17.3 ± 1.9	0.034
Anxious temperament (mean ± SD)	20.1 ± 2.3	17.5 ± 1.6	0.040	22.1 ± 2.6	18.2 ± 1.5	0.014

Table 2: Comparing of MetS (+) and (–) patients.

depressive disorder (MDD) [16]. Differences in MetS prevalences were not mediated by age, gender, geographical area, smoking, antidepressant use, presence of psychiatric co-morbidity. In another study, there was some mediating role for tricyclic and non-selective serotonin-reuptake inhibitor antidepressant use but overall, the mediating role of clinical differences were limited [17]. When Margary et al. evaluated 83 psychiatric inpatients diagnosed with schizophrenia, bipolar disoreder and MDD they found a positive association between antidepressant drug treatment with triglycerides, and triglycerides/HDL ratio levels and antipsychotics drugs with the HOMA and Framingham index [18].

In Perugi et al.'s study, duration of pharmacological treatment and age at onset of first major episode were associated with the presence of comorbid MetS [8]. Specific features of MetS in psychiatric population are mainly represented by young age of onset, hyperinsulinemia, increased abdominal adiposity, and low HDL cholesterol whose common denominator may be insulin-resistance [18]. In our study, when tested between patients with or without MetS, mean of age of MetS (+) patients was lower in FME with PDE group while mean of age of MetS (+) patients was higher in FME without PDE group. In another words, onset of bipolar disorder is earlier in MetS (+) subjects of FEM with PED group. However, MetS (+) subjects of FEM without PED group is older. It means that, onset of bipolar disorder is relatively late in patients with MetS of this group. In accordance with this result, in one of our previous studies in which we investigated the incidence of diabetes in first episode mania patients, late onset was found as one of the predictors of diabetes development [19]. Also in one of our more recent studies in which we studied cellular adhesion molecules as a component of proinflammatory processes in first episode mania without previous depressive episode, the age of onset was found as 30.5

± 9.9 and this result could be considered as relatively old for the onset of bipolar disorder [4].

It is an important but yet unanswered question whether there is a relation of time or phase between bipolar disorder and MetS as both disorders has negative effects on the prognosis of one another and on selection and application of treatment modalities for both disorders. Soreca et al. suggested that comorbid medical conditions were independent of age but related to duration of bipolar disorder and they were related to some shaed mechanisms and biological determinants [20]. In one of our prospective studies in which we evaluated 2000 consecutive patients who were admitted to our outpatient clinic and gave their informed consent, we investigated the process of diagnosis and treatment of MetS according to NCEP ATP III criteria in patients who were diagnosed as schizophrenia, bipolar disorder, recurrent major depressive disorder and anxiety disorder (generalized anxiety disorder, panic disorder, obsessive compulsive disorder) according to the DSM-IV [21]. In aforementioned study, assessments of 1816 patients were considered reliable and included in statistical analysis. When correlations of time elapsed since onset of Axis I psychiatric disorder and onset of MetS were tested, although these durations were found similar in affective disorders group (6.19 ± 7.55 and 7.12 ± 8.15) (r=0.912), value of r was 0.265 for anxiety disorders group (3.21 ± 3.15 and 8.34 ± 5.71) and 0.425 for schizophrenia group (13.82 ± 11.36 ve 8.21 ± 8.55) respectively. This results means that time of onset for affective disorders and medical conditions were relatively concurrent.

When comorbidity of medical conditions were evaluated in terms of phases of bipolar disorder, possibly they are more prevalent at onset and earlier episodes. This is because early mortality is observed more in patients with earlier onset [22]. Comorbid medical conditions that emerge in middle stages of bipolar disorder would possibly be related to the effect of treatment and effects of patient's habits and lifestyle. However it was showed that even in these circumstances they emerge one decade earlier than the age-matched subjects without bipolar disorder. When all these findings are taken together, it seems that MetS is one of the variables which is in a position as both an initiator and an outcome of bipolar disorder.

Negative family history of BD was related to MetS for the first time in this study. It was suggested as one of the predictive variables of MetS in patients with first episode mania. This result is very important as it suggests possible alternative etiological links apart from MetS and genetic factors for BD whose monozygotic concordance is 70%. Molecular genetic studies showed that, BD shares similar conversions and deletions in same loci with some general medical conditions including coronary artery disease, hypertension, diabetes mellitus type I and II [23]. However genetic association can only explain 10% of total variance of clinical co-existance [24]. This outcome, which researchers call "missing heritability", means that interactions with environmental influences have absolute role both in etiology and resilience in accordance with epigenetic principles. In this study childhood trauma is found as another predictive factor for MetS. This mentioned relationship was also suggested earlier by McIntry et al. [25]. Acute stress prompts a response by an inflammatory reaction in the brain [21]. Autonomic nervous system is directly activated. Release of adrenaline and noradrenaline is end up with their binding to alpha and beta adrenergic receptors on cytokine cells. Subsequently, nuclear factor kappa-beta mediated proinflammatory cytokine release starts. On the other hand, chronical stress leads to HPA axis disorders and consequent hypercortisolism, so childhood traumas are frequently associated with obesity, diabetes, coronary artery disease, chronic obstructive pulmonary disease and autoimmune diseases. At this point abnormal stress response could play a role in the etiology of both a chronic psychiatric disorder and a comorbid medical condition. Hypertension and obesity are the medical conditions that are associated with childhood trauma in bipolar disorder [25]. Additionally, early menarche and EEG abnormalities are found as the projections of childhood trauma on bipolar disorder [25-27].

Although it's genetic aspects are set forth more clearly in recent years, seasonality is a variable which can also be evaluated in the context of epigenetic principles, and according to our results it is a predictor clinical factor for MetS in first episode manic patients. Environmental factors as seasonality affect susceptibility to allostatic load. It is amply documented that bipolar symptoms or episodes are affected by seasonality in susceptible subsets. It could be conceptualized that MetS is a phenotypic manifestation of an abnormal stress response with somatic manifestations [28]. It would be interesting to know whether individuals with MetS syndrome seasonality are more or less likely to also experience breakthrough symptomatology. The principal circadian clock generates seasonal variations in behavior as well. Seasonality elevates the risk for metabolic syndrome, and evidence suggests that disruption of the clockwork can lead to alterations in metabolism. Englund et al.'s findings support that relationship between circadian clocks and the MetS [29]. Circadian gene variants associate to the risk factors of MetS, that they were associated with hypertension and high fasting blood glucose.

Temperament originates in the brain structure, and individual differences are attributable to neural and physiological function differences. It has been suggested that temperament is associated with metabolic syndrome (MetS) markers, which may be partly mediated by lifestyle and socioeconomic status. Altınbaş et al. suggest that depressive temperament profiles may predispose an individual to the development of MetS in the winter [30]. In their study the proportions of MetS were 19.2, 23.1, 34.6, and 38.5% in the summer, fall, spring, and winter, respectively. Only depressive temperament scores were higher during the winter in patients with MetS.

Temperamental factors were related cross-sectionally to, as well as predicted for, the metabolic syndrome precursors over the 3-year period [31]. Mental vitality and positive emotionality were likely to be related and positive emotionality were likely to be related to a low MetS risk level, whereas hyperactivity, negative emotionality, responsivity to others, and cooperativeness were related to a high level of MetS risk. Same group's results showed that a temperament profile characterized by a high level of persistence and reward dependence, an average level of novelty seeking, and a low level of harm avoidance was related to a high level of MetS risk factors [32]. In a systematic review with thirteen cross-sectional analyses, and ten longitudinal analyses, hostility, anger, type A behavior and neuroticism and type D personality were associated with an increased prevalence of metabolic syndrome and its development over time [33]. In our study, two types of affective temperament were differantiated between MetS (+) and (-) subjects: Anxious and irritable temperaments. Hyperactivity, high level of persistence and reward dependence, average level of novelty seeking, and low level of harm avoidance which were reported in earlier studies are similar to the features defined for irritable temperament. Additionally, negative emotionality, responsivity to others and cooperativeness are features consistent with the properties defined for the anxious temperament. Anxious temperament overlaps with depressive temperament in terms of responsivity to others and cooperativeness. In this context, our findings are consistent with Altınbaş et al.'s results as well.

There are also studies that emphasizes the role of gender in the relationship between temperament and MetS. Rejave et al. stated that the relationship between MetS and hyperactivity and negative emotionality was more prominent in men. Sovio et al. assessed the association between temperament and metabolic syndrome in Northern Finland 1966 Birth Cohort [34]. According to their results novelty seeking was positively associated with waist circumference in both genders. However, systolic blood pressure was highest in men with high harm avoidance and low persistence scores, a profile consistent with anxious temperament and lowest in women with high reward dependence and high persistence scores, a profile consistent with irritable temperament. In one of our previous studies we detected an association between impulsivity and triglyceridemia spesific for the anxious temperament [35]. When assessed separately for genders, the relationship between impulsivity and triglyceride levels was detected only in female bipolar patients [36]. In one of our following studies in which we investigated MetS components by gender in first episode subjects, we found triglyceride levels of female patients different from healthy controls [37]. In this study, gender difference between MetS(+) and (-) patients is close to statistical significance only in FME with PDE group and is more prominent in female gender. We know that anxious temperament is more common in females and irritable temperament is more common in males [14]. Anxious temperament differantiates in favor of MetS(+) in the FME with PDE group where female gender is predominant. In addition to this result, irritable temperament differantiates in favor of MetS as well in the FME without PDE group where gender distribution is similar between MetS(+) and (-) patients. We think that the reason for irritable temperament scores' undifferantiation in favor of MetS in FME with PDE group could be the presence of predominantly female gender distribution in this group. Female gender is a risk factor for MetS [7]. According to our results, the same applies to FME with PDE.

Affective temperament is a suggested endophenotype for BD as well. Cyclothymic ve hyperthymic temperaments are the ones that are found to be genetically associated with BD and different in patients and their healthy relatives from healthy controls [38]. In this study anxious and irritable temperaments which differantiate in MetS(+) patients, underlines the effect of environmental influences on the development of MetS once more. Irritable temperament was associated with mixed episodes in patients with BD [39]. According to McIntyre, obesity may affect the symptomatic presentation of BD, by increasing the likelihood that these patients will present with mixed episodes [28]. We think this is applicable not only to obesity but also to MetS. Inappropriate psycopharmacological antidepressant use may contribute to this situation directly by increasing the risk of mixed episode and indirectly by increasing the risk of MetS. On the other hand, there was no clear association between temperament measures and the occurrence and development of the metabolic syndrome. There is, however, a cluster of risk factors that include the presence of the metabolic syndrome, as well as a more negative prone temperament profile, that both predispose to the development of coronary heart disease and diabetes.

In conclusion, there is multidimensional explanation for bipolar disorders that is coherent, comprehensive, and explanatory. The presence of MetS seems to be correlated with the onset and progression of BD. It is possible that common risk factor are present in the onset of both metabolic syndrome and BD. This link could provide an interesting new paradigm for the study of the "systemic" nature of BD and the other mood disorders. This may also contribute to the discovery of biological markers, increase in our diagnostic tools, development of protective and individual-spesific treatment options.

Acknowledgment

The authors have not any conflicts of interest and financial disclosures. Funding or support was not used for this investigation.

References

1. Evans DL, Charney DS, Lewis L (2005) Mood disorders in the medically ill: scientific review and recommendations. Biol Psychiatry 158: 175-189.

2. Fagiolini A, Goracci A (2009) The effects of undertreated chronic medical illnesses in patients with severe mental disorders. J Clin Psychiatry 70: 22-29.

3. Vancampfort D, Vansteelandt K, Correll CU (2013) Metabolic syndrome and metabolic abnormalities in bipolar disorder: a meta-analysis of prevalence rates and moderators. Am J Psychiatry 170: 265-274.

4. Turan Ç, Kesebir S, Süner Ö (2014) Are ICAM, VCAM and E-selectin levels different in first manic episode and subsequent remission? J Affect Disord 163: 76-80.

5. Kesebir S, Yaylacı ET, Süner Ö, Gültekin BK (2014) Uric acid levels May be a biological marker for the differentiation of unipolar and bipolar disorder: The role of affective temperament. J Affect Disord 165: 131-134.

6. Jerrell JM, McIntyre RS, Tripathi A (2010) A cohort study of the prevalence and impact of comorbid medical conditions in pediatric bipolar disorder. J Clin Psychiatry 71: 1518-1525.

7. Maina G, Bechon E, Rigardetto S, Salvi V (2013) General medical conditions are associated with delay to treatment in patients with bipolar disorder. Psychosomatics 54: 437-442.

8. Perugi G, Quaranta G, Belletti S, Casalini F, Mosti N, et al. (2015) General medical conditions in 347 bipolar disorder patients: clinical correlates of metabolic and autoimmune-allergic diseases. J Affect Disord 170: 95-103.

9. Özkürkçügil A, Aydemir Ö, Yıldız M (1999) DSM-IV Eksen I bozuklukları icin yapılandırılmış klinik görüşmenin Türkçe'ye uyarlanması ve güvenilirlik calısması. İlac ve Tedavi Dergisi 12: 233-236.

10. Özerdem A, Yazici O, Tunca Z, Tirpan K (2004) Establishment of computerized registry program for bipolar illness in Turkey: SKIP-TURK. J Affect Disord 84: 82-86.

11. Young RC, Biggs JT, Ziegler VE (1978) A rating scale for mania: reliability, validity and sensitivity. Br J Psychiatry 133: 429-435.

12. Karadag F, Oral ET, Yalcın F (2001) Young Mani Derecelendirme Ölçeği'nin Türkiye'de geçerlik ve güvenirligi. Türk Psikiyatri Dergisi 13: 107-114.

13. Akiskal HS, Akiskal KK, Haykal RF, Manning JS, Connor PD (2005) TEMPS-A: progress towards validation of a self-rated clinical version of the Temperament Evaluation of the Memphis, Pisa, Paris, and San Diego Autoquestionnaire. J Affect Disord 85: 3-16.

14. Vahip S, Kesebir S, Alkan M, Yazıcı O, Akiskal KK, et al. (2005) Affective Temperaments in clinically-well subjects in Turkey: initial psychometric data on the TEMPS-A. J Affect Disord 85: 113-125.

15. Expert Panel on Detection, Evaluation, and Treatment of High Blood Cholesterol in Adults (2001) Executive Summary of The Third Report of The National Cholesterol Education Program (NCEP) Expert Panel on Detection, Evaluation, And Treatment of High Blood Cholesterol In Adults (Adult Treatment Panel III). JAMA 285: 2486-2497.

16. Vancampfort D, Correll CU, Wampers M, Sienaert P, Mitchell AJ, et al. (2013) Metabolic syndrome and metabolic abnormalities in patients with major depressive disorder: a meta-analysis of prevalences and moderating variables. Psychol Med 21: 1-12.

17. Luppino FS, Bouvy PF, Giltay EJ, Penninx BW, Zitman FG (2014) The metabolic syndrome and related characteristics in major depression: inpatients and outpatients compared: metabolic differences across treatment settings. Gen Hosp Psychiatry 36: 509-515.

18. Margari F, Lozupone M, Pisani R, Pastore A, Todarello O, et al. (2013) Metabolic syndrome: differences between psychiatric and internal medicine patients. Int J Psychiatry Med 45: 203-226.

19. Gençer AG, Kesebir S (2012) Diabetes in first episode mania: relations with clinical and the other endocrinological and metabolic parameters. Bipolar Disord 14: 90.

20. Soreca I, Fagiolini A, Frank E, Houck PR, Thompson WK (2008) Relationship of general medical burden, duration of illness and age in patients with bipolar I disorder. J Psychiatr Res 42: 956-961.

21. Kesebir S (2014) Metabolic syndrome and childhood trauma: Also comorbidity and complication in mood disorder. World J Clin Cases 2: 332-337.

22. Goldstein BI, Kemp DE, Soczynska JK, McIntyre RS (2009) Inflammation and the phenomenology, pathophysiology, comorbidity, and treatment of bipolar disorder: a systematic review of the literature. J Clin Psychiatry 70: 1078-1090.

23. So HC, Gui AH, Cherny SS, Sham PC (2011) Evaluating the heritability explained by known susceptibility variants: a survey of ten complex diseases. Genet Epidemiol 35: 310-317.

24. Lee SH, Wray NR, Goddard ME, Visscher PM (2011) Estimating missing heritability for disease from genome-wide association studies. Am J Hum Genet 88: 294-305.

25. McIntyre RS, Soczynska JK, Liauw SS, Woldeyohannes HO, Brietzke E, et al. (2012) The association between childhood adversity and components of metabolic syndrome in adults with mood disorders: results from the international mood disorders collaborative project. Int J Psychiatry Med 43: 165-177.

26. Kesebir S, Şair BY, Unübol B, Yaylacı ET (2013) Is there a relationship between age at menarche and clinical and temperamental characteristics in bipolar disorder? Ann Clin Psychiatry 25: 121-124.

27. Kesebir S, Güven S, Yaylacı ET, Topçuoğlu ÖB, Altıntaş M (2013) EEG Abnormality in first episode mania: is it trait or state? Psychol Res 3: 563-570.

28. McIntyre RS (2013) Seasonal and temperamental contributions in patients with bipolar disorder and metabolic syndrome. Rev Bras Psiquiatr 35: 210.

29. Englund A, Kovanen L, Saarikoski ST, Haukka J, Reunanen A, et al. (2009) NPAS2 and PER2 are linked to risk factors of the metabolic syndrome. J Circadian Rhythms 26: 5-7.

30. Altinbas K, Guloksuz S, Oral ET (2013) Metabolic syndrome prevalence in different affective temperament profiles in bipolar-I disorder. Rev Bras Psiquiatr 35: 131-135.

31. Ravaja N, Keltikangas-Järvinen L (1995) Temperament and metabolic syndrome precursors in children: a three-year follow-up. Prev Med 24: 518-527.

32. Keltikangas-Järvinen L, Ravaja N, Viikari J (1999) Identifying Cloninger's temperament profiles as related to the early development of the metabolic cardiovascular syndrome in young men. Arterioscler Thromb Vasc Biol 19: 1998-2006.

33. Mommersteeg PM, Pouwer F (2012) Personality as a risk factor for the metabolic syndrome: a systematic review. J Psychosom Res 73: 326-333.

34. Sovio U, King V, Miettunen J, Ek E, Laitinen J, et al. (2007) Cloninger's Temperament dimensions, socio-economic and lifestyle factors and metabolic syndrome markers at age 31 years in the Northern Finland Birth Cohort 1966. J Health Psychol 12: 371-382.

35. Yaylacı ET, Kesebir S, Güngördü O (2014) The relationship between impulsivity and lipid levels in bipolar patients: does temperament explain it? Compr Psychiatry 55: 883-886.

36. Kesebir S, Yaylacı ET, Demirkan AK, Altıntaş M (2014) The relationship of impulsivity and lipid levels in bipolar patients: gender effect. Bipolar Disord 16: 126.

37. Kesebir S, Yaylacı ET, Atgüden N, Altıntaş M (2014) Metabolic parameters in first episode mania. Bipolar Disord 16: 110.

38. Kesebir S, Vahip S, Akdeniz F, Akiskal H, Yüncü Z, et al. (2005) Affective Temperaments as measured by TEMPS-A in patients with Bipolar I disorder and their First Degree Relatives. J Affect Disord 85: 127-133.

39. Kesebir S, Vahip S, Akdeniz F, Yüncü Z (2005) The relationship of affective temperament and clinical features in bipolar disorder. Türk Psikiyatri Dergisi 16: 164-169.

19

Hepatic Gene Expression Associated With Macrophage and Oxidative Stress of Simple Steatosis and Non-Alcoholic Steatohepatitis Model Rats Using DNA Microarray Analysis

Keiichiro Ohba[1,3]*, Toshio Kumai[3], Shinichi Iwai[1], Minoru Watanabe[4], Go Koizumi[1,3], Masayuki Arai[1], Kanji Furuya[1], Go Oda[3], Naoki Matsumoto[2], Shinichi Kobayashi[1] and Katsuji Oguchi[1]

[1]Department of Pharmacology, Showa University School of Medicine, 1-5-8 Hatanodai, Shinagawa-ku, Tokyo 142-8555, Japan
[2]Department of Pharmacology, St. Marianna University School of Medicine, 2-16-1 Sugao, Miyamae-ku, Kawasaki, Kanagawa 216-8511, Japan
[3]Department of Pharmacogenomics, St. Marianna University Graduate School of Medicine, 2-16-1 Sugao, Miyamae-ku, Kawasaki, Kanagawa 216-8511, Japan
[4]Institute for Animal Experimentation, St. Marianna University Graduate School of Medicine, 2-16-1 Sugao, Miyamae-ku, Kawasaki, Kanagawa 216-8511, Japan

Abstract

Aim: To clarify the mechanism governing progression of Non-Alcoholic Steatohepatitis (NASH), we examined hepatic gene expression associated with macrophage and oxidative stress/inflammation, which plays an important role in the progression of Non-Alcoholic Fatty Liver Disease (NAFLD) in simple steatosis (SS) model and NASH model rats.

Methods: Four-month-old male Spontaneously Hypertensive Hyperlipidemic Rats (SHHR) and Sprague-Dawley (SD) rats were each divided into two groups: SD rats received a high-fat diet and 30% sucrose solution (HFDS) as SS model rats and SHHR received the HFDS as NASH model rats. Microarray analysis was performed on the liver of these rats at eight months of age to select those gene sets, e.g., "genes correlated with progression of NAFLD" and "genes expressed exclusively in NASH", which are related to macrophage or oxidative stress/inflammation.

Results: Thirteen genes were selected from the microarray analysis data. Four genes were associated with macrophage: acid phosphatase 5, tartrate-resistant (Acp5), a member of the RAS oncogene family (Rab8a), scavenger receptor class B, member 2 (Scarb2) and CD36 molecule (Cd36). Nine genes were associated with oxidative stress/inflammation: translocator protein (Tspo), prostaglandin I2 synthase (Ptgis), tumor necrosis factor receptor superfamily, member 9 (Tnfrsf9), glutathione S-transferase alpha 5 (Gsta5), regucalcin (Rgn), glutathione S-transferase kappa 1 (Gstk1), disabled homolog 2, mitogen-responsive phosphoprotein (Dab2), glutathione S-transferase mu 5 (Gstm5) and flavin-containing monooxygenase 5 (Fmo5). Acp5, Tspo, Ptgis, Tnfrsf, Gsta5 (up-regulated) and Rab8a, Rgn, Gstk1 (down-regulated) were included in genes correlated with progression of NAFLD. Scarb2, Cd36, Dab2 Gstm5 (up-regulated) and Fmo5 (down-regulated) were included in genes expressed in only NASH model rats.

Conclusion: We hypothesized that scavenger receptor class B and glutathione S-transferase play an important role in the progression from simple NAFLD to NASH. Our results afford beneficial data regarding therapeutic targets of progression of NAFLD/NASH.

Keywords: Spontaneously hypertensive hyperlipidemic rats (SHHR)(SHHR); Non-alcoholic steatohepatitis (NASH); Non-alcoholic fatty liver disease (NAFLD); Microarray

Introduction

Non-alcoholic Fatty Liver Disease (NAFLD) is defined as the accumulation of lipid, primarily triacylglycerols, in individuals who do not consume large quantities of alcohol. NAFLD encompasses a spectrum of disease ranging from Simple Steatosis (SS) to inflammatory steatohepatitis with increasing levels of fibrosis and ultimately cirrhosis [1]. NAFLD, which is strongly correlated with obesity and insulin resistance, is recognized as representing the hepatic manifestation of the metabolic syndrome [2]. Non-Alcoholic Steatohepatitis (NASH) is a progressive form of NAFLD that is diagnosed on the basis of histopathological features [3]. The prevalence of the metabolic syndrome, which is rapidly increasing due to hyperalimentation and a sedentary lifestyle [4], is reflected by the increasing prevalence of NAFLD and associated complications [5]. NAFLD can be quite unobtrusive; in contrast, NASH is a serious condition, with nearly one quarter of affected patients developing cirrhosis, which, in turn, increases the risk of subsequent progression to hepatocellular carcinoma [6]. Despite recent advances in the elucidation of the complex metabolic and inflammatory pathways involved in NAFLD, the pathogenesis of steatosis and progression to steatohepatitis and fibrosis/cirrhosis remains incompletely understood [2,7].

Few rat models lend themselves to the evaluation of atherosclerosis; as a result, Spontaneously Hypertensive Hyperlipidemic Rats (SHHRs) were developed as a stable model of early vascular degeneration [8], SHHRs display persistently high systolic blood pressure (above 150 mmHg) and plasma total cholesterol levels exceeding 150 mg/dL. In addition, vascular intimal lesions and lipid deposits have been observed under endothelial cells in the aorta of SHHRs, but not in spontaneously hyperlipidemic rats or controls [9]. Moreover, invasive changes occur in the subendothelium of SHHR when nitric oxide production is inactivated, followed by a high fat diet and sucrose water treatment (HFDS) [10]; moreover, a previous study noted visceral fat accumulation and increased oxidative stress in SHHR-HFDS [11,12].

Corresponding author: Keiichiro Ohba, Department of Pharmacology, Showa University School of Medicine, 1-5-8, Hatanodai, Shinagawa-ku, Tokyo 142-8555, Japan, E-mail: kei@oba.name

We detected hepatocyte ballooning and steatosis with HFDS feeding for 9-13 months. Severe fibrosis and cell inflammation around the central vein were observed in SHHR-HFDS but were only slightly detectable in SD-HFDS [13]; thus, SD-HFDS and SHHR-HFDS were employed as rat models of simple steatosis and NASH, respectively.

Numerous researchers have applied microarray analysis in order to clarify the underlying mechanism governing NAFLD; however, these investigations noted only the genes correlated with lipid metabolism. The metabolic abnormalities and gene expressions of liver in terms of the pathological progression of early stage NASH remain unclear.

Microarray analysis was performed in the current study to clarify the pathogenetic mechanisms governing early stage NASH and to evaluate SD-HFDS and SHHR-HFDS as models of simple steatosis and NASH, respectively.

Materials and Methods

Animals and samples

Four-month-old male SHHRs and SD rats were divided into two groups each: a control group, which received a regular diet (ND; CE2; CLEA Japan Inc., Tokyo, Japan), and a HFDS-fed group. The regular diet consisted of 8.9% water, 25.4% protein, 4.4% fat, 4.1% fiber, 6.9% carbohydrate and 50.3% nitrogen-free extracts (caloric value: 342.2 kcal/100 g). The high-fat diet (HFD) consisted of 8.2% water, 23.4% protein, 11.0% fat, 3.8% fiber, 6.3% carbohydrate and 46.3% nitrogen-free extracts (caloric value: 378.0 kcal/100 g). The regular diet was available to all groups ad libitum until the age of four months; subsequently, the two HFDS groups received the high-fat diet with 30% sucrose solution ad libitum for four months. Thus, rats of 8 months of age were obtained. This study utilized SHHRs characterized by systolic blood pressure over 150 mmHg, as determined by the tailcuff method (PS-100; Riken Kaihatsu, Tokyo, Japan). The rats were housed in a semi-barrier system under controlled room temperature (23 ± 1°C), humidity (55 ± 5%) and lighting (lights on from 6 AM to 6 PM). All experiments were conducted according to the "Guiding Principles for the Care and Use of Laboratory Animals" of Showa University [12].

Statistical analysis

Data were analyzed employing the Mann-Whitney U-test. Correlations were calculated with the Pearson's product moment correlation coefficient. All data are expressed as mean ± S.E.M. $p < 0.05$ was considered significant.

Preparation and biochemical determination of plasma samples

Blood samples, which were obtained from the inferior vena cava under pentobarbital anesthesia (35 mg/kg, intraperitoneal administration), were mixed with 3.2% sodium citrate solution in a volume ratio of 9:1. After 15 minutes of centrifugation at 3,000 rpm, the supernatant, as citrated plasma, was analyzed. Rats were sacrificed by decapitation, after which the liver and visceral fat (VisF) were isolated and weighed under the pentobarbital anesthesia.

Plasma levels of total cholesterol and total triglycerides were determined employing commercially available kits (Cholesterol E-test and Triglyceride E-test, respectively; Wako Pure Chemical Industries Ltd., Tokyo, Japan). Plasma levels of Aspartate Aminotransferase (AST) and Alanine Aminotransferase (ALT) were determined with the Transaminase CII-test (Wako) [11]. Oxidative stress was measured in rat plasma utilizing the d-ROMs test (Free Radical Elective Evaluator; Wismerll Co. Ltd., Tokyo, Japan) by gently mixing 20 μl of plasma sample and 1 mL of buffer solution in a cuvette, prior to the addition of 10 μL of the chromogenic substrate. After mixing, the cuvette was incubated immediately in the thermostatic block of the analyzer for 5 minutes at 37°C; subsequently, the absorbance at 505 nm was recorded. Measurements are expressed as Carr units, with 1 Carr corresponding to 0.8 mg/L H_2O_2 [12].

Morphological study

The fresh left lobe of liver was harvested from all rats and stored in

	N	BW(g)	LW(g)	Vis Fat(g)	LW/100gBW	Vis Fat/100gBW	d-ROMS
SD-ND	8	574.1 ± 8.5	14.7 ± 0.3	17.3 ± 0.3	2.6 ± 0.0	3.0 ± 0.1	281.8 ± 8.7
SD-HFDS	8	590 ± 12.1	38.2 ± 1.4	19.3 ± 1.4	6.5 ± 0.1	3.3 ± 0.2	482.0 ± 35.0
SHHR-ND	6	565 ± 7.7	16.3 ± 0.5	14.7 ± 1.1	2.9 ± 0.1	2.6 ± 0.2	360.7 ± 13.0
SHHR-HFDS	6	671.2 ± 14.9	48.3 ± 0.5	50.4 ± 3.8	7.2 ± 0.1	7.5 ± 0.4	616.8 ± 23.4
		*3*5*6	*1*2*3 *4*5*6	*2*3 *4*5*6	*1*2*3 *4*5*6	*2*3 *4*5*6	*1*2*3 *4*5*6

Body weight (BW), visceral fat (VisF), plasma glucose (Glu), hemoglobin A1c (HbA1c), total cholesterol (TC), total triglycerides (TG), aspartate aminotransferase (AST), alanine aminotransferase (ALT) and diacron reactive oxidative metabolites (d-ROMs) in Sprague-Dawley rats receiving normal diet (SD-ND) and SD-high-fat diet with sucrose (SD-HFDS) as well as in spontaneously hypertensive hyperlipidemic rats (SHHR-ND and SHHR-HFDS) at 8 months of age. The results are presented as mean ± S.E.M.
Student t test unpaired p<0.05 for *1, SD-ND vs. SD-HFDS ; *2, SD-ND vs. SHHR-ND ; *3, SD-ND vs. SHHR-HFDS ; *4, SD-HFDS vs. SHHR-ND ; *5, SD-HFDS vs. SHHR-HFDS ; *6, SHHR-ND vs. SHHR-HFDS

Table 1a: Biochemical characteristics of SD-ND, SD-HFDS, SHHR-ND and SHHR-HFDS at 8 months of age.

	N	Glu(mg/dl)	HbA1c	T-Cho(mg/dl)	TG(mg/dl)	AST	ALT
SD-ND	8	150.9 ± 7.9	2.7 ± 0.1	65.8 ± 4.9	77.0 ± 8.2	141.9 ± 15.3	53.9 ± 8.9
SD-HFDS	8	162.6 ± 5.1	2.8 ± 0.1	109.9 ± 10.3	72.8 ± 5.4	264.1 ± 46.9	71.1 ± 10.0
SHHR-ND	6	135.8 ± 8.9	2.6 ± 0.1	140.2 ± 9.9	125.0 ± 9.2	140.3 ± 9.2	47.5 ± 4.8
SHHR-HFDS	6	162.8 ± 3.6	2.9 ± 0.1	457.3 ± 42.5	84.7 ± 6.6	170.7 ± 12.0	62.2 ± 18.0
		*4*6	*1*2	*3*5*6	*2*4*6	*1*4	

Body weight (BW), visceral fat (VisF), plasma glucose (Glu), hemoglobin A1c (HbA1c), total cholesterol (TC), total triglycerides (TG), aspartate aminotransferase (AST), alanine aminotransferase (ALT) and diacron reactive oxidative metabolites (d-ROMs) in Sprague-Dawley rats receiving normal diet (SD-ND) and SD-high-fat diet with sucrose (SD-HFDS) as well as in spontaneously hypertensive hyperlipidemic rats (SHHR-ND and SHHR-HFDS) at 8 months of age. The results are presented as mean ± S.E.M.
Student t test unpaired p<0.05 for *1, SD-ND vs. SD-HFDS ; *2, SD-ND vs. SHHR-ND ; *3, SD-ND vs. SHHR-HFDS ; *4, SD-HFDS vs. SHHR-ND ; *5, SD-HFDS vs. SHHR-HFDS ; *6, SHHR-ND vs. SHHR-HFDS

Table 1b: Biochemical characteristics of SD-ND, SD-HFDS, SHHR-ND and SHHR-HFDS at 8 months of age.

saline on ice, after which it was dissected from the surrounding tissues and fixed in 10% neutral buffered formalin (pH 7.4; Wako). Sections of the liver were stained with Hematoxylin-Eosin (HE) and Masson Trichrome (MT).

RNA extraction and microarray hybridization

A sample of each liver specimen was stored at -80°C until the microarray analysis.

Total RNA was purified using an RNeasy Kit (Qiagen, Germany) per the manufacturer's manual. Cy3-labeled cRNA was obtained from 200 ng total RNA with the Agilent Low Input Quick Amp Labeling Kit. Cy3-labeled cRNA was hybridized to Whole Rat genome Oligo Microarray ver 3.0 (4×44 k) according to the manufacturer's hybridization protocol. After the washing step, microarray slides were analyzed with an Agilent Microarray scanner B version; the default settings were applied for all parameters. Microarray expression data were obtained utilizing Agilent Feature Extraction software ver 10.5.1; the default settings were applied for all parameters. The raw data and associated sample interpretation were loaded and processed by GeneSpring ver11 (Tomy Digital Biology). Four experiments were performed; data were expressed as mean values.

Results

Comparison of the four groups

Tables 1a and 1b displays body weight and Liver Weight (LW) as well as the levels of VisF, plasma glucose, hemoglobin A1C, total cholesterol, total triglycerides, AST, ALT and d-ROMs in SD-ND, SD-HFDS, SHHR-ND and SHHR-HFDS. In both the SD and SHHR groups, VisF and LW were elevated significantly or tended to be elevated following ingestion of HFDS. VisF and LW in SHHR-ND and SHHR-HFDS increased markedly in comparison with SD-ND and SD-HFDS, respectively. The level of oxidative stress (d-ROMs) demonstrated meaningful elevation after ingestion of HFDS. The level of d-ROMs in SHHR-ND and SHHR-HFDS increased significantly in comparison with SD-ND and SD-HFDS, respectively. Plasma hemoglobin A1C, AST and ALT levels were unchanged among the SD and SHHR groups.

Morphological study

Figures 1 and 2 presents the results of the morphological study

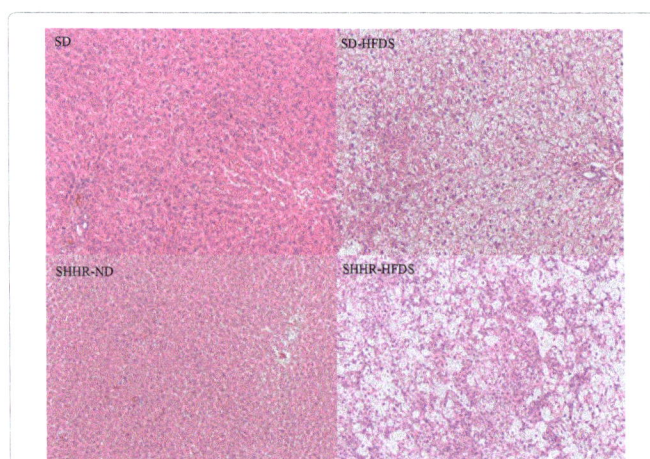

Figure 1: Effects of high fat diet and 30% sucrose on the liver of Spontaneously Hypertensive Hyperlipidemic Rats (SHHR) and SD rats (Hematoxylin -eosin stain) SD-ND; SD rats fed with normal diet (ND), SD-HFDS; SD rats fed with high fat diet and 30% sucrose (HFDS), SHHR-ND; SHHR fed with ND, SHHR-HFDS; SHHR fed with HFDS.

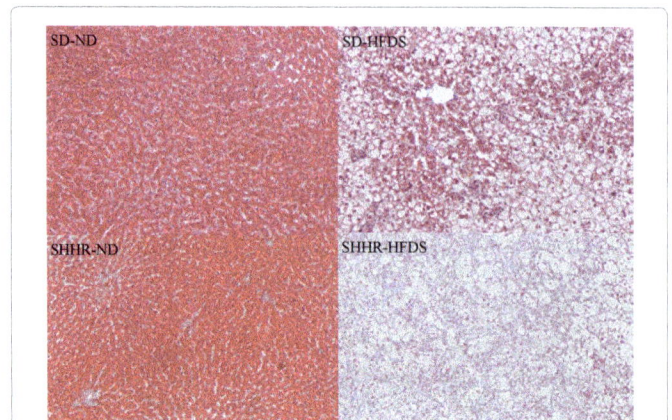

Figure 2: Effects of high fat diet and 30% sucrose on the liver of Spontaneously Hypertensive Hyperlipidemic Rats (SHHR) and SD rats (Masson trichrome stain) SD-ND; SD rats fed with Normal Diet (ND), SD-HFDS; SD rats fed with high fat diet and 30% sucrose (HFDS), SHHR-ND; SHHR fed with ND, SHHR-HFDS; SHHR fed with HFDS.

with a representative sample of liver from each group of SHHR and SD rats at eight months stained with HE and MT. Hepatocyte ballooning and steatosis are well recognized with HFDS feeding. Fibrosis and cell inflammation, which were observed in SHHR-HFDS, were slightly detectable in SD-HFDS.

DNA microarray analysis

On the basis of quality control, 8388 genes were detected. Genes were analyzed statistically employing Student T test unpaired (p-value computation; asymptotic, multiple testing correction; Benjamini-Hochberg, p-value cut off; <0.05) to select pathophysiologically important genes: "Genes correlated with progression of NAFLD", which met all criteria; p<0.05 for SD-ND vs. SD-HFDS, SHHR-ND vs. SHHR-HFDS, SD-ND vs. SHHR-ND, SD-HFDS vs. SHHR-HFDS. "Genes expressed exclusively in NASH", which met all criteria; p<0.05 for SD-ND vs. SD-HFDS, p<0.05 for SHHR-ND vs. SHHR-HFDS, SD-ND vs. SHHR-ND, SD-HFDS vs. SHHR-HFDS. Subsequently, those genes demonstrating identical regulation among all four criteria were obtained as up-regulated or down-regulated. Forty-four and 49 genes were correlated with up-regulation and down-regulation, respectively, in terms of NAFLD progression. Seventy-seven and 32 genes were correlated with up-regulation and down-regulation, respectively, in NASH. Finally, 13 genes were selected from the macrophage infiltration- and oxidative stress-related genes per microarray analysis data.

Discussion

Several earlier studies have established a relationship between obesity and lifestyle-related diseases. In particular, visceral obesity is directly correlated with the clustering of lifestyle-related diseases, leading to various ailments [14-16]. Our previous report demonstrated that visceral fat accumulation is closely associated with increased oxidative stress [12]. We disclosed that oxidative stress, matrix metalloproteinases (MMPs) and tissue inhibitors of metalloproteinases (TIMPs) play an important role in NASH progression in the liver of NASH model rats fed HFDS for 9-13 months. We also determined that hepatocyte ballooning and steatosis are well recognized with HFDS feeding for 9-13 months; moreover, severe fibrosis and cell inflammation were readily apparent around the central vein in SHHR-HFDS but only slightly detectable in SD-HFDS [13]. This study examined hepatic gene expression profiles in the early stage of NASH in the liver of NASH model rats receiving the HFDS for 8 months.

The most accepted theory regarding the explanation of progression from simple steatosis to NASH is the "two-hit hypothesis" wherein fat accumulation is sufficient to induce progression to steatohepatitis, rendering the liver more susceptible to a "second hit" that, once imposed upon the steatotic liver, causes further aberrations that culminate in the development of NASH [17,18]. A key factor in this "second hit" is oxidative stress [13]. Biochemical characteristics of SHHR-HFDS indicate that SHHR-HFDS at 8 months of age may develop metabolic syndrome leading to NAFLD.

A second feature of this study was the statistical method utilized to clarify the pathophysiological mechanism governing progression from simple steatosis to NASH. Based on our previous report, e.g., severe fibrosis and cell inflammation around the central vein were readily apparent in SHHR-HFDS but only slightly detectable in SD-HFDS [13], two groups of genes were extracted: "Genes correlated with progression of NAFLD" and "Genes expressed exclusively in NASH". The former category contained those genes changed in expression, correlated with liver steatosis, oxidative stress and visceral fat accumulation; in other words, "first-hit" induced the gene expressions and "second-hit" enhanced them. The latter category consisted of those genes induced not by "first-hit" but by "second-hit", associated with the aforementioned background. Recently, it was reported that macrophage infiltration and oxidative stress are an initiating event in NASH [19,20]. Therefore, 13 genes were selected from the candidate genes per microarray analysis data and classified as macrophage-related or oxidative stress/inflammation-related genes (Tables 2a-2c). Four genes were associated with macrophage: acid phosphatase 5, tartrate-resistant (Acp5), a member of the RAS oncogene family (Rab8a), scavenger receptor class B, member 2 (Scarb2) and CD36 molecule (Cd36). Furthermore, nine genes were associated with oxidative stress/inflammation: translocator protein (Tspo), prostaglandin I2 synthase (Ptgis), tumor necrosis factor receptor superfamily, member 9 (Tnfrsf9), glutathione S-transferase alpha 5 (Gsta5), regucalcin (Rgn), glutathione S-transferase kappa 1

	Genes correlated with progression of NAFLD		Genes expressed exclusively in NASH	
	Up-regulated	Down-regulated	Up-regulated	Down-regulated
macrophage	Acp5	Rab8a	Scarb2 Cd36	
oxidative stress inflammation	Tspo Ptgis Tnfrsf Gsta5	Rgn Gstk1	Dab2 Gstm5	Fmo5

Table 2a: Macrophage- and oxidative stress/inflammation-related genes acid phosphatase 5, tartrate resistant (Acp5), translocator protein (Tspo), prostaglandin I2 synthase (Ptgis), tumor necrosis factor receptor superfamily, member 9 (Tnfrsf,), glutathione S-transferase alpha 5 (Gsta5), member RAS oncogene family (Rab8a), regucalcin (Rgn), glutathione S-transferase kappa 1 (Gstk1), scavenger receptor class B, member 2 (Scarb2), CD36 molecule (Cd36), disabled homolog 2, mitogen-responsive phosphoprotein (Dab2), glutathione S-transferase mu 5 (Gstm5), flavin-containing monooxygenase 5 (Fmo5).

Gene Symbol	SD-HFDS vs. SD-ND	SHHR-ND vs. SD-ND	SHHR-HFDS vs. SD-HFDS	SHHR-HFDS vs. SHHR-ND
Up-regulated genes				
Acp5	2.21	2.38	3.26	3.02
Tspo	2.29	2.17	2.11	2.22
Gsta5	4.00	6.34	3.44	1.84
Ptgis	1.90	4.84	13.50	5.30
Tnfrsf9	6.51	7.75	4.25	3.57
Down-regulated genes				
Rgn	-2.31	-3.32	-2.51	-1.75
Rab8a	-1.31	-1.31	-1.22	-1.22
Gstk1	-1.97	-1.64	-1.68	-2.02

Table 2b: Changed genes correlated with steatosis HFDS treatment significantly increased or decreased gene expression in SD and SHHR. Meaningful differences were observed between comparison groups. Each mean fold value is presented.

Gene Symbol	SD-HFDS vs. SD-ND	SHHR-ND vs. SD-ND	SHHR-HFDS vs. SD-HFDS	SHHR-HFDS vs. SHHR-ND
Up-regulated genes				
Scarb2	1.07	1.02	1.12	1.18
Dab2	1.58	2.14	3.05	2.25
Gstm5	1.22	1.79	3.36	1.54
Cd36	1.21	1.73	4.57	2.19
Down-regulated genes				
Fmo5	-1.52	-2.17	-3.09	-2.17

Table 2(c): Changed genes correlated with steatohepatitis HFDS treatment significantly increased or decreased gene expression in only SHHR. HFD treatment did not lead to meaningful differences between the SD HFDS and SD ND groups. Each mean fold value is presented.

(Gstk1), disabled homolog 2, mitogen-responsive phosphoprotein (Dab2), glutathione S-transferase mu 5 (Gstm5) and flavin-containing monooxygenase 5 (Fmo5). Acp5, Tspo, Ptgis, Tnfrsf, Gsta5 (up-regulated) as well as Rab8a, Rgn and Gstk1 (down-regulated) were included in the group of genes correlated with progression of NAFLD. Scarb2, Cd36, Dab2 Gstm5 (up-regulated) and Fmo5 (down-regulated) were included in the group of genes expressed exclusively in NASH.

Acp5, Tspo, Ptgis, Tnfrsf and Gsta5 expression increased among genes correlated with the progression of NAFLD. Acp5 is also known as TRACP 5a, which is the novel marker of macrophage activation and inflammatory disease processes [21,22]. TRACP mRNA and a monomeric TRACP protein, equivalent to serum TRACP 5a, demonstrated more abundant expression in adipose-derived macrophages of obese adults in comparison with those of lean individuals [23]. Therefore, elevated Acrp5 may be representative of macrophage infiltration in the liver of SS and NASH model rats.

Tspo is involved in the regulation of cholesterol transport into mitochondria in relation to bile production and steroidogenesis as well as in oxidative stress, apoptosis and inflammatory and immune responses [24-32]. Interestingly, Kugler et al. found that Tspo appears to be an active participant in the generation of Reactive oxygen Species (ROS) at mitochondrial levels and in the modulation of the mitochondrial membrane potential, thereby playing a role in the induction of the mitochondrial apoptosis cascade [33,34]. Increased Tspo may be a key factor in oxidative stress in the liver of SS and NASH model rats. The 4-1BB (also known as ILA; 4-1BB; CD137; CDw137) receptor, a recently identified molecule of the tumor necrosis factor-receptor (Tnfr) superfamily, is a type I membrane protein expressed on activated cytolytic and helper T cells [35]. The 4-1BB receptor ligand (4-1BBL) is expressed on APCs including B cells, macrophages and dedritic cells [36,37]. Ligation of 4-1BB with 4-1BBL plays an important role in sustaining T cell activation and amplifying Cytotoxic T Lymphocyte (CTL) response [38]. Enhanced Tnfr may be related to cytokine signal in the liver of SS and NASH model rats. These data suggested that Acrp5, Tspo and Tnfr were already elevated in liver at the SS stage, which may initiate macrophage infiltration and oxidative stress in the liver. Prostacyclin (PGI2) inhibits platelet aggregation and vasoconstriction. PGI2 synthase (Ptgis), which is widely distributed, occurs predominantly in vascular endothelial and smooth muscle cells [39]. Ptgis is over-expressed and exhibits a strong protective effect against cytokine toxicity, which is correlated with decreased activation of the transcription factor NFkB and the inducible NO synthase promoter as well as reduced inducible NO synthase protein expression and nitrite production. Reduction in the cytokine-stimulated endoplasmic reticulum and mitochondrial stress was also observed in the Ptgis-over-expressing cells. As a result, increased Ptgis may function as a protection system in the liver of SS and NASH model rats. The Glutathione-S-transferases (GST) comprise a major group of detoxification enzymes, which are ubiquitous in all eukaryotic species [40]. GST is responsible for catalyzing the conjugation of Glutathione (GSH) to a wide spectrum of electrophilic compounds including endogenous substances and xenobiotics [41]. Increased expression of GST in response to exposure to xenobiotics is thought to constitute an adaptive response by the exposed cells to chemical or oxidative stress [42]. Gsta5 may also play a role in the protection system in the NAFLD model liver. It is possible that Ptgis and Gsta5 are up-regulated in compensatory fashion in NAFLD liver as a protective mechanism. Rab8, Rgn and Gstk1 decreased among genes correlated with progression of NAFLD.

Rab8, which regulates endosomal cholesterol removal to apoA-I in human fibroblasts, is abundantly expressed in human atherosclerotic lesion macrophages and up-regulated on lipid loading of macrophages *in vitro*; additionally, Rab8 reduces foam cell formation by facilitating ABCA1 surface expression and stimulating endosomal cholesterol efflux to apoA-I in primary human macrophages [43]. Rab8 redistributes cholesterol from late endosomes to the cell periphery and stimulates cholesterol efflux to the ABCA1-ligand apolipoprotein A-I (apoA-I) without increasing cholesterol esterification. Depletion of Rab8 from wild-type fibroblasts results in cholesterol deposition within late endosomal compartments [44]. Diminished Rab8 expression may be related to lipid deposition in the liver of SS and NASH model rats.

Rgn (also known as Senescence Marker Protein-30 (SMP30)) acts as an antioxidant and anti-apoptotic protein. Hepatic SMP30 is closely associated with the pathogenesis of NAFLD [45]; over-expression of SMP30/GNL in Hep G2 cells contributes to decreased ROS formation accompanied by declines in lipid peroxidation, SOD activity and GSH levels [46]. SMP30, which is a potential biomarker for the diagnosis and prognosis of acute liver failure, also plays a very important role in a self-protective mechanism in survival and participates in the pathophysiological processes of acute liver failure [47]. Therefore, the down-regulation of Rgn may be representative of increased oxidative stress in the liver of SS and NASH model rats.

The kappa class GST, which occurs specifically within mitochondria and peroxisomes [48], conjugates glutathione to the classic xenobiotic substrate 1-chloro-2,4-dinitrobenzene. Detection of mGstk1 in the mitochondria of hepatic and renal tissue suggests that this kappa class transferase likely functions as an antioxidant in this organelle [49]. These data suggested that the anti-lipid deposition and antioxidant systems are diminished in the liver of SS and NASH model rats. Scarb2, Cd36, Dab2 and Gstm5 increased among genes expressed exclusively in NASH. Scarb2 is also known as AMRF, EPM4, LGP85, CD36L2, HLGP85, LIMP-2, LIMPII and Scavenger receptors type II (SR-BII). Ishikawa et al. [50] previously reported that SR-B type I and II are expressed in macrophages. Foam cell formation of macrophages is mediated by the uncontrolled uptake of modified and oxidized Low-Density Lipoprotein (LDL) via scavenger receptors, which produces excessive lipoprotein-derived Cholesteryl Ester (CE) accumulation [51]. Elevated scarb2 may be indicative of macrophage infiltration in the liver of NASH model animals.

Cd36 was described as a transporter governing the rate-limiting steps of fatty acid uptake on the plasma membrane of hepatocytes [52]. Involvement of the Cd36 antigen has been demonstrated in phagocytosis of apoptotic cells [53] as well as in the endocytosis of long-chain fatty acids, anionic phospholipids and oxidized lipoproteins [54]; moreover, Cd36 is a class B scavenger receptor. High LDL levels have been shown to become atherogenic when oxidized to modify LDL (Ox-LDL) by inducing foam cell formation via enhanced Cd36 expression on

macrophages. In addition to Ox-LDL, elevated levels of glucose, insulin resistance, low HDL cholesterol and increased levels of free fatty acid (FFA) all result in enhanced expression of CD36, thereby contributing to type 2 diabetes mellitus (T2DM) and related atherosclerosis. Therefore, up-regulation of Cd36 may lead to progression of lipid deposition in the liver of SS and NASH model rats. The cytokine TGF-beta acts as a tumor suppressor in normal epithelial cells during the early stages of tumorigenesis. It was suggested that down-regulation of Dab2 blocks TGF-beta-mediated inhibition of cell proliferation and migration and enables TGF-beta promotion of cell motility, anchorage-independent growth and tumor growth *in vivo* [55]. Up-regulation of Dab2 may be related to cytokine signaling in the liver of SS and NASH model rats.

Members of the GST isoenzyme families, alpha, mu and pi, are elevated in response to chemical and oxidative stress [56]. An increasing volume of data suggests that African-Americans with NAFLD tend to display less progressive liver disease. In comparison to Caucasian NASH patients, African-American NASH patients exhibit over-expression of GSTM 2, GSTM4, GSTM5, FH and ASCL4 [57]. Over-expression of glutathione S-transferase mu transcripts (GSTM1, GSTM3, GSTM4 and GSTM5) may contribute to a decrease in oxidative stress [58]. These findings suggested that increased Scarb2, Cd36 and Dab2 may be related to pathogenesis of NASH and that GSTm5 may be enhanced in compensatory fashion.

Fmo5, which belongs to a family of enzymes that catalyzes the oxygenation of nucleophilic N- and S-containing compounds, decreased among genes expressed exclusively in NASH. The FMO enzyme family consists of five forms (FMOs1-5) that share approximately 50-60% sequence identity with one another [59]. Fmo1, Fmo3 and Fmo5 mRNAs were also found to be down-regulated in LPS models of inflammation [60]. Toll-Like Receptor (TLR) 4 is responsible for LPS signaling in association with several proteins. The down-regulation of Fmo3 and Fmo5 in this model is TLR4-dependent [61]. These data suggested that decreased Fmo5 may be related to inflammation of NASH liver.

Conclusion

Hepatic gene expressions in NAFLD and NASH model rats were elucidated. We hypothesized that scavenger receptor class B and Glutathione S-transferase (GST) play important roles in the progression from simple NAFLD to NASH. The current data afford beneficial information regarding therapeutic targets of NAFLD/NASH progression. Additional studies are necessary in order to confirm the role of these genes.

Acknowledgement

We are grateful for the support from the Showa University Research Grant for Young Researchers.

References

1. McCullough AJ (2004) The clinical features, diagnosis and natural history of nonalcoholic fatty liver disease. Clin Liver Dis 8: 521-533.

2. Dowman JK, Tomlinson JW, Newsome PN (2011) Systematic review: the diagnosis and staging of non-alcoholic fatty liver disease and non-alcoholic steatohepatitis. Aliment Pharmacol Ther 33: 525-540.

3. Brunt EM, Janney CG, Di Bisceglie AM, Neuschwander-Tetri BA, Bacon BR (1999) Nonalcoholic steatohepatitis: a proposal for grading and staging the histological lesions. Am J Gastroenterol 94: 2467-2474.

4. Edmison JM, Kalhan SC, McCullough AJ (2009) Obesity, hepatic metabolism and disease. Nestle Nutr Workshop Ser Pediatr Program 63: 163-172.

5. Siegel AB, Zhu AX (2009) Metabolic syndrome and hepatocellular carcinoma: two growing epidemics with a potential link. Cancer 115: 5651-5661.

6. Adams LA, Lymp JF, St Sauver J, Sanderson SO, Lindor KD, et al. (2005) The natural history of nonalcoholic fatty liver disease: a population-based cohort study. Gastroenterology 129: 113-121.

7. Petta S, Muratore C, Craxi A (2009) Non-alcoholic fatty liver disease pathogenesis: the present and the future. Dig Liver Dis 41: 615-625.

8. Dowman JK, Tomlinson JW, Newsome PN (2010) Pathogenesis of non-alcoholic fatty liver disease. QJM 103: 71-83.

9. Kumai T, Oonuma S, Kitaoka Y, Tadokoro M, Kobayashi S (2003) Biochemical and morphological characterization of spontaneously hypertensive hyperlipidaemic rats. Clin Exp Pharmacol Physiol 30: 537-544.

10. Kumai T, Oonuma S, Matsumoto N, Takeba Y, Taniguchi R, et al. (2004) Anti-lipid deposition effect of HMG-CoA reductase inhibitor, pitavastatin, in a rat model of hypertension and hypercholesterolemia. Life Sci 74: 2129-2142.

11. Saiki R, Okazaki M, Iwai S, Kumai T, Kobayashi S, et al. (2007) Effects of pioglitazone on increases in visceral fat accumulation and oxidative stress in spontaneously hypertensive hyperlipidemic rats fed a high-fat diet and sucrose solution. J Pharmacol Sci 105: 157-167.

12. Tomita Y, Iwai S, Kumai T, Ohnuma S, Kurahashi C, et al. (2010) Visceral fat accumulation is associated with oxidative stress and increased matrix metalloproteinase-9 expression in atherogenic factor-overlapped model rats. Showa Univ J Med Sci 22: 27-40.

13. Tsuchiya H, Iwai S, Kumai T, Ohnuma S, Tsuboi A, et al. (2011) Increase in matrix metalloproteinase-2 and 9 in the liver of nonalcoholic steatohepatitis (NASH) model rats. Showa Univ J Med Sci 23: 37-50.

14. Matsuzawa Y (1997) Pathophysiology and molecular mechanisms of visceral fat syndrome: the Japanese experience. Diabetes Metab Rev 13: 3-13.

15. Kurukulasuriya LR, Govindarajan G, Sowers J (2006) Stroke prevention in diabetes and obesity. Expert Rev Cardiovasc Ther 4: 487-502.

16. Eguchi Y, Mizuta T, Sumida Y, Ishibashi E, Kitajima Y, et al. (2011) The pathological role of visceral fat accumulation in steatosis, inflammation, and progression of nonalcoholic fatty liver disease. J Gastroenterol 46: 70-78.

17. Sakaguchi S, Takahashi S, Sasaki T, Kumagai T, Nagata K (2011) Progression of alcoholic and non-alcoholic steatohepatitis: common metabolic aspects of innate immune system and oxidative stress. Drug Metab Pharmacokinet 26: 30-46.

18. Day CP, James OF (1998) Steatohepatitis: a tale of two "hits"? Gastroenterology 114: 842-845.

19. Bieghs V, Rensen PC, Hofker MH, Shiri-Sverdlov R (2012) NASH and atherosclerosis are two aspects of a shared disease: central role for macrophages. Atherosclerosis 220: 287-293.

20. Koek GH, Liedorp PR, Bast A (2011) The role of oxidative stress in non-alcoholic steatohepatitis. Clin Chim Acta 412: 1297-1305.

21. Shidara K, Inaba M, Okuno S, Yamada S, Kumeda Y, et al. (2008) Serum levels of TRAP5b, a new bone resorption marker unaffected by renal dysfunction, as a useful marker of cortical bone loss in hemodialysis patients. Calcif Tissue Int 82: 278-287.

22. Janckila AJ, Slone SP, Lear SC, Martin A, Yam LT (2007) Tartrate-resistant acid phosphatase as an immunohistochemical marker for inflammatory macrophages. Am J Clin Pathol 127: 556-566.

23. Lang P, van Harmelen V, Ryden M, Kaaman M, Parini P, et al. (2008) Monomeric tartrate resistant acid phosphatase induces insulin sensitive obesity. PLoS One 3: e1713.

24. Gavish M, Bar-Ami S, Weizman R (1992) The endocrine system and mitochondrial benzodiazepine receptors. Mol Cell Endocrinol 88: 1-13.

25. Knudsen J, Mandrup S, Rasmussen JT, Andreasen PH, Poulsen F, et al. (1993) The function of acyl-CoA-binding protein (ACBP)/diazepam binding inhibitor (DBI). Mol Cell Biochem 123: 129-138.

26. Krueger KE, Papadopoulos V (1990) Peripheral-type benzodiazepine receptors mediate translocation of cholesterol from outer to inner mitochondrial membranes in adrenocortical cells. J Biol Chem 265: 15015-15022.

27. Kunduzova OR, Escourrou G, De La Farge F, Salvayre R, Seguelas MH, et al. (2004) Involvement of peripheral benzodiazepine receptor in the oxidative stress, death-signaling pathways, and renal injury induced by ischemia-reperfusion. J Am Soc Nephrol 15: 2152-2160.

28. Papadopoulos V, Baraldi M, Guilarte TR, Knudsen TB, Lacapere JJ, et al. (2006) Translocator protein (18kDa): new nomenclature for the peripheral-type benzodiazepine receptor based on its structure and molecular function. Trends Pharmacol Sci 27: 402-409.

29. Veenman L, Gavish M (2006) The peripheral-type benzodiazepine receptor and the cardiovascular system. Implications for drug development. Pharmacol Ther 110: 503-524.

30. Veenman L, Papadopoulos V, Gavish M (2007) Channel-like functions of the 18-kDa translocator protein (TSPO): regulation of apoptosis and steroidogenesis as part of the host-defense response. Curr Pharm Des 13: 2385-2405.

31. Veenman L, Shandalov Y, Gavish M (2008) VDAC activation by the 18 kDa translocator protein (TSPO), implications for apoptosis. J Bioenerg Biomembr 40: 199-205.

32. Veenman L, Alten J, Linnemannstons K, Shandalov Y, Zeno S, et al. (2010) Potential involvement of F0F1-ATP(synth)ase and reactive oxygen species in apoptosis induction by the antineoplastic agent erucylphosphohomocholine in glioblastoma cell lines : a mechanism for induction of apoptosis via the 18 kDa mitochondrial translocator protein. Apoptosis 15: 753-768.

33. Kugler W, Veenman L, Shandalov Y, Leschiner S, Spanier I, et al. (2008) Ligands of the mitochondrial 18 kDa translocator protein attenuate apoptosis of human glioblastoma cells exposed to erucylphosphohomocholine. Cell Oncol 30: 435-450.

34. Zeno S, Zaaroor M, Leschiner S, Veenman L, Gavish M (2009) CoCl(2) induces apoptosis via the 18 kDa translocator protein in U118MG human glioblastoma cells. Biochemistry 48: 4652-4661.

35. Kwon BS, Weissman SM (1989) cDNA sequences of two inducible T-cell genes. Proc Natl Acad Sci U S A 86: 1963-1967.

36. Pollok KE, Kim YJ, Hurtado J, Zhou Z, Kim KK, et al. (1994) 4-1BB T-cell antigen binds to mature B cells and macrophages, and costimulates anti-mu-primed splenic B cells. Eur J Immunol 24: 367-374.

37. DeBenedette MA, Shahinian A, Mak TW, Watts TH (1997) Costimulation of CD28- T lymphocytes by 4-1BB ligand. J Immunol 158: 551-559.

38. Chu NR, DeBenedette MA, Stiernholm BJ, Barber BH, Watts TH (1997) Role of IL-12 and 4-1BB ligand in cytokine production by CD28+ and CD28- T cells. J Immunol 158: 3081-3089.

39. Nakayama T (2010) Genetic polymorphisms of prostacyclin synthase gene and cardiovascular disease. Int Angiol 29: 33-42.

40. Kazi S, Ellis EM (2002) Expression of rat liver glutathione-S-transferase GSTA5 in cell lines provides increased resistance to alkylating agents and toxic aldehydes. Chem Biol Interact 140: 121-135.

41. Booth J, Boyland E, Sims P (1961) An enzyme from rat liver catalysing conjugations with glutathione. Biochem J 79: 516-524.

42. Hayes JD, Ellis EM, Neal GE, Harrison DJ, Manson MM (1999) Cellular response to cancer chemopreventive agents: contribution of the antioxidant responsive element to the adaptive response to oxidative and chemical stress. Biochem Soc Symp 64: 141-168.

43. Linder MD, Mayranpaa MI, Peranen J, Pietila TE, Pietiainen VM, et al. (2009) Rab8 regulates ABCA1 cell surface expression and facilitates cholesterol efflux in primary human macrophages. Arterioscler Thromb Vasc Biol 29: 883-888.

44. Linder MD, Uronen RL, Holtta-Vuori M, van der Sluijs P, Peranen J, et al. (2007) Rab8-dependent recycling promotes endosomal cholesterol removal in normal and sphingolipidosis cells. Mol Biol Cell 18: 47-56.

45. Park H, Ishigami A, Shima T, Mizuno M, Maruyama N, et al. (2010) Hepatic senescence marker protein-30 is involved in the progression of nonalcoholic fatty liver disease. J Gastroenterol 45: 426-434.

46. Handa S, Maruyama N, Ishigami A (2009) Over-expression of Senescence Marker Protein-30 decreases reactive oxygen species in human hepatic carcinoma Hep G2 cells. Biol Pharm Bull 32: 1645-1648.

47. Lv S, Wang JH, Liu F, Gao Y, Fei R, et al. (2008) Senescence marker protein 30 in acute liver failure: validation of a mass spectrometry proteomics assay. BMC Gastroenterol 8: 17.

48. Morel F, Rauch C, Petit E, Piton A, Theret N, et al. (2004) Gene and protein characterization of the human glutathione S-transferase kappa and evidence for a peroxisomal localization. J Biol Chem 279: 16246-16253.

49. Thomson RE, Bigley AL, Foster JR, Jowsey IR, Elcombe CR, et al. (2004)

Tissue-specific expression and subcellular distribution of murine glutathione S-transferase class kappa. J Histochem Cytochem 52: 653-662.

50. Ishikawa Y, Kimura-Matsumoto M, Murakami M, Yamamoto K, Akasaka Y, et al. (2009) Distribution of smooth muscle cells and macrophages expressing scavenger receptor BI/II in atherosclerosis. J Atheroscler Thromb 16: 829-839.

51. de Villiers WJ, Smart EJ (1999) Macrophage scavenger receptors and foam cell formation. J Leukoc Biol 66: 740-746.

52. Stahlberg N, Rico-Bautista E, Fisher RM, Wu X, Cheung L, et al. (2004) Female-predominant expression of fatty acid translocase/CD36 in rat and human liver. Endocrinology 145: 1972-1979.

53. Ren Y, Silverstein RL, Allen J, Savill J (1995) CD36 gene transfer confers capacity for phagocytosis of cells undergoing apoptosis. J Exp Med 181: 1857-1862.

54. Rigotti A, Acton SL, Krieger M (1995) The class B scavenger receptors SR-BI and CD36 are receptors for anionic phospholipids. J Biol Chem 270: 16221-16224.

55. Hannigan A, Smith P, Kalna G, Lo Nigro C, Orange C, et al. (2010) Epigenetic downregulation of human disabled homolog 2 switches TGF-beta from a tumor suppressor to a tumor promoter. J Clin Invest 120: 2842-2857.

56. Hayes JD, Wolf CR (1990) Molecular mechanisms of drug resistance. Biochem J 272: 281-295.

57. Stepanova M, Hossain N, Afendy A, Perry K, Goodman ZD, et al. (2010) Hepatic gene expression of Caucasian and African-American patients with obesity-related non-alcoholic fatty liver disease. Obes Surg 20: 640-650.

58. Raza A, Dikdan G, Desai KK, Shareef A, Fernandes H, et al. (2010) Global gene expression profiles of ischemic preconditioning in deceased donor liver transplantation. Liver Transpl 16: 588-599.

59. Motika MS, Zhang J, Ralph EC, Dwyer MA, Cashman JR (2012) pH dependence on functional activity of human and mouse flavin-containing monooxygenase 5. Biochem Pharmacol 83: 962-968.

60. Zhang J, Chaluvadi MR, Reddy R, Motika MS, Richardson TA, et al. (2009) Hepatic flavin-containing monooxygenase gene regulation in different mouse inflammation models. Drug Metab Dispos 37: 462-468.

61. Koutoulaki A, Langley M, Sloan AJ, Aeschlimann D, Wei XQ (2010) TNFalpha and TGF-beta1 influence IL-18-induced IFNgamma production through regulation of IL-18 receptor and T-bet expression. Cytokine 49: 177-184.

20

Inter-patient Variability in Clinical Efficacy of Metformin in Type 2 Diabetes Mellitus Patients

Biswabandhu Bankura[1], Madhusudan Das[1], Arup Kumar Pattanayak[1], Bidisha Adhikary[1], Rana Bhattacharjee[2], Soumik Goswami[2], Subhankar Chowdhury[2] and Ajitesh Roy[2]*

[1]Department of Zoology, University of Calcutta, 35 Ballygunge Circular Road, Kolkata-700 019, West Bengal, India
[2]Department of Endocrinolgy, Institute of Post Graduate Medical Education & Research, 244 A J C Bose Road, Kolkata-700 020, West Bengal, India

Abstract

Background and objective: Metformin is often used as a first-line therapy for Type 2 diabetes mellitus (T2DM), but the glycemic response to metformin is variable in patients. Here, we aimed to assess the inter-patient variability in terms of glycemic response to metformin in the state of West Bengal, India.

Material and methods: We enrolled newly diagnosed treatment naïve 113 patients with T2DM. Patients were subjected to assay of glycated hemoglobin (HbA1c), fasting blood glucose (FBG), postprandial blood glucose (PP) and measurement of body mass index (BMI), waist circumstances (WC) before and after the end of 3 months of immediate release metformin (2000mg/day) therapy.

Results: Out of 113 patients, 111 (58 male and 53 female; average age 43.13 years) were provided with 3 months of metformin therapy. 102 individuals responded to metformin, but HbA1c levels of 9 patients did not improve after 3 months of drug therapy.

Conclusions: In the present study, metformin lead to improvements in glycemic control in 92% of newly diagnosed T2DM patients but in 8% does not which is much less in this part of India.

Keywords: Type 2 diabetes mellitus; Metformin; Glycemic response; Glycated hemoglobin; Non-responder

Introduction

Type 2 diabetes mellitus (T2DM) is a major health problem in worldwide [1]. T2DM is a multifactorial, heterogeneous group of disorder with varying prevalence among different ethnic groups [2]. The disease is affecting at an alarming rate to both rural and urban populations in India [3-6]. Recent epidemiologic studies have shown more than 62 million diabetic individuals currently diagnosed with the disease in India [7]. The prevalence of diabetes in West Bengal state, India, is in between 2.7% - 13.2% [6].

The pathophysiology of T2DM is characterized by peripheral insulin resistance, impaired regulation of hepatic glucose production, and declining beta cell function. It can now be treated with several classes of approved drugs, in addition to diet and exercise regimens [8]. Among them, metformin, a biguanide is one of the most widely prescribed oral anti-hyperglycemic drugs. It ameliorates hyperglycemia by decreasing hepatic glucose output, gastrointestinal glucose absorption, improving insulin sensitivity and improvement of peripheral glucose uptake in skeletal muscle and fat [9-11]. Metformin is slowly absorbed in the Gastrointestinal (GI) tract and not bound with any protein and also remained intact during the process of metabolism. The drug is mainly eliminated by renal excretion with renal clearance 4-5 times greater than glomerular filtration rate [12]. It is effective as monotherapy or in combination with other agents, such as insulin secretagogues, other insulin-sensitizing drugs, or inhibitors of glucose absorption. The anti-diabetic drug metformin has attracted much attention for several reasons. Metformin does not cause weight gain, may lead to weight loss. Metformin also has beneficial effects on several cardiovascular risk factors such as dyslipidemia elevated plasma plasminogen activator inhibitor, other fibrinolytic abnormalities and insulin resistance [13].

The antidiabetic response to metformin differs significantly from patients to patients. Based on clinical trial experience, patients using metformin monotherapy as their first-ever anti hyperglycemic drug, less than two-thirds of patients achieve a desired fasting glucose level or the HbA1c goal of <7% [14]. The non-response rate to metformin may be upwards to 50% [15]. This incomplete response rate of metformin coupled with waning effectiveness over time, highlights the need for personalized medications to maintain tight glycemic control [16]. To date, no such studies in patients with T2DM have shown that glycemic response to metformin is variable in subpopulation of West Bengal, India. Thus, we have conducted an open-label study for 12 months with a course of metformin in 111 patients with well characterized T2DM.

Materials and Methods

Study sample

The 113 subjects were recruited from the diabetes out-patient department of Seth Sukhlal Karnani Memorial Hospital (SSKM) & Institute of Post Graduate Medical Education & Research (IPGME&R), Kolkata, West Bengal, India in the period of November, 2013-September, 2014. Patients were diagnosed based on the American diabetes association criteria [17].

We excluded those patients from our study who had i) glomerular filtration rates (GFRs) less than 60 ml. min^{-1}.1.73 m^{-2} ii) Severe cardiovascular, malignant or chronic inflammatory diseases iii) active infection iv) metabolic decompensation or HbA1c>12% and

---

*Corresponding author: Dr. Ajitesh Roy, Department of Endocrinolgy, Institute of Post Graduate, Medical Education & Research, J C Bose Road, Kolkata, West Bengal, India, E-mail: ajiteshmd@yahoo.com

v) pregnant patients or women hoping to conceive. We also excluded patients who were co-prescribed acarbose, glitazone, sulfonylurea, or insulin at the time of one of the two Hb_{A1C}, FBS and PPBS measurements. There are no generally accepted criteria in the clinical cut-off point to divide patients into metformin responder and non-responder. Thus we selected the criteria, based on clinical experience and previous reports [10, 18]. 1) Responder: Where HbA1c levels had decreased more than 1% from the baseline within 3 months of metformin therapy. 2) Non-responder: decrease in HbA1c levels less than 1% from the baseline or another hypoglycemic drug has been added to the therapy because of poor glycemic status. The study had been started after obtaining informed consents of the participants. The experimental protocol was approved by the Institutional Ethical Committee of *IPGME&R, Kolkata*. All the participants were instructed to maintain appropriate lifestyle habits during the course of the study.

Baseline evaluation

Patients were initially screened during an outpatient clinic visit with brief medical history, review of outside medical records, physical examination, information about demographic parameters and routine blood test in collaboration with the physician. None of the patients were taking antidiabetic medication prior to their diabetes diagnosis.

HbA1c was analyzed using the high-pressure liquid chromatography (BioRad D 10, Hercules, CA). Blood glucose was determined by a glucose oxidase method (Roche, Basel, Switzerland).

Therapy and monitoring

After complete medical evaluation and HbA1c, FBS and PPBS tests, patients who qualified for the therapy were treated with metformin at an initial dose of 500 mg once daily and then rapidly upgraded to full dose (2000 mg/day) with following schedule: 500 mg once a day for 5 days followed by 1000 mg once a day for 5 days and finally 1000 mg twice daily, if no side effects were observed. Patients were monitored for a 12-week period. Patients were asked to come after 6 week to see compliances. Also they are asked to bring used medicine strips. The HbA1c, FBS and PPBS tests were repeated again after 3 months of therapy. Metformin treatment was well tolerated. 10 (9%) patients had mild gastrointestinal symptoms in the form of abdominal discomfort with increase bile motion, which subsided with few weeks. Two patients stopped therapy because of severe gastrointestinal side effects.

Statistical analyses

Two tailed paired and unpaired *t*-tests were performed to test the statistical significance among the data for each group and between two groups before and after treatment measures. We analysed non-parametric variables by Mann-Whitney test and Wilcoxon matched pairs test. Statistical analysis was performed using Graphpad Prism 4 software (Graphpad Software Inc., San Diego, CA, USA).

Results

Patients enrolled

113 adult patients with T2DM were enrolled in the study and 111 completed the 3 months of therapy and underwent follow-up testing. The 2 been excluded (a 45 years and 53 years old women) as they stopped therapy after 12 days. These two patients were not included for further analyses.

Baseline features

The 111 patients included 58 male and 53 female with an average age was 44.91 years. No patient was treated for diabetes at the time of the enrolment. The baseline demographic characteristics (Table 1) and the anthropometric characteristics of all patients were presented in Table 1. Indeed there was almost two times increase in the prevalence of diabetes with age group 40-60 years compare to 20-40 years age and almost ten times increase compare to age above 60 years (Table 1). The prevalence of overweight and obesity in the entire study population were almost 20% and 45%. Furthermore, central obesity was observed in 57% in patients with diabetes. Approximately 61% patients were family history positive for diabetes. Comparison of presenting symptoms was shown in Table 1. Osmotic symptoms was most common (51.3%) followed by general weakness (22.2%), Polyphagia (15.3%), weight loss (7.2%), Burning sensation in feet and palm (7.2%), Blurring of vision (4.5%), Pruritus (3.6%), Balanoposthitis (3.6%), Numbness in feet (2.7%) and Vaginitis(1.8%). We also found 21 (18.9%) patients without any symptoms.

The responder and non-responder groups did not differ significantly in term of age (45.23 ± 10.49 in the responder group, 41.33 ± 10.55 in the non-responder group, p = 0.50). At baseline, also the difference of average BMI, WC, FBS, PPBS and HbA1c values between responder and non-responder group were insignificant (Table 2).

Metformin responder and non-responder

Responder: Number of patients: 102

Characteristic	Patients (n-111)
Men:Women	58:53
Age (years)	n (%)
20-40	36 (32.4)
41-60	69 (62.1)
61 above	7 (6.3)
Family history of Diabetes	68 (61.2)
BMI (kg/m²)	
<18.5 (underweight)	7 (6.3)
18.5-22.9 (normal range)	32 (28.8)
23-24.9 (overweight)	22 (19.8)
25-29.9 (obese)	50 (45.0)
Abdominal obesity	
Waist <80 cm (female), <90 (male)	48 (43.2)
Waist> 80-89 cm (female), >90-99 cm (male)	32 (28.8)
Waist>90 cm (female), >100 cm (male)	31 (27.9)
Occupation	
Unskilled/skilled worker	45 (40.54)
Entrepreneur	14 (12.61)
Farmer	11 (9.9)
Housewife	36 (32.4)
Retired	5 (4.5)
Smoking	22 (19.8)
Smoking + alcohol	13 (11.7)
Oral tobacco	17 (15.3)
Hypertension	26 (23.4)
Osmotic symptoms	57 (51.3)
Polyphagia	17 (15.3)
Gen weakness	25 (22.2)
Weight loss	8 (7.2)
Burning sensation in feet and palm	8 (7.2)
Numbness in feet	3 (2.7)
Pruritus	4 (3.6)
Balanoposthitis	4 (3.6)
Vaginitis	2 (1.8)
Blurring of vision	6 (4.5)
Asymptomatic	21 (18.9)

Table 1: Baseline demographic characteristics of patients.

Parameters	Baseline			After 3 months		
	Responder (n-102)	Non- responder (n-9)	P-value	Responder (n-102)	Non- responder (n-9)	P-value
BMI (kg/m²)	25.01 (4.47)	24.38 (4.68)	0.995*	23.91 (3.71)	24.10 (4.48)	0.364
WC (cm)	91.95 (12.03)	88.67 (13.58)	0.439	90.45 (10.78)	87.98 (13.27)	0.519
FBS (mg/dL)	182.13 (40.01)	185.67 (50.41)	0.837	114.73(18.85)	186.89 (34.06)	**<0.001**
PPBS (mg/dL)	277.28 (63.53)	283.44 (71.01)	0.782	156.55 (30.79)	294.11 (63.29)	**<0.001**
HbA1c%	9.36 (1.19)	9.07 (1.20)	0.402	6.72 (0.85)	9.21 (1.04)	**<0.001**

P-value based on 2 tailed unpaired t-test and
*P-value based on Mann-Whitney test
Values are given as mean (s.d.)

Table 2: Comparisons between metformin responder and non-responder at baseline.

Parameter	Baseline	After 3 months	P-value	Baseline	After 3 months	P-value
		Responder (n-102)			Non-responder (n-9)	
BMI (kg/m²)	25.01 (4.47)	23.91 (3.71)	**<0.001***	24.38 (4.68)	24.10 (4.48)	0.08
WC (cm)	91.95 (12.03)	90.45 (10.78)	**<0.001**	88.67 (13.58)	87.98 (13.27)	0.126
FBS (mg/dL)	182.13 (40.01)	114.73(18.85)	**<0.001**	185.67 (50.41)	186.89 (34.06)	0.906
PPBS (mg/dL)	277.28 (63.53)	156.55 (30.79)	**<0.001**	283.44 (71.01)	294.11 (63.29)	0.53
HbA1c%	9.36 (1.19)	6.72 (0.85)	**<0.001**	9.07 (1.20)	9.21 (1.04)	0.428

P-value based on 2 tailed paired t-test and
*P-value based on Wilcoxon matched pairs test
Values are given as mean (s.d.)

Table 3: Comparison of clinical parameters at baseline and after 3 months of metformin therapy of responder and non-responder patients.

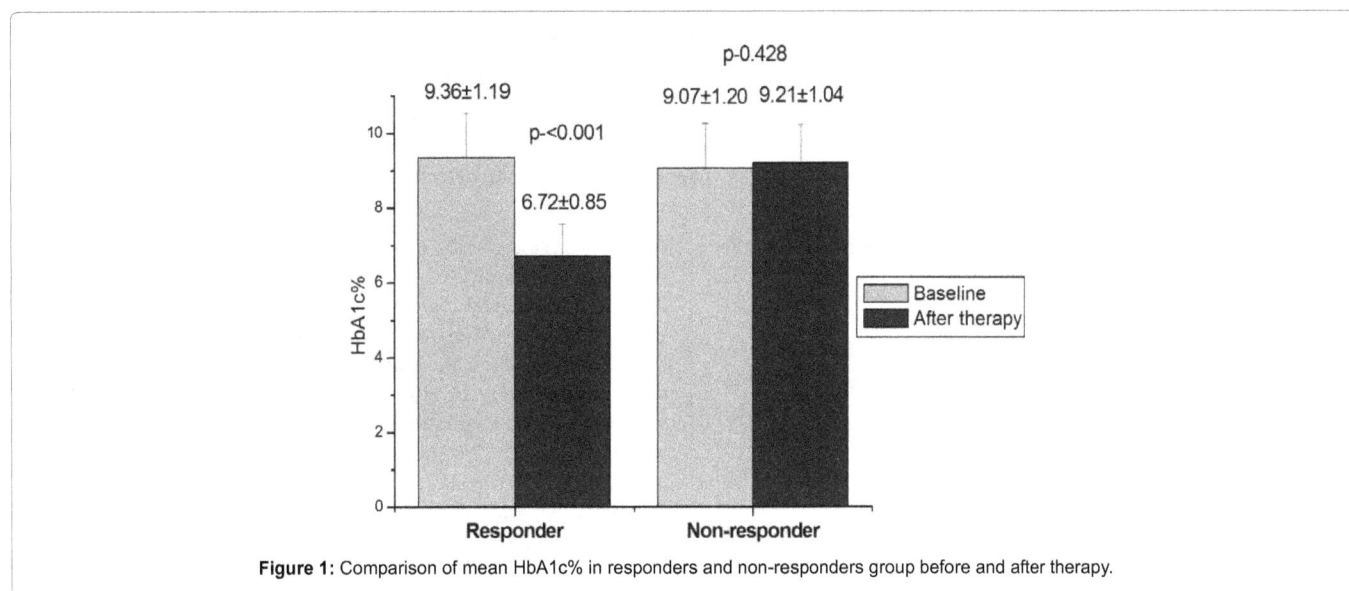

Figure 1: Comparison of mean HbA1c% in responders and non-responders group before and after therapy.

Gender a) Male–56(55%)

b) Female - 46 (45%)

According to the selection criteria, 102 patients were responders, among them 56% were male and 46% female. Improvements in BMI, WC, FBS, PPBS and HbA1c were observed during metformin treatment in 102 patients (responder). After therapy, the average BMI decreased from 25.01 kg/m⁻² to 23.91 kg/m⁻² (P = <0.001), was statistically significant and the changes in average WC, FBS, PPBS and HbA1c values were significantly decreased from baseline (Table 3). The histogram shows average changes in HbA1c% in responders before and after therapy (Figure 1).

Non-responder: Number of patients: 9

Gender a) Male - 2 (22%)

b) Female - 7 (78%)

According to the selection criteria, 9 patients were non responders, among them 22% were male and 78% female. The average BMI, WC, FBS, PPBS and HbA1c levels did not improve in nine patients (non-responder) (Table 4) out of 102 patients after therapy. The average HbA1c level was increased from 9.07% to 9.21% after metformin monotherapy. The graph shows average changes in HbA1c% in non-responders before and after therapy group (Figure 1). The HbA1c levels of six non-responders were increased from baseline and the value was decreased (~0.4%) in three non-responders (Figure 2).

After completion of metformin therapy, FBS, PPBS and HbA1c levels were significantly different between responders and non-responders (Table 2).

Discussion

We conducted this open-label trial study to determine the inter-patient variability in the clinical efficacy of metformin in patients

Parameter	Baseline	After 3 months	P-value
BMI (kg/m²)	24.38 (4.68)	24.10 (4.48)	0.08
WC (cm)	88.67 (13.58)	87.98 (13.27)	0.126
FBS (mg/dL)	185.67 (50.41)	186.89 (34.06)	0.906
PPBS (mg/dL)	283.44 (71.01)	294.11 (63.29)	0.53
HbA1c%	9.07 (1.20)	9.21 (1.04)	0.428

P-value based on 2 tailed paired t-test.
Values are given as mean (s.d)

Table 4: Comparison of clinical parameters at baseline and after 3 months of metformin therapy of non-responder patients.

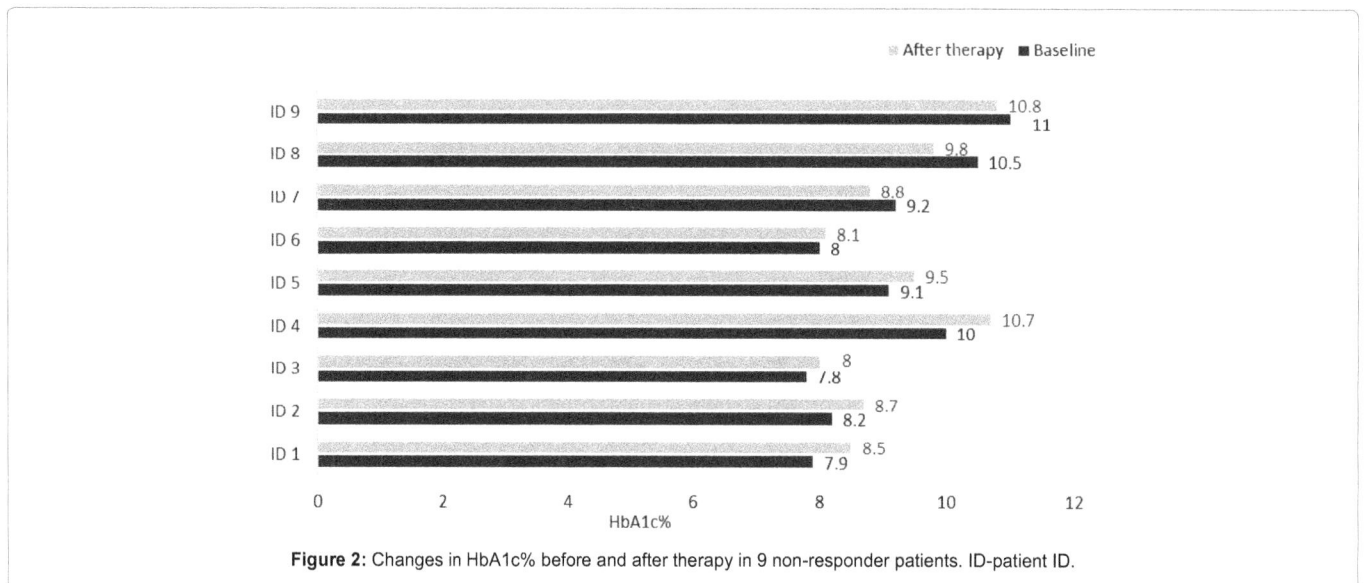

Figure 2: Changes in HbA1c% before and after therapy in 9 non-responder patients. ID-patient ID.

with T2DM in the state of West Bengal, India. Our data suggest that 8% T2DM patients are not able to improved glycemic response with metformin therapy.

Our study was designed to assess glycemic control of metformin as measured by changes in HbA1c from baseline to week 12. Three months course of metformin in dose of 2000 mg/day was associated with improvements in HbA1c, FBS and PPBS in over one third of (92%) patients with T2DM. 8% of patients did not show improvement in the HbA1c, FBS and PPBS levels. All the guidelines advocates use of metformin as 1st line agent for most T2DM therapy. Nevertheless, metformin is known to cause variable glycemic response. In responders, the improvements in average HbA1c, FBS, PPBS, BMI and WC values were significant before and after the therapy, but in non-responders group these levels did not improve after the therapy. It was previously reported that metformin was effective in a smaller dose (500 mg) in the Asian Indian population [19]. In our study, we used metformin in doses of 2000 mg/day to optimize treatment. However, some patients may not need 2000 mg/day dose but to assess a proper glycemic response, we used to increase the dose to a best possible dose.

Earlier studies reported that oral antidiabetic drug sufficiently decrease HbA1c levels by 0.5–1.5% [18]. A very recent study conducted by Mahrooz et al. showed that, decrease in HbA1c levels by more than 1% from baseline may possibly a criterion for classifying diabetic patients as metformin responders or non-responders [20]. In our study, we showed that, after metformin therapy the average decrease in HbA1c levels reached 2.41% (2.41 ± 1.17%). In addition, the mean decrease was 2.64% (2.64 ± 0.92%) among responders, whereas the value was increased 0.13% (0.13 ± 0.47%) in non-responders. The

average decrease in HbA1c levels in our study is higher compare to previous study conducted by Mahrooz et al. [20]. Mahrooz et al. used metformin dose 1000 mg/day in their study whereas in our study we used 2000 mg/day. The simultaneous use of metrormin and dietary and life style modification and ethnic variation may be the probable reason for greater decrease of HbA1c level. However there is considerable variation in response to metformin, with about 35% of patients failing to achieve initial glycemic control on metformin monotherapy as reported [21,22] whereas, we found 8% (n=9) of patients were non-responder to metformin. Many questions remain regarding metformin response, which may be due to genetic or non-genetic. Till now most reproducible associations have been in known transporter genes. As we learn more about the genetics of drug response, we are finding a number of circumstances in which genetic differences can influence both the likelihood of responding and the likelihood of having a severe side effect to medication.

This study enrolled patients with well characterized T2DM. The strength of this study was selection of drug naïve patients (who never took anti-diabetic drugs), careful follow up, and ensuring drug compliance. The major limitations of this study were small number of patients and conducted in small area. Further large replicating study is needed to support our result.

Conclusions

In summary, this is the first study regarding the glycemic efficacy of metformin in treatment naïve T2DM patients from West Bengal, India. Our study revealed that, decrease in HbA1c levels by more than 1% from baseline could be considered a criterion for response to metformin. In addition, few patients were non responders to metformin therapy, which may be combined effects of multiple gene variants in the same or converging pathways and their interaction with non-genetic factors.

Acknowledgements

We thank Prof. Partha P. Majumder, Director, National Institute of Biomedical Genomics, Kalyani, West Bengal, India for his guidance. The study was funded by the Department of Biotechnology, Govt. of India [Sanction No-BT/PR5917/MED/12/568/2012-20/2007 dt-06.08.2013].

Disclosures

The authors declare that they have no conflict of interest.

References

1. Hundal RS, Inzucchi SE (2003) Metformin: new understandings, new uses. Drugs 63: 1879-1894.

2. Harris MI, Couric CC, Reiber G, Boyko E, Stern M, et al (1995) Diabetes in America. 2nd ed. Washington DC: National Institutes of Health.

3. Mohan V, Shanthirani S, Deepa R, Premalatha G, Sastry NG, et al. (2001) Intra-urban differences in the prevalence of the metabolic syndrome in southern India -- the Chennai Urban Population Study (CUPS No. 4). Diabet Med 18: 280-287.

4. Ramachandran A, Snehalatha C, Kapur A, Vijay V, Mohan V, et al. (2001) High prevalence of diabetes and impaired glucose tolerance in India: National Urban Diabetes Survey. Diabetologia 44: 1094-1101.

5. Ramachandran A, Chamukuttan S, Viswanathan V (2003) Explosion of type 2 diabetes in the Indian subcontinent. International Diabetes Monitor 15: 1-6.

6. Pradhan R, Kumar BD, Mitra A (2009) Some Salient Points in Type 2 Diabetes Prevalence in Rural Bengal. Ethno-Medicine 3: 127-131.

7. Kaveeshwar SA, Cornwall J (2014) The current state of diabetes mellitus in India. Australas Med J 7: 45-48.

8. Reitman ML, Schadt EE (2007) Pharmacogenetics of metformin response: a step in the path toward personalized medicine. J Clin Invest 117: 1226-1229.

9. Mohan V, Vijayaprabha R, Rema M (1996) Vascular complications in long-term south Indian NIDDM of over 25 years' duration. Diabetes Res Clin Pract 31: 133-140.

10. Shikata E, Yamamoto R, Takane H, Shigemasa C, Ikeda T, et al. (2007) Human organic cation transporter (OCT1 and OCT2) gene polymorphisms and therapeutic effects of metformin. J Hum Genet 52: 117-122.

11. Distefano JK, Watanabe RM (2010) Pharmacogenetics of Anti-Diabetes Drugs. Pharmaceuticals (Basel) 3: 2610-2646.

12. Scheen AJ (1996) Clinical pharmacokinetics of metformin. Clin Pharmacokinet 30: 359-371.

13. Cusi K, Defronzo RA (1998) Metformin: a review of its metabolic effects. Diab Rev 6: 89-131.

14. Kahn SE, Haffner SM, Heise MA, Herman WH, Holman RR, et al. (2006) Glycemic durability of rosiglitazone, metformin, or glyburide monotherapy. N Engl J Med 355: 2427-2443.

15. Pearson ER, Donnelly LA, Kimber C, Whitley A, Doney AS, et al. (2007) Variation in TCF7L2 influences therapeutic response to sulfonylureas: a GoDARTs study. Diabetes 56: 2178-2182.

16. Zolk O (2012) Disposition of metformin: variability due to polymorphisms of organic cation transporters. Ann Med 44: 119-129.

17. American Diabetes Association (2013) Standards of medical care in diabetes--2013. Diabetes Care 36 Suppl 1: S11-66.

18. Sherifali D, Nerenberg K, Pullenayegum E, Cheng JE, Gerstein HC (2010) The effect of oral antidiabetic agents on A1C levels: a systematic review and meta-analysis. Diabetes Care 33: 1859-1864.

19. Ramachandran A, Snehalatha C, Mary S, Mukesh B, Bhaskar AD, et al (2006) The Indian Diabetes Prevention Programme shows that lifestyle modification and metformin prevent type 2 diabetes in Asian Indian subjects with impaired glucose tolerance (IDPP-1). Diabetologia 49: 289-297.

20. Barthel W, Markwardt F (1975) Aggregation of blood platelets by adrenaline and its uptake. Biochem Pharmacol 24: 1903-1904.

21. Mahrooz A, Parsanasab H, Hashemi-Soteh MB, Kashi Z, Bahar A, et al. (2015) The role of clinical response to metformin in patients newly diagnosed with type 2 diabetes: a monotherapy study. Clin Exp Med 15: 159-165.

22. Pawlyk AC, Giacomini KM, McKeon C, Shuldiner AR, Florez JC (2014) Metformin pharmacogenomics: current status and future directions. Diabetes 63: 2590-2599.

21

Maternal Serum Leptin at 11-13 Weeks Gestation in Normal 1 and Pathological Pregnancies

Surabhi Nanda[1,2], Ranjit Akolekar[1,2], Isabela C Acosta[1,3], Dorota Wierzbicka[1,3] and Kypros H Nicolaides[1,2,3]*

[1]Harris Birthright Research Centre for Fetal Medicine, King's College Hospital, London, UK
[2]Department of Fetal Medicine, Medway Maritime Hospital, Gillingham (Kent), UK
[3]Department of Fetal Medicine, University College Hospital, London, UK

Abstract

Objective: To examine maternal serum levels of leptin at 11-13 weeks gestation in normal and pathological pregnancies.

Methods: Serum leptin, PAPP-A and uterine artery pulsatility index (PI) at 11-13 weeks were measured in 480 singleton pregnancies, including 240 with normal outcome, 60 that subsequently developed preeclampsia (PE), 60 that developed Gestational Diabetes Mellitus (GDM), 60 that delivered Large for Gestational Age (LGA) neonates and 60 that delivered small(SGA) neonates. Regression analysis was used to determine factors affecting maternal serum leptin concentration and from this model each value was expressed as Multiples of the Median (MoM). The median MoM values in the outcome groups were compared.

Results: In the normal group serum leptin levels increased with maternal weight and decreased with maternal height. In the PE group, the median leptin (1.18 MoM, p=0.027) and uterine artery PI (1.25 MoM, p<0.0001) were increased and serum PAPP-A (0.72 MoM, p<0.0001) was decreased. There was no significant association between serum leptin and either uterine artery PI (p=0.983) or serum PAPP-A (p=0.403). In the SGA, LGA and GDM groups serum leptin MoM was not significantly different from the controls (p=0.621, p=0.385 and p=0.722, respectively).

Conclusion: In conclusion, in pregnancies that develop PE, maternal serum leptin concentration at 11-13 weeks is increased in a manner not related to altered placental perfusion or function. In pregnancies complicated by the development of GDM or delivery of SGA or LGA neonates, serum leptin is not significantly altered.

Keywords: Preeclampsia; Gestational Diabetes Mellitus (GDM); Small for gestational age; Large for gestational age; First-trimester screening

Abbreviations: β-HCG: β- Human Chorionic Gonadotrophin; CRL: Crown-rump length; CV: Coefficient of Variation; ELISA: Enzyme-linked Immunosorbent Assay; GDM: Gestational Diabetes Mellitus; LGA: Large for gestational age; MoM: Multiples of Median; NT: Nuchal Translucency; PAPP-A: Pregnancy-associated Plasma Protein A; PE: Preeclampsia; PI: Pulsatility Index; SGA: Small for Gestational age

Introduction

Leptin, an adipose tissue derived polypeptide hormone, is thought to play an important role in metabolism by reducing insulin secretion and through an action on hypothalamic receptors to decrease food intake and increase energy expenditure [1,2]. 75 Additionally, leptin has anti-inflammatory and angiogenic properties and is involved in immune response and T cell activation [3].

In pregnancy the maternal serum levels of leptin start rising in the first trimester prior to significant maternal weight gain, increase with gestation to reach a peak during the second or third trimester and decline shortly after delivery [4]. Although the main determinant of circulating maternal leptin is visceral fat [5], an additional source is the placenta [6]. Indeed, studies at 7-10 weeks' gestation reported that the concentration of leptin is four times higher in coelomic fluid than maternal serum reflecting the high production of the protein by trophoblast [7].

Previous studies have reported that levels of maternal serum or plasma leptin are altered in pathological pregnancies, including Gestational Diabetes Mellitus (GDM), Preeclampsia (PE) and pregnancies delivering Small for Gestational Age (SGA) neonates.

Although most studies have reported on pregnancies with established disease some have also examined circulating levels in the first and second trimester before the clinical onset of the disease and reported contradictory results [8-14].

The aim of our study was to establish a normal range of maternal serum levels of leptin at 11-13 weeks' gestation and to examine whether the levels are altered in pregnancies that subsequently develop PE or GDM and those resulting in delivery of SGA and Large for Gestational Age (LGA) neonates.

Methods

Study population

This study was drawn from a large prospective observational study for early prediction of pregnancy complications in women attending for their routine first hospital visit in pregnancy at King's College Hospital, London, UK. In this visit, which was held at 11+0-13+6 104 weeks of gestation, we recorded maternal characteristics and medical history and performed combined screening for aneuploidies by measurement of the fetal Crown-Rump Length (CRL) and Nuchal Translucency (NT) thickness and maternal serum free ß-hCG and PAPP-A [15,16]. In addition, transabdominal Doppler studies were carried out and the mean uterine artery pulsatility index (PI) was measured [17]. Women

***Corresponding authors:** Kypros H Nicolaides, Harris Birthright Research Centre for Fetal Medicine, King's College Hospital, Denmark Hill, London SE5 9RS, E-mail: kypros@fetalmedicine.com

attending for this visit were invited to participate in research and from those who agreed serum and plasma samples were stored at -80°C for subsequent biochemical analysis. The study was approved by King's College Hospital Ethics Committee (02-03-033).

Women were asked to complete a questionnaire on maternal age, racial origin (Caucasian, African, South Asian and East Asian), parity (nulliparous, parous), cigarette smoking during pregnancy (yes or no), mode of conception (spontaneous or after use of assisted reproduction technologies), medical history, including chronic hypertension and diabetes mellitus. The questionnaire was then reviewed by a doctor together with the patient and the maternal weight and height were measured.

In this study we measured maternal serum leptin concentration in 240 singleton pregnancies with no medical complications, such as hypertensive disorders or diabetes mellitus, resulting in the birth after 37 weeks' gestation of a phenotypically normal neonate with birth weight between the 5th and 95th 124 percentiles for gestational age [18]. The values were compared to those from 60 pregnancies that subsequently developed PE, 60 that developed 125 GDM, 60 that delivered LGA neonates with birth weight above the 95th 126 percentile and 60 that delivered SGA neonates with birth weight below the 5th 127 percentile. The cases of PE, GDM, SGA and LGA were selected at random from our database of stored samples for these conditions. Each case was matched to one control that was sampled on the same day.

Preeclampsia was defined according to the criteria by the International Society for the Study of Hypertension in Pregnancy [19]. Screening for GDM in our hospital is based on a two-step approach. In all women random plasma glucose is measured at 24-28 weeks of gestation and if the concentration is more than 6.7 mmol/l, a 100 g oral glucose tolerance test is carried out within the subsequent 2 weeks. The diagnosis of GDM is made if the fasting plasma glucose level is at least 6 mmol/L or the plasma glucose level 2-hours after the oral administration of 75 g glucose is 7.8 mmol/l or more [20].

Sample analysis

Maternal serum leptin was measured by a quantitative Enzyme-Linked Immunoassay (ELISA) technique using Quantikine Human Leptin ELISA kit (Catalogue no. DLP000, R and D Systems Europe Ltd., Abingdon, UK). The lower limit of detection of the assay was 0.01 ng/ml. The intra assay and inter-assay coefficient of variation (CV) varied from 3.0% to 3.3% and 3.5% to 5.4%, respectively. All samples were done in duplicates and samples with a CV exceeding 10% were reanalyzed. None of the samples in this study were previously thawed and refrozen.

Statistical analysis

Comparisons between outcome groups were by X^2-test or Fisher's exact test for categorical variables and by Mann Whitney-U test for continuous variables. Data are presented as median and Interquartile Range (IQR).

The distribution of serum leptin, PAPP-A and uterine artery PI were logarithmically transformed and probability plots and Kolmogorov-Smirnov test (p=0.153, p=0.061 and p=0.075, respectively) were used to confirm Gaussian normality. In the normal outcome group, multiple regression analysis was used to determine the factors from maternal characteristics and gestation that provided significant contribution in the prediction of log10 leptin. Each value in both the normal and pathological outcome groups was expressed as a multiple of the normal median (MoM), after adjustment for those characteristics found to be significant in the multiple regression analysis. Similarly, the measured values of uterine artery PI and serum PAPP-A were converted into MoMs as previously described [21,22]. The median MoM values of serum leptin, serum PAPP-A and uterine artery PI in the outcome groups were compared. The statistical software package SPSS 16.0 (SPSS Inc., Chicago, IL) was used for data analyses.

Literature search

We searched MEDLINE and EMBASE from 1994, when leptin was first described [23], to July 2012 to identify English language articles reporting on circulating maternal levels of leptin in pregnancy. We included case-control and cohort studies, which reported data regarding the outcome measures of PE, GDM, and birth of SGA or LGA neonates. We used the reported data in each paper and excluded duplicate publications.

Two independent reviewers extracted the data from each article, which was then examined by a third reviewer. Standardized Mean Difference (SMD) with 95% Confidence Intervals (CI) was calculated

Maternal	Characteristics	Control PE	GDM	LGA	SGA
Sample size, n	240	60	60	60	60
Maternal age in years, median (IQR)	33.0 (27.3-35.9)	32.9 (27.4-37.0)	32.0 (28.5-35.6)	32.5 (29.0-36.9)	30.4 (24.8-35.8)
Maternal weight in kg, median (IQR)	64.0 (58.9-70.0)	71.5 (63.0-85.7)*	76.5 (64.3-94.0)*	75.5 (69.0-89.2)*	63.0 (54.3-77.3)
Maternal height in cm, median (IQR)	165 (159-169)	162 (158-167)	163 (159-168)	167 (163-172)*	162 (157-165)*
Crown rump length in mm, median (IQR)	63.2 (58.5-69.7)	59.8 (55.4-65.4)	63.7 (58.1-71.6)	65.1 (60.1-71.7)	60.7 (56.0-67.4)
Gestation at sampling in days, median (IQR)	88.9 (86.1-91.2)	87.1 (84.8-90.0)	89.1 (86.2-93.1)	89.9 (87.3-93.2)	87.6 (85.1-91.0)
Racial origin					
Caucasian, n (%)	172 (71.7)	31 (51.7)*	30 (50)*	32 (53.3)*	33 (55.0)
African, n (%)	51 (21.3)	21 (35.0)	19 (31.7)	28 (46.7)*	22 (36.7)
Asian, n (%)	17 (7.1)	8 (13.3)	11 (28.3)	0	5 (8.3)
Parity					
Nulliparous, n (%)	102 (42.5)	39 (65.0)*	19 (31.7)	24 (40.0)	36 (60.0)
Parous, n (%)	138 (57.5)	21 (35.0)*	41 (68.3)	36 (60.0)	24 (40.0)
Cigarette smoker, n (%)	22 (9.2)	2 (3.3)	2 (3.3)	2 (3.3)	20 (33.3)*
Chronic hypertension, n (%)	1 (0.4)	11 (18.3)*	0 (0)	1 (1.7)	1 (1.7)
Birth weight percentile, median (IQR)	50.6 (30.9-67.0)	15.4 (6.21-46.3)*	67.9 (38.3-89.2)*	97.8 (96.7-98.9)*	0.5 (0.0-2.2)*

Table 1: Maternal and pregnancy characteristics in the outcome groups.
 Comparison between outcome groups by Mann-Whitney U-test with post hoc Bonferroni correction and 2-test or Fisher's exact test for categorical variables; Adjusted significance level p=0.0125.

for each outcome in each study. Forest plots were constructed and a random-effects model, which takes into account the random variation within studies [24], was used to calculate weighted summary SMDs by taking into account the weight of each study. Forest plots were generated using Medcalc software version 9.6.2.0 (MedCalc Software, Mariakerke, Belgium).

Results

The maternal characteristics of the study groups are presented in table 1.

Normal controls

In the normal outcome group multiple regression analysis demonstrated that serum leptin increased with maternal weight and decreased with maternal height but there was no significant association with fetal CRL (p=0.652), maternal age (p=0.196), racial origin (p=0.081), cigarette smoking (p=0.558), mode of conception (p=0.606) or parity (p=0.597). Log10 leptin expected=1.264 + 0.017 × maternal weight in kg – 0.007 × maternal height in cm;

$R^2196 =0.298$, p<0.0001.

Preeclampsia

In the PE group, compared to the unaffected controls, there was a significant increase in median serum leptin (1.18, IQR 0.75-1.84 MoM vs 1.00, IQR 0.68-1.37 MoM, p=0.027) and uterine artery PI (1.25, IQR 1.05-1.48 MoM vs 1.00, IQR 0.83-1.15 MoM, p<0.0001) and decrease in serum PAPP-A (0.72, IQR 0.46-1.14 MoM vs 1.01, IQR 0.76-11.35 MoM, p<0.0001) (Figure 1).

The median gestation at delivery of the PE group was 36.0 (range 206, 28-41) weeks. There was a significant association between gestation at delivery and uterine artery PI (r=-0.289, p=0.038) and serum PAPP-A (r=0.274, p=0.036) but not serum leptin (p=0.868). There was no significant association between serum leptin and either uterine artery PI (p=0.983) or serum PAPP-A (p=0.403).

Gestational diabetes mellitus

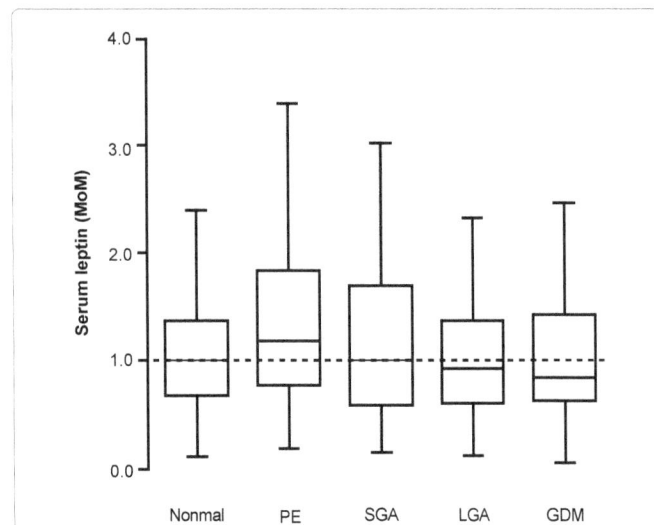

Figure 1: Box (median, interquartile range) and whisker (range) plot of maternal serum leptin Multiple of the Median (MoM) in normal and pathological pregnancies.

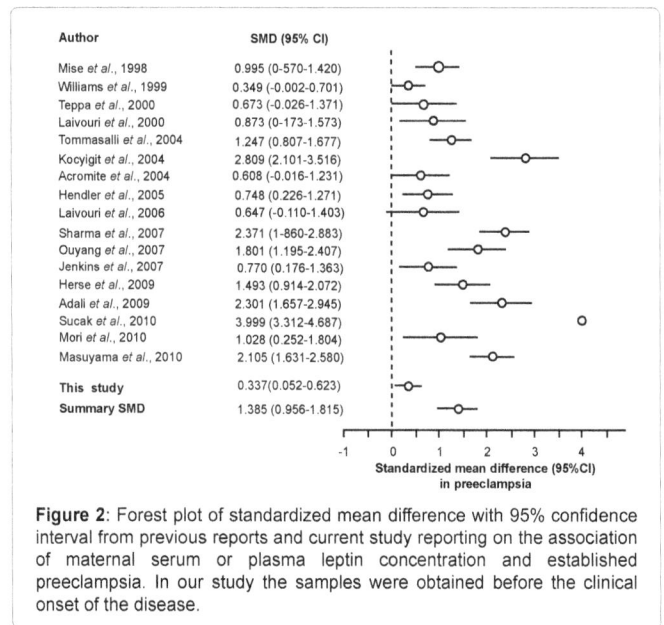

Figure 2: Forest plot of standardized mean difference with 95% confidence interval from previous reports and current study reporting on the association of maternal serum or plasma leptin concentration and established preeclampsia. In our study the samples were obtained before the clinical onset of the disease.

In the GDM group, compared to the unaffected controls, there was no significant difference in median serum leptin (0.89, IQR 0.62-1.45 MoM vs 1.00, IQR 0.68-1.37 MoM, p=0.722), uterine artery PI (0.96, IQR 0.86-1.22 MoM vs 1.00, IQR 0.83-1.15 MoM, p=0.535) or serum PAPP-A (0.99, IQR 0.75-1.41 MoM vs 1.01, IQR 0.76-11.35 MoM, p=0.779) (Figure 1).

Small for gestational age

In the SGA group, compared to the unaffected controls, the median serum PAPP-A was decreased (0.70, IQR 0.44-0.89 MoM vs 1.01, IQR 0.76-11.35 MoM, p<0.0001) and uterine artery PI was increased (1.24, IQR 0.94-1.49 MoM vs 1.00, IQR 0.83-1.15 MoM, p<0.0001) but there was no significant difference in median serum leptin (1.02, IQR 0.58-1.71 MoM vs 1.00, IQR 0.68-1.37 MoM, p=0.621) (Figure 1).

Large for gestational age

In the LGA group, compared to the unaffected controls, the median serum PAPP-A was increased (1.26, IQR 0.92-1.77 MoM vs 1.01, IQR 0.76-11.35 MoM, p=0.003) but there was no significant difference in median serum leptin (0.92, IQR 0.59-1.38 MoM vs 1.00, IQR 0.68-1.37 MoM, p=0.385) or uterine artery PI (0.95, IQR 0.68-1.19 MoM vs 1.00, IQR 0.83-1.15 MoM, p=0.280) (Figure 1).

Literature search

Forest plots of SMDs from previous reports and our study for PE, GDM, and delivery of SGA-neonates are shown in figures 2-4. PE [25-42]; GDM [11,12,43-50]; SGA [13,33,36,51-55].

Discussion

This study has demonstrated that maternal serum leptin concentration at 11-13 weeks' gestation in pregnancies that subsequently develop PE is increased. In pregnancies that develop GDM and those that result in delivery of SGA and LGA neonate's serum leptin is not significantly different from pregnancies with normal outcome.

In normal pregnancies, serum leptin concentration increased with maternal weight and decreased with maternal height but was not affected by other maternal factors including age, racial origin, and

Author	SMD (95% CI)
Qiu et al., 2004	0.649 (0.353 to 0.946)
Gao et al., 2008	4.005 (2.887 to 5.123)
Chen et al., 2010	1.640 (0.890 to 2.390)
Mokhtari et al., 2010	-0.426 (-1.017 to 0.164)
Yilmaz et al., 2010	0.406 (-0.004 to 0.815)
Gao et al., 2008	2.988 (2.055 to 3.920)
McLachlan et al., 2005	-0.646 (-1.323 to 0.031)
Cseh et al., 2002	0.309 (-0.191 to 0.809)
Kautzky-Willer et al., 2001	0.620 (0.129 to 1.110)
Vitoratos et al., 2001	1.546 (0.738 to 2.354)
Festa et al., 2001	-0.229 (-0.536 to 0.077)
This study	-0.109 (-0.393 to 0.175)
Summary SMD	0.782 (0.291 to 1.274)

Standardized mean difference (95% CI) in gestational diabetes mellitus

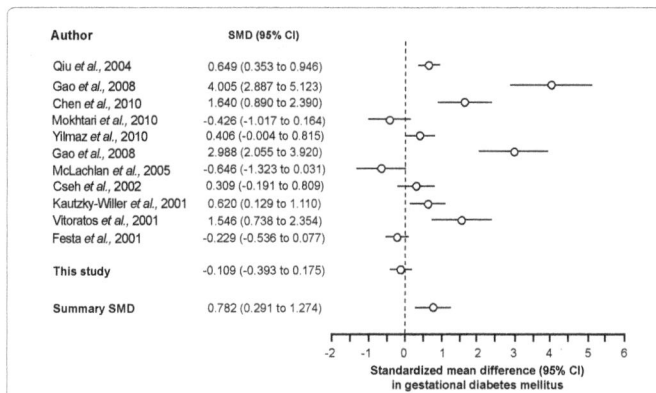

Figure 3: Forest plot of standardized mean difference with 95% confidence interval from previous reports and current study reporting on the association between maternal serum or plasma leptin concentration and gestational diabetes mellitus. In the top two studies and in our study the samples were obtained before the clinical onset of the disease.

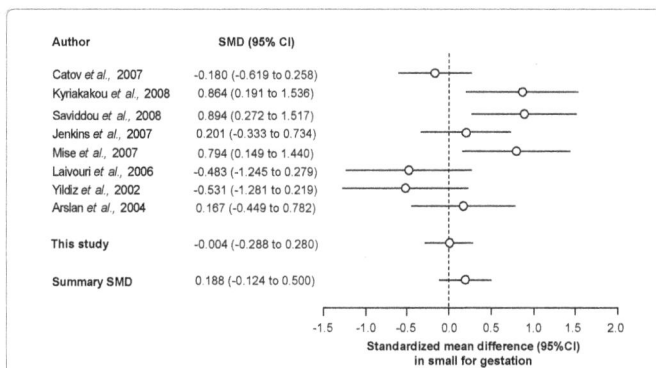

Author	SMD (95% CI)
Catov et al., 2007	-0.180 (-0.619 to 0.258)
Kyriakakou et al., 2008	0.864 (0.191 to 1.536)
Savidou et al., 2008	0.894 (0.272 to 1.517)
Jenkins et al., 2007	0.201 (-0.333 to 0.734)
Mise et al., 2007	0.794 (0.149 to 1.440)
Laivouri et al., 2006	-0.483 (-1.245 to 0.279)
Yildiz et al., 2002	-0.531 (-1.281 to 0.219)
Arslan et al., 2004	0.167 (-0.449 to 0.782)
This study	-0.004 (-0.288 to 0.280)
Summary SMD	0.188 (-0.124 to 0.500)

Standardized mean difference (95%CI) in small for gestation

Figure 4: Forest plot of standardized mean difference with 95% confidence interval from previous reports and current study reporting on the association between delivery of small for gestational age neonates and maternal serum or plasma leptin concentration. In the top study and in our study the samples were obtained before the clinical onset of the disease.

parity, smoking status or mode of conception. The association with maternal weight is the inevitable consequence of the main source of this adipocytokine, which is fat tissue, and is compatible with the results of previous studies in both pregnant and non-pregnant individuals[56].

Previous studies in pregnancies with established PE have consistently reported that maternal circulating leptin concentration is increased (Figure 2). It was suggested that leptin is a marker of placental hypoxia [25] and the increased serum levels observed in PE may be due to the underlying impaired placental perfusion and oxygenation. Our findings indicate that the increased leptin precedes the clinical onset of the disease and is apparent from the first trimester of pregnancy. Previous studies in pregnancies before the onset of PE provided conflicting results. Samolis et al. [8] reported that the median maternal plasma leptin concentration at 13 weeks' gestation was approximately twice as high in 37 pregnancies that subsequently developed PE than in normotensive controls. In contrast, two other studies reported no significant differences in leptin levels at 7-13 and 18 weeks' gestation in 30 and 71 cases, respectively, that subsequently developed PE compared to controls [9,10]. In our study the increase in serum leptin concentration was unrelated to the severity of PE, reflected in the gestational age at delivery and was also unrelated to biophysical and biochemical evidence of impaired placentation reflected in increased uterine artery PI and decreased serum PAPP-A [57]. Two previous

studies examining serum leptin levels in patients with established PE reported that the levels were higher in those with severe than mild disease [38,39] but in two other studies the opposite was true [41,42].

In pregnancies that developed GDM the serum concentration of leptin at 11-13 weeks was not significantly different from normal controls. Previous studies in patients with established disease reported contradictory results with levels that were either increased or not significantly altered (Figure 3). Our findings did not confirm the results of two previous studies, which reported increased leptin levels at 13 and 14-20 weeks' gestation, respectively, in women that subsequently developed GDM [11,12].

In the pregnancies delivering SGA neonates, there was evidence of impaired placentation reflected in increased uterine artery PI and decreased serum PAPP-A but serum levels of leptin at 11-13 weeks were not altered. Previous studies in pregnancies with SGA fetuses reported contradictory results with levels that were either increased or not significantly altered (Figure 4).

Our findings are consistent with one of the two studies examining serum leptin levels prior to the onset of SGA, in the absence of PE. In one study, there was no significant difference in leptin levels at 8-13 weeks between pregnancies delivering SGA and non-SGA neonates [14] but another longitudinal study reported decreased levels of leptin at 18 weeks' gestation in pregnancies that subsequently delivered SGA neonates [13]. In pregnancies delivering LGA neonates, there was a significant increase in serum PAPP-A at weeks' gestation as reported previously [58], but maternal serum levels of leptin were not altered. These findings are consistent with those of Horosz et al. [59] who reported that maternal serum leptin levels at 27 and 32 weeks' gestation in pregnancies delivering macrosomic neonates were not altered in either diabetic or non-diabetic women.

Conclusion

The findings of this study indicate that the reported altered maternal levels of leptin in pregnancies with established GDM and those delivering SGA neonates are not apparent at 11-13 weeks' gestation and therefore measurement of this adipocytokine is unlikely to be useful in early screening for these pregnancy complications. In the case of PE we found that increased levels of leptin, previously reported in cases of established disease, are apparent from early pregnancy but the levels are unrelated to the severity of PE.

Acknowledgments

The assay for leptin was performed by Ms. Tracy Dew at the Department of Biochemistry, King's College Hospital, London, UK.

Funding

This study was supported by a grant from the Fetal Medicine Foundation (United Kingdom Charity No. 1037116).

References

1. Wauters M, Considine RV, Van Gaal LF (2000) Human leptin: from an adipocyte hormone to an endocrine mediator. Eur J Endocrinol 143: 293-311.

2. Mantzoros CS, Magkos F, Brinkoetter M, Sienkiewicz E, Dardeno TA, et al. (2011) Leptin in human physiology and pathophysiology. Am J Physiol Endocrinol Metab 301: E567-E584.

3. Sennello JA, Fayad R, Morris AM, Eckel RH, Asilmaz E, et al. (2005) Regulation of T cell-mediated hepatic inflammation by adiponectin and leptin.

Endocrinology 146: 2157-2164.

4. Highman TJ, Friedman JE, Huston LP, Wong WW, Catalano PM (1998) Longitudinal changes in maternal serum leptin concentrations, body composition, and resting metabolic rate in pregnancy. Am J Obstet Gynecol 178: 1010-1015.

5. Fattah C, Barry S, O'Connor N, Farah N, Stuart B, et al. (2011) Maternal leptin and body composition in the first trimester of pregnancy. Gynecol Endocrinol 27: 263-266.

6. Sagawa N, Yura S, Itoh H, Kakui K, Takemura M, et al. (2002) Possible role of placental leptin in pregnancy: a review. Endocrine 19: 65-71.

7. Makrydimas G, Vandecruys H, Sotiriadis A, Lakasing L, Spencer K, et al. (2005) Coelomic fluid leptin concentration in normal first-trimester pregnancies and missed miscarriages. Fetal Diagn Ther 20: 406-409.

8. Samolis S, Papastefanou I, Panagopoulos P, Galazios G, Kouskoukis A, et al. (2010) Relation between first trimester maternal serum leptin levels and body mass index in normotensive and pre-eclamptic pregnancies--role of leptin as a marker of pre-eclampsia: a prospective case-control study. Gynecol Endocrinol 26: 338-343.

9. Salomon LJ, Benattar C, Audibert F, Fernandez H, Duyme M, et al. (2003) Severe preeclampsia is associated with high inhibin A levels and normal leptin levels at 7 to 13 weeks into pregnancy. Am J Obstet Gynecol 189: 1517-1522.

10. Clausen T, Djurovic S, Reseland JE, Berg K, Drevon CA, et al. (2002) Altered plasma concentrations of leptin, transforming growth factor-beta(1) and plasminogen activator inhibitor type 2 at 18 weeks of gestation in women destined to develop pre-eclampsia. Circulating markers of disturbed placentation? Placenta 23: 380-385.

11. Qiu C, Williams MA, Vadachkoria S, Frederick IO, Luthy DA (2004) Increased maternal plasma leptin in early pregnancy and risk of gestational diabetes mellitus. Obstet Gynecol 103: 519-525.

12. Gao XL, Yang HX, Zhao Y (2008) Variations of tumor necrosis factor-alpha, leptin and adiponectin in mid-trimester of gestational diabetes mellitus. Chin Med J (Engl) 121: 701-705.

13. Catov JM, Patrick TE, Powers RW, Ness RB, Harger G, et al. (2007) Maternal leptin across pregnancy in women with small-for-gestational-age infants. Am J Obstet Gynecol 196: 558.e1-558.e8.

14. Hedley P, Pihl K, Krebs L, Larsen T, Christiansen M (2009) Leptin in first trimester pregnancy serum: no reduction associated with small-for-gestational-age infants. Reprod Biomed Online 18: 832-837.

15. Snijders RJ, Noble P, Sebire N, Souka A, Nicolaides KH (1998) UK multicentre project on assessment of risk of trisomy 21 by maternal age and fetal nuchal-translucency thickness at 10-14 weeks of gestation. Fetal Medicine Foundation First Trimester Screening Group. Lancet 352: 343-346.

16. Kagan KO, Wright D, Baker A, Sahota D, Nicolaides KH (2008) Screening for trisomy 21 by maternal age, fetal nuchal translucency thickness, free beta-human chorionic gonadotropin and pregnancy-associated plasma protein-A. Ultrasound Obstet Gynecol 31: 618-624.

17. Plasencia W, Maiz N, Bonino S, Kaihura C, Nicolaides KH (2007) Uterine artery Doppler at 11 + 0 to 13 + 6 weeks in the prediction of pre-eclampsia. Ultrasound Obstet Gynecol 30: 742-749.

18. Poon LC, Karagiannis G, Staboulidou I, Shafiei A, Nicolaides KH (2011) Reference range of birth weight with gestation and first-trimester prediction of small-for-gestation neonates. Prenat Diagn 31: 58-65.

19. Brown MA, Lindheimer MD, de Swiet M, Van Assche A, Moutquin JM (2001) The classification and diagnosis of the hypertensive disorders of pregnancy: statement from the International Society for the Study of Hypertension in Pregnancy (ISSHP). Hypertens Pregnancy 20: IX-XIV.

20. World Health Organisation (2006) Definition and diagnosis of diabetes mellitus and intermediate hyperglycaemia. Report of a WHO/IDF consultation 1-50.

21. Kagan KO, Wright D, Spencer K, Molina FS, Nicolaides KH (2008) First-trimester screening for trisomy 21 by free beta-human chorionic gonadotropin and pregnancy-associated plasma protein-A: impact of maternal and pregnancy characteristics. Ultrasound Obstet Gynecol 31: 493-502.

22. Akolekar R, Syngelaki A, Sarquis R, Zvanca M, Nicolaides KH (2011) Prediction of early, intermediate and late pre-eclampsia from maternal factors, biophysical and biochemical markers at 11-13 weeks. Prenat Diagn 31: 66-74.

23. Zhang Y, Proenca R, Maffei M, Barone M, Leopold L, et al. (1994) Positional cloning of the mouse obese gene and its human homologue. Nature 372: 425-432.

24. DerSimonian R, Laird N (1986) Meta-analysis in clinical trials. Control Clin Trials 7: 177-188.

25. Mise H, Sagawa N, Matsumoto T, Yura S, Nanno H, et al. (1998) Augmented placental production of leptin in preeclampsia: possible involvement of placental hypoxia. J Clin Endocrinol Metab 83: 3225-3229.

26. Williams MA, Havel PJ, Schwartz MW, Leisenring WM, King IB, et al. (1999) Pre-eclampsia disrupts the normal relationship between serum leptin concentrations and adiposity in pregnant women. Paediatr Perinat Epidemiol 13: 190-204.

27. Teppa RJ, Ness RB, Crombleholme WR, Roberts JM (2000) Free leptin is increased in normal pregnancy and further increased in preeclampsia. Metabolism 49: 1043-1048.

28. Laivuori H, Kaaja R, Koistinen H, Karonen SL, Andersson S, et al. (2000) Leptin during and after preeclamptic or normal pregnancy: its relation to serum insulin and insulin sensitivity. Metabolism 49: 259-263.

29. Tommaselli GA, Pighetti M, Nasti A, D'Elia A, Guida M, et al. (2004) Serum leptin levels and uterine Doppler flow velocimetry at 20 weeks' gestation as markers for the development of pre-eclampsia. Gynecol Endocrinol 19: 160-165.

30. Kocyigit Y, Bayhan G, Atamer A, Atamer Y (2004) Serum levels of leptin, insulin-like growth factor-I and insulin-like growth factor binding protein-3 in women with pre-eclampsia, and their relationship to insulin resistance. Gynecol Endocrinol 18: 341-348.

31. Acromite M, Ziotopoulou M, Orlova C, Mantzoros C (2004) Increased leptin levels in preeclampsia: associations with BMI, estrogen and SHBG levels. Hormones (Athens) 3: 46-52.

32. Hendler I, Blackwell SC, Mehta SH, Whitty JE, Russell E, et al. (2005) The levels of leptin, adiponectin, and resistin in normal weight, overweight, and obese pregnant women with and without preeclampsia. Am J Obstet Gynecol 193: 979-983.

33. Laivuori H, Gallaher MJ, Collura L, Crombleholme WR, Markovic N, et al. (2006) Relationships between maternal plasma leptin, placental leptin mRNA and protein in normal pregnancy, pre-eclampsia and intrauterine growth restriction without pre-eclampsia. Mol Hum Reprod 12: 551-556.

34. Sharma A, Satyam A, Sharma JB (2007) Leptin, IL-10 and inflammatory markers (TNF-alpha, IL-6 and IL-8) in pre-eclamptic, normotensive pregnant and healthy non-pregnant women. Am J Reprod Immunol 58: 21-30.

35. Ouyang Y, Chen H, Chen H (2007) Reduced plasma adiponectin and elevated leptin in pre-eclampsia. Int J Gynaecol Obstet 98: 110-114.

36. Jenkins LD, Powers RW, Adotey M, Gallaher MJ, Markovic N, et al. (2007) Maternal leptin concentrations are similar in African Americans and Caucasians in normal pregnancy, preeclampsia and small-for-gestational-age infants. Hypertens Pregnancy 26: 101-109.

37. Herse F, Bai Youpeng, Staff AC, Yong-Meid J, Dechend R, et al. (2009) Circulating and uteroplacental adipocytokine concentrations in preeclampsia. Reprod Sci 16: 584-590.

38. Adali E, Yildizhan R, Kolusari A, Kurdoglu M, Bugdayci G, et al. (2009) Increased visfatin and leptin in pregnancies complicated by pre-eclampsia. J Matern Fetal Neonatal Med 22: 873-879.

39. Sucak A, Kanat-Pektas M, Gungor T, Mollamahmutoglu L (2010) Leptin levels and antihypertensive treatment in preeclampsia. Singapore Med J 51: 39-43.

40. Mori T, Shinohara K, Wakatsuki A, Watanabe K, Fujimaki A (2010) Adipocytokines and endothelial function in preeclamptic women. Hypertens Res 33: 250-254.

41. Masuyama H, Segawa T, Sumida Y, Masumoto A, Inoue S, et al. (2010) Different profiles of circulating angiogenic factors and adipocytokines between early- and late-onset pre-eclampsia. BJOG 117: 314-320.

42. Dalamaga M, Srinivas SK, Elovitz MA, Chamberland J, Mantzoros CS (2011) Serum adiponectin and leptin in relation to risk for preeclampsia: results from a large case-control study. Metabolism 60: 1539-1544.

43. Chen D, Xia G, Xu P, Dong M (2010) Peripartum serum leptin and soluble leptin receptor levels in women with gestational diabetes. Acta Obstet Gynecol Scand 89: 1595-1599.

44. Mokhtari M, Hashemi M, Yaghmaei M, Naderi M, Shikhzadeh A, et al. (2011) Evaluation of the serum leptin in normal pregnancy and gestational diabetes mellitus in Zahedan, southeast Iran. Arch Gynecol Obstet 284: 539-542.

45. Yilmaz O, Kucuk M, Ilgin A, Dagdelen M (2010) Assessment of insulin sensitivity/ resistance and their relations with leptin concentrations and anthropometric measures in a pregnant population with and without gestational diabetes mellitus. J Diabetes Complications 24: 109-114.

46. McLachlan KA, O'Neal D, Jenkins A, Alford FP (2006) Do adiponectin, TNFalpha, leptin and CRP relate to insulin resistance in pregnancy? Studies in women with and without gestational diabetes, during and after pregnancy. Diabetes Metab Res Rev 22: 131-138.

47. Cseh K, Baranyi E, Melczer Z, Csakany GM, Speer G, et al. (2002) The pathophysiological influence of leptin and the tumor necrosis factor system on maternal insulin resistance: negative correlation with anthropometric parameters of neonates in gestational diabetes. Gynecol Endocrinol 16: 453-460.

48. Kautzky-Willer A, Pacini G, Tura A, Bieglmayer C, Schneider B, et al. (2001) Increased plasma leptin in gestational diabetes. Diabetologia 44: 164-172.

49. Vitoratos N, Chrystodoulacos G, Salamalekis E, Kassanos D, Kouskouni E, et al. (2002) Fetoplacental leptin levels and their relation to birth weight and insulin in gestational diabetic pregnant women. J Obstet Gynaecol 22: 29-33.

50. Festa A, Shnawa N, Krugluger W, Hopmeier P, Schernthaner G, et al. (1999) Relative hypoleptinaemia in women with mild gestational diabetes mellitus. Diabet Med 16: 656-662.

51. Kyriakakou M, Malamitsi-Puchner A, Militsi H, Boutsikou T, Margeli A, et al. (2008) Leptin and adiponectin concentrations in intrauterine growth restricted and appropriate for gestational age fetuses, neonates, and their mothers. Eur J Endocrinol 158: 343-348.

52. Mise H, Yura S, Itoh H, Nuamah MA, Takemura M, et al. (2007) The relationship between maternal plasma leptin levels and fetal growth restriction. Endocr J 54: 945-951.

53. Savvidou MD, Sotiriadis A, Kaihura C, Nicolaides KH, Sattar N (2008) Circulating levels of adiponectin and leptin at 23-25 weeks of pregnancy in women with impaired placentation and in those with established fetal growth restriction. Clin Sci (Lond) 115: 219-224.

54. Yildiz L, Avci B, Ingec M (2002) Umbilical cord and maternal blood leptin concentrations in intrauterine growth retardation. Clin Chem Lab Med 40: 1114-1117.

55. Arslan M, Yazici G, Erdem A, Erdem M, Arslan EO, et al. (2004) Endothelin 1 and leptin in the pathophysiology of intrauterine growth restriction. Int J Gynaecol Obstet 84: 120-126.

56. Margetic S, Gazzola C, Pegg GG, Hill RA (2002) Leptin: a review of its peripheral actions and interactions. Int J Obes Relat Metab Disord 26: 1407-1433.

57. Poon LC, Stratieva V, Piras S, Piri S, Nicolaides KH (2010) Hypertensive disorders in pregnancy: combined screening by uterine artery Doppler, blood pressure and serum PAPP-A at 11-13 weeks. Prenat Diagn 30: 216-223.

58. Poon LC, Karagiannis G, Stratieva V, Syngelaki A, Nicolaides KH (2011) First-trimester prediction of macrosomia. Fetal Diagn Ther 29: 139-147.

59. Horosz E, Bomba-Opon DA, Szymanska M, Wielgos M (2011) Third trimester plasma adiponectin and leptin in gestational diabetes and normal pregnancies. Diabetes Res Clin Pract 93: 350-356.

22

Effects of Polymorphism rs3123554 in the Cannabinoid Receptor Gene Type 2 (*Cnr2*) on Body Weight and Insulin Resistance after Weight Loss with a Hypocaloric Mediterranean Diet

de Luis DA*, Aller R, Primo D, Izaola O, Fuente B and Romero E

Center of Investigation of Endocrinology and Nutrition, Medicine School and Dpt of Endocrinology and Investigation, Hospital Clinico Universitario, University of Valladolid, Valladolid, Spain

Abstract

Background: There is few evidence of CNR2 SNPs and obesity. The role of CNR2 gene variants on weight loss after a dietary intervention remained uninvestigated.

Objective: Our aim was to analyze the effects of rs3123554) of *CNR2* receptor gene polymorphism on body weight, metabolic parameters and serum adipokine levels after a Mediterranean hypocaloric diet.

Design: A Caucasian population of 82 obese patients was analyzed before and after 3 months on a Mediterranean hypocaloric diet.

Results: In non A allele carriers, the decrease in weight -3.2 ± 1.9 kg (-2.2 ± 1.0 kg : p=0.02), BMI -1.0 ± 0.1 kg (-1.2 ± 0.5 kg : p=0.01), fat mass -2.5 ± 1.0 kg (-1.2 ± 0.8 kg : p=0.003), waist circumference -2.9 ± 1.1 cm (-2.1 ± 3.1 cm : p=0.004), systolic blood pressure were -5.9 ± 3.9 mmHg (-2.9 ± 2.2 mmHg), total cholesterol -25.1 ± 5.3 mg/dl (-6.4 ± 4.7 mg/dl : p=0.005), LDL- cholesterol -19.1 ± 9.5 mg/dl (-6.2 ± 8.5 mg/dl : p=0.003), glucose -5.2 ± 2.5 mg/dL (-0.1 ± 1.1 mg/dL : p=0.004), insulin -2.8 ± 1.3 mUI/L (-0.2 ± 1.0 mUI/L:p=0.01), HOMA-IR -0.9 ± 0.3 (± 0.1 ± 0.1 : p=0.01), IL-6 -0.7 ± 0.5 ng/dL (-0.1 ± 0.4 ng/dL:p=0.02) and CRP -2.8 ± 1.5 ng/dL (± 0.1 ± 0.2 ng/dL:p=0.02) were higher than A allele carriers.

Conclusion: Non A allele carriers has a better improvement after a Mediterranean hypocaloric diet in body weight, fat mass, waist circumference, level of insulin, HOMA-IR, total cholesterol, LDL cholesterol, IL-6 and CRP than A allele carriers.

Keywords: Adipokines; Cannabinoid receptor gene type 2; Obesity; Mediterranean diet; Rs3123554

Introduction

Obesity is a major health problem in industrialized countries, leading to increased morbidity from metabolic syndrome, diabetes mellitus type 2, stroke, coronary heart disease and cancer [1]. Genetic and environmental factors play important roles in the development of obesity. The increasing prevalence of obesity is caused by the excessive calorie intake and diminished physical activity in our modern environment. However, available evidence also suggests a significant genetic contribution to adiposity [2]. During the last decades, increasing numbers of genetic loci associated with obesity and/or body mass index (BMI) have been identified as a result of the genome-wide association study (GWAS). These loci include; fat related obese gene (FTO), melanocortin receptor subtype 4 (Mc4R), brain derived neutrophic factor (BDNF), cannabinoid receptors (CNRs) and so on [3].

The important role played by the endocannabinoid system is an interesting area of investigation. The cannabinoid receptor system consists of two receptors (CNR1 and CNR2). CNR1 is mainly located in the brain: its role in eating behavior is well-established [4]. In contrast, CNR2 has been referred to as the peripheral cannabinoid receptor isoform that is mainly expressed in cells of the immune system. This endogenous cannabinoid system consists of endogenous ligands 2-arachidonoylglycerol (2-AG) and anandamide (ADA), and the above-mentioned two types of G-protein-coupled cannabinoid receptor. A greater insight into the endocannabinoid system has been derived from studies in animals with a genetic deletion of the CNR1 receptor, which have a lean phenotype and are resistant to

diet-induced obesity [5]. Otherwise, a single nucleotid polymorphism (SNP) rs1049353 of the *CNR1* gene resulting in the substitution of the G to A at nucleotide position 1359 in codon 435 (Thr), was reported as a common SNP in Caucasian population [6], with metabolic implications. Few SNPs have been described in *CNR2* gene [7]. For example, Ketterer et al. [7] have found that carriers of minor allele (A) of this SNP showed an inverse relation with body weight. As far as we know the role of *CNR2* gene variants on weight loss after a dietary intervention remained uninvestigated.

Our aim was to analyze the effects of rs3123554) of *CNR2* receptor gene polymorphism on body weight, metabolic parameters and serum adipokine levels after a Mediterranean hypocaloric diet in obese subjects.

Subjects and Methods

Subjects and procedure

This study was conducted according to the guidelines laid down in the Declaration of Helsinki and our Hospital ethics committee approved all procedures involving patients. All participants provided

*Corresponding author: Dr. D.A de Luis, Professor Associated of Nutrition, Executive Director of Institute of Endocrinology and Nutrition, Medicine School, Valladolid University, Valladolid, Spain, E-mail: dadluis@yahoo.es

informed consent. A population of 82 Caucasians subjects with obesity (body mass index >30) and without diabetes mellitus was analyzed in an interventional study. The recruitment of subjects was a non-probabilistic method of sampling among patients send from Primary Care Physicians with obesity. Inclusion criteria were body mass index > 30 and absence of a diet during the 6 months previously to the study. Exclusion criteria included history of cardiovascular disease or stroke during the previous 24 months, total cholesterol > 200 mg/dl, triglycerides > 250 mg/dl, blood pressure > 140/90 mmHg, as well as the use of metformin, sulfonylurea, dypeptidil type IV inhibitors drugs, thiazolidinedions, insulin, glucocorticoids, antineoplasic agents, angiotensin receptor blockers, angiotensin converting enzyme inhibitors, psychoactive medications, statins and other lipid drugs.

Procedure

Basal fasting glucose, c-reactive protein (CRP), insulin, insulin resistance (HOMA-IR), total cholesterol, LDL-cholesterol, HDL-cholesterol, plasma triglycerides concentration and adipokines (leptin, adiponectin, resistin, interleukin 6 and TNF-alpha) were measured within the start of the trial and repeated after 3 months of dietary intervention. Weight, height, and blood pressure measures were measured within the start of the trail and repeated 3 months of intervention. A tetrapolar bioimpedance was realized in order to measure fat mass. These measures were realized at same time of the day (morning). Genotype of CNR2 receptor gene polymorphism was studied.

Dietary intervention: The lifestyle modification program was a Mediterranean hypocaloric diet (1508 calories per day) during three months, the distribution of macronutrient was; 52% of carbohydrates, 25% of lipids and 23% of proteins. Distribution of fats was: 50.7% of monounsaturated fats, 38.5% of saturated fats and 11.8% of polyunsaturated fats. Diet was enriched with olive oil (30 ml per day), 3 servings of oily fish a week, 30-40 g 3 servings nuts days a week, vegetables 3-4 servings per day. The adherence of this diet was assessed each 14 days with a phone call by a dietitian in order to improve compliment of the calorie restriction, macronutrient distribution and Mediterranean diet recommendations. All enrolled subjects received instruction to record their daily dietary intake for three days including a weekend day. Records were reviewed by a dietitian and analysed with a computer-based data evaluation system. National composition food tables were used as reference [8].

Biochemical assays: Serum total cholesterol and triglyceride concentrations were determined by enzymatic colorimetric assay (Technicon Instruments, Ltd., New York, N.Y., USA), while HDL cholesterol was determined enzymatically in the supernatant after precipitation of other lipoproteins with dextran sulfate-magnesium. LDL cholesterol was calculated using Friedewald formula [9]. Plasma glucose levels were determined by using an automated glucose oxidase method (Glucose analyser 2, Beckman Instruments, Fullerton, California).

Insulin was measured by RIA (RIA Diagnostic Corporation, Los Angeles, CA) with a sensitivity of 0.5 mUI/L (normal range 0.5-30 mUI/L) [10] and the homeostasis model assessment for insulin resistance (HOMA-IR) was calculated using these values [11]. CRP was measured by immunoturbimetry (Roche Diagnostics GmbH, Mannheim, Germany), with a normal range of (0-7 mg/dl) and analytical sensivity 0.5 mg/dl.

Adipokine assays: Resistin was measured by ELISA (Biovendor Laboratory, Inc., Brno, Czech Republic) with a sensitivity of 0.2 ng/

ml with a normal range of 4-12 ng/ml [12]. Adiponectin was measured by ELISA (R&D systems, Inc., Mineapolis, USA) with a sensitivity of 0.246 ng/ml and a normal range of 8.65-21.43 ng/ml [13]. Leptin was measured by ELISA (Diagnostic Systems Laboratories, Inc., Texas, USA) with a sensitivity of 0.05 ng/ml and a normal range of 10-100 ng/ml [14]. Interleukin 6 and TNF alpha were measured by ELISA (R&D systems, Inc., Mineapolis, USA) with a sensitivity of 0.7 pg/ml and 0.5 pg/ml, respectively. Normal values of IL6 was (1.12-12.5 pg/ml) and TNF-alpha (0.5-15.6 pg/ml) [15].

Genotyping: Oligonucleotide primers and probes were designed with the Beacon Designer 5.0 (Premier Biosoft International *, LA, CA). The polymerase chain reaction (PCR) was carried out with 50 ng of genomic DNA, 0.5 uL of each oligonucleotide primer (primer forward: 5'- ACGTTGGATGATTGTACCGAGGAGGGAACT-3' and reverse 5'- ACGTTGGATGGAGACACGTATTCTAGTCCC-3' in a 2 uL final volume (Termociclador Life Tecnologies, LA, CA). DNA was denaturated at 95ºC for 3 min; this was followed by 45 cycles of denaturation at 95ºC for 15 s, and annealing at 59.3º C for 45 s). The PCR were run in a 25 uL final volume containing 12.5 uL of IQTM Supermix (Bio-Rad®, Hercules, CA) with hot start Taq DNA polymerase Hardy Weimberg equilibrium was assessed with a statistical test (Chi-square) to compare our expected and observed counts. The two variants were in Hardy Weimberg equilibrium (p=0.03).

Blood pressure determination and anthropometric measurements: The same investigator evaluated all patients. Blood pressure was measured twice after a 10 minutes rest with a random zero mercury sphygmomanometer, and averaged (Omrom, LA, CA). Body weight was measured to an accuracy of 0.1 Kg and body mass index computed as body weight/(height^2). Waist (narrowest diameter between xiphoid process and iliac crest) and hip (widest diameter over greater trochanters) circumferences to derive waist-to hip ratio (WHR) were measured, too. Tetrapolar body electrical bioimpedance was used to determine body composition with an accuracy of 50 g [16].

Statistical analysis

Sample size was calculated to detect differences over 3 kg in body weight loss with 90% power and 5% significance (n=80). The Kolmogorov–Smirnov test was used to determine variable distribution. The results were expressed as average ± standard deviation. Quantitative variables with normal distribution were analyzed with a two-tailed Student's-t test. Non-parametric variables were analyzed with the U-Mann-Whitney test. Qualitative variables were analyzed with the chi-square test, with Yates correction as necessary, and Fisher's test. A Chi square test was used to evaluate the Hardy–Weinberg equilibrium. The statistical analysis was performed for the combined *AA* and *AG* as a group (mutant) and GG genotype as second group (wild), with a dominant model. A p-value <0.05 was considered significant.

Results

Eighty-two obese subjects gave informed consent and were enrolled in the study. The mean age was 49.1 ± 7.3 years and the mean body mass index (BMI) 34.8 ± 4.1 kg/m². Thirty five patients (42.7%) had the genotype *GG* and 47 (57.3%) subjects had the next genotypes; *GA* (29 patients, 35.4%) or *GG* (18 study subjects, 22.0%) (second group). Age was similar in both groups (49.3 ± 8.2 years vs 48.9 ± 4.2 years: ns). Sex distribution was similar in both groups, males (20.0% vs 27.7%) and females (80.0% vs 72.3%). All patients completed the 3-month follow-up period without drop-outs.

After 3 months of intervention, all patients achieved dietary recommendations in both genotype groups without statistical differences between calorie intake (wild genotype: 1503.1 ± 287.1 kcal/day vs mutant genotype: 1490.3 ± 212.8 kcal/day). Macronutrient intakes were similar; (wild genotype: 50.4% from carbohydrates vs 50.6% mutant genotype), (wild genotype: 25.2% from fats (50.1% of monounsaturated fats, 37.9% of saturated fats and 13.0% of polyunsaturated fats) vs 25.1% mutant genotype (50.2% of monounsaturated fats, 39.0% of saturated fats and 11.8% of polyunsaturated fats) and (wild genotype: 24.4% from proteins vs 24.3% mutant genotype).

Anthropometric characteristics of participants at baseline and at month 3 of intervention are shown in Table 1. In wild and mutant genotype groups, body weight, body mass index (BMI), fat mass, waist circumference and systolic blood pressure decreased. Before and after dietary intervention, body weight, BMI, fat mass and waist circumference were higher in A allele carriers than non A allele carriers. In non A allele carriers, the decrease in body weight was -3.2 ± 1.9 kg (A allele group -2.2 ± 1.0 kg:p=0.02), BMI -1.0 ± 0.1 kg (A allele group -1.2 ± 0.5 kg:p=0.01), fat mass -2.5 ± 1.0 kg (A allele group -1.2 ± 0.8 kg : p=0.003) and waist circumference -2.9 ± 1.1 cm (A allele group -2.1 ± 3.1 cm : p=0.004). These improvements were higher in non A allele carriers than A allele carriers. In non A allele carriers, the decrease in systolic blood pressure were -5.9 ± 3.9 mmHg (A allele carriers -2.9 ± 2.2 mmHg). These improvements were higher in non A allele carriers than A allele carriers, too. No differences were detected among other variables after weight loss.

Table 2 shows the classic cardiovascular risk factors. No differences were detected among baseline and post-treatment values of variables between both genotypes. In non A allele carriers and after dietary treatment, glucose, total cholesterol, LDL cholesterol, insulin and HOMA-IR decreased. Total Cholesterol and LDL cholesterol improved in A allele carriers, too. In non A allele carriers, the decrease in total cholesterol was -25.1 ± 5.3 mg/dl (A allele carriers -6.4 ± 4.7 mg/dl:p=0.005) and LDL- cholesterol decrease was -19.1 ± 9.5 mg/dl (A allele carriers -6.2 ± 8.5 mg/dl:p=0.003). Glucose -5.2 ± 2.5 mg/dL (A allele group -0.1 ± 1.1 mg/dL:p=0.004), insulin -2.8 ± 1.3 mUI/L (in A allele -0.2 ± 1.0 mUI/L:p=0.01) and HOMA-IR -0.9 ± 0.3 (A allele group ± 0.1 ± 0.1:p=0.01) improvement was higher in non A allele carriers than A allele carriers, too.

Table 3 shows levels of adipokines and inflammatory status. No differences were detected among baseline and post-treatment values of adipokines and inflammatory parameters between both genotypes. Leptin levels decrease in both genotypes after dietary treatment. IL-6 (-0.7 ± 0.5 ng/dL in non A allele carriers vs -0.1 ± 0.4 ng/dL in A allele carriers:p=0.02) and CRP (-2.8 ± 1.5 ng/dL in non A allele carriers vs ± 0.1 ± 0.2 ng/dL in A allele carriers:p=0.02) improvement were higher in non A allele carriers than A allele carriers. Other adipokines and inflammatory parameters remained unchanged in both groups.

Discussion

To the best of our knowledge, this is the first study that analyzes the effects of a Mediterranean hypocaloric diet and the *CNR2* gene variant rs3123554 on body weight loss and subsequent changes of metabolic parameters and adipokines. In addition, non A-allele carriers showed a better response of glucose, total cholesterol, LDL cholesterol, HOMA-IR, insulin, IL-6 and CRP levels than A-carriers. Secondly, A allele carriers had higher body weight, fat mass and waist circumference than non-carriers.

The observed percentage of minor allele carriers over 50% was similar than other studies [7]. Actually, the scientific evidence supports that endocannabinoid system with both receptors (CNR1 and CNR2)

is been positioned for regulation of endocannabinoid levels that could influence craving and reward behaviors through the relevant neuronal circuitry and metabolic parameters [17]. CNR2 has long been referred to as the peripheral cannabinoid receptor isoform. Interestingly, there is now evidence of CNR2 expression in different areas of the brain [18]. In our interventional study, we found the significant association of the SNP with obesity and metabolic parameters in the cross sectional cohort. Recently, a potential role of cerebral CNR2 receptors has been hypothesized in the modulation of body weight. For example, central CNR2 over expression leads to a lean phenotype in mice [19] and secondly, CNR2 activation in humans seems to influence eating behavior [20].

Surprisingly, we found that the minor allele of rs31235554 – that was associated with higher body weight in the baseline- led to a significantly reduced loss of body weight during dietary intervention, and this effect was independent of the body weight at baseline. Perhaps, the effect of this SNP on central insulin action could explain our results

Parameters	GG		(GA or AA)	
	0 time	At 3 months	0 time	At 3 months
BMI(kg/m²)	34.3 ± 5.5	32.8 ± 5.1*	35.0 ± 4.9$	33.7 ± 4.2*$
Weight (kg)	87.6 ± 18.7	84.2 ± 17.3*	90.1 ± 16.1$	88.4 ± 16.8*$
Fat mass (kg)	37.2 ± 11.2	35.9 ± 10.8*	38.3 ± 16.1$	36.8 ± 11.8*$
WC (cm)	105.8 ± 15.4	102.1 ± 15.3*	106.4 ± 9.6$	104.3 ± 9.1*$
WHR	0.92 ± 0.08	0.91 ± 0.09	0.90 ± 0.1	0.89 ± 0.1
SBP (mmHg)	131.9 ± 9.9	128.6 ± 10.3*	133.5 ± 11.7	126.7 ± 12.5*
DBP (mmHg)	82.4 ± 7.5	80.4 ± 9.1	84.4 ± 7.0	84.2 ± 9.3

SBP: Systolic Blood pressure. DBP: Diastolic Blood Pressure. WC: Waist circumference. Waist to hip ratio ($) (p<0.05) Statistical differences between genotype groups. (*) (p<0.05) Statistical differences in the same genotype group after dietary intervention.

Table 1: Changes in anthropometric variables after a hypocaloric meditteranean diet.

Parameters	GG		(GA or AA)	
	0 time	At 3 months	0 time	At 3 months
Glucose (mg/dl)	100.6 ± 9.5	95.1 ± 8.8*	92.3 ± 8.4	92.1 ± 7.2
Total ch. (mg/dl)	212.5 ± 40.6	188.3 ± 21.3*	218.8 ± 31.7	212.4 ± 20.1*
LDL-ch. (mg/dl)	129.5 ± 24.7	103.1 ± 21.8*	146.0 ± 33.2	139.1 ± 21.3*
HDL-ch. (mg/dl)	53.5 ± 10.1	54.0 ± 9.8	53.9 ± 12.4	54.1 ± 11.5
TG (mg/dl)	130.5 ± 30.3	128.1 ± 23.4	127.5 ± 22.1	116.9 ± 31.3
Insulin (mUI/L)	13.6 ± 7.2	10.8 ± 7.1*	14.5 ± 6.2	14.3 ± 8.1
HOMA-IR	3.5 ± 2.0	2.6 ± 1.8'	3.8 ± 2.1	3.9 ± 2.0

Ch: Cholesterol. TG: Triglycerides CRP: C reactive protein. HOMA-IR: Homeostasis model assessment. (*) (p<0.05) Statistical differences in the same genotype group after dietary intervention. No statistical differences between genotype groups.

Table 2: Clasical cardiovascular risk factors after a hypocaloric meditteranean diet.

Parameters	GG		GA or AA	
	0 time	At 3 months	0 time	At 3 months
IL 6 (pg/ml)	1.50 ± 1.2	0.68 ± 0.9 *	1.31 ± 1.1	1.33 ± 1.2
TNF-œ (pg/ml)	7.01 ± 3.0	7.11 ± 2.1	7.12 ± 3.1	7.34 ± 2.2
CRP (mg/dl)	8.9 ± 1.1	6.1 ± 1.0*	5.3 ± 2.0	5.5 ± 1.1
Adiponectin (ng/ml)	26.7 ± 10.4	22.4 ± 9.8	26.1 ± 11.3	25.9 ± 11.3
Resistin (ng/ml)	4.1 ± 1.2	3.8 ± 1.2	4.20 ± 1.2	4.42 ± 1.3
Leptin (ng/ml)	81.9 ± 32.4	62.1 ± 23.1*	80.7 ± 19.8	69.9 ± 30.6

IL6: Interleukin 6, CRP: C reactive protein. TNF-œ: Tumor necrosis factor alpha (*) (p<0.05) Statistical differences in the same genotype group after dietary intervention. No statistical differences between genotype groups.

Table 3: Circulating adypocitokines and inflammatory status after a hypocaloric meditteranean diet.

[7], because insulin action is an important regulator of body weight [21]. Ketterer et al. [7] have found that carriers of minor allele of this SNP showed lower cerebral insulin sensitivity. In contrast of the insulin effects on peripheral tissues, cerebral insulin sensitivity rather facilities body weight loss during dietary interventions [22]. One could speculate that altered cerebral insulin sensitivity in carriers of the minor allele of rs3123554 may be responsible for lower body weight loss than non-carriers.

The different metabolic response in our study after body weight could be explained by a double mechanism. First of them, it is the better body weight loss in subjects without minor allele after a hypocaloric Mediterranean diet. Interactions between weight loss secondary to a hypocaloric Mediterranean diet and other polymorphism has been yet described [23]. A second hypothesis could be due to peripheral metabolic mechanisms, because CNR2 has been isolated in organs important for the control of metabolism like adipose tissue, liver and skeletal muscle [24]. Only one previous study has explored relation of rs3123554 with body weight or metabolic parameters [7]. Ketterer et al. [7] showed an inverse relation of minor allele of this SNP with body weight. However, this relationship has been described only in females and in a population of obese subjects for high risk for diabetes mellitus type 2 or diagnosis of impaired fasting glycaemia). Our sample has male, females, and diabetes/impaired glycaemia was an exclusion criterion.

In order to show the complex relationships of this receptor with metabolism and the inconsistent results in the literature in this topic area. Recently, the CNR2 rs35761398 polymorphism revealed a significantly earlier age of menarche in subjects carrying the Q63 allele, which was also found after adjusting for BMI. This study reported that patients homozygous for the Q allele had a 2.2-fold higher risk of presenting with an early menarche (age at menarche <12 years) [25]. Finally, rs3003336, rs2501431, rs2502992, rs2501432 SNPs of *CNR2* genes are related in the etiology of osteoporosis and suggest that it may be a genetic risk factor for bone density and osteoporosis in postmenopausal women [26].

Limitations of our study include the lack of a control group without intervention, however strengths are many others as the design of intervention and evaluate a healthy diet as it is a low calorie Mediterranean diet pattern.

In conclusion, our data showed an association between the rs3123554 polymorphism of (*CNR2*) gene and metabolic response after weight loss. Non A allele carriers has a better improvement after a Mediterranean hypocaloric diet in body weight, fat mass, waist circumference, level of insulin, HOMA-IR, total cholesterol, LDL cholesterol, IL-6 and CRP than A allele carriers. Further studies will be needed to explore the relationship of this SNP with the response to other interventions in obese subject such as drugs or bariatric surgery.

References

1. Guh DP, Zhang W, Bansback N, Amarsi Z, Birmingham CL, et al. (2009) The incidence of co-morbidities related to obesity and overweight: a systematic review and meta-analysis. BMC Public Health 9: 88.

2. Loos RJ, Bouchard C (2003) Obesity--is it a genetic disorder? J Intern Med 254: 401-425.

3. Thorleifsson G, Walters GB, Gudbjartsson DF, Steinthorsdottir V, Sulem P, et al. (2009) Genome-wide association yields new sequence variants at seven loci that associate with measures of obesity. Nat Genet 41: 18-24.

4. Burch J, McKenna C, Palmer S, Norman G, Glanville J, et al. (2009) Rimonabant for the treatment of overweight and obese people. Health Technol Assess 13 Suppl 3: 13-22.

5. Ravinet Trillou C, Delgorge C, Menet C, Arnone M, Soubrié P (2004) CB1 cannabinoid receptor knockout in mice leads to leanness, resistance to diet-induced obesity and enhanced leptin sensitivity. Int J Obes Relat Metab Disord 28: 640-648.

6. de Luis DA, Ballesteros M, Lopez Guzman A, Ruiz E, et al. (2016) Polymorphism G1359A of the cannabinoid receptor gene (CNR1): allelic frequencies and influence on cardiovascular risk factors in a multicentre study of Castilla-Leon. J Hum Nutr Diet 29: 112-117.

7. Ketterer C, Heni M, Stingl KM, Tschitter O, Linder K, Wagner R, Machicao F, Haring H. Polymorphism rs3123554 in CNR2 reveals gender specific effects on body weight and affects loss of body weight and cerebra insulin action. Obesity 2014;22:925-931.

8. Mataix J, MaÃnas M. (2003) Tablas de composiciÃon de alimentos espaÃnoles. Ed: University of Granada.

9. Friedewald WT, Levy RI, Fredrickson DS (1972) Estimation of the concentration of low-density lipoprotein cholesterol in plasma, without use of the preparative ultracentrifuge. Clin Chem 18: 499-502.

10. Duart Duart MJ, Arroyo CO, Moreno Frígols JL (2002) Validation of a kinetic model for the reactions in RIA. Clin Chem Lab Med 40: 1161-1167.

11. Matthews DR, Hosker JP, Rudenski AS, Naylor BA, Treacher DF, et al. (1985) Homeostasis model assessment: insulin resistance and beta-cell function from fasting plasma glucose and insulin concentrations in man. Diabetologia 28: 412-419.

12. Pfützner A, Langenfeld M, Kunt T, Löbig M, Forst T (2003) Evaluation of human resistin assays with serum from patients with type 2 diabetes and different degrees of insulin resistance. Clin Lab 49: 571-576.

13. Suominen P (2004) Evaluation of an enzyme immunometric assay to measure serum adiponectin concentrations. Clin Chem 50: 219-221.

14. Lubrano V, Cocci F, Battaglia D, Papa A, Marraccini P, et al. (2005) Usefulness of high-sensitivity IL-6 measurement for clinical characterization of patients with coronary artery disease. J Clin Lab Anal 19: 110-114.

15. Khan SS, Smith MS, reda D, Suffredini AF, Mc Coy JP (2004) Multiplex bead array assays for detection of soluble cytokines: comparisons of sensitivity and quantitative values among kits from multiple manufactures. Cytometry B Clin Cytom61:35-39.

16. Lukaski HC, Johnson PE, Bolonchuk WW, Lykken GI (1985) Assessment of fat-free mass using bioelectrical impedance measurements of the human body. Am J Clin Nutr 41: 810-817.

17. Di Marzo V, Goparaju SK, Wang L, Liu J, Bátkai S, et al. (2001) Leptin-regulated endocannabinoids are involved in maintaining food intake. Nature 410: 822-825.

18. Morgan NH, Stanford IM, Woodhall GL (2009) Functional CB2 type cannabinoid receptors at CNS synapses. Neuropharmacology 57: 356-368.

19. Romero-Zerbo SY, Garcia-Gutierrez MS, Suárez J, Rivera P, Ruz-Maldonado I, et al. (2012) Overexpression of cannabinoid CB2 receptor in the brain induces hyperglycaemia and a lean phenotype in adult mice. J Neuroendocrinol 24: 1106-1119.

20. Onaivi ES, Carpio O, Ishiguro H, Schanz N, Uhl GR, et al. (2008) Behavioral effects of CB2 cannabinoid receptor activation and its influence on food and alcohol consumption. Ann N Y Acad Sci 1139: 426-433.

21. Hallschmid M, Schultes B (2009) Central nervous insulin resistance: a promising target in the treatment of metabolic and cognitive disorders? Diabetologia 52: 2264-2269.

22. Tschritter O, Preissl H, Hennige AM, Sartorius T, Stingl KT, et al. (2012) High cerebral insulin sensitivity is associated with loss of body fat during lifestyle intervention. Diabetologia 55: 175-182.

23. Garaulet M, Smith CE, Hernández-González T, Lee YC, Ordovás JM (2011) PPARÎ³ Pro12Ala interacts with fat intake for obesity and weight loss in a behavioural treatment based on the Mediterranean diet. Mol Nutr Food Res 55: 1771-1779.

24. Cavuoto P, McAinch AJ, Hatzinikolas G, Janovská A, Game P, et al. (2007) The expression of receptors for endocannabinoids in human and rodent skeletal muscle. Biochem Biophys Res Commun 364: 105-110.

23

MicroRNA-150 Regulates Lipid Metabolism and Inflammatory Response

Nanlan Luo[1], W. Timothy Garvey[1,2], Da-Zhi Wang[3] and Yuchang Fu[1]*

[1]*Department of Nutrition Sciences, University of Alabama at Birmingham, Birmingham, AL 35294-3360, USA*
[2]*Birmingham VA Medical Center, Birmingham, AL 35233, USA*
[3]*Department of Cardiology, Boston Children's Hospital, Harvard Medical School, Boston, MA 02115, USA*

Abstract

Background: MicroRNAs (miRNAs) have emerged as an important class of small molecules that regulate a spectrum of biological processes. However, their roles in the regulation of lipid metabolism and inflammatory response in metabolic syndrome are not completely known. To identify miRNAs and investigate how they are involved in lipid metabolism and inflammatory response in cells and animals and define the function and regulatory mechanism of these microRNAs.

Methods and results: We stimulated human THP-1 macrophages with oxLDL and found that one of the miRNAs, miR-150, strongly responded to the lipid accumulation and inflammatory response in these cells. Overexpression of miR-150 in macrophage cells resulted in an increase in lipid accumulation, accompanying with a high expression of several pro-inflammatory cytokines. Conversely, when miR-150 knockout mice were challenged with a high fat diet, these mice presented reduced whole body weight with less fat accumulation, improved systemic glucose tolerance and insulin sensitivity. The expression of pro-inflammatory cytokines in the insulin target adipose tissues was reduced in miR-150 null mice. We identified Adiponectin receptor 2 (AdipoR2) as a potential miR-150 target gene and suggested it may play an important role in miR-150-mediated lipid metabolism and inflammatory response.

Conclusions: These results uncovered novel functions for miR-150 in modulating lipid metabolism and inflammatory response by regulating genes linked to lipid accumulation and related inflammation and provided a firm mechanistic explanation with characterization and determination of critical miR-150 for its associations with the metabolic diseases. These studies will highly impact and benefit metabolic disease research both *in vitro* and *in vivo*.

Keywords: MiR-150; Macrophage foam cells; Lipid metabolism; Inflammation

Introduction

Metabolic syndrome is a powerful risk factor not only for the future development of type 2 diabetes but also cardiovascular disease [1-3]. Alterations of lipid metabolism and inflammatory response in macrophage cells represent a complex pathophysiological process that plays a crucial role in development of metabolic syndrome because macrophage cells accumulate large amounts of lipid and convert to foam cells, which both initiate and actively participate in atherosclerotic lesion development and insulin resistance, as well as other metabolic disorders [4]. Thus, the transformation of macrophages into foam cells is a critical component in the pathophysiological process. A well characterized model system to study the transformation of macrophages to foam cells is the THP-1 human monocytic cell line [5]. THP-1 monocytic cells can be induced to differentiate into macrophages by administration of Phorbol Myristate Acetate (PMA), and resulting macrophages can then be converted to foam cells following treatment with oxidized Low-Density Lipoprotein (oxLDL). The molecular determinants responsible for the transformation of macrophages to foam cells have not been fully elucidated. Here, we decided to capitalize on the advantages of this model system to identify microRNA molecules that are differentially expressed during this cell transformation [6,7]. Toward this end, we performed a microRNA qPCR array utilizing microRNAs isolated from oxLDL-treated and control THP-1 macrophages. One of the microRNA genes which we defined in this screen as being significantly up-regulated in oxLDL-treated macrophage foam cells is microRNA-150 (miR-150).

MiR-150 has been reported mainly expressing in the lymph nodes and spleen and is highly upregulated during the development of mature T and B cells; over expression of miR-150 in hematopoietic stem cells had little effect on the formation of either mature T cells or granulocytes or macrophages, but the formation of mature B cells was greatly impaired [8]. Studies have found that opposite expression pattern of miR-150 and c-Myb, a transcription factor controlling multiple steps of lymphocyte development, was detected during B cell differentiation and miR-150 could inhibit c-Myb gene expression and function *in vitro* [9,10]. Furthermore, studies have also shown that deletion of miR-150 in mice caused increased c-Myb expression and B1 cell expansion, conversely, overexpression of miR-150 in mice would reduce c-Myb expression levels and B1 cell population *in vivo* [11]. These results from both loss- and gain-of-function of miR-150 clearly indicate that miR-150 is responsible for B1 cell differentiation *in vivo* through c-Myb regulation [12].

Recent studies have shown that in human blood cells and cultured THP-1 cells, miR-150 is selectively packaged into microvesicles (MVs) and actively secreted into the blood or the culture medium; and these THP-1-derived MVs can enter and deliver miR-150 into Human Microvascular Endothelial Cells (HMEC-1), effectively reducing c-Myb expression and enhancing cell migration in HMEC-1 cells [13]. Moreover, these studies have found that MVs isolated from the plasma of patients with atherosclerosis contained higher levels of miR-150, and they more effectively promoted HMEC-1 cell migration by blood circulation than MVs from healthy donors.

Our present studies demonstrate for the first time that miR-150 can physiologically modulate metabolic activities and inflammatory

*Corresponding author: Yuchang Fu, Department of Nutrition Sciences, The University of Alabama at Birmingham, Shelby Building/1213, 1825 University Boulevard, Birmingham, AL 35294-0012, USA, E-mail: yfu@uab.edu

response both in cells and animals by regulating lipid metabolism and inflammatory response. These current studies have revealed a new regulatory role of miR-150 which is related to the mechanism for lipid metabolism and inflammation.

Methods

Human THP-1 cell culture

Human monocytic leukemia THP-1 cells were purchased from the American Type Culture Collection (ATCC, Manassas, VA). These cells were cultured in RPMI 1640 medium supplemented with 10% fetal calf serum (Tissue Culture Biologicals, Tulare, CA), penicillin (100 U/ml) and streptomycin (100 mg/ml) at 37°C in 5% CO_2. THP-1 monocytes were treated with 100 nm PMA for 24 hr to facilitate differentiation into macrophages. After treatment, the adherent macrophages were washed three times with Phosphate-Buffered Saline (PBS) and incubated with cell culture medium for 24 hr at 37°C until addition of 100 µg/mL oxLDL which was purchased from Kalen Biomedical (Montgomery Village, MD).

MicroRNA qPCR array

Human THP-1 macrophage foam cells (treated with 100 µg/ml of oxLDL for 24 hr) were harvested for microRNA isolation using a complete miRNA qPCR Array System from Qiagen (Austin, TX). Three RT2 miRNA PCR Arrays were performed and analyzed according to the manufacturer's protocols and software. The selected miRNA molecules were confirmed in oxLDL treated THP-1 macrophage foam cells and the control cells using the real-time PCR methods.

Determination of cholesterol and triglyceride concentrations in THP-1 macrophage foam cells

The concentrations of cholesterol and triglyceride in THP-1 macrophages foam cells were determined using enzymatic colorimetric assays (Wako, Richmond, VA) according to the manufacturer's protocols. The concentrations of cellular proteins from these macrophage cells were measured with a protein assay kit from Bio-Rad (Hercules, CA).

Overexpression and knockdown of miR-150 in THP-1 cells

GFP hsa-mir-150 microRNA and inhibitory hsa-mir-150 microRNA lentiviruses (10^6 pfu/ml) were purchased from the Applied Biological Materials (ABM) (Richmond, BC, Canada). These LentimiRa-GFP-hsa-mir-150 and LentimiRa-Off-hsa-miR-150 lentivirus were used to infect 2×10^5 THP-1 cells/well for 24 hr according to the manufacturer's protocols with 53% to 62% of efficiency for the infection of cells. These infected THP-1 cells were then treated with 100 nm PMA for 24 h to differentiate into macrophages. Then, these macrophages were treated with 100 µg/mL oxLDL for 24 hr to transform them into macrophage foam cells for using in the experiments.

Experimental animals

Wild type and whole body miR-150 knockout mice were purchased from the Jackson Laboratory for the experiments. To investigate the metabolism of these mice, a chow diet or a high fat diet (60% kcal% fat) from the Research Diets Company (New Brunswick, NJ) was fed to these mice from 4 weeks to 20 weeks for measuring mouse body weight and analyzing lipid accumulation and gene expression in adipose tissues.

All of these animals were housed in a specific pathogen-free facility with 12-hours light/dark cycles and received a standard laboratory chow diet except for the high fat diet experiments. Only male mice were used for the experiments. All animal procedures were approved by the Institutional Animal Care and Use Committee (IACUC) of the Animal Resources Program (ARP) at the University of Alabama at Birmingham.

Mouse glucose and insulin tolerance testing

Glucose Tolerance Testing (GTT) and Insulin Tolerance Testing (ITT) in miR-150 knockout and control mice were performed as described previously [14]. Mice were injected with glucose or insulin at 20 or 22 weeks of age after consuming the high fat diet for 16 or 18 weeks. To determine glucose tolerance, animals were first fasted overnight and then given an intraperitoneal injection of glucose solution with 1.0 ml/kg (1M glucose solution) and glucose concentration was determined in mouse tail blood collected at baseline (prior to injection), and at 30, 60, 90 and 120 minutes post-injection using a HemoCue glucose 201 glucometer (HemoCue USA). To determine insulin tolerance, mice were fasted for 6 hours in the morning of the measurement and then administered an intraperitoneal injection of insulin solution (0.5U insulin/kg body weight). Glucose levels were measured in blood samples collected as above described for the glucose tolerance testing.

Gene expression in THP-1 macrophage foam cells and mouse adipose tissues

To determine the expression levels of genes coding for lipid metabolism and inflammatory cytokines, total RNA was extracted from THP-1 foam cells or wild type and transgenic mouse adipose tissues using a commercially available TRIzol reagent from Invitrogen (Carlsbad, CA) according to the manufacturer's instructions. The quantitative real-time PCR analysis was using an ABI StepOnePlus Real-Time PCR System. Reactions were carried out in triplicate in a total volume of 20 µl using and a SYBR Green QPCR Master Mix (Applied Biosystems). Quantification was calculated using the starting quantity of the cDNA of interest relative to that of 18S ribosomal cDNA in the same sample.

Statistics

Experimental results are reported as the mean ± SEM. Statistical analyses were conducted using the unpaired Students's t-test assuming unequal variance unless otherwise indicated. Significance was defined as the $p < 0.05$.

Results

MiR-150 is highly induced by oxLDL in macrophage foam cells

To identify miRNAs and investigate their functional roles in lipid accumulation and inflammatory response in macrophage cells, we treated human THP-1 macrophages with 100 µg/ml of oxLDL to transform these cells into macrophage foam cells with accumulated lipid content inside of these cells. We performed miRNA PCR arrays to identify miRNA molecules that are induced by the lipid accumulation and inflammatory stimulation. Our experimental results showed that miR-150 (average over 4-fold levels, $p < 0.01$) was one of the miRNAs which were significantly induced by oxLDL treatment in macrophage foam cells (Figure 1). Increased miR-150 expression was further confirmed with real-time PCR (data not shown).

Overexpression and knockdown of miR-150 in THP-1 cells

To study biological functions of miR-150, we over express or knockdown miR-150 in THP-1 macrophage cells using lenti viruses. We verified the over expression or knockdown of miR-150 by quantitative RT-PCR (Figure 2A). We found that lipid accumulation

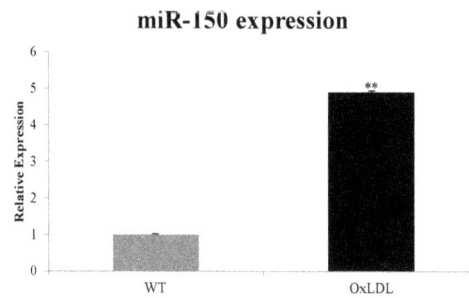

Figure 1: miR-150 is highly induced by oxLDL in THP-1 macrophage foam cells.
Human monocytic leukemia THP-1 cells were treated with 100 nM PMA for 24 h to facilitate differentiation into macrophages and the macrophages were then treated with 100 µg/mL oxLDL for 24 h to transform into foam cells. MicroRNAs were isolated by using an RT2 miRNA First Strand Kit (Qiagen) from control THP-1 macrophages (WT) and THP-1 macrophage foam cells (OxLDL) to convert to cDNAs and three RT2 miRNA PCR arrays were performed and analyzed using the complete miRNAqPCR Array System from Qiagen. The expression of miR-150 represented as three separate experiments. Error bars represented the ± SEM, **p<0.01.

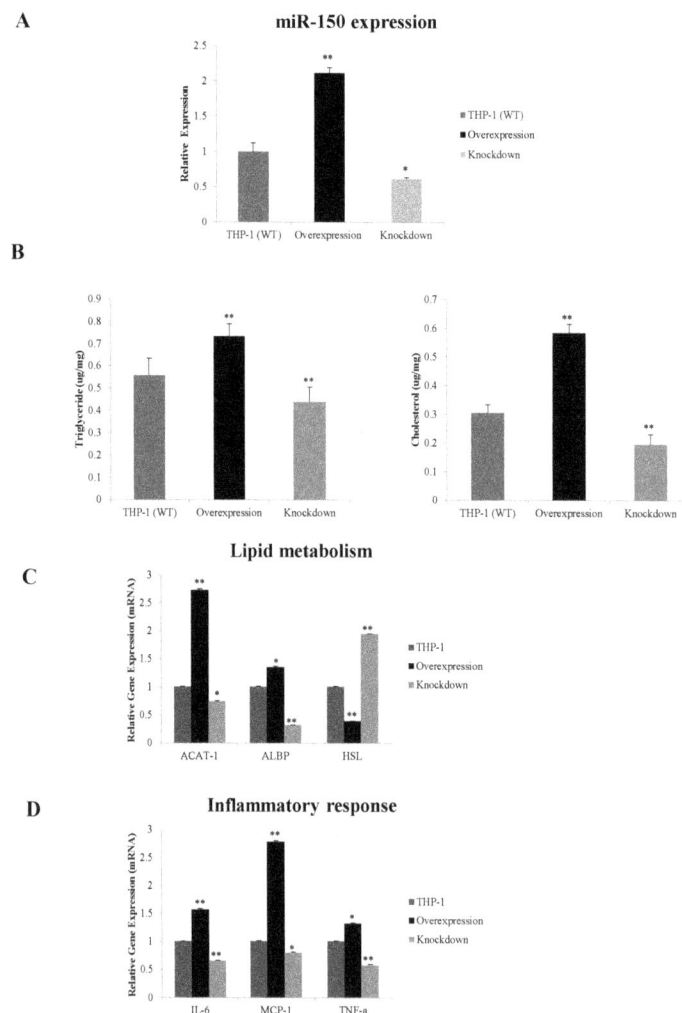

Figure 2: (A) Overexpression and knockdown of miR-150 gene in macrophage cells
 LentimiRa-GFP-hsa-mir-150 and LentimiRa-Off-hsa-miR-150 lentiviruues were used to infect 2×10^5 THP-1 cells/well for 24 h and treated with 100 nM PMA for another 24 h. These macrophages were transformed into foam cells by adding 100 µg/mL oxLDL for 24 h. **(A)** Expression of miR-150 gene were examined by QPCR analyses in control THP-1 macrophage foam cells (WT), overexpression and knockdown of miR-150 macrophage foam cells. Error bars represented the ± SEM, *p<0.05, **p<0.01.
(B) Determination of triglyceride and cholesterol concentrations in macrophage foam cells
The concentrations of triglyceride and cholesterol in THP-1 (WT), overexpression and knockdown of miR-150 macrophages foam cells were determined using enzymatic colorimetric assays. The concentrations of cellular proteins from these macrophage foam cells were measured with protein assay kits. Error bars represented the ± SEM, **p<0.01.
(C) and (D) Gene expression related to lipid metabolism and inflammatory response in macrophage foam cells
Total RNA was isolated from control THP-1, overexpression and knockdown of miR-150 macrophages foam cells, cDNAs were synthesized, and QPCR was performed with ACAT-1, ALBP, and HSL gene primers for lipid metabolism; IL-6, MCP-1, and TNF- µfor inflammatory response. Mean ± SEM from three separate experiments with triplicate samples were presented, *p<0.05 and **p<0.01.

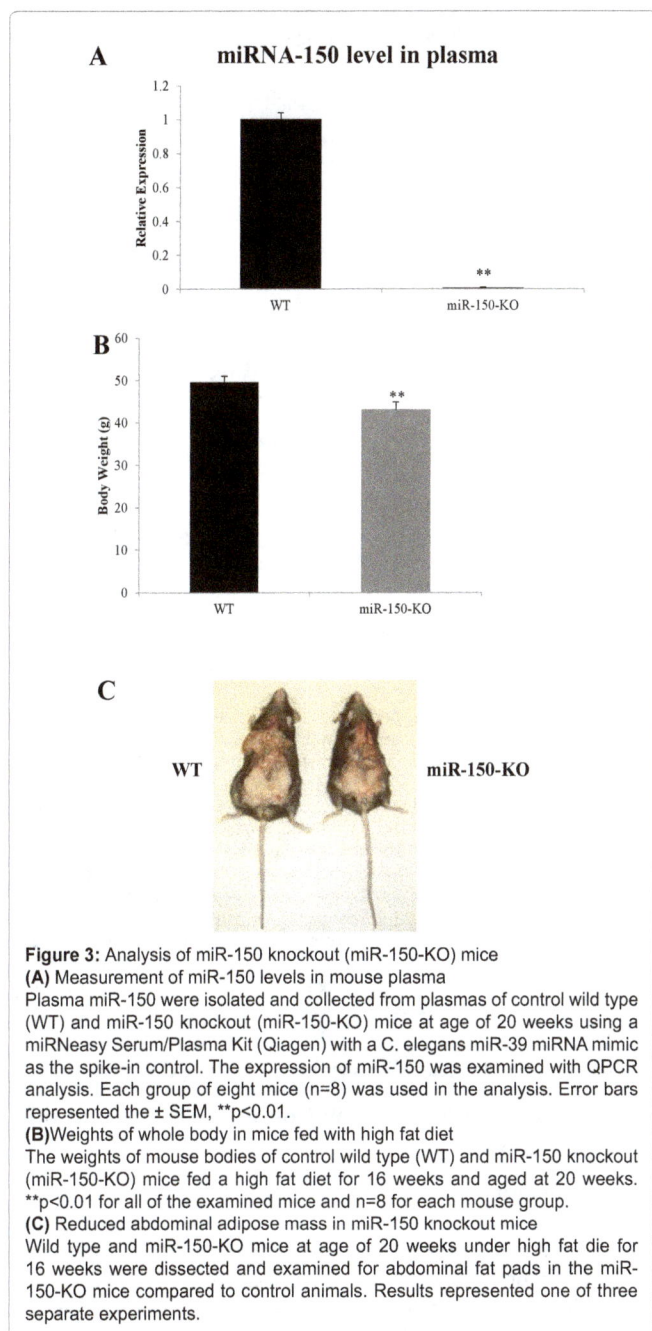

Figure 3: Analysis of miR-150 knockout (miR-150-KO) mice
(A) Measurement of miR-150 levels in mouse plasma
Plasma miR-150 were isolated and collected from plasmas of control wild type (WT) and miR-150 knockout (miR-150-KO) mice at age of 20 weeks using a miRNeasy Serum/Plasma Kit (Qiagen) with a C. elegans miR-39 miRNA mimic as the spike-in control. The expression of miR-150 was examined with QPCR analysis. Each group of eight mice (n=8) was used in the analysis. Error bars represented the ± SEM, **p<0.01.
(B) Weights of whole body in mice fed with high fat diet
The weights of mouse bodies of control wild type (WT) and miR-150 knockout (miR-150-KO) mice fed a high fat diet for 16 weeks and aged at 20 weeks. **p<0.01 for all of the examined mice and n=8 for each mouse group.
(C) Reduced abdominal adipose mass in miR-150 knockout mice
Wild type and miR-150-KO mice at age of 20 weeks under high fat die for 16 weeks were dissected and examined for abdominal fat pads in the miR-150-KO mice compared to control animals. Results represented one of three separate experiments.

(triglyceride and cholesterol) was significantly increased in the miR-150 overexpressed macrophage foam cells. In contrast, in the miR-150 knockdown cells, the lipid accumulation was significantly decreased when compared to control THP-1 macrophage foam cells (Figure 2B). We further examined the expression of several key genes related to lipid metabolism, such as, acyl-coenzyme A: Cholesterol acyl transferase 1 (ACAT-1), Adipocyte Lipid-Binding Protein (ALBP/aP2/FABP4) and Hormone Sensitive Lipase (HSL), and to inflammation, including Interleukin 6 (IL-6), Monocyte Chemoatractant Protein 1 (MCP-1) and Tumor Necrosis Factor alpha (TNF-α) in miR-150 overexpressed or knockdown cells. Our data demonstrated that miR-150 strongly induced the expression of pro-inflammatory cytokines and increased the expression of lipid accumulation genes in the THP-1 macrophage foam cells (Figures 2C and 2D).

MiR-150 knockout mice display reduction of whole body and fat mass

The above observations prompted us to investigate the *in vivo* function of miR-150 in lipid metabolism and inflammatory response. MiR-150 has been implicated in the regulation of B and T cell development and function and miR-150 knockout mice have been reported viable and fertile [11]. We first examined the levels of miR-150 in plasma of wild type and miR-150 knockout mice and we confirmed the absence of miR-150 expression in knockout mice (Figure 3A). Next, we assessed whether growth and development were affected in miR-150 knockout mice compared to wild type mice. There were no significant differences in reproduction, food consumption, or development between control and knockout mice when these animals were fed normal chow or the high fat diet (data not shown). However, compared to wild type mice, miR-150 knockout mice had significantly lower body weight (average 12%) when these mice fed with a high fat diet (60% kcal% fat) for 16 weeks at age of 20 weeks (Figure 3B).

To confirm these data, we dissected wild type and miR-150 knockout mice and found significantly reduced abdominal adipose masses in knockout mice when compared to control wild type animals (Figure 3C). Our results suggest that deficiency of miR-150 in mice can significantly affect adiposity, especially adipose tissue accumulation under the high fat diet condition.

Decreased lipid accumulation and pro-inflammatory gene expression in miR-150 knockout mice

To determine the function of miR-150 on lipid metabolism and inflammatory response, mouse adipose tissues were isolated from

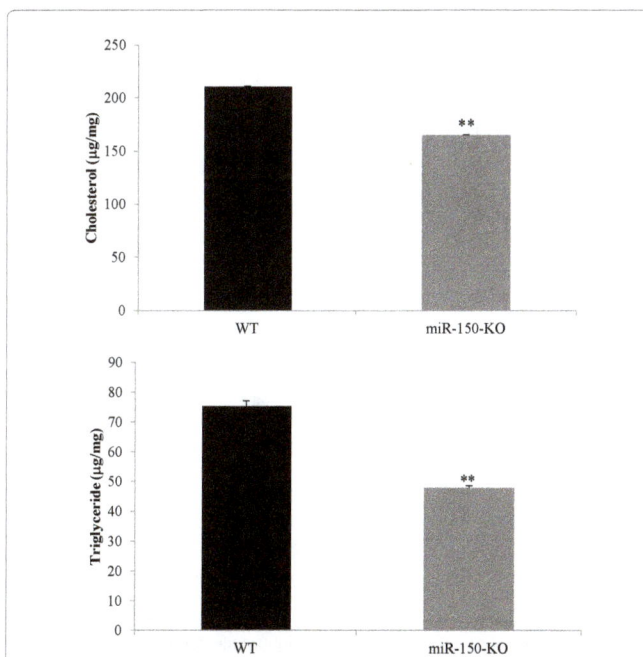

Figure 4: Changes of lipid accumulation in mouse adipose tissues
Mouse abdominal fat tissue masses from 20-week-old control wild type (WT) and miR-150 knockout (miR-150-KO) mice fed the high fat diet for 16 weeks were isolated. Cellular accumulation of cholesterol and triglyceride was assessed in the WT and miR-150-KO adipose tissues using enzymatic colorimetric kits from Wako Company. Cellular lipid mass was normalized using cellular protein levels which were determined using a protein analysis kit from the Bio-Rad. Mean ± SEM from three separate experiments with triplicate samples (n=9 for each group) were examined, **p<0.01.

20-week-old control (WT) and miR-150 knockout (miR-150-KO) mice and the cellular contents of cholesterol and triglyceride were determined. Both cholesterol (maximal average 16%) and triglyceride (maximal average 33%) levels in adipose tissues were significantly reduced (p<0.01) in miR-150 knockout mice under high fat feeding condition for 16 weeks (Figures 4A and 4B). We also examined the impact of miR-150 gene knockout on lipid metabolism and inflammatory response gene expression in adipose tissues and we found a reduced expression of ALBP, which is for lipid loading and pro-inflammatory cytokines, IL-6, MCP-1 and TNF-α, in miR-150 knockout in mice. However, we observed an increased expression of HSL, which is for lipid hydrolyzing and anti-inflammatory cytokine IL-10 in adipose tissues of miR-150 knockout mice (Figure 5A).

To further investigate whether the reduced lipid accumulation in the metabolically active adipose tissues of miR-150 knockout mice could influence the change of macrophage subtype specific markers, we next examined the expression of macrophage-specific F4/80, macrophage galactose N-acetyl-galactosamine specific lectin 1 (Mgl 1), a marker for alternatively activated Macrophage (M2) phenotype, and Chemokine Receptor 2 (CCR2), a marker for classically activated macrophage (M1) phenotype, in adipose tissues of miR-150 knockout mice. As expected, the percentage of these pro-inflammatory markers, F4/80 (average 26%, p<0.05) and CCR2 (average 61%, p<0.01), were markedly lower in adipose tissues of miR-150 knockout mice (Figure 5B). In contrast, the anti-inflammatory marker, Mgl 1, was significantly higher (average 82%, p<0.01) in adipose tissues of miR-150-KO mice than those from control wild type mice. Thus, elimination of miR-150

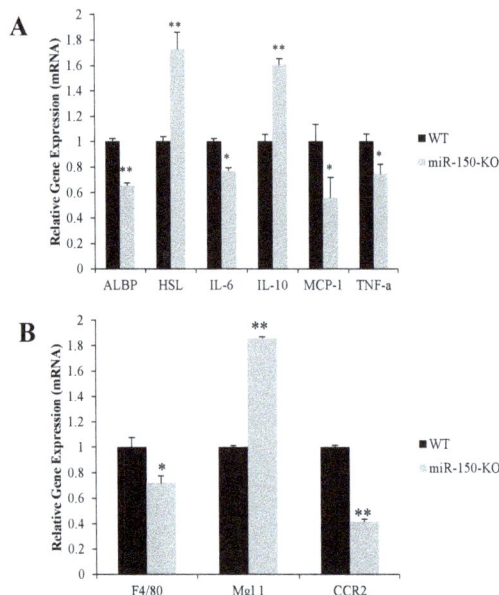

Figure 5: Effects of miR-150 deficiency on gene expression in mouse adipose tissues
Total RNA was isolated from adipose tissues of control wild type (WT) and miR-150 knockout (miR-150-KO) mice fed with high fat diet for 16 weeks at age of 20 weeks, cDNAs were synthesized, and QPCR was performed and analyzed.
(A) Gene expression linked to lipid metabolism and inflammatory response
ALBP and HSL gene primers for lipid metabolism; and IL-6, IL-10, MCP-1, and TNF-μ for inflammatory response were used in the QPCR experiments.
(B) Changed expression pattern of macrophage-specific markers
Expression of macrophage-specific markers, F4/80, Mgl 1, and CCR2, in adipose tissues from the control (WT) and miR-150 knockout (miR-150-KO) mice were examined by using QPCR analysis. All of experiments are mean ± SEM from three separate samples with triplicate sets (n=12 for each group) were examined, *p<0.05 and **p<0.01.

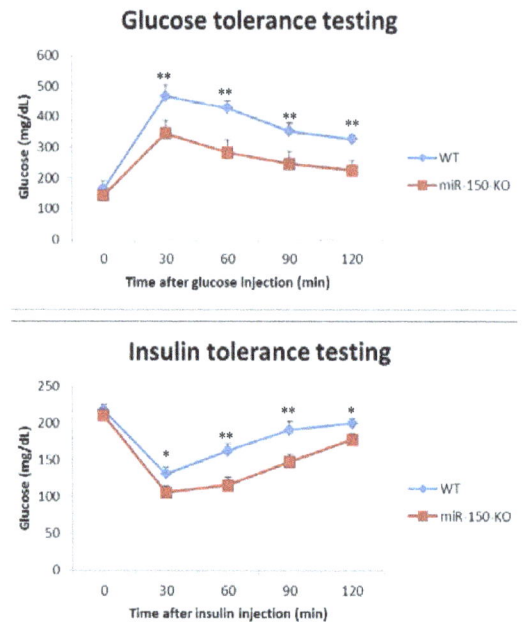

Figure 6: Glucose tolerance tests (GTT) and insulin tolerance tests (ITT) in mice
Glucose tolerance tests were performed on control wild type (WT) and miR-150 knockout (miR-150-KO) mice fed with high fat diet for 16 weeks at age of 20 weeks. Experiments were performed in fasting overnight male mice. Glucose solutions were injected into peritoneal cavity at the dose of 1.0 ml/kg (1M glucose solution). Blood was collected via tail vein at the indicated time points. Glucose concentration in plasma was measured using a glucometer (Precision); n=10 in each group of mice. Insulin tolerance tests were performed on control wild type and miR-150 knockout mice under high fat diet condition for 18 weeks at age of 22 weeks. Experiments were conducted similar as the described above for the glucose tolerance tests but fasting 6 hours before the injections and insulin solutions were injected into peritoneal cavity at the dose of 0.5 U/kg body weight. Blood was collected via tail vein at the indicated time points, and glucose levels were measured; n=10 in each group of animals, Error bars represented the ± SEM, *p<0.05 and **p<0.01.

resulted in favorable metabolic macrophage subtype changes *in vivo*.

Improved glucose tolerance and insulin sensitivity in miR-150 knockout mice

To investigate the function of miR-150 in systemic insulin sensitivity *in vivo*, we performed Glucose Tolerance Tests (GTT) and Insulin Tolerance Tests (ITT) in control and miR-150-KO mice fed with high fat diet for 16 weeks at age of 20 weeks. We found that plasma glucose levels were consistently lower (p<0.01) during the glucose tolerance tests in miR-150-KO mice when compared to that of control wild type animals (Figure 6A). Similarly, the plasma glucose levels were also consistently lower (p<0.05 or 0.01) when insulin was injected for the insulin tolerance tests than the levels in miR-150-KO mice (Figure 6B). We conclude that knockout of miR-150 gene in mice influences systemic metabolism in distal tissues as demonstrated by improved glucose tolerance and insulin sensitivity in these animals.

AdipoR2 is a miR-150 target in mouse adipose tissues

Finally, we attempted to determine miR-150 targets in adipose tissues. Based on the miRDB database for miRNA target prediction and functional annotations [15,16], AdipoR2 is one of the miR-150 target genes in both human and mouse. We experimentally examined adiponectin receptor 2 (AdipoR2) expression in adipose tissues of both miR-150 knockout and wild type control mice. AdipoR2 expression was significant increased (average 33%, p<0.01) in adipose tissues of

AdipoR2 expression

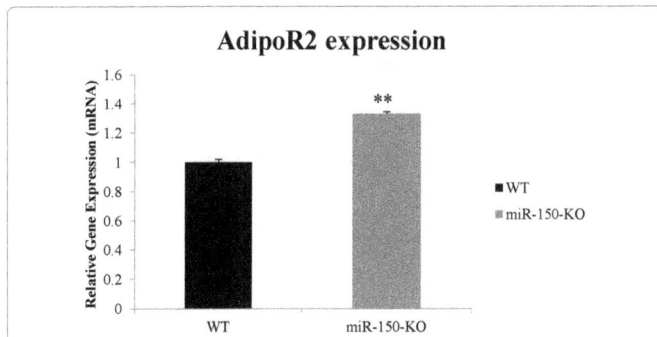

Figure 7: Analysis of adiponectin receptor 2 (AdipoR2) gene expression in mouse adipose tissues
Control wild type (WT) and miR-150 knockout (miR-150-KO) mice were fed with the high fat diet for 18 weeks at age of 22 weeks; abdominal adipose tissues were dissected from these mice and total RNA was isolated from these tissues; cDNAs were synthesized, and QPCR was performed with AdipoR2 gene primers for gene expression. Mean ± SEM from three separate experiments with triplicate samples (n=9 for each group) were presented, **p<0.01.

miR-150 knockout mice when compared to those in control wild type mice (Figure 7). Thus, the knockout of miR-150 in mice altered the expression of one important adiponectin receptor gene in metabolically active adipose tissues in a manner that would tend to promote lipid metabolism and reduce inflammation in these tissues.

Discussion

As previously demonstrated, miR-150 was involved in regulating B cell development [8] and megakaryocyte differentiation [17,18]; although the evidence has shown that except of lymphocytes miR-150 does not influence on the formation of either mature T cells or granulocytes or macrophages in hematopoietic stem cells, considering that interactions among these immune cells to respond to pathogens, miR-150 should have a vital role in the immune system [19]. Since lymphoid blood cells tightly are correlated with corresponding white blood cell counts, as one of the cancer biomarkers which have high stability in plasma, association with disease states, and ease of sensitive measurement, miR-150 has been investigated in numerous cancer studies [20,21]. In addition of cancer, disorders of the immune system can also result in autoimmune and inflammatory diseases [22,23].

It is well known that overnutrition or high fat diets are associated with autoimmune and inflammatory diseases such as diabetes and obesity; here, high fat diets exert multiple deleterious effects to key metabolic tissues *in vivo*, and immune cells, such as macrophages, T cells, and B cells, have all been implicated to play prominent roles in the inflammatory processes [24]. Recent studies have revealed that miR-150 secretion was significantly increased in ob/ob diabetic mice to promote angiogenesis in these animals [25]. Recent studies have also suggested that microRNAs play an important role in regulating lipid and glucose metabolism [26].

Previous studies have identified two cell-surface trans-membrane receptors, AdipoR1 and AdipoR2, for adiponectin action [27], and the adiponectin action is known to signal through these receptors and the docking protein APPL1 [28]. Simultaneous disruption of both AdipoR1 and AdipoR2 abolished adiponectin binding and actions, resulting in increased triglyceride content, inflammation and oxidative stress in adipose tissue, and thus leading to insulin resistance and marked glucose intolerance [29]. Although recent studies have indicated that microRNAs play an important role in metabolic syndrome [26], currently, the interactions among microRNAs and AdipoR2 are completely undefined yet. Here, we have demonstrated that AdipoR2

was regulated by miR-150 as its one of the potential target genes and the interactions between miR-150 and AdipoR2 may play a critical role in physiological metabolic activities in cells/tissues; further investigations should reveal more detailed regulatory mechanism of the function of miR-150 involved in metabolism and inflammation.

Our current studies have for the first time identified that miR-150 was highly induced by oxLDL stimulation in human THP-1 macrophage foam cells; and its expression and function were related to lipid accumulation in these cells by regulating genes that are involved in lipid metabolism, such as, ACAT-1, ALBP, and HSL. Since the lipid metabolic activity and miR-150 itself are highly related to immune/inflammatory response in cells, cytokines, including IL-6, IL-10, MCP-1, and TNF-α, are also regulated by the expression of miR-150 in these cells. We have further used miR-150 knockout mice to confirm the important roles of miR-150 in regulating these key gene expression related to lipid metabolism, inflammatory response, glucose tolerance and insulin resistance *in vivo*. Our results have indicated that miR-150 was involved in high fat diet induced obesity/diabetes through regulating lipid metabolism and inflammatory response, probably through one of its target genes, AdipoR2, *in vivo*.

In conclusion, our current studies suggest that miR-150 can physiologically modulate metabolic activities and inflammatory response both in cells and animals by mainly regulating lipid metabolism and inflammatory response. These studies have revealed a new regulatory role of miR-150 and the related mechanism for lipid metabolism and inflammation, suggesting that miR-150 maybe a potential pharmaceutical candidate for prevention and therapy of metabolic disorders in the future.

Acknowledgments

We thank the UAB Diabetes Research and Training Center for providing outstanding core services (NIH P30 DK-56336). This work was supported by grants from American Diabetes Association (1-13-IN-19) to YF, a grant from NIH (DK-083562) to TG and a grant from NIH (HL085635) to DZW.

Reference

1. Reaven GM (1988) Banting lecture 1988. Role of insulin resistance in human disease. Diabetes 37: 1595-1607.

2. Reaven GM (1991) Insulin resistance, hyperinsulinemia, hypertriglyceridemia, and hypertension. Parallels between human disease and rodent models. Diabetes Care 14: 195-202.

3. Nigro J, Osman N, Dart AM, Little PJ (2006) Insulin resistance and atherosclerosis. Endocr Rev 27: 242-259.

4. Steinberg D (1997) Low density lipoprotein oxidation and its pathobiological significance. J Biol Chem 272: 20963-20966.

5. Auwerx J (1991) The human leukemia cell line, THP-1: a multifacetted model for the study of monocyte-macrophage differentiation. Experientia 47: 22-31.

6. Wang N, Tabas I, Winchester R, Ravalli S, Rabbani LE, et al. (1996) Interleukin 8 is induced by cholesterol loading of macrophages and expressed by macrophage foam cells in human atheroma. J Biol Chem 271: 8837-8842.

7. Jang MK, Choi MS, Park YB (1999) Regulation of ferritin light chain gene expression by oxidized low-density lipoproteins in human monocytic THP-1 cells. Biochem Biophys Res Commun 265: 577-583.

8. Zhou B, Wang S, Mayr C, Bartel DP, Lodish HF (2007) miR-150, a microRNA expressed in mature B and T cells, blocks early B cell development when expressed prematurely. Proc Natl Acad Sci U S A 104: 7080-7085.

9. Monticelli S, Ansel KM, Xiao C, Socci ND, Krichevsky AM, et al. (2005) MicroRNA profiling of the murine hematopoietic system. Genome Biol 6: R71.

10. Thomas MD, Kremer CS, Ravichandran KS, Rajewsky K, Bender TP (2005) c-Myb is critical for B cell development and maintenance of follicular B cells. Immunity 23: 275-286.

11. Xiao C, Calado DP, Galler G, Thai TH, Patterson HC, et al. (2007) MiR-150 controls B cell differentiation by targeting the transcription factor c-Myb. Cell 131: 146-159.

12. Park CY, Choi YS, McManus MT (2010) Analysis of microRNA knockouts in mice. Hum Mol Genet 19: R169-175.

13. Zhang Y, Liu D, Chen X, Li J, Li L, et al. (2010) Secreted monocytic miR-150 enhances targeted endothelial cell migration. Mol Cell 39: 133-144.

14. Maeda K, Cao H, Kono K, Gorgun CZ, Furuhashi M, et al. (2005) Adipocyte/macrophage fatty acid binding proteins control integrated metabolic responses in obesity and diabetes. Cell Metab 1: 107-119.

15. Wang X, El Naqa IM (2008) Prediction of both conserved and nonconserved microRNA targets in animals. Bioinformatics 24: 325-332.

16. Wang X (2008) miRDB: a microRNA target prediction and functional annotation database with a wiki interface. RNA 14: 1012-1017.

17. Lu J, Guo S, Ebert BL, Zhang H, Peng X, et al. (2008) MicroRNA-mediated control of cell fate in megakaryocyte-erythrocyte progenitors. Dev Cell 14: 843-853.

18. Barroga CF, Pham H, Kaushansky K (2008) Thrombopoietin regulates c-Myb expression by modulating micro RNA 150 expression. Exp Hematol 36: 1585-1592.

19. Tsitsiou E, Lindsay MA (2009) microRNAs and the immune response. Curr Opin Pharmacol 9: 514-520.

20. Garzon R, Croce CM (2008) MicroRNAs in normal and malignant hematopoiesis. Curr Opin Hematol 15: 352-358.

21. Pritchard CC, Kroh E, Wood B, Arroyo JD, Dougherty KJ, et al. (2012) Blood cell origin of circulating microRNAs: a cautionary note for cancer biomarker studies. Cancer Prev Res (Phila) 5: 492-497.

22. Coussens LM, Werb Z (2001) Inflammatory cells and cancer: think different! J Exp Med 193: F23-26.

23. O'Byrne KJ, Dalgleish AG (2001) Chronic immune activation and inflammation as the cause of malignancy. Br J Cancer 85: 473-483.

24. Swindell WR, Johnston A, Gudjonsson JE (2010) Transcriptional profiles of leukocyte populations provide a tool for interpreting gene expression patterns associated with high fat diet in mice. PLoS One 5: e11861.

25. Li J, Zhang Y, Liu Y, Dai X, Li W, et al. (2013) Microvesicle-mediated transfer of microRNA-150 from monocytes to endothelial cells promotes angiogenesis. J Biol Chem 288: 23586-23596.

26. Fernández-Hernando C, Ramírez CM, Goedeke L, Suárez Y (2013) MicroRNAs in metabolic disease. Arterioscler Thromb Vasc Biol 33: 178-185.

27. Yamauchi T, Kamon J, Ito Y, Tsuchida A, Yokomizo T, et al. (2003) Cloning of adiponectin receptors that mediate antidiabetic metabolic effects. Nature 423: 762-769.

28. Mao X, Kikani CK, Riojas RA, Langlais P, Wang L, et al. (2006) APPL1 binds to adiponectin receptors and mediates adiponectin signalling and function. Nat Cell Biol 8: 516-523.

29. Yamauchi T, Nio Y, Maki T, Kobayashi M, Takazawa T, et al. (2007) Targeted disruption of AdipoR1 and AdipoR2 causes abrogation of adiponectin binding and metabolic actions. Nat Med 13: 332-339.

24

Links between Autonomic Dysfunction and Metabolic Syndrome

Federica Giampetruzzi and Gabriella Garruti*

Section of Internal Medicine, Endocrinology, Andrology and Metabolic Diseases, Department of Emergency and Organ Transplantation (DETO), University of Bari "Aldo Moro", School of Medicine, Bari, Italy

Abstract

The autonomic nervous system (ANS) plays a key role in the control of a number of vital functions including cardiovascular, endocrine/neurovascular, gastrointestinal, genitourinary, pupil and thermoregulatory functions. Its abnormalities have been associated with early mortality, sudden death, silent myocardial infarction, gastrointestinal diseases.

The manifestation of the ANS dysfunction in several human diseases is underestimated. Evidences exist on the important role of ANS dysfunctions in different clinically relevant conditions, including diabetes mellitus, chronic functional constipation, scleroderma, thalassemia major.

Beside the classical evaluation in patients with diabetes mellitus, little is known about the effects of metabolic factors on ANS dysfunction. The metabolic syndrome (MetS) includes a cluster of frequent abnormalities (impaired fasting glycaemia, dyslipidemia, arterial hypertension and increased visceral adiposity) predisposing to the atherosclerotic changes and increased cardiovascular mortality. Early signs of autonomic dysfunction are often found in subjects with MetS even in the absence of diabetes. Epidemiological studies demonstrated that diabetics display a cardiovascular risk which is twice that of sex- and age-matched non-diabetic population. Manifestations of such a high cardiovascular risk of subjects with DM are the frequent silent myocardial infarctions (MI)s of diabetics which are often due to impaired cardiovascular autonomic function. Only recently major attention has been given to the interactions between impaired glucose tolerance (IGT) and cardiovascular autonomic dysfunctions. When increased waist circumference (one of the features of the MetS) and IGT are both present, cardiovascular autonomic dysfunction also occurs. Some adipokines (e.g. adiponectin) seem to play a role in cardiovascular risk and autonomic dysfunction. This review will therefore focus on some subtle aspects linking ANS dysfunction and MetS.

Keywords: Cardiovascular; Metabolic syndrome; Autonomic neuropathy; Adipokines

List of Abbreviations: ANS: Autonomic Nervous System; CAF: Cardiovascular Autonomic Function; CAN: Cardiovascular Autonomic Neuropathy; CT: Cough Test; CVD: Cardiovascular Disease; DB: Deep Breathing; DCCT: The Diabetes Control and Complications Trial; DM: Diabetes Mellitus; EDIC: Epidemiology of Diabetes Interventions and Complications; IGT: Impaired Glucose Tolerance; HRV: Heart Rate Variability; LS: Lying to Standing; MI: Myocardial Infarction; MetS: Metabolic Syndrome; OSAS: Obstructive Sleep Apnea Syndrome; PH: Postural Hypotension; PNS: Parasympathetic Nervous System; SNS: Sympathetic Nervous System; SST: Sweat Spot Test; VS: Valsalva Manouvre

Introduction

Epidemiological studies unequivocally show that subjects with metabolic syndrome (MetS) as well as subjects with Diabetes Mellitus (DM) are at increased risk of cardiovascular diseases (CVD).

Subjects displaying a cluster of factors predisposing to the Atherosclerotic Cardiovascular Disease might be included in the syndrome named Syndrome X [1-3], (Table 1) and show a risk for stroke and coronary heart disease which is threefold higher as compared with that of controls [4]. Diabetics display a risk for CVD which is twice that of sex- and age-matched non-diabetic population and they frequently experience silent myocardial infarctions (MI) s [5,6]. Clinically unrecognized MIs might be the consequence of an impaired cardiovascular autonomic function which finally evolves to an overt cardiovascular autonomic neuropathy (CAN).

As far as the links between DM and MetS are concerned, subjects with Type 2 DM obligatory have one of the diagnostic criteria of MetS (glycaemia ≥ 100 mg/dl), but they do not always show the other diagnostic features for the MetS. However, in subjects with DM, cardiovascular risk becomes higher when clinical features of the MetS are present along with DM [7,8]. When an impaired balance between the sympathetic and parasympathetic regulation of the cardiovascular function arises, a worsening of the prognosis of Diabetes already occurs.

In this review we will report recent updates on the link between autonomic dysfunction and the presence of MetS with respect to screening tests, and coexistence of several metabolic abnormalities.

Screening Tests for Autonomic Dysfunction

In the Rochester Diabetic Neuropathy study no correlation was often found between autonomic symptoms and autonomic cardiovascular tests in subjects with Type 2 Diabetes [9,10]. Therefore an analysis of cardiovascular reflexes with tests which are sensitive, and non-invasive represent the only way to confirm the diabetic CAN. The cardiovascular reflexes are automatic responses in which heart and vascular functions are modified by stimulating different receptors involved in the control of heart rate, circulating blood volume, blood vessel diameter (vasodilation and vasoconstriction).

***Corresponding author:** Gabriella Garruti, MD PhD, Assistant Professor, Section of Internal Medicine, Endocrinology, Andrology and Metabolic Diseases, Department of Emergency and Organ Transplantation (DETO), University of Bari "Aldo Moro", Policlinico, Piazza G. Cesare 1170124 Bari, Italy, E-mail: gabriella.garruti@uniba.it

Central obesity (necessary)
Plus any two of the following conditions:
2. Elevated triglycerides (>150 mg/dl)
3. Decreased HDL cholesterol (<40 mg/dl in males: <50 mg/dl in females)
4. Elevated arterial blood pressure (>130/85 mmHg)
5. Elevated fasting blood glucose (>100 mg/dl)

Table 1: Diagnostic criteria for the metabolic syndrome according to International Diabetes Federation.

Test	PNS	SNS	Both PNS/SNS
CT	+		
DB	+		
HRV			+
LS	+		
PH		+	
SST	+		
VS			+

Abbreviations: CT: Cough Test; DB: Deep Breathing; HRV: Heart Rate Variability; LS: Lying To Standing; PH: Postural Hypotension; PNS: Parasympathetic Nervous System; SNS: Sympathetic Nervous System; SST: Sweat Spot Test; VS: Valsalva Manouvre;

Table 2: Sympathetic and parasympathetic screening tests.

The tests based on cardiovascular reflexes include Beat-to-beat heart rate variation (DB), heart rate changes after standing (LS), heart rate response to Valsalva maneuver (Vs), heart rate changes induced by cough (cough test, CT), systolic blood pressure response to upright position (PH) [11,6,12-14], (Table 2). All tests are usually performed with portable computerized systems that are used for step-by-step performance of several cardiovascular tests for autonomic neuropathy. Tests are performed after an overnight fast but never after overnight hypoglycaemia. It was unequivocally demonstrated that hypoglycaemia blunts vagal baroreflex sensitivity and sympathetic response to hypotension.

Before each test, subjects are instructed to refrain from smoking and drinking coffee for at least 8 h, to lying in the supine position for at least 30 minutes and a basal ECG is registered.

For DB, a parasympathetic function test, a 1min-ECG is performed when the subject is lying supine and deeply breathes 6 times per minute. The expiration/inspiration R-R ratio is calculated and compared with that found in age-matched control subjects.

For LS, a parasympathetic function test, the patient is invited to stand suddenly and the R-R interval is measured at beats 15 and 30 after standing and the 30/15 ratio is calculated.

For VS, the patient exhales for 15 min into the mouthpiece of a manometer exerting a pressure of 40 mmHg and the ratio between the longest and the shortest R-R interval is measured.

For PH assessment, supine systolic blood pressure is measured after the patient is lying down for 30 min and orthostatic blood pressure after the patient is suddenly standing for 2 minutes. Orthostatic hypotension is diagnosed when the fall in systolic blood pressure levels is ≥30 mmHg or that of diastolic BP fall was ≥10 mmHg in response to the postural change from the supine to the upright position [15]. Orthostatic hypotension is known to reflect sympathetic dysfunction [16] (Table 2).

CT, a parasympathetic test function, evaluates the cough-mediated increase in heart rate. During the test the patient is in the supine position, ECG is performed when patient breathed for 15 seconds (basal) and again when he coughed 3 times. The R-R ratio between the shortest R-R interval after the last cough and the mean R-R interval during regular respiration is calculated [13]. For each test the range of normal values is changing with age.

Another method to screen autonomic dysfunctions is to analyze heart rate variability [17]. It is measured in the resting position either over a period or for 24 hours. The time-domain and frequency-domain indices of heart rate variability are usually analyzed and power spectral analysis in the low frequency spectrum (0.05-0.15 Hz) and in the high frequency spectrum (0.15-0.5 Hz) and then the low frequency/ high frequency ratio might be calculated by specific software. In normal subjects the LF components prevail during the day while the components of the HF spectrum are predominant during the night. The explanation is that the sympathetic activity (responsible for the low frequency components), is mainly present during the day, while the vagal activity is predominant during night [7].

Sympathetic skin response (SSR) and Quantitative pupillography have been also recently used to screen autonomic fuction in children and adults, as elsewhere reported [18-22].

Impaired Autonomic Function in Metabolic Syndrome and Diabetes

Because of CAN, diabetics might not only experience silent myocardial infarctions but also silent hypoglycaemia and a high ASA risk during major surgery. Autonomic nervous system is anatomically poorly accessible and few direct physiological tests are available to study cardiovascular autonomic function (CAF). Therefore, some indirect clinical tests are used as screening tests which detect impaired CAF on the basis of heart responses to a simple stimulus [23]. In subjects with abnormal screening tests, the diagnosis might be completed with more sensitive techniques, but indirect screening tests help to select candidate subjects for more sophisticated analyses [23]. The diagnosis of CAN is usually made on the basis of the criteria of Ewing recently revised by Spallone et al. [17], but often when two tests are already impaired and the diagnosis of CAN is made might be too late to reverse the prognosis. Viceversa, sometimes early parasympathetic neuropathy may improve. Of note, in a longitudinal study [24], Gottsäter et al. demonstrated that after 7-10 years a subgroup of patients who were diagnosed with parasympathetic neuropathy, did not fulfil the criteria for the diagnosis anymore because of improved metabolic control. Therefore in a recent study, we thought to consider as an early deficit of CAF the detection of at least one pathological test. CAF was analysed by utilizing five different tests in a cohort of relatively young subjects with T2D. To each abnormal test we gave a score to establish a grading of severity of impaired CAF. In our cohort, the occurrence of 2 abnormal tests was rare, but the prevalence of at least one abnormal test was as high as 33.9%. In two multicenter studies and a population study of type 2 diabetics, the prevalence of CAN was 16-22% [25,26], and slightly lower than the prevalence found in our study. A plausible explanation is that the authors used only 2 (i.e., DB, LS) or 3 (i.e., DB, LS. PH) screening tests, whereas in our cohort, 5 tests (i.e., DB, LS, CT, VS, PH) were invariably performed in triplicate, likely increasing the sensitivity of tests. Concerning MetS in our young cohort, 65% subjects had MetS according to IDF, but the prevalence of MetS among subjects showing at least one abnormal test for CAF was more than 85%. A significant positive correlation between impaired CAF and MetS was confirmed with two different models of multivariate analysis. It was previously assessed an association between parasympathetic dysfunction (pathologic cardiac response to DB) and some features of the MetS according to WHO [27]. However, our report demonstrates that, MetS according to the criteria of IDF, is associated with a higher occurrence of an early deficit of CAF in a relatively young cohort of type 2 diabetics. In the same cohort we also analyzed the possible associations between the single components of MetS and the detection of an early deficit of CAF.

We found a significant correlation between the occurrence of at least one pathologic test for CAF and overweight (BMI >25), which supports the negative role played by the excess of body fat on cardiovascular risk. Overweight also has a negative effect on glycaemic control. In this line of evidence in our study we demonstrate a significant association between high HbA1c values (HbA1c >7.0%) and the occurrence of at least one abnormal test [8]. HbA1c is an established parameter to assess mean glycemia over the preceding 3 months.

Many studies have already demonstrated that either an acute or a chronic poor glycaemic control might facilitate the appearance of CAN [28-30]. These data suggest a long term benefit of intensive therapy on microvascular complication explained by the treatment group differences in mean HbA1c levels over time. Moreover, in EDIC study patient with CAN showed an increase in left ventricular mass and mass-to-volume ratios compared with diabetics without CAN (p 0.0001 for each), changes consistent with left ventricular concentric remodeling that were independent of age, sex, and other traditional cardiovascular risk factors. From different meta-analysis the median value of mortality after 5 years was around 25% in diabetics with CAN and 4% in diabetics without CAN. If the diagnosis of CAN was based on the occurrence of 2 abnormal tests the relative risk of mortality was 3.5 [31,32]. Subjects from EDIC were recently analysed to test the association between testosterone levels and CAN, but "Testosterone levels" were not "associated with CAN among men with type1 diabetes" [33].

Interestingly, improving the glycaemic control also counteracts the early deficit of CAF or stops its progression (DCCT 1993). In studies utilizing heart rate variability as an index of CAF, mild CAF abnormalities improved if HbA1c values decreased from 9.5% to 8.4% [34,35].

A strong association was found between the duration of Diabetes and CAN [36]. Both PH and decreased heart rate variability are more frequent and severe 5 years after the diagnosis of Diabetes [36]. Unexpectedly, we found no association between CAF score and the duration of Diabetes, however, the subjects of our cohort [8], probably had a better metabolic memory than that of subjects from previous studies, not only because they were younger than those considered in previous studies, but also because they experienced a program of education to healthy life-style together with insulin and /or oral anti-diabetic agents of last generation since the onset of Diabetes.

Several factors associated with MetS might account for sympathetic over-activity. Excess of abdominal body (central obesity) is one of the obligatory component of MetS and increased central/visceral fat results in overproduction of inflammatory adipokines which also play a role in some pathogenic pathways inducing autonomic impaired balance and enhancing cardiovascular risk. The two hormones leptin and adiponectin (both originating from visceral adipose tissue),appear to be involved as well, since increased circulating levels of leptin and decreased circulating levels of adiponectin stimulate sympathetic overflow.

Several reports show that a higher cardiovascular risk is present in subjects displaying a cluster of factors predisposing to the Atherosclerotic Cardiovascular Disease and included in the syndrome named MetS(Table 1) [2,3]. Subjects with T2D always have one of the diagnostic criteria of (glycaemia ≥ 100 mg/dl), but do not obligatory show other diagnostic features for MetS. Interleukin-6 is a multifunctional cytokine that plays a central role in inflammatory responses.

In both MetS and Diabetes C-reactive protein (CRP) and interleukin-6 (IL-6) play a pathogenetic role. C-reactive protein (CRP) and interleukin-6 (IL-6) are strongly interrelated since CRP is produced in the liver in response to IL-6 in the acute-phase of inflammation. Both CRP and IL-6 are inflammatory markers and they have been found to be inversely related with reduced heart rate variability in a study concerning more than 200 male twins who had never had any symptom of coronary artery disease. Nonetheless, diabetic polyneuropathy correlates with CRP and IL-6 levels [36], the possibility exists that impaired autonomic function might induce chronic low-grade inflammation, but it has also been suggested that inflammation might induce cardiovascular dysfunction [36].

Early in the development of autonomic dysfunction, there was loss of heart rate variability (HRV), and this correlated with an increase in circulating markers of inflammation, such as C-reactive protein (CRP) and IL-6. Of great interest to us was the loss of HRV as well as the loss of sympathetic/parasympathetic balance, even before the advent of inflammation. Cardiac autonomic imbalance also correlated with markers of adipose tissue-derived inflammation (adiponectin-to-leptin ratio) and this was seen early in type 2 diabetes patients.

An increased sympathetic tone and decreased vagal response usually account for an impaired autonomic balance. In isolated adipocytes, an increased sympathetic tone is usually associated with inflammation since after β-adrenergic stimulation the levels of IL-6 are increased [37]. In several studies increased levels of acetylcholine and/or electrical stimulation of vagal nerve endings were associated with a reduced release of cytokines from inflammatory cells (macrophages) [38].

In central Obesity increased circulating leptin levels are present which might account for the activation of sympathetic nervous system found in MetS. Human leptin is a protein of 167 amino acids. It is mainly synthesized in the adipocytes of white adipose tissue, and there is a direct correlation between the total amount of fat in the body and the circulating levels of leptin [39,40].

Very recently it was unequivocally demonstrated that Leptin responsive neurons exists in the nucleus of the solitary tract (NTS) which is one of the main regulatory sites of the sympathetic nervous system. Interestingly, the long form of the leptin receptor (Ob-Rb) has been detected in NTS of Sprague–Dawley rats and leptin injection in NTS elicits sympathoexicitatory responses through the stimulation of Ob-Rb and mediate chemoreceptor afferent information to specific areas of the rostral ventrolateral medulla (RVLM) which are involved in the reflex control of arterial blood pressure [41]. Hyperleptinemia is associated with increased fat mass and human obesity. Interestingly, leptin is known to play a role in food intake regulation and energy balance at the level of several areas of the hypothalamus which are also involved in the switching on of the sympathetic nervous system. In animal models displaying leptin-resistance (db/db mice), diabetes and obesity are associated with distraught circadian rhythm of blood pressure [42], To support the idea that leptin effects were mediated by the activation of the sympathetic nervous system there are studies demonstrating that intravenous infusion of leptin induces an increase in both arterial blood pressure and heart rate which is completely blunted by β-adrenergic blockers [43,44].

However, hyperleptinemia can be considered a marker of increased sympathetic tone and leptin insufficiency is associated with reduced sympathetic activity.

Not only low-grade inflammation but also hypo-adiponectinemia ensure in MetS and obesity. Adiponectin is a secretory protein uniquely encoded by adipocytes in different mammal species. Adipose tissue is richly innervated by both sympathetic and parasympathetic nerve endings and an impaired balance between the two autonomic branches has been claimed to influence adiponectin and cytokine secretion thus changing the inflammatory state of pathologic conditions characterized by visceral fat accumulation (e.g. metabolic syndrome, diabetes) [45].

Little is known about the effect of adiponectin in the regulation of sympathetic nervous system. However Adiponectin injection in the hypothalamic paraventricular nucleus depolarizes parvocellular neurons controlling both autonomic function and endocrine pathways [46]. Adiponectin plays an hypotensive effect either by modulating the NPY neurons of the NTS or stimulating the renal sympathetic nerve endings [46, 47]. By contrast in conditions characterized by an increased sympathetic tone (e.g. cold exposure) serum adiponectin levels are suppressed [48]. In subjects with Type 2 Diabetes a direct correlation exists between increased vagal activity and adiponectin circulating levels [49].

Recent evidences suggest that a transient autonomic imbalance occurs before diabetes and/or overt autonomic neuropathy. New insights in the relationships between glucose tolerance and autonomic function have been recently pointed out. In subjects with impaired glucose tolerance (IGT), heart rate variability is already impaired. Heart rate analysis represents a non-invasive method to test cardiovascular autonomic function. However, some other studies demonstrate that in subjects with impaired glucose tolerance neither heart rate variability nor cardiovascular reflex tests (deep breathing, heart rate response to Valsalva maneuver, blood pressure response to standing up quickly) are sometimes able to discover a mild initial form of autonomic neuropathy which might be early detected with sympathetic skin response (SSR) that evaluates postganglionic sympathetic sudomotor function. In patients with IGT the amplitude of the SSR of two different limbs (right arm and leg) is often lower than that found in healthy subjects [50]. These data support the view that sympathetic sudomotor function might be impaired before cardiovascular autonomic function but unfortunately the above mentioned studies did not directly analysed the cardiovascular risk in subjects showing impaired SSR and it is possible that impaired SSR does not correlate with any other metabolic abnormality except for glucose tolerance.

In normalweight and normotensive individuals short-term hyperinsulinemia, which is one of the features of pre-diabetes, was already able to induce a decrease in heart rate variability [53]. Hyperinsulinemia is one of the features of pre-diabetes and the possibility exists that the early impairment of the cardiovascular reflex function occurring in both IGT and hyperinsulinemia/insulin-resistance may be the cross-bridge between the increased cardiovascular disease risk and the early changes in glucose tolerance [53].

Autonomic Imbalance associated with Cardiovascular Risk, Metabolic Syndrome and Obstructive Sleep Apnea Syndrome

Subjects with MetS show an impaired function of the autonomic system. In different reports central obesity, insulin resistance and increased levels of high blood pressure which represent the features of the MetS, are accompanied by an increased sympathetic tone [54,55].

Before overt diabetes, several subjects might experience pre-diabetes such as impaired glucose tolerance and hyperinsulinemia. In both conditions circadian regulation of cardiac autonomic function is compromised. In lean normotensive individuals [56], demonstrated that 2-day hyperinsulinemia reduced heart rate variability during night and blunted the nocturnal lowering of the arterial blood pressure.

It might be argued that the early impairement of the cardiovascular reflex function may represent the link between cardiovascular disease and early changes in glucose tolerance [55]. The cardiovascular reflex function includes a group of reflexes in which heart and circulatory functions changes in response to variations in heart rate, vascular tone, blood volume, or other variables.

Several studies demonstrate an increased activity of the sympathetic nervous system (SNS) in hypertension and insulin resistance which are components of the metabolic syndrome and/or Syndrome X. Central obesity is an obbligatory component of the MetS according to the International Diabetes Federation (IDF) and it is also associated with SNS hyperactivity. However, it is difficult to establish whether the impaired function of SNS is one of the causes of or one of the comorbidities of such a syndrome.

In a study involving more than 1000 subjects, an impaired function of the ANS seemed to be already present in subjects showing only one of the abnormalities of the MetS, even before the appearance of insulin resistance [56].

Therefore it is reasonable to believe that an impaired autonomic balance might be associated with the early negative changes of gluco-metabolic control and might play a potential role in switching on the pathogenic pathways which lastly produce diabetes [57].

Very often the excess of central fat is not only associated with diabetes and/or but also with obstructive sleep apnea syndrome (OSAS). This feature is clarly evident in subjects with severe forms of obesity undergoing bariatric surgery. The increased circulating levels of CO_2 which are present in subjects with OSAS might be themselves responsible for an increased low-grade inflammatory state which favor sympathetic overactivity. To support the idea that fat excess is associated with autonomic dysfunction, Blüher's group recently demonstrated that overweight and obese children without diabetes or impaired glucose tolerance already showed a decrease in both parasympathetic and sympathetic activity.

Lifestyle and Sympathetic Autonomic Dysfunction

Few studies considered the dietary habits of subjects showing impaired cardiovascular autonomic function (CAF). In a recent paper from our group we screened for cardiovascular autonomic neuropathy 180 subjects with type 2 diabetes with mean age of 48 years and we also analyzed whether any relationship existed between the nutritional habits of our cohort and the occurrence of any deficit of the autonomic function [8]. Interestingly, subjects with impaired CAF more often had MetS as compared with subjects with normal CAF but also eat a higher amount of saturated fat (higher amount of cheese and fat meet) as compared with diabetics who did not show any sign of abnormal CAF and MetS Unexpectedly, subjects with impaired CAF and MetS chose a western-style diet even if they were living in a mediterranean area [8]. Some data already exist about subjects with MetS who showed an improvement in their chronic low-grade inflammatory state (reduction in serum concentrations of C-reactive protein, interleukin-6, insulin-resistance, and improved endothelial function score) after experiencing a mediterranean-style diet (high content of whole grains, fruits, vegetables, nuts, and olive oil). This dietary model seems to be more effective than a balanced low-fat diet [58]. These data support the idea that lifestyle intervention program might reduce the risk of impaired autonomic function as already demonstrated by the Diabetes Prevention Program (DPP) where a low-glycaemic index and low-fat diet plus moderate exercise reduced the risk of autonomic neuropathy of one forth [59]. Regular exercise as well as dietary intervention program might also prevent autonomic dysfunction. In type 2 Diabetes, chronic aerobic activity (three-month exercise) restored heart rate variability, barorecptor sensitivity and vagal activity [60]. However exercise can be significantly increased only in early cardiac autonomic neuropathy, by contrast dietary intervention might be applied in any kind of autonomic dysfunctions and also in the presence of resting tachycardia, which is the extreme manifestation of severe autonomic neuropathy.

Conclusion

In conclusion, cardiovascular autonomic dysfunction is usually considered as a complication of diabetes, by contrast recent data point out its role at the very begininnig of the cascade of events inducing the chronic low-grade inflammation which represents the "primum movens" of both pre-diabetes and MetS. An emerging insight is the early impairement of autonomic function in childhood obesity in the absence either of overt diabetes or impaired glucose tolerance. However lifestyle intervention might improve and/or delay autonomic neuropathy and/or MetS either in childhood or adulthood.

Acknowledgements

The authors are grateful to Prof. Francesco Giorgino for precious suggestions.

References

1. Reaven GM (1993) Role of insulin resistance in human disease (syndrome X): an expanded definition. Annu Rev Med 44: 121-131.

2. Grundy SM, Cleeman JI, Daniels SR, Donato KA, Eckel RH, et al. (2005) American Heart Association; National Heart, Lung, and Blood Institute, 2005. Diagnosis and management of the Metabolic Syndrome: An American Heart Association/National Heart, Lung and Blood Institute Scientific Statement. Circulation 112: 2735-2752.

3. Zimmet P, Magliano D, Matsuzawa Y, Alberti G, Shaw J (2005) The metabolic syndrome: a global public health problem and a new definition. J Atheroscler Thromb 12: 295-300.

4. Isomaa B, Almgren P, Tuomi T, Forsén B, Lahti K, et al. (2001) Cardiovascular morbidity and mortality associated with the metabolic syndrome. Diabetes Care 24: 683-689.

5. Langer A, Freeman MR, Josse RG, Steiner G, Armstrong PW (1991) Detection of silent myocardial ischemia in diabetes mellitus. Am J Cardiol 67: 1073-1078.

6. Vinik AI, Erbas T (2001) Recognizing and treating diabetic autonomic neuropathy. Cleve Clin J Med 68: 928-930, 932, 934-44.

7. Vinik AI, Maser RE, Ziegler D (2011) Autonomic imbalance: prophet of doom or scope for hope? Diabet Med 28: 643-651.

8. Garruti G1, Giampetruzzi F, Vita MG, Pellegrini F, Lagioia P, et al. (2012) Links between metabolic syndrome and cardiovascular autonomic dysfunction. Exp Diabetes Res 2012: 615835.

9. Low PA, Benrud-Larson LM, Sletten DM, Opfer-Gehrking TL, Weigand SD, et al. (2004) Autonomic symptoms and diabetic neuropathy: a population-based study. Diabetes Care 27: 2942-2947.

10. Church TS, Thompson AM, Katzmarzyk PT, Sui X, Johannsen N, et al. (2009) Metabolic syndrome and diabetes, alone and in combination, as predictors of cardiovascular disease mortality among men. Diabetes Care 32: 1289-1294.

11. Vespasiani G, Bruni M, Meloncelli I, Clementi L, Amoretti R, et al. (1996) Validation of a computerised measurement system for guided routine evaluation of cardiovascular autonomic neuropathy Comput. Methods Programs Biomed 51: 211-216

12. Portincasa P, Moschetta A, Berardino M, Di Ciaula A, Vacca M, et al. (2004) Impaired gallbladder motility and delayed orocecal transit contribute to pigment gallstone and biliary sludge formation in beta-thalassemia major adults. World J Gastroenterol 10: 2383-2390.

13. Cardone C, Bellavere F, Ferri M, Fedele D (1987) Autonomic mechanisms in the heart rate response to coughing. Clin Sci (Lond) 72: 55-60.

14. Cardone C, Paiusco P, Marchetti G, Burelli F, Feruglio M, et al. (1990) Cough test to assess cardiovascular autonomic reflexes in diabetes. Diabetes Care 13: 719-724.

15. Freeman R, Landsberg L, Young J (1999) The treatment of neurogenic orthostatic hypotension with 3,4-DL-threo- dihydroxyphenylserine: a randomized, placebo-controlled, crossover trial. Neurology 53: 2151- 2157.

16. Low PA, Walsh JC, Huang CY, McLeod JG (1975) The sympathetic nervous system in diabetic neuropathy. A clinical and pathological study. Brain 98: 341-356.

17. Spallone V, Bellavere F, Scionti L, Maule S, Quadri R, et al. (2011) on behalf of the Diabetic Neuropathy Study Group of the Italian Society of Diabetology. Recommendations for the use of cardiovascular tests in diagnosing diabetic autonomic neuropathy. Nutr Metab Cardiovas Dis 21: 69-78.

18. Arunodaya GR, Taly AB (1995) Sympathetic skin response: a decade later. J Neurol Sci 129: 81-89.

19. Baum P, Petroff D, Classen J, Kiess W, Blüher S (2013) Dysfunction of autonomic nervous system in childhood obesity: a cross-sectional study. PLoS One 8: e54546.

20. Altomare DF, Portincasa P, Rinaldi M, Di Ciaula A, Martinelli E, et al. (1999) Slow-transit constipation: solitary symptom of a systemic gastrointestinal disease. Dis Colon Rectum 42: 231-240.

21. Portincasa P, Moschetta A, Berardino M, Di Ciaula A, Vacca M, et al. (2004) Impaired gallbladder motility and delayed orocecal transit contribute to pigment gallstone and biliary sludge formation in beta-thalassemia major adults. World J Gastroenterol 10: 2383-2390.

22. Heller PH, Perry F, Jewett DL, Levine JD (1990) Autonomic components of the human pupillary light reflex. Invest Ophthalmol Vis Sci 31: 156-162.

23. Freeman R (2006) Assessment of cardiovascular autonomic function. Clin Neurophysiol 117: 716-730.

24. Töyry JP, Niskanen LK, Mäntysaari MJ, Länsimies EA, Haffner SM, et al. (1997) Do high proinsulin and C-peptide levels play a role in autonomic nervous dysfunction?: Power spectral analysis in patients with non-insulin-dependent diabetes and nondiabetic subjects. Circulation 96: 1185-1191.

25. [No authors listed] (1994) Microvascular and acute complications in IDDM patients: the EURODIAB IDDM Complications Study. Diabetologia 37: 278-285.

26. Neil H AW, Thompson AV, John S, McCarthy ST, Mann JI (1989) Diabetic autonomic neuropathy: the prevalence of impaired heart rate variability in a geographically defined Population. Diabetic Medicine 6: 20-24.

27. Takayama S, Sakura H, Katsumori K, Wasada T, Iwamoto Y (2001) A possible involvement of parasympathetic neuropathy on insulin resistance in patients with type 2 diabetes. Diabetes Care 24: 968-969.

28. [No authors listed] (1993) The effect of intensive treatment of diabetes on the development and progression of long-term complications in insulin-dependent diabetes mellitus. The Diabetes Control and Complications Trial Research Group. N Engl J Med 329: 977-986.

29. Burger AJ, Weinrauch LA, D'Elia JA, Aronson D (1999) Effect of glycemic control on heart rate variability in type I diabetic patients with cardiac autonomic neuropathy. Am J Cardiol 84: 687-691.

30. Gaede P, Vedel P, Parving HH, Pedersen O (1999) Intensified multifactorial intervention in patients with type 2 diabetes mellitus and microalbuminuria: the Steno type 2 randomised study. Lancet 353: 617-622.

31. Shaw JE, Zimmet PZ, Gries FZ, Ziegler D (2003) Epidemiology of diabetic neuropathy. In: Griesw FA, Cameron NE, Low PA, and Ziegler D, (eds), Textbook of Diabetic Neuropathy, Thieme Medical Publishers, New York, NY, USA.

32. Vinik A, Erbas T, Casellini CM (2013) Diabetic cardiac autonomic neuropathy, inflammation and cardiovascular disease. J Diabetes Investig 4: 4-18.

33. Kim C, Pop-Busui R, Braffett B, Cleary PA, Bebu I, et al. (2015) Testosterone Concentrations and Cardiovascular Autonomic Neuropathy in Men with Type

1 Diabetes in the Epidemiology of Diabetes Interventions and Complications Study (EDIC). J Sex Med 11: 2153-2159.

34. Szelag, B, Wroblewski M, Castenfors J, Henricsson M, Berntorp K, et al. (1999) Obesity, microalbuminuria, hyperinsulinemia, and increased plasminogen activator inhibitor 1 activity associated with parasympathetic neuropathy in type 2 diabetes. Diabetes Care 22: 1907-1908.

35. Herder C, Lankisch M, Ziegler D, Rathmann W, Koenig W, et al. (2009) Subclinical inflammation and diabetic polyneuropathy: MONICA/KORA Survey F3 (Augsburg, Germany). Diabetes Care 32: 680- 682.

36. Lampert R, Bremner JD, Su S, Miller A, Lee F, et al. (2008) Decreased heart rate variability is associated with higher levels of inflammation in middle-aged men. Am Heart J 156: 759.

37. Mohamed-Ali V, Flower L, Sethi J, Hotamisligil G, Gray R, et al. (2001) beta-Adrenergic regulation of IL-6 release from adipose tissue: in vivo and in vitro studies. J Clin Endocrinol Metab 86: 5864-5869.

38. Borovikova LV, Ivanova S, Zhang M, Yang H, Botchkina GI, et al. (2000) Vagus nerve stimulation attenuates the systemic inflammatory response to endotoxin. Nature 405: 458-462.

39. Margetic S, Gazzola C, Pegg GG, Hill RA (2002) Leptin: a review of its peripheral actions and interactions. Int J Obes Relat Metab Disord 26: 1407-1433.

40. Bado A, Levasseur S, Attoub S, Kermorgant S, Laigneau JP, et al. (1998) The stomach is a source of leptin. Nature 394: 790-793.

41. Ciriello J, Moreau JM (2013) Systemic administration of leptin potentiates the response of neurons in the nucleus of the solitary tract to chemoreceptor activation in the rat Neuroscience 229: 88-99.

42. da Costa Goncalves AC, Tank J, Diedrich A, Hilzendeger A, Plehm R, et al. (2009) Diabetic hypertensive leptin receptor-deficient db/db mice develop cardioregulatory autonomic dysfunction. Hypertension 53: 387- 392.

43. Paolisso G, Manzella D, Montano N, Gambardella A, Varricchio M (2000) Plasma leptin concentrations and cardiac autonomic nervous system in healthy subjects with different body weights. J Clin Endocrinol Metab 85: 1810-1814.

44. Carlyle M, Jones OB, Kuo JJ, Hall JE (2002) Chronic cardiovascular and renal actions of leptin: role of adrenergic activity. Hypertension 39: 496-501.

45. Kreier F, Fliers E, Voshol PJ, Van Eden CG, Havekes LM, et al. (2002) Selective parasympathetic innervation of subcutaneous and intra-abdominal fat--functional implications. J Clin Invest 110: 1243-1250.

46. Hoyda TD, Samson WK, Ferguson AV (2009) Adiponectin depolarizes parvocellular paraventricular nucleus neurons controlling neuroendocrine and autonomic function. Endocrinology 150: 832- 840.

47. Tanida M, Shen J, Horii Y, Matsuda M, Kihara S, et al. (2007) Effects of adiponectin on the renal sympathetic nerve activity and blood pressure in rats. Exp Biol Med (Maywood) 232: 390-397.

48. Imai J, Katagiri H, Yamada T, Ishigaki Y, Ogihara T, et al. (2006) Cold exposure suppresses serum adiponectin levels through sympathetic nerve activation in mice. Obesity (Silver Spring) 14: 1132-1141.

49. Wakabayashi S, Aso Y (2004) Adiponectin concentrations in sera from patients with type 2 diabetes are negatively associated with sympathovagal balance as evaluated by power spectral analysis of heart rate variation. Diabetes Care 27: 2392- 2397.

50. Smith AG, Russell J, Feldman EL, Goldstein J, Peltier A, et al. (2006) Lifestyle intervention for pre-diabetic neuropathy. Diabetes Care 29: 1294-1299.

51. Grandinetti A, Chow DC, Sletten DM, Oyama JK, Theriault AG, et al. (2007) Impaired glucose tolerance is associated with postganglionic sudomotor impairment. Clin Auton Res 17: 231-233.

52. Isak B, Oflazoglu B, Tanridag T, Yitmen I, Us O (2008) Evaluation of peripheral and autonomic neuropathy among patients with newly diagnosed impaired glucose tolerance. Diabetes Metab Res Rev 24: 563-569.

53. Petrova M, Townsend R, Teff K L (2006) Prolonged (48-h) modest hyperinsulinemia decreases nocturnal heart rate variability and attenuates the nocturnal decrease in blood pressure in lean, normotensive humans. J. Clin. Endocrinol. Metab 91: 851-859.

54. Ziegler D, Zentai C, Perz S, Rathmann W, Haastert B, et al. (2006) Selective contribution of diabetes and other cardiovascular risk factors to cardiac autonomic dysfunction in the general population. Exp Clin Endocrinol Diabetes 114: 153-159.

55. Licht CM, Vreeburg SA, van Reedt Dortland AK, Giltay EJ, Hoogendijk WJ, et al. (2010) Increased sympathetic and decreased parasympathetic activity rather than changes in hypothalamica "pituitarya" adrenal axis activity is associated with metabolic abnormalities. J Clin Endocrinol Metab 95: 2458-2466.

56. Chang CJ, Yang YC, Lu FH, Lin TS, Chen JJ, et al. (2010) Altered cardiac autonomic function may precede insulin resistance in metabolic syndrome. Am J Med 123: 432-438.

57. Carnethon MR, Jacobs DR Jr, Sidney S, Liu K; CARDIA study (2003) Influence of autonomic nervous system dysfunction on the development of type 2 diabetes: the CARDIA study. Diabetes Care 26: 3035-3041.

58. Esposito K, Marfella R, Ciotola M, Di Palo C, Giugliano F, et al. (2004) Effect of a mediterranean-style diet on endothelial dysfunction and markers of vascular inflammation in the metabolic syndrome: a randomized trial. JAMA 292: 1440-1446.

59. Carnethon MR, Prineas RJ, Temprosa M, Zhang ZM, Uwaifo G, et al. (2006) The association among autonomic nervous system function, incident diabetes, and intervention arm in the Diabetes Prevention Program. Diabetes Care 29: 914- 919.

60. Michalsen A, Knoblauch NT, Lehmann N, Grossman P, Kerkhoff G, et al. (2006) Effects of lifestyle modification on the progression of coronary atherosclerosis, autonomic function, and anginaa"the role of GNB3 C825T polymorphism. Am. Heart J 151: 870-877.

25

Nonalcoholic Fatty Liver Disease Alone Is a Better Predictor of Metabolic Syndrome and Insulin Resistance than Existing ATP-III Criteria

Shivaram Prasad Singh[1]*, Preetam Nath[1], Ayaskanta Singh[1], Jimmy Narayan[1], Prasant Parida[1], Pradeep Kumar Padhi[1], Girish Kumar Pati[1], Chudamani Meher[2] and Omprakash Agrawal[2]

[1]Department of Gastroenterology, S.C.B. Medical College, 753007 Cuttack, India
[2]Department of Radiology, Beam Diagnostics Centre, Bajrakabati Road, 753001 Cuttack, India

Abstract

Objective: Metabolic syndrome (MS) also known as insulin resistance syndrome is a surrogate marker of insulin resistance (IR). Traditionally this is being diagnosed by Adult Treatment Panel III (ATP-III) and International Federation of Diabetes (IDF) criteria. Despite mounting evidence in favor of non-alcoholic fatty liver disease (NAFLD), this has not been yet included as a component of either ATP-III or IDF criteria. We conducted this study to evaluate if NAFLD could be used as a criterion for identifying metabolic syndrome.

Methods: Setting: Single center observational study in Gastroenterology OPD at SCB Medical College, Cuttack.

Subjects: Consecutive subjects presenting with functional bowel disease were included; these included 68 NAFLD subjects and 200 subjects with normal liver on ultrasonography.

Investigations: All 268 subjects were evaluated for the presence of metabolic syndrome by ATP-III and insulin resistance by HOMA IR method. NAFLD subjects were compared with those with metabolic syndrome for presence of insulin resistance

Results: Patients with NAFLD had higher HOMA-IR than those with metabolic syndrome (2.34±1.01 vs. 1.79±1.01; p<0.000). Presence of NAFLD can detect insulin resistance with a sensitivity of 78.0% and specificity of 86.3 % with an odds ratio of 25.55 (95%CI: 11.51-56.70) which is better than that of metabolic syndrome diagnosed by ATP-III criteria (sensitivity 71.43%, specificity 70.32%; OR: 5.92, 95%CI: 2.99-11.74). Multivariate logistic regression analysis showed that fatty liver was an independent predictor for insulin resistance and metabolic syndrome.

Conclusion: NAFLD alone is a better predictor for insulin resistance than existing ATP-III criteria. Hence NAFLD should be used as a surrogate marker for metabolic syndrome.

Keywords: Metabolic syndrome; Criterion; Fatty liver; NAFLD; Insulin resistance

Abbreviations: MS: Metabolic Syndrome; NAFLD: Nonalcoholic Fatty Liver Disease; CVD: Cardio Vascular Disease; DM: Diabetes Mellitus; NCEP: National Cholesterol Education Program; ATP-III: Adult Treatment Panel III; IDF: International Federation of Diabetes; HDL: High-Density Lipoprotein; IR: Insulin Resistance; HOMA: Homeostatic Model Assessment; SBP: Systolic Blood Pressure; DBP: Diastolic Blood Pressure; FBG: Fasting Blood Glucose; BMI: Body Mass Index; 95% CI: 95%Confidence Interval; PPV: Positive Predictive Value; NPV: Negative Predictive Value; LR+: Positive Likelihood Ratio; LR-: Negative Likelihood Ratio

Introduction

Metabolic syndrome is defined as a constellation of certain metabolic abnormalities that render an individual at higher risk for subsequent development of cardiovascular disease (CVD) and diabetes mellitus (DM) [1]. The concept and criteria for this syndrome were evolved by the World Health Organization in 1998 [2]. This was later modified by National Cholesterol Education Program (NCEP): Adult Treatment Panel III (ATP-III) [3] and International Federation of Diabetes (IDF) [4]. The major features of the metabolic syndrome are central obesity, hypertriglyceridemia, low high-density lipoprotein (HDL) cholesterol, hyperglycemia and hypertension. All the components of this syndrome share insulin resistance (IR) which is the common denominator and is responsible for the vascular and metabolic sequelae. Despite the

increase in the prevalence of the components of the metabolic syndrome in obesity [5], all obese subjects do not develop the syndrome, and on the contrary, even some lean individuals can be insulin resistant [6,7]. It has been observed that the liver, once fatty, is insulin resistant [8,9] and overproduces both glucose [9] and VLDL [10] leading to hyperglycemia, hypertriglyceridemia, and low HDL cholesterol concentration. Nonalcoholic fatty liver disease (NAFLD) which is considered as the hepatic manifestation of metabolic syndrome is defined as fat accumulation in the liver exceeding 5% to 10% by weight [11], as determined from the percentage of fat-laden hepatocytes by light microscopy, absence of significant alcohol abuse (not exceeding 20 g/day) and other viral, toxic and autoimmune etiologies. NAFLD confers upon the patient increased risk for ischemic heart disease and diabetes mellitus [11]. Inclusion of NAFLD as a criterion for metabolic syndrome has been proposed [12] but has not yet been incorporated into any criteria. Therefore, this study was planned to assess the possibility of NAFLD as a criterion to diagnose metabolic syndrome. Also, the aim of the study was to assess the validity of NAFLD alone and in combination with existing criteria to diagnose individuals with metabolic syndrome.

***Corresponding author:** Shivaram Prasad Singh, Department of Gastroenterology, SCB Medical College, Cuttack 753007, Orissa, India, E-mail: spsingh.cuttack@gmail.com

Subjects and Methods

It was a single center observational study conducted in SCB Medical College. The subjects were the consecutive outpatients who attended Gastroenterology OPD for functional bowel disease from January 2012 to December 2012.

Inclusion Criteria

Consecutive outpatients who presented with functional abdominal pain (ROME III criteria) [13], functional dyspepsia (ROME III criteria) [14] and/or irritable bowel syndrome (ROME III criteria) [15] were included in this study. All these patients were in good general health, and with normal findings on medical history, physical examination, blood counts, and ultrasonography (except for fatty liver).

Exclusion Criteria- Patients who had organic gastrointestinal disease revealed by ultrasonography or gastro-duodenoscopy were excluded. Participants consuming alcohol >20 g /day, having other known liver diseases (hepatitis viruses A to E, autoimmune disease, Wilson's disease) and those on medications known to induce fatty liver or insulin sensitization such as estrogens, amiodarone, methotrexate, tamoxifen, glitazones and metformin were excluded.

An informed consent was taken from each subject. The anthropometric assessment included measurements of weight, height, and waist circumference (WC) and hip circumference (HC). The WC and HC were measured at the level midway between the lowest rib and the iliac crest and at the level of the great trochanter respectively. Body mass index (BMI) was calculated as weight (kg)/height^2 (m^2).

The measurements of fasting glucose, triglycerides, cholesterol, and high-density lipoprotein (HDL) cholesterol and liver function tests were performed by standard laboratory methods. Serum insulin level was estimated by electrochemiluminescence using standard kit (Roche-Diagnostics, USA) with autoanalyser Elecsys 2010 (Roche-Hitachi, Japan). IR was calculated using the homeostatic model assessment (HOMA) method using a mathematical model derived from FBG and plasma insulin. The value of HOMA was calculated by the following equation: (fasting insulin (µU/ml) X FBG (mg/dl))/405, and depicted as HOMA-IR value [16]. For the purpose of calculation HOMA-IR value above 2 was considered insulin resistance in our study.

The ATP III criteria [3] were used for diagnosis of metabolic syndrome (Table 1). Three or more of the five criteria were needed to be present for diagnosis of metabolic syndrome. The cut off for waist circumference taken were 80 cm for males and 90 cm for females as per the Asian population criteria [17]. Other parameters were fasting blood glucose ≥ 110 mg/dl, blood pressure ≥ 130/85 mmHg or treatment with antihypertensives, serum HDL cholesterol < 40 mg/dl for males and < 50 mg/dl for females and serum triglycerides ≥ 150 mg/dl or patients on treatment with hypolipidemic drugs.

Trans abdominal ultrasonography was done to see fatty changes in liver. Fatty liver was defined according to the standard criteria accepted by the American Gastroenterology Association [18] i.e., an increase in hepatic echogenicity with renal echogenicity as a reference, the presence of enhancement and lack of differentiation in periportal intensity and the vascular wall due to great hyperechogenicity of the parenchyma. Ethical clearance was taken from the Institutional Ethic Committee of SCB Medical College.

Statistical Analysis

Normally distributed continuous variables were expressed as mean ± SD. Student's t-test for unpaired data was used to compare groups when variables are normally distributed. Chi square test was used to compare differences in categorical variables. All analysis was done in software, SPSS version 16. P value of less than 0.05 was taken as significant. Logistic regression analysis was performed to assess the ability of ultrasonographic fatty liver to predict metabolic syndrome / insulin resistance after adjustment for individual ATP III criteria.

Results

A total of 316 participants were screened for the study, out of which 48 were excluded. A total of 268 subjects participated in this study, out of which 170 were males and 98 females. Metabolic syndrome was detected in 100 subjects. NAFLD was diagnosed in 68 participants.

The baseline demographic, clinical, and anthropometric and biochemical characteristics of participants having NAFLD and metabolic syndrome were compared as shown in Table 2. Patients with metabolic syndrome (n=100) and NAFLD (n=68) had similar gender ratio, mean age, BMI, waist circumference, blood pressure, fasting blood glucose, serum triglycerides and serum HDL cholesterol. Mean serum insulin was quite higher in NAFLD group (9.90 ± 3.27) than that of metabolic syndrome group (7.35 ± 3.41). The patients with NAFLD also had higher mean HOMA IR (2.34 ± 1.01 versus 1.79 ± 1.01).

Patients were classified into two groups as per their HOMA IR values. Participants with HOMA IR < 2 were kept in first group (insulin sensitive) where as those with HOMA IR ≥ 2 were placed in the second group (insulin resistant). 49 subjects belonged to the Insulin Resistant group and the rest to the Insulin Sensitive group. The baseline demographic, anthropometric, biochemical and sonographic characteristics between the two groups were compared in the Table 3. There was male predominance (79.59% versus 51.89%, p=0.006) in the insulin resistant group. Insulin resistant group had significantly higher mean BMI, waist and hip circumference, fasting blood glucose and serum triglycerides.

Metabolic syndrome was present in 35 (71.43%) whereas NAFLD was detected in 38 (77.55%) of patients with insulin resistance (IR ≥

Risk Factor	Defining Level
Waist Circumference	Men >102 cm Women >88 cm
Triglycerides	≥150 mg/dL
HDL cholesterol	Men <40 mg/dL Women <50 mg/dL
Blood pressure	≥130/85 mmHg
Fasting glucose	≥110 mg/dL

Table 1: Clinical identification of the metabolic syndrome.

	METABOLIC SYNDROME (n=100)	NAFLD (n=68)
Male (%)	60 (60%)	44 (64.7%)
Age	44.26 ± 12.75	43.32 ± 1.14
BMI	28.41 ± 4.13	28.47 ± 4.02
WAIST	92.58 ± 9.03	95.21 ± 7.98
Waist Hip Ratio	0.71 ± 0.41	0.95 ± 0.06
SBP	133.68 ± 14.59	127.47 ± 7.98
DBP	86.98 ± 9.41	83.00 ± 7.37
FPG	96.94 ± 17.64	94.73 ± 19.87
Triglycerides	194.14 ± 67.79	185.71 ± 66.69
HDL	40.65 ± 6.40	43.95 ± 8.92
INSULIN	7.35 ± 3.41	9.90 ± 3.27
HOMA IR	1.79 ± 1.01	2.34 ± 1.01

Table 2: Baseline characteristics in participants with nafld & metabolic syndrome.

Variables	IR<2 (n=219)	IR≥2(n=49)	P Value
Male (%)	131(51.89%)	39(79.59%)	0.006
Age	41.27 ± 14.37	43.48 ± 13.71	0.316
BMI	22. 07± 4.63	26.74 ± 4.68	<0.001
WAIST	83.17 ±10.07	93.69 ± 11.52	<0.001
HIP	90.58 ± 10.37	100.65 ± 9.09	<0.001
Waist Hip Ratio	0.89 ± 0.07	0.96 ± 0.07	<0.001
Weight Height Ratio	0.51 ± 0.09	0.57 ± 0.15	0.001
SBP	125.51 ± 15.46	129.04 ± 13.37	0.143
DBP	81.34 ± 10.22	84.62 ± 7.54	0.036
FPG	89.25 ± 10.43	101.23 ± 21.79	<0.001
Triglycerides	137.85 ± 51.35	199.69 ± 73.47	<0.001
AST	29.16 ± 7.77	30.87 ± 16.00	0.355
ALT	33.37 ± 12.06	39.29 ± 19.61	0.025
HDL	44.95 ± 8.05	42.21 ± 8.12	0.031
INSULIN	5.21 ± 2.19	11.13 ± 3.12	<0.001
MS (ATP III)	65 (27.39%)	35 (71.43%)	<0.001
Fatty Liver	30 (13.69%)	38 (77.55%)	<0.001

Table 3: Baseline characteristics of study subjects according to homa-ir index.

	METABOLIC SYNDROME	NAFLD	NAFLD + 2 METABOLIC SYNDROME Criteria	NAFLD + 1 METABOLIC SYNDROME Criteria
Sensitivity (95% CI)	71.43 % (56.74-83.40)	78.00 % (64.03-88.46)	67.35 % (52.46-80.04)	73.47 % (58.92-85.04)
Specificity (95% CI)	70.32 % (63.79-76.29)	86.30 % (81.02-90.56)	89.11 % (83.97-93.05)	86.63 % (81.15-91.00)
PPV (95% CI)	35.00 % (25.73-45.19)	56.52 % (44.04-68.42)	60.00 % (45.91-72.97)	57.14 % (44.05-69.54)
NPV (95% CI)	91.67 % (86.41-95.37)	94.50 % (90.37-97.22)	87.08 % (87.08-95.26)	93.09 % (88.46-96.26)
LR+ (95% CI)	2.41 (1.84-3.15)	5.69 (3.96-8.19)	6.18 (3.98-9.60)	5.50 (3.72-8.11)
LR- (95% CI)	0.41 (0.26-0.64)	0.25 (0.15-0.43)	0.37 (0.24-0.55)	0.31 (0.19-0.49)

CI: Confidence Interval, PPV: Positive Predictive Value, NPV: Negative Predictive Value,
LR+: Positive Likelihood Ratio, LR-: Negative Likelihood Ratio

Table 4: Diagnostic ability of metabolic syndrome criteria and nafld to detect ir (ir ≥ 2).

2). 35% of participants with metabolic syndrome had IR ≥ 2 where as 55.9% of participants who had NAFLD were insulin resistant (IR ≥ 2). This reflects higher diagnostic ability of NAFLD in predicting IR than metabolic syndrome. To assess the validity of employing NAFLD to detect IR, we compared the diagnostic abilities of ATP III criteria for metabolic syndrome and presence of NAFLD for detection of Insulin Resistance (IR ≥ 2) (Table 4). NAFLD with any one or two of these criteria were also compared with existing ATP III criteria of metabolic syndrome and with NAFLD alone. While the sensitivity and specificity of ATP III criteria for metabolic syndrome to detect insulin resistance were 71.43% and 70.32% respectively, NAFLD alone had a sensitivity of 78.00% and specificity of 86.30% which was quite higher than that of ATP III criteria. Addition of one ATP III criterion to NAFLD increased specificity slightly but at a lower sensitivity. Addition of two metabolic syndrome criteria to NAFLD resulted in further decline in sensitivity with additional improvement in specificity (Table 4).

Out of 49 subjects with insulin resistance, 38 had NAFLD. Insulin Resistant participants with and without NAFLD were compared in Table 5. The baseline demographic, clinical, and anthropometric and biochemical characteristics were compared between these two groups

(Table 3). No statistical significance was observed between the two groups except BMI.

The odds ratio for ATP III criteria, NAFLD alone, NAFLD with any one of the ATP III criteria and NAFLD with any two ATP III criteria for detection of IR was calculated (Table 6). NAFLD alone had a higher odds ratio of detecting insulin resistance (25.55, 95%CI:11.51–56.70) than NAFLD + 1 ATP III criterion (22.89, 95%CI:10.6 –49.39) followed by NAFLD + 2 ATP III criteria (21.37, 95%CI:10.03–45.51) and ATP III criteria (5.92, 95%CI:2.99–11.74).

Multivariate logistic regression was done to assess the adjusted odds ratio for detection of insulin resistance (Table 7). After adjustment for blood pressure, fasting plasma glucose, serum triglycerides, serum HDL and waist circumference, fatty liver was found to be an independent predictor for insulin resistance.

Discussion

Metabolic syndrome is a cluster of metabolic factors which has increased cardiovascular risk and shares the hallmark of insulin resistance. Identification and early treatment of insulin resistance is important because it is an independent predictor of cardiovascular disease and type 2 diabetes mellitus [19-21]. NAFLD predicted incident diabetes independent of classic risk factors in large prospective cohort studies and may therefore be an early marker of mechanism predisposing to future metabolic events [22,23]. NAFLD is also being recognized as an indicator of early atherosclerosis. Elevated liver enzymes and hepatic steatosis on liver histology predict incident

Variables	IR>2 with NAFLD (n=38)	IR>2 without NAFLD (n=11)	P Value
Male (%)	28 (73.68%)	11 (100%)	0.058
Age	43.36 ± 11.87	43.27 ± 19.30	0.984
BMI	28.13 ± 3.75	21.03 ± 3.55	<0.001
SBP	129.05 ± 14.05	130.00 ± 10.95	0.838
DBP	84.00 ± 7.33	87.27 ± 7.86	0.206
FPG	101.34 ± 23.73	99.72 ± 13.41	0.831
Triglycerides	199.50 ± 72.22	196.73 ± 78.86	0.913
HDL	42.50 ± 8.69	40.81 ± 5.43	0.548
INSULIN	11.36 ± 3.44	10.56 ± 1.33	0.456
HOMA IR	2.84 ± 1.08	2.57 ± 0.35	0.423
MS (ATP III)	29 (76.32%)	6 (54.55%)	0.152

Table 5: Comparison of IR participants with or without NAFLD.

	Odds Ratio	95% CI	P Value
METABOLIC SYNDROME	5.92	2.99 – 11.74	<0.001
NAFLD	25.55	11.51 – 56.70	<0.001
NAFLD + 1 ATP III Criteria	22.89	10.61 – 49.39	<0.001
NAFLD + 2 ATP III Criteria	21.37	10.03 – 45.51	<0.001

Table 6: Odds ratio for detection of insulin resistance.

	Odds Ratio (P Value)	Adjusted Odds Ratio* (P Value)
Blood pressure	0.541 (0.069)	0.643 (0.313)
FPG	0.260 (<0.001)	0.187 (0.001)
TG	0.197 (<0.001)	0.363 (0.030)
HDL	0.519 (0.055)	0.856 (0.716)
Waist Circumference	0.263 (<0.001)	1.619 (0.364)
Fatty Liver	17.914 (<0.001)	1.847 (<0.001)

*Calculated by Logistic Regression analysis

Table 7: Odds ratio of individual atp iii criteria and fatty liver for detection of insulin resistance.

cardiovascular disease independent of traditional risk factors and metabolic syndrome. It is being increasingly postulated that the vessels and the liver share common inflammatory mediators [24,25] which leads to atherosclerosis and cardiovascular disease.

It can be interpreted from our observations that individuals with insulin resistance are more likely to have central obesity, hyperglycemia, hypertriglyceridemia, hypertension and low serum HDL cholesterol. Incidence of NAFLD and metabolic syndrome are higher in insulin resistant persons.

The objective of the ATP III criteria [3] is to identify the individuals at increased risk for development of cardiovascular disease and diabetes. The current ATP III criteria were selected because they tend to cluster together, share insulin resistance as the common denominator and are individually associated with an increased coronary risk. Due to the low sensitivity, some cases of insulin resistance remain undiagnosed, especially in nonobese nondiabetic subjects, in whom the diagnosis of metabolic syndrome is less assisted by obesity and plasma glucose criteria. Our study has shown that fatty liver is an excellent marker of metabolic syndrome and insulin resistance. Fatty liver alone was superior to ATP-III criteria in diagnosing insulin resistance. The sensitivity and specificity of ATP III criteria for metabolic respectively, NAFLD alone had a sensitivity of 78.00% and specificity of 86.30% which was quite higher than that of ATP III criteria. Thus inclusion of fatty liver into the existing criteria is strongly suggested, which can help to identify more patients who are at increased risk for the consequences of metabolic syndrome. An earlier study by Musso et al. had assessed the strength of the associations of ATP III criteria and of NAFLD to insulin resistance, oxidative stress, and endothelial dysfunction in nonobese nondiabetic subjects and showed that NAFLD was more tightly associated with insulin resistance and with markers of oxidative stress and endothelial dysfunction than ATP III criteria [26].

Marchesini et al. showed that insulin resistance was the most important finding, closely associated with the presence of NAFLD in a large series of patients, irrespective of BMI, fat distribution or glucose tolerance [27]. A study from coastal eastern India has shown that both in NAFLD patients, insulin resistance was closely associated not only with fatty liver but also histologically severe disease [28]. Thus, NAFLD might represent another feature of the metabolic syndrome, with decreased insulin sensitivity being the common factor [29]. The strong association of NAFLD with other features of the metabolic syndrome (obesity, central fat distribution, diabetes, dyslipidemia, hypertension, and atherosclerotic cardiovascular disease) further supports this hypothesis [30,31]. Various pathogenic mechanism(s) has been postulated regarding this association between NAFLD and insulin resistance. Impaired hepatic lipid and lipoprotein handling and increased oxidative stress may enhance liver fat accumulation and lead to insulin resistance by nuclear factor-κB pathway activation [32-34]. The findings of the study suggest that hepatic fat accumulation is more tightly related to insulin resistance than visceral adiposity, as estimated by waist circumference or any other feature of the metabolic syndrome, as defined by ATP III criteria.

A Japanese study conducted on 4401 employees without liver disease or drug treatment (mean age 48 years, BMI 23 kg/m2) revealed that the odds ratios of men and women with NAFLD to develop the metabolic syndrome (ATP III criteria) during the follow-up were 4.0 and 11.2 after adjustment for age, alcohol intake, and changes in body weight [35]. Similar data have been reported by Schindhelm et al and Hanley et al. [36,37]. Likewise, in a study of 2839 type 2 diabetic outpatients with NAFLD, the risk of cardiovascular disease was significantly increased in NAFLD patients after adjustment for all

components of the metabolic syndrome [38]. In a Swedish study of 129 consecutive biopsy-proven NAFLD patients followed for 13.7 years, mortality from cardiovascular (15.5% versus 7.5%) and liver-related (2.8% versus 0.2%) causes was significantly higher compared with a matched reference-population (control) [39].

Early identification of subjects with insulin resistance, a high cardiometabolic risk factor, may facilitate earlier lifestyle modifications and pharmacological interventions. Consistently, therapeutic measures in NAFLD improve insulin sensitivity and cardiovascular risk profile, the ultimate goal of a diagnosis of metabolic syndrome [40,41].

The study is not without limitations. As an observational study, this study is limited by selection and confounding bias. Presence of an age sex matched control could have strengthened the study. Markers of inflammation like Adipokines and cytokines and markers of endothelial dysfunction like carotid intima thickness were not measured due to resource constraint setting. Liver histopathological study was also not done in the NAFLD patients, which could have shown whether simple steatosis or necroinflammation or fibrosis were risk factors for decrease in insulin sensitivity.

Conclusion

Direct comparison between NAFLD and ATP III criteria revealed that the former is better indicator for detection of insulin resistance. Addition of one or two ATP criteria to NAFLD does not add much to the diagnostic accuracy. It can be concluded that NAFLD should not be considered as a mere hepatic manifestation of metabolic syndrome. It is an important predictor of insulin resistance. It should be included as a criterion along with the existing criteria to identify metabolic syndrome.

References

1. Haffner SM (2000) Obesity and the metabolic syndrome: the San Antonio Heart Study. Br J Nutr 83: 67-70.
2. Alberti KG, Zimmet PZ (1998) Definition, diagnosis and classification of diabetes mellitus and its complications, part 1: diagnosis and classification of diabetes mellitus provisional report of a WHO consultation. Diabet Med 15: 539-553.
3. National Cholesterol Education Program (NCEP) Expert Panel on Detection, Evaluation, and Treatment of High Blood Cholesterol in Adults (Adult Treatment Panel III) (2002) Third Report of the National Cholesterol Education Program (NCEP) Expert Panel on Detection, Evaluation, and Treatment of High Blood Cholesterol in Adults (Adult Treatment Panel III) final report. Circulation 106: 3143-3421A.
4. Alberti KG, Zimmet P, Shaw J, IDF Epidemiology Task Force Consensus Group (2005) The metabolic syndrome: a new worldwide definition. Lancet 366: 1059-1062.
5. Singh SP, Kar SK, Panigrahi MK, Misra B, Pattnaik K, et al. (2013) Profile of patients with incidentally detected nonalcoholic fatty liver disease (IDNAFLD) in coastal eastern India. Trop Gastroenterol 34: 144-152.
6. Bhat G, Baba CS, Pandey A, Kumari N, Choudhuri G (2013) Insulin resistance and metabolic syndrome in nonobese Indian patients with non-alcoholic fatty liver disease. Trop Gastroenterol 34: 18-24.
7. Masharani UB, Maddux BA, Li X, Sakkas GK, Mulligan K, et al. (2011) Insulin Resistance in Non-Obese Subjects Is Associated with Activation of the JNK Pathway and Impaired Insulin Signaling in Skeletal Muscle . PLoS ONE 6: e19878.
8. Ryysy L, Hakkinen AM, Goto T, Vehkavaara S, Westerbacka J, et al. (2000) Hepatic fat content and insulin action on free fatty acids and glucose metabolism rather than insulin absorption are associated with insulin requirements during insulin therapy in type 2 diabetic patients. Diabetes 49: 749-758.
9. Seppala-Lindroos A, Vehkavaara S, Hakkinen AM, Goto T, Westerbacka J, et al. (2002) Fat accumulation in the liver is associated with defects in insulin suppression of glucose production and serum free fatty acids independent of obesity in normal men. J Clin Endocrinol Metab 87: 3023-3028.

10. Adiels M, Taskinen MR, Packard C, Caslake MJ, Soro-Paavonen A, et al. (2006) Overproduction of large VLDL particles is driven by increased liver fat content in man. Diabetologia 49: 755-765.

11. Chalasani N, Younossi Z, Lavine JE, Diehl AM, Brunt EM, et al. (2012) The Diagnosis and Management of Non-Alcoholic Fatty Liver Disease: Practice Guideline by the American Association for the Study of Liver Diseases, American College of Gastroenterology, and the American Gastroenterological Association. Hepatology 55: 2005-2023.

12. Giovanni M, Roberto G, Simona B, Barbara U, Giampaolo B, et al. (2008) Should Nonalcoholic Fatty Liver Disease Be Included in the Definition of Metabolic Syndrome? A cross-sectional comparison with Adult Treatment Panel III criteria in nonobese nondiabetic subjects. Diabetes Care 31: 562-568.

13. Drossman D, Li Z, Andruzzi E, Temple RD, Talley NJ, et al. (1993) U.S. householder survey of functional gastrointestinal disorders: Prevalence, sociodemography, and health impact. Dig Dis Sci 38: 1569-1580.

14. Tack J, Talley NJ, Camilleri M, Holtmann G, Hu P, et al. (2006) Functional gastroduodenal disorders. Gastroenterology 130: 1466-1479.

15. Longstreth GF, Thompson WG, Chey W, Houghton LA, Mearin F, et al. (2006) Functional bowel disorders. Gastroenterology 130: 1480-1491.

16. Matthews DR, Hosker JP, Rudenski AS, Naylor BA, Treacher DF, et al. (1985) Homeostasis Model Assessment: Insulin Resistance and Beta Cell Function from Fasting Plasma Glucose and Insulin Concentrations in Man. Diabetologia 28: 412-419.

17. Misra A, Vikram NK, Gupta R, Pandey RM, Wasir JS, et al. (2006) Waist circumference cutoff points and action levels for Asian Indians for identification of abdominal obesity. Int J Obes (Lond) 30: 106-111.

18. Gore RM (1994) Diffuse liver disease. In: Gore RM, Levine MS, Laufer.I, eds. Textbook of gastrointestinal radiology. WB Saunders, Philadelphia.

19. Saely CH, Aczel S, Marte T, Langer P, Hoefle G, et al. (2005) The metabolic syndrome, insulin resistance, and cardiovascular risk in diabetic and nondiabetic patients. J Clin Endocrinol Metab 90: 698-703.

20. Resnick HE, Jones K, Ruotolo G, Jain AK, Henderson J, et al. (2003) Strong Heart Study: insulin resistance, the metabolic syndrome, and risk of incident cardiovascular disease in nondiabetic American Indians: the Strong Heart Study. Diabetes Care 26: 861-867.

21. Bonora E, Kiechl S, Willeit J, Oberhollenzer F, Egger G, et al. (2007) Insulin resistance as estimated by homeostasis model assessment predicts incident symptomatic cardiovascular disease in Caucasian subjects from the general population: the Bruneck study. Diabetes Care 30: 318-324.

22. Yokoyama H, Emoto M, Fujiwara S, Motoyama K, Morioka T, et al. (2003) Quantitative insulin sensitivity check index and the reciprocal index of homeostasis model assessment in normal range weight and moderately obese type 2 diabetic patients. Diabetes Care 26: 2426-2432.

23. Sattar N, Scherbakova O, Ford I, O'Reilly DSJ, Stanley A, et al. (2004) Elevated alanine aminotransferase predicts new-onset type 2 diabetes independently of classical risk factors, metabolic syndrome, and C-reactive protein in the West of Scotland Coronary Prevention Study. Diabetes 53: 2855-2860.

24. Schindhelm RK, Dekker JM, Nijpels G, Bouter LM, Stehouwer CD, et al. (2007) Alanine aminotransferase predicts coronary heart disease events: a 10-year follow-up of the Hoorn Study. Atherosclerosis 191: 391-396.

25. Targher G, Bertolini L, Poli F, Rodella S, Scala L, et al. (2005) Nonalcoholic fatty liver disease and risk of future cardiovascular events among type 2 diabetic patients. Diabetes 54: 3541-3546.

26. Musso G, Gambino R, Bo S, Uberti B, Biroli G, et al. (2008) Should Nonalcoholic Fatty Liver Disease Be Included in the Definition of Metabolic Syndrome? A cross-sectional comparison with Adult Treatment Panel III criteria in nonobese nondiabetic subjects. Diabetes Care 31:562-568.

27. Marchesini G, Brizi M, Morselli-Labate AM, Bianchi G, Bugianesi E, et al. (1999) Association of non-alcoholic fatty liver disease to insulin resistance. Am J Med 107: 450-455.

28. Singh SP, Singh A , Pati G , Misra B , Misra D, et al. (2014) A Study of Prevalence of Diabetes and Prediabetes in Patients of Non-Alcoholic Fatty Liver Disease and the Impact of Diabetes on Liver Histology in Coastal Eastern India. Journal of Diabetes Mellitus 4: 290-296.

29. Cortez-Pinto H, Camilo ME, Baptista A, De Oliveira AG, De Moura MC (1999) Non-alcoholic fatty liver: another feature of the metabolic syndrome? Clin Nutr 18: 353-358.

30. DeFronzo RA, Ferrannini E (1991) Insulin resistance: a multifaceted syndrome responsible for NIDDM, obesity, hypertension, dyslipidemia, and atherosclerotic cardiovascular disease. Diabetes Care 14: 173-194.

31. Musso G, Gambino R, Durazzo M, Biroli G, Carello M, et al. (2005) Adipokines in NASH: postprandial lipid metabolism as a link between adiponectin and liver disease. Hepatology 42: 1175-1183.

32. Musso G, Cassader M, Gambino R, Durazzo M, Pagano G (2006) Association between postprandial LDL conjugated dienes and the severity of liver fibrosis in NASH. Hepatology 43: 1169-1170.

33. Pan M, Cederbaum AI, Zhang YL, Ginsberg HW, Williams KJ, et al. (2004) Lipid peroxidation and oxidant stress regulate hepatic apolipoprotein B degradation and VLDL production. J Clin Invest 113: 1277-1287.

34. Gambino R, Cassader M, Pagano G, Durazzo M, Musso G (2007) Polymorphism in microsomal triglyceride transfer protein: a link between liver disease and atherogenic postprandial lipid profile in NASH? Hepatology 45: 1097-1107.

35. Hamaguchi M, Kojima T, Takeda N, Nakagawa T, Taniguchi H, et al. (2005) The metabolic syndrome as a predictor of nonalcoholic fatty liver disease. Ann Intern Med 143: 722-728.

36. Schindhelm RK, Diamant M, Dekker JM, Tushuizen ME, Teerlink T, et al. (2006) Alanine aminotransferase as a marker of non-alcoholic fatty liver disease in relation to type 2 diabetes mellitus and cardiovascular disease. Diabetes Metab Res Rev 22: 437-443.

37. Hanley AJ, Williams K, Festa A, Wagenknecht LE, D'Agostino RB Jr, et al. (2005) Liver markers and development of the metabolic syndrome: the insulin resistance atherosclerosis study. Diabetes 54: 3140-3147.

38. Targher G, Bertolini L, Padovani R, Rodella S, Tessari R, et al. (2007) Prevalence of nonalcoholic fatty liver disease and its association with cardiovascular disease among type 2 diabetic patients. Diabetes Care 30: 1212-1218.

39. Ekstedt M, Franzen LE, Mathiesen UL, Thorelius L, Holmqvist M, et al. (2006) Long-term follow-up of patients with NAFLD and elevated liver enzymes. Hepatology 44: 865-873.

40. Gerstein HC, Yusuf S, Bosch J, Pogue J, Sheridan P, et al. (2006) Effect of rosiglitazone on the frequency of diabetes in patients with impaired glucose tolerance or impaired fasting glucose: a randomised controlled trial. Lancet 368: 1096-1105.

41. Huang MA, Greenson JK, Chao C, Anderson L, Peterman D, et al. (2005) One-year intense nutritional counseling results in histological improvement in patients with non-alcoholic steatohepatitis: a pilot study. Am J Gastroenterol 100: 1072-1081.

26

Inflammatory Cytokines Link Obesity and Breast Cancer

Nalin Siriwardhana[1], Rett Layman[2], Ayub Karwandyar[2], Shiwani Patel[2], Blair Tage[2], Matthew Clark[2], Jessica Lampley[2], Courtney Rhody[2], Erica Smith[2], Arnold M Saxton[1], Naima Moustaid-Moussa[1]* and Jay Wimalasena[2]*

[1]*Department of Animal Science and Obesity Research Center, University of Tennessee, Knoxville, Tennessee 37996*
[2]*Department of Obstetrics and Gynecology, Graduate School of Medicine, University of Tennessee Medical Center, Knoxville, Tennessee 37920*

Abstract

The risk of postmenopausal breast cancer is significantly increased by obesity. Further, low grade chronic inflammation, a hallmark of obesity, can contribute to detrimental health effects including high cancer incidence. Our goal is to understand the molecular basis for obesity-breast cancer interactions and dissect the role of inflammatory mediators secreted by adipocytes and breast cancer cells. Accordingly, we developed a three-dimensional (3D) co-culture system to facilitate direct cell-cell interactions and also performed media transfer from adipocyte cultures to growing breast cell cultures. The co-culture system will facilitate both adipocyte and breast cell growth in an environment closely mimicking *in-vivo* tumor microenvironment. Co-cultures of human primary adipocytes obtained from lean and obese women with MCF10A, MCF7 and MDAMB231 breast cells (non-cancerous epithelial cells, cancerous and invasive breast cancer cells, respectively), led to cell type specific changes in secretion of several pro-inflammatory cytokines, such as IL-6 and TNFα, compared to monocultures. Regulation of cytokine secretion of breast cells by adipocytes and vice versa indicates the two-way communication between breast cells and adipocytes. Further, 3D co-culture and adipocyte conditioned media transfer experiments demonstrated that obese adipocyte-derived conditioned media can promote higher growth of breast cancer cells compared to that from lean adipocytes. Moreover, obese adipocyte conditioned media increased the activation of nuclear factor-κB (NF-κB) family members in breast cells, compared to lean adipocyte-derived media. Our results provide a novel model system to study adipocyte-breast cancer cell interactions which may underlie the link between breast cancer and obesity and also demonstrate that inflammatory cytokines and other secreted factors are important in this interaction.

Keywords: Obesity; Breast cancer; Adipocytes; Inflammation; Cy-tokines

Introduction

Obesity has become a critical problem in the US and worldwide and results in a variety of chronic diseases including diabetes, cardiovascular disease and cancer [1]. Clinical evidence directly suggests that obesity has a significant impact on breast cancer progression and specifically that obesity in postmenopausal women doubles their risk for developing breast cancer and also acts as a risk factor for metastasis [2-5]. Recent clinical evidence also suggests that not only obesity but also other metabolic diseases such as the metabolic syndrome or type 2 diabetes can increase the risk of breast cancer. Additionally metformin, an AMPK activator, has been found to improve the survival of breast cancer in patients with type 2 diabetes [6,7]. These studies indicate the importance of metabolic/hormonal imbalances such as those observed in obesity in breast cancer. Of particular interest to us, very few studies have addressed the mechanisms by which obesity enhances breast cancer occurrence and progression. It has been proposed that adipocyte-derived estradiol may induce breast cancer [2,8]. Further, adipocyte-derived inflammatory cytokine profiles exhibit significant differences between lean and obese individuals and this unbalanced inflammatory profile (increased pro-inflammatory cytokine and decreased anti-inflammatory cytokine secretion) in the obese condition may play a role in worsening both metabolic disorders and breast cancer progression [9-13]. Since the breast stroma is mostly constituted of adipocytes and their precursors, it is logical to propose that there are molecular interactions between breast cells and adipose tissue components which may underlie promotion of tumorigenesis. Chronic inflammation is associated with both obesity and breast cancer progression [8] and visceral adipose tissue is a major source of inflammatory mediators, and these may exert profound effects on breast cancer cells [12,13]. In this communication we have co-cultured human visceral adipocytes isolated from lean or obese women together with cancerous and non-cancerous breast epithelial cells in three dimensional (3D) co-cultures to dissect molecular and cellular interactions between adipocyte and breast cancer cells. This system facilitates direct cell-cell interactions mimicking *in-vivo* conditions and allows investigation of the effects of adipocytes and their secretory cytokines on breast cell biology and vice versa. Our results demonstrate the two-way communication between the adipocytes and breast cancer cells in 3D co-cultures and further support the role for adipocyte-derived adipokines in modulating breast cancer cell growth and metabolism.

Methods and Procedures

Age-matched visceral preadipocytes from lean and obese women were obtained from Zenbio (Research Triangle Park, NC). The preadipocytes were cultured and differentiated in monolayer cultures according to supplier's procedures. After differentiation, cells were maintained in adipocyte maintenance media purchased from the supplier. Conditioned media (1 day old) obtained from differentiated mature adipocytes were mixed with standard MCF10A culture media at a 1:1 ratio and used for media transfer experiments. Prepared media mixtures were added into 1-day-old growing breast cell cultures seeded at the concentration of 5,000 cells / well of 96-well plates. This experimental setup was used to measure cell growth differences assayed

*Corresponding authors: Dr. Jay Wimalasena, University of Tennessee Medical Center, 1924 Alcoa Highway, Knoxville, TN, 37920 USA,
E-mail: jwimalas@utmck.edu

Dr. Naima Moustaid-Moussa, University of Tennessee Institute of Agriculture, 201L McCord Hall, 2640 Morgan Circle Drive, Knoxville, TN 37996, USA; E-mail: E-mail: moustaid@utk.edu

by MTT assay and cell lysates prepared for TNFα and NF-κB assays. ELISA assays, including multiplex cytokine ELISAs, were performed according to manufacturer's guidelines.

Three dimensional (3D) cultures and 3D co-cultures were performed with additional modifications of previously described 3D breast epithelial culture methods [14,15]. Briefly, 400 µl of Growth Factor-Reduced Matrigel Matrix (BD Biosciences, Bedford, MA) was added into each well of 24-well culture plates and placed in the cell culture incubator for 20 min. Five thousand breast cells and/or 45,000 adipocytes were mixed with breast cell adipocyte culture media (MCF10A media and adipocyte culture media at a 1:1 ratio) and plated on top of the base layer of Matrigel. Cultures were maintained in 5% CO_2 at 37°C. Media were carefully replaced every 2 days, and conditioned media were collected and stored at -80°C for cytokine assays. Growing co-cultures were photographed every 3 days at our microscopic image facility and the diameters of acini-like spheroids were recorded. All experiments were conducted in triplicate and repeated two times to verify the results. Cell lysates in Figure 4B were prepared according to instructions of RayBiotech (Atlanta, GA) and Active Motif (Carlsbad, CA), respectively.

Results and Discussion

We co-cultured pre-adipocytes derived from either lean or obese women with MCF10A, MCF7, and MDAMB231 breast epithelial cells in 3D co-cultures in Matrigel. As shown in Figure 1A, MCF10A cells formed round, growth restricted spheroids, while MCF7 cells formed growth unrestricted irregular structures (Figure 1B). MDAMB231 cells formed mixed cellular masses with elongated extensions (Figure 1C). Figure 1D shows differentiated obese adipocytes grown in 3D culture with inter cellular connections. In the MCF10A, MCF7 and MDAMB231/adipocyte co-cultures, there appeared to be structural connections between the two cell types, as represented in Figure 1E. The diameters of these cellular structures in the co-cultures were measured microscopically. The diameter of MCF7 structures increased when co-cultured with obese adipocytes compared to co-cultures with lean adipocytes (Figure 2B). This increase, suggestive of a greater cell number, was not observed with MCF10A cells. Since MDAMB231 cells did not form compact structures, their diameters could not be ascertained. In conditioned media transfer experiments, we tested effects of lean and obese adipocyte-conditioned media on the growth of monolayers of breast cancer cells. When compared to lean derived adipocyte-conditioned media, obese adipocyte media induced time-dependent increases in cell number in all three breast epithelial cell types (Figure 2A). The increases in cell number, although relatively modest, were statistically significant for MCF7 cells from 24-72 h following addition of conditioned media. Similar results were observed for MDAMB231cells at 72 h. Studies have shown that obese adipocyte-derived adipokines and growth factors may regulate breast cell growth, as previously reviewed [16]. Thus, further studies are needed to identify specific factors derived from adipocytes which affect tumor growth and invasion.

It is well known that adipocytes secrete a variety of cytokines, and in the case of obese women, there is a significant increase in secretion of several pro-inflammatory adipokine compared to adipocytes from lean women [9,10]. Therefore, we measured levels of secreted inflammatory cytokines, which may regulate the cellular behavior of breast epithelial cells in the co-cultures. In our study, secretion of granulocyte colony stimulation factor (G-CSF) was higher in obese vs. lean monocultures (Figure 3). G-CSF secretion was greatly increased in cancer cells when compared to MCF10A cells. Co-culture changed G-CSF secretion in all

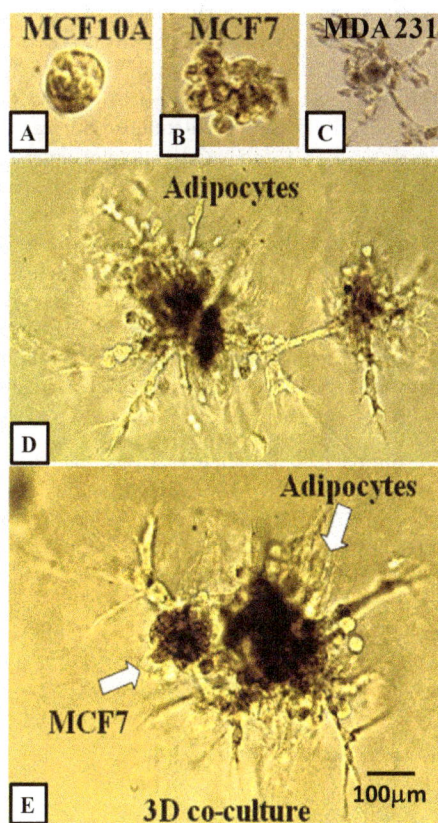

Figure 1: Representative 3D cultures and co-cultures of differentiated adipocytes and breast cancer cells. Adipocytes from age-matched women were co-cultured with MCF10A, MCF7 and MDA 231 cells at a 9:1 ratio, respectively, in 3D Matrigel cultures. MCF10A cells formed size-restricted, regular round spheroids (A), and MCF7 cells formed size-unrestricted irregular spheroids (B), while invasive MDA 231 cells formed elongated cell clusters or interconnected cellular structures (C), but not spheroids like MCF10A cells. D and E show connections between adipocytes and MCF7 cells. Arrows indicates the respective cell populations.

three breast cell lines. In MCF10A-lean adipocyte co-cultures, G-CSF secretion from lean adipocytes was increased several fold, compared to obese adipocytes. By contrast, in MDAMB231 cells, both lean and obese co-cultures suppressed G-CSF. In MCF7 co-cultures, G-CSF secretion from obese adipocytes was significantly increased compared to lean adipocytes. The order of G-CSF secretion in monoculture was MDAMB231 > MCF7 > MCF10A.

IL-6 secretion (Figure 3B) was also up-regulated in MCF10A and MCF7 co-cultures with obese adipocytes, but was highly repressed in MDAMB231 co-cultures with lean or obese adipocytes, with a larger inhibitory effect seen with obese adipocytes. IL-6 secretion was 2-3-fold higher in obese adipocytes compared to lean adipocytes, consistent with previous reports [17] and neither MCF10A nor MCF7 secreted detectable levels of IL-6 in 3D monocultures. The decrease in IL-6 in adipocytes and MDAMB231 co-cultures was over five-fold with obese adipocytes, while the reverse effects with less fold changes were observed with MCF10A and MCF7 cells.

IL-8 secretion from obese-derived adipocytes was significantly lower compared to lean adipocytes in 3D monocultures (Figure 3C). Furthermore, MCF10A cells did not secrete detectable IL-8; however, when co-cultured with adipocytes from lean or obese subjects, IL-8 secretion was significantly reduced from adipocytes, and this reduction was more pronounced in co-cultures of MCF 10A with obese adipocytes, compared to adipocytes alone. This decrease is possibly due to MCF10A cells inhibiting secretion of IL-8 by adipocytes. It could also result from uptake of IL-8 by MCF10A cells. MCF7 cells secreted low quantities of IL-8 and in co-cultures with lean adipocytes, there was a decrease in IL-8 compared to monocultures. However, in the presence of obese adipocytes, there was a significant increase in secreted IL-8, which suggests that MCF7 cells were stimulated to secrete IL-8 by obese adipocytes or that IL-8 secreted by obese adipocytes was stabilized by MCF7 cells, resulting in higher IL-8 in the medium. It is also possible that MCF7 cells stimulated obese adipocytes to secrete more IL-8. MDAMB231 cells secreted large quantities of IL-8, consistent with other reports on breast cancer cells [18]. IL-8 levels were significantly decreased when these cells were co-cultured with lean or obese adipocytes.

MCP-1 secretion by obese adipocytes was significantly higher than lean adipocytes (Figure 3D). This is in line with previous studies demonstrating higher MCP-1 production in obese vs. lean human subjects and from visceral vs. subcutaneous adipose tissue [19]. Breast cell lines secreted relatively lower MCP-1; in co-cultures with lean adipocytes and MCF10A or MCF7 cells, MCP-1 was relatively unchanged. In both MCF7 and MCF10A cell co-cultures with obese adipocytes, there was a large reduction in MCP-1 levels, suggesting that these two cell types may have decreased MCP-1 secretion by

Cytokine	Adipocyte	Media	MCF10A	MCF7	MDAMB231
Eotaxin	Control		5.65	10.325	14.335
	Lean	15.08	7.065	12.995	32.23
	Obese	**35.865**	7.755	13.33	**23.715**
GM-CSF	Control		2.495	6.05	64.525
	Lean	5.855	11.96	20.085	14.225
	Obese	3.94	**6.875**	**13.145**	11.15
IFNα2	Control		5.945	8.98	11.53
	Lean	26.605	15.565	19.26	9.485
	Obese	**13.05**	12.04	**14.555**	9.485
IL1α	Control		104.03	27.56	22.315
	Lean	1.495	4.42	8.68	24.185
	Obese	2.38	**11.78**	10.255	**10.57**
IL-7	Control		2.94	4.59	27.855
	Lean	10.45	7.33	8.735	9.79
	Obese	8.735	7.335	10.14	8.035
IP-10	Control		26.895	51.225	73.44
	Lean	5.6	16.115	14.325	19.005
	Obese	**15.31**	**21.715**	**30.175**	13.32
MIP1α	Control		4.77	4.78	7.045
	Lean	4.945	4.955	6.36	7.705
	Obese	3.88	6.36	5.31	**3.7**

Table 1: Cytokines differentially expressed in 3D co-cultures of adipocytes and breast cells.
Breast cancer cells were either maintained in Matrigel as mono-cultures (control designation), or co-cultured with adipocytes from lean or obese women. Cytokines secreted by monocultures of lean or obese adipocytes only, in Matrigel, are shown in the column labeled "Media". Values are in pg/ml. All the **bolded** values are significantly different compared to the lean adipocyte co-culture (P<0.05).

obese adipocytes, or that the MCF7 or MCF10A cells bound and/or metabolized MCP-1 rendering it unavailable in the medium. In contrast to G-CSF, IL-6 and IL-8, MDAMB231 cells did not secrete detectable MCP-1 and these cells were much more efficient in inhibiting lean or obese adipocyte MCP-1 secretion and/or binding/metabolizing MCP-1 than the other two cell lines. In this respect, co-culture of either lean or obese adipocytes with MDAMB231 cells showed a similar trend in secreted G-CSF, IL-6 and IL-8, in that co-culture with either lean or obese adipocytes significantly reduced secretion of these cytokines by MDAMB231 cells.

Of the twenty six cytokines measured in this study using 3D mono- and co-culture media, 11 cytokines showed differential and significant changes (selected cytokines are shown in Figure 3 and others are shown in Table 1) . Of the cytokines significantly changed, GM-CSF secretion was increased in monocultures in the order MCF10A < MCF7 < MDAMB231. In co-cultures with lean adipocytes, GM-CSF secretion from both MCF10A and MCF7 cells was increased. By contrast, GM-CSF secretion was significantly reduced from MDAMB231 cells in co-cultures with lean or obese adipocytes. Furthermore, compared to lean-derived adipocytes, obese adipocytes decreased secretion of GM-CSF in co-cultures with all the breast cell lines. GM-CSF secretion by lean adipocytes was similar to that of obese adipocytes; however, compared to lean adipocytes, obese adipocytes were less stimulatory towards GM-CSF secretion by MCF10A and MCF7 cells in co-cultures. Both lean and obese adipocytes in co-cultures with MDAMB231 cells drastically reduced the GM-CSF secretion by the latter.

Obese adipocytes secreted significantly more eotaxin (CCL11) than lean adipocytes in monoculture and Vasudevan et al. (2006) [20] reported that obesity promote the secretion of eotaxin. Similar to other cytokines/ interleukins, there was an increase in eotaxin secretion from MCF10A to MDMBA231 cells in monocultures. In lean

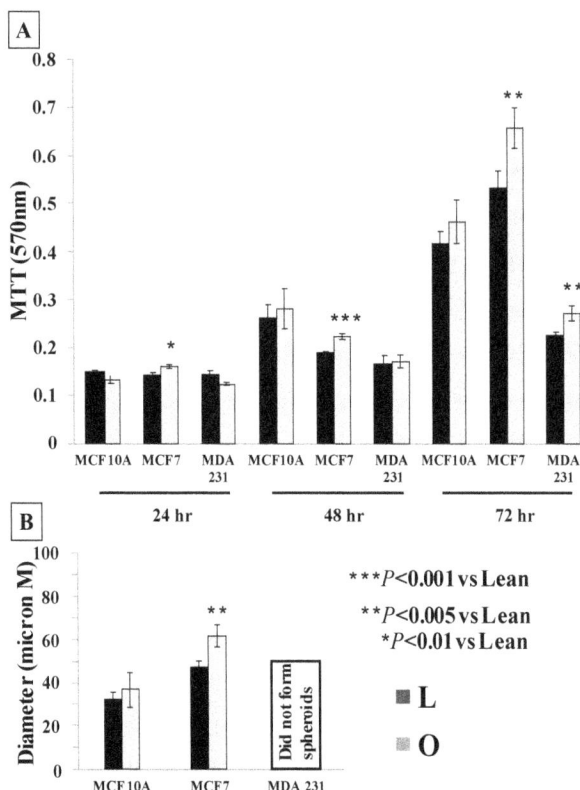

Figure 2: Effect of lean and obese adipocytes on breast cell growth. A. Lean and obese adipocytes from age-matched women were individually cultured, and the conditioned media was transferred to growing breast cell cultures. Cell growth was measured by MTT assay at 24, 48 and 72 h. B. Diameter of the structures shown in Figure 1 is shown (data are from triplicate cultures, mean +/- SE). L=Lean O = Obese

adipocyte/MDAMB231 co-cultures, there was a significant (P<0.05) increase in eotaxin, suggesting a positive mutual interaction between the two cell types in secretion of eotaxin. On the other hand, in obese adipocyte/MDAMB231 cell co-cultures, there was a negative influence of the MDAMB31 cells on obese adipocyte secretion of eotaxin and/or metabolism of eotaxin by MDAMB231 cells. Co-cultures did not change secretion of eotaxin by MCF10A and MCF7.

Secretion of IFNα2 also increased in monocultures (from MCF10A to MDAMB231 cells). Secretion of IFNα2 was higher in lean adipocyte than in obese adipocyte monocultures. In co-cultures with lean adipocytes, there were increased levels in MCF10A and MCF7 cells; the magnitude of changes was less in obese adipocyte co-cultures compared to lean adipocyte co-cultures. Interestingly, there was no effect of lean adipocytes or obese adipocytes on the MDAMB231 secretion of IFNα2 compared to highly significant effects of lean or obese adipocytes on secretion of other cytokines or interleukins from MDAMB231 cells. However, MDAMB231 cells decreased the quantity of IFNα2 secreted by adipocytes in monoculture, similar to effects of MCF10A and MCF7 cells on lean adipocytes IFNα2 secretion.

In contrast to all other cytokines, secretion of IL1α was higher in MCF10A monocultures, compared to MCF7 and MDAMB231 cancer cells. In monoculture, lean and obese adipocytes secreted only small quantities of IL1α. However, both types of adipocytes drastically reduced secretion of this interleukin by MCF10A as well as MCF 7. In MDAMBA231 co-cultures, only adipocytes from obese women reduced IL1α secretion.

IP-10 (CXCL10) secretion by monocultures of obese adipocytes was higher compared to lean adipocytes. However, both obese and lean adipocytes reduced IP-10 secretion from MCF10A and MDAMB231 cells. Adipocytes from lean subjects exerted a more pronounced decrease in IP-10 secretion from MCF10A and MCF7 cells, while obese adipocytes exerted larger inhibition in MDAMB231 cells. The secretion of IP-10 was in the order MDAMB231 > MCF7 > MCF10A in monocultures. In addition, in co-cultures of obese (but not lean) adipocytes with MDAMB231 cells, MIP 1α secretion was significantly reduced.

Secretion of a variety of cytokines/interleukins is regulated by TNFα [11] and both adipocytes and breast cancer cells can secrete TNFα. The concentrations of TNFα in mono- and co-culture media are shown in Figure 4A,B. Obese adipocyte monocultures secreted more TNFα than lean adipocytes, as previously observed [21]. All the breast cell lines secreted TNFα, with MCF7 cells secreting the largest quantity in monoculture. In MCF10A cells co-cultured with lean adipocytes, the secretion of TNFα was similar compared to that by lean adipocytes alone. In MCF7 co-culture with lean adipocytes or obese adipocytes, there was a significant reduction in secreted TNFα (P<0.05). Interestingly, in all three cell types, obese adipocyte co-cultures accumulated significantly more TNFα than lean adipocyte co-cultures. Data in Figure 4B depicts TNFα levels in cell lysates in breast cells. Concentrations of TNFα in cell lysates were approximately ten-fold that of media in monocultures, and all three breast cell types had similar TNFα concentrations (normalized to total cell protein) in lysates. In co-cultures, both lean and obese adipocyte-conditioned media increased MCF10A and MCF7 cells cellular TNFα; lean adipocyte-conditioned medium induced significantly higher MCF10A TNFα than obese adipocyte-conditioned medium. Obese adipocyte-conditioned media significantly increased TNFα content in MDAMB231 and MCF7 cultures.

One of the well-known downstream targets of TNFα is the NF-κB pathway [22,23]. Using the nucleotide sequence to which all members

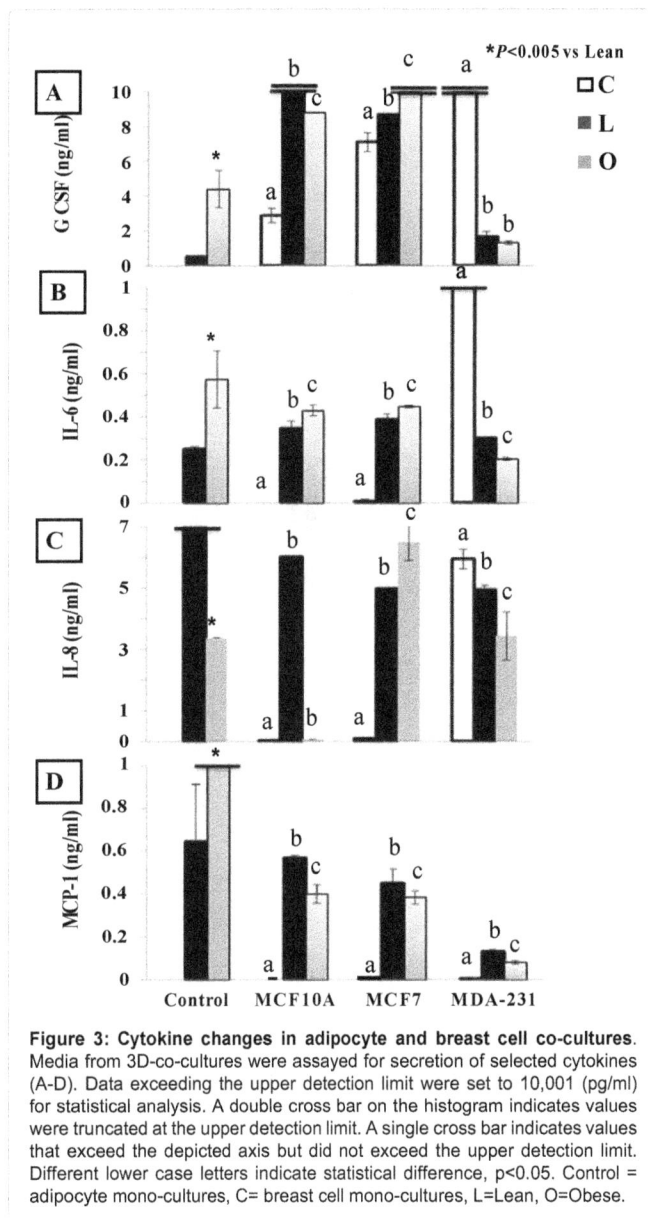

Figure 3: Cytokine changes in adipocyte and breast cell co-cultures. Media from 3D-co-cultures were assayed for secretion of selected cytokines (A-D). Data exceeding the upper detection limit were set to 10,001 (pg/ml) for statistical analysis. A double cross bar on the histogram indicates values were truncated at the upper detection limit. A single cross bar indicates values that exceed the depicted axis but did not exceed the upper detection limit. Different lower case letters indicate statistical difference, p<0.05. Control = adipocyte mono-cultures, C= breast cell mono-cultures, L=Lean, O=Obese.

of the NF-κB family bind and specific antibodies against individual members of the NF-κB family, oligonucleotide-bound NF-κB was measured by a commercial ELISA kit. As shown in Figure 5, all five family members are present in all of the breast cell types. Using the same conditioned media transfer technique as in Figure 4B, we measured the effects of adipocyte-conditioned media on the activity of all five NF-κB family members. Conditioned media regulated activities in a cell-specific manner. The most prominent effects of obese vs. lean adipocyte media transfer were observed with MDAMD231 cells, where a significant increase in active p65, p50, p52, Rel B and Rel C was observed with obese adipocyte-conditioned media compared to lean adipocyte-conditioned media. In MCF7 cells, a similar pattern was observed for p65, p50, p52, and Rel C. However, the changes in MCF7 cells were relatively modest. In MCF10A cells, which had lower NF-κB family member concentrations compared to cancer cells except for Rel C, both obese and lean adipocyte-conditioned media exerted similar positive effects. Clearly, obese adipocyte-conditioned media had a larger stimulatory effect than lean adipocyte-conditioned media

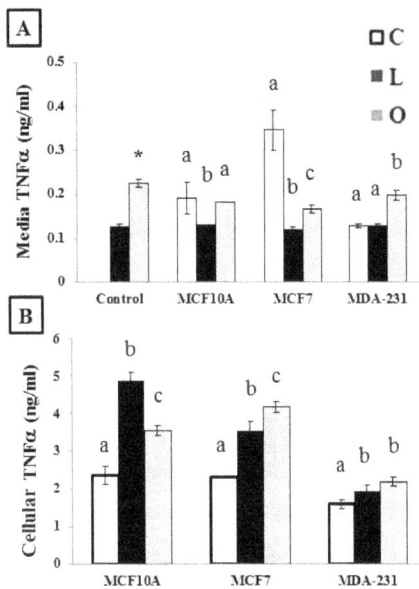

Figure 4:TNFα changes in co-culture media and adipocyte conditioned media transferred to breast cell cultures. Media and cell lysates were assayed for TNFα (A & B) following adipocyte conditioned media transfer to breast cell monocultures. Different lower case letters indicate statistical difference, *p<0.05. C= breast cell mono-cultures, Control = adipocyte mono-cultures, C= breast cell mono-cultures, L=Lean, O=Obese.

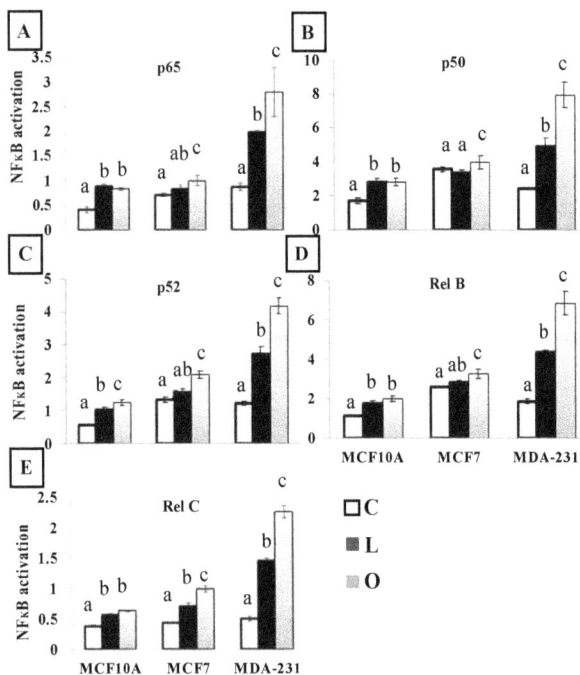

Figure 5: NF-kB activation changes in adipocyte conditioned media transferred to breast cell cultures. Adipocyte conditioned media-exposed breast cells were assayed for NFκB activation using an ELISA assay. Different lower case letters indicate statistical difference, p<0.05. C = Breast cell mono-cultures, L=Lean, O=Obese.

on NF-κB family member activities in MDAMB231 cancer cells.

Our results demonstrate that co-culturing breast cell lines with

adipocytes had significant effects on their growth. Further, obese adipocytes had a greater effect on breast cancer cells, especially on MCF7 cells. It is possible that cell-to-cell contact had a potential role here and/or that adipocyte secretions (such as cytokines) may have produced these effects. Our data suggests that the breast cell growth and metabolism is regulated by adipocyte-secreted cytokines. Although, we have not identified specific factors secreted by adipocytes which regulate breast cancer cell growth and NF-κB expression in these cells, the methods we have developed can be utilized to identify the molecules which mediate the two way communication between adipocytes and breast cells.

The effects of co-cultures on cytokine secretion are highly complex. We identified 11 cytokines that changed out of the twenty six measured. Lean and obese adipocytes exhibited substantial differences in secretion of many of these cytokines in 3D monocultures, except for GM-CSF, IL1a, IL-7 and MIP1a. In general, MDMBA231 cells produced greater amounts of cytokines (except IL1a and MCP-1) than either cancerous MCF7 or non-cancerous MCF10A cells. There was an increase in secretion in the order MCF10A < MCF7 < MDAMB231 cells, which is also the order of the malignant nature in the three breast cell lines.

The interaction between lean or obese adipocytes and the breast cells are highly complex, with both lean and obese adipocytes decreasing secretion of several cytokines from MDAMB231 cells (except for eotaxin and IL1a). In contrast, co-cultures enhanced secretion of some other cytokines from MCF10A (e.g., G CSF) and MCF7 cells, with notable exceptions such as IL1-α and IP-I0. In some cases, such as with IL-8, MCF7 cells appeared to decrease IL-8 secretion by lean and obese adipocytes. For obese adipocytes /MCF7 co-cultures, there was a significantly higher secretion of IL-8 than in either obese adipocytes or MCF7 cells alone. These data strongly suggest mutual interaction between adipocytes and breast cells in regulating these cytokines.

What is remarkable is that the highly malignant MDAMB231 cell line behaves differently in this interaction, compared to the less malignant MCF7 cells. In general, we observed a significant difference between lean and obese adipocyte co-cultures with breast cells (cell growth, secretion of the majority of cytokines, as well as activation of the NF-κB family of transcription factors). Remarkably, there were significant increases in activation of all NF-κB family members in MDAMB231 cells after conditioned media transferred from obese adipocytes compared to the lean counterparts. These increases were even higher than when obese adipocyte conditioned media was transferred to MCF7 or MCF10A cultures.

NF-κB activation is known to modulate several different cellular processes in cancer cells leading to cell growth, as pharmacological inhibition of NF-κB in cell lines suppresses proliferation and leads to apoptosis [24,25]. In agreement with our data that the invasive MDAMB231cells showed higher NF-κB activation, Spiller et al. (2011) [24] showed that NF-κB is activated and required for medulloblastoma tumor growth. Further, it has been shown that anti-inflammatory treatments that suppresses NF-κB activation are promising anti-cancer agents [26-28]. We observed that conditioned media derived from obese adipocytes significantly increased MDAMB 231 cell growth compared to the lean counterpart [Figure 2] and this is in agreement with Park et al. (2007) [29] where they showed that NF-κB activation in breast cancer cells promote bone metastasis and obesity increases metastasis in patients and our data suggest that increased NF-κB activation due to obese condition media transfer can promote MDAMB 231 growth.

Our novel studies on the co-culture of lean /obese adipocytes with breast epithelial cells in a 3D matrix demonstrates two-way direct communication between adipocytes and breast cells, as occurs naturally in the human breast. These interactions appear to be specific for each breast cell type (non-cancerous, cancerous and invasive) and lean vs. obese adipocytes. Therefore, our technique provides novel tools to elucidate the molecular interactions between adipocytes and breast cancer cells; these interactions may contribute to the increased incidence and poorer prognosis of breast cancer in post-menopausal, obese women. Furthermore, separation of breast cells from adipocytes and monoculture of the breast cells following co-culture may reveal molecular changes in breast cells that occurred during the co-culture. Finally, the system we developed would be highly suitable for testing effects of dietary interventions that may lessen the effects of fat cell inflammation on breast cancer cells and ultimately decrease the risk of breast cancer in obesity.

Acknowledgement

We acknowledge the grant support by University of Tennessee (UT) Obesity Research Center and UT Graduate School of Medicine. Further, we extend our thanks to Misty Bailey for technical editing of the manuscript. Authors 2-9 are undergraduate research trainees.

References

1. (1998) Clinical Guidelines on the Identification, Evaluation, and Treatment of Overweight and Obesity in Adults--The Evidence Report. National Institutes of Health. Obes Res 2: 51S-209S.

2. Roberts DL, Dive C, Renehan AG (2010) Biological Mechanisms Linking Obesity and Cancer Risk: New Perspectives. Annu Rev Med 61: 301-316.

3. Conroy SM, Maskarinec G, Wilkens LR, White KK, Henderson BE, et al. (2011) Obesity and breast cancer survival in ethnically diverse postmenopausal women: the Multiethnic Cohort Study. Breast Cancer Res Treat 129: 565-574.

4. Gu JW, Young E, Patterson SG, Makey KL, Wells J, et al. (2011) Postmenopausal obesity promotes tumor angiogenesis and breast cancer progression in mice. Cancer Biol Ther 11: 910-917.

5. Healy L, Ryan A, Rowley S, Boyle T, Connolly E, et al. (2010) Obesity Increases the Risk of Postmenopausal Breast Cancer and is Associated with More Advanced Stage at Presentation But no Impact on Survival. Breast J 16: 95-97.

6. Goodwin P, Ligibel J, Stambolic V (2009) Metformin in Breast Cancer: time for action. J Clin Oncol 27: 3271-3273.

7. Bosco J, Antonsen S, Sorensen H, Pedersen L, Lash T (2011) Metformin and Incident Breast Cancer among Diabetic Women: A Population-Based Case-Control Study in Denmark. Cancer Epidemiol Biomarkers Prev 20: 101-111.

8. Brow K, Simpson E (2010) Obesity and Breast Cancer: Progress to Understanding the Relationship. Cancer Res 70: 4-7.

9. Kalupahana NS, Claycombe K, Moustaid-Moussa N (2011) (n-3) Fatty Acids Alleviate Adipose Tissue Inflammation and Insulin Resistance: Mechanistic Insights. Adv Nutr 2: 304-316.

10. Ouchi N, Parker JL, Lugus JJ, Walsh K (2011) Adipokines in inflammation and metabolic disease. Nat Rev Immunol 11: 85-97.

11. Goldberg J, Schwertfeger K (2010) Proinflammatory Cytokines in Breast Cancer: Mechanisms of Action and Potential Targets for Therapeutics. Curr Drug Targets 11: 1133-1146.

12. Nicolini A, Carpi A, Rossi G (2006) Cytokines in breast cancer. Cytokine Growth Factor Rev 17: 325-337.

13. Lyon DE, McCain NL, Walter J, Schubert C (2008) Cytokine comparisons between women with breast cancer and women with a negative breast biopsy. Nurs Res 57: 51-58.

14. Song X, Siriwardhana N, Rathore K, Lin D, Wang HC (2010) Grape Seed Proanthocyanidin Suppression of Breast Cell Carcinogenesis Induced by Chronic Exposure to Combined 4-(Methylnitrosamino)-1-(3-Pyridyl)-1-Butanone and Benzo[a]Pyrene. Mol Carcinog 49: 450-463.

15. Siriwardhana N, Choudhary S, Wang HC (2008) Precancerous model of human breast epithelial cells induced by NNK for prevention. Breast Cancer Res Treat 109:427-441.

16. Vona-Davis L, Rose D P (2007) Adipokines as endocrine, paracrine, and autocrine factors in breast cancer risk and progression. Endocr Relat Cancer 14: 189-206.

17. Yudkin JS, Kumari M, Humphries SE, Mohamed-Ali V (2000) Inflammation, obesity, stress and coronary heart disease: is interleukin-6 the link? Atherosclerosis 148: 209-214.

18. Freund A, Jolivel V, Durand S, Kersual N, Chalbos D, et al. (2004) Mechanisms underlying differential expression of interleukin-8 in breast cancer cells. Oncogene 23: 6105-6114.

19. Bruun JM, Lihn AS, Pedersen SB, Richelsen B (2005) Monocyte chemoattractant protein-1 release is higher in visceral than subcutaneous human adipose tissue (AT): implication of macrophages resident in the AT. J Clin Endocrinol Metab 90: 2282-2289.

20. Vasudevan AR, Wu H, Xydakis AM, Jones PH, Smith EO, et al. (2006) Eotaxin and obesity. J Clin Endocrinol Metab 91: 256-261.

21. Cottam D, Fisher B, Ziemba A, Atkinson J, Grace B, et al. (2010) Tumor growth factor expression in obesity and changes in expression with weight loss: another cause of increased virulence and incidence of cancer in obesity. Surg Obes Relat Dis 6: 538-541.

22. Van Laere SJ, Van der Auwera I, Van den Eynden GG, Elst HJ, Weyler J, et al. (2006) Nuclear factor-kappa B signature of inflammatory breast cancer by cDNA microarray validated by quantitative real-time reverse transcription-PCR, immunohistochemistry, and nuclear factor-kappa B DNA-binding. Clin Cancer Res 12: 3249-3256.

23. Vanden Berghe W, Vermeulen L, De Wilde G, De Bosscher K, Boone E, et al. (2000) Signal transduction by tumor necrosis factor and gene regulation of the inflammatory cytokine interleukin-6. Biochem Pharmacol 60: 1185-1195.

24. Spiller SE, Logsdon NJ, Deckard LA, Sontheimer H (2011) Inhibition of nuclear factor kappa-B signaling reduces growth in medulloblastoma in vivo. BMC Cancer 11: 136.

25. Demchenko YN, Kuehl WM (2010) A critical role for the NFκB pathway in multiple myeloma. Oncotarget 1: 59-68.

26. Peralta EA, Murphy LL, Minnis J, Louis S, Dunnington GL (2009) American Ginseng inhibits induced COX-2 and NFKB activation in breast cancer cells. J Surg Res 157: 261-267.

27. Spencer L, Mann C, Metcalfe M, Webb M, Pollard C, et al. (2009) The effect of omega-3 FAs on tumour angiogenesis and their therapeutic potential. Eur J Cancer 45: 2077-2086.

28. Antoon JW, White MD, Slaughter EM, Driver JL, Khalili HS, et al. (2011) Targeting NFκB mediated breast cancer chemoresistance through selective inhibition of sphingosine kinase-2. Cancer Biol Ther 11: 678-689.

29. Park BK, Zhang H, Zeng Q, Dai J, Keller ET, et al. (2007) NF-kappaB in breast cancer cells promotes osteolytic bone metastasis by inducing osteoclastogenesis via GM-CSF. Nat Med 13: 62-69.

27

Effects of Malaria on Iron Stores in the Pregnant Women of Buea and Tiko Health District, South West Region, Cameroon

Nfor O Nlinwe*

Department of Medical Laboratory Science, University of Bamenda, Cameroon

Abstract

Malaria infection has a complex effect on iron metabolism that may affect the interpretation of haemoglobin, serum ferritin, serum transferrin and serum iron. The main objective of this study was to determine the effect of malaria parasitaemia on the iron store forms of pregnant women in the Buea and Tiko health districts of the S.W Region of Cameroon. This investigation was carried out from the 3rd of August 2011 to the 30th of April 2012. The non-probabilistic sampling method was used to recruit a total of 377 pregnant women into the study. Questionnaires were used for the collection of secondary data. The microscopy method was used to detect the presence of malaria infection. A total of 41.4% (156/377) of the pregnant women were infected with Plasmodium falciparum. Of the infected cases; 32.1% had low levels of serum ferritin (<20 µg/L), 10.9% had high levels of serum transferrin (>360 mg/dl), and 45.5% had low levels of serum iron (<9.0 µmol/l). The quantitative results using regression analysis justified that 88% variation in serum ferritin, transferrin and iron were accounted for by variation in malaria parasitaemia during the second and the third trimesters. Serum iron, ferritin and transferrin measurements should be incorporated as one of the routine laboratory tests during the regular antenatal care visits.

Keywords: Anaemia; Pregnancy; Low birth weight; Malaria; Cameroon

Introduction

Severe anaemia in pregnancy is an important direct and indirect cause of maternal death, and for the foetus, severe maternal anaemia may result in intra-uterine growth retardation, stillbirth and low birthweight [1,2]. Malaria infection has a complex effect on iron metabolism that may affect the interpretation of haemoglobin, serum ferritin, serum transferrin and serum iron [1].

In 1999, a special symposium entitled "Improving Adolescent Iron status before childbearing" was convened in Washington D.C. The resolution adopted from the symposium was that, emphasis needs to be placed on pre-pregnancy programmes to increase body iron stores [3]. In spite of this, severe anaemia continues to increase the risk for maternal mortality. Worse of all, malaria anaemia is estimated to affect up to 16 million women and children by the year 2015 [4]. In September 2000, the largest gathering of world leaders in human history convened for the Millenium Summit on the Millenium Development Goals (MDGs) in which a plan was adopted to achieve eight anti-poverty goals by the year 2015. As one of the steps to achieving the goals, stakeholders committed 40 billion US dollars in resources to a global effort to save the lives of the 16 million women and children who are likely to be affected by malaria induced anaemia by the year 2015.

In line with the MDG, this work was designed to investigate into the insidious effect of malaria on the iron stores of the pregnant women in Buea and Tiko Health Districts of the Fako Division in the South West Region of Cameroon. In order to achieve this objective, attempts will be made to answer the following question:

What is the insidious effect of malaria on the iron status of the pregnant women in the Buea and Tiko Health Districts?

Materials and Methods

Study area

The study was conducted in the Buea and Tiko Health Districts located in the Fako division of the South West Region of Cameroon. Both districts are located between Longitude 8.6°10'E and Latitude 4°5.2'N. The climate alternates from the hot humid coastline, the Tiko plain, to the temperate climate on the mountain slopes where Buea is situated [4].

The mount Cameroon region is hyper-endemic for malaria, with Plasmodium falciparum being the predominant malaria parasite species [5]. Fako division is divided into four health districts; Buea, Limbe, Muyuka and Tiko Health District. In these health districts, there are health units, district hospitals and a regional hospital which offer services of antenatal care to pregnant women. The inhabitants of this region are of the English speaking Cameroonians and their occupations vary from farmers, business personnel and public servants.

Ethical clearance

Ethical Clearance and authorization to collect specimens for this research was obtained from the Ethical Committee Board of the Ministry of Public Health, Regional Delegation for the South West Region, Cameroon. Informed consent was handed to the prospective research subjects on recruitment.

Experimental design

Sample size determination: The sample size for this work was determined based on the Yaro Yamane's approach for finite population [6]. This was made possible by using the formula;

$$n = N/ 1 + N (e)^2$$

Where;

n = the expected sample size,

Corresponding author: Nfor O Nlinwe, Department of Medical Laboratory Science, University of Bamenda, Cameroon; E-mail: omarinenlinwe@yahoo.ca

N = the finite population out of which the sample was drawn.

e = the level of significance (or limit of tolerable error) [6].

For this work, the estimated population size (N) from the 2010 population statistics was 11047 [7] (Regional Delegation of Public Health, SW Region, 2010), and the level of significance (e) is 0.05 or 5%. So:

Estimated Sample Size = $11047/1 + 11047(0.05)^2$

$= 11047/28.6175 \approx 386$

From the above calculation, the estimated sample size was 386 pregnant women. To make for attrition, a total of 482 pregnant women were recruited for this study, from five different centres.

Scope of study: This cohort (longitudinal) study recruited pregnant women at the time of registration for antenatal care visits. This intensive field research was carried out within a period of nine months, from the 3rd of August 2011 to 30th of April 2012.

Population sampled: Samples were drawn from the Cameroon Development Coorperation (CDC) Central Clinic Tiko (CCT), Mutengene Baptist Hospital (MBH), Buea Regional Hospital (BRH), Government Health Center Muea (GHCM) and the Buea Road Integrated Health Center (BIH). Newly registered pregnant women for antenatal clinic were considered eligible for recruitment as research participants. The sampling method which was used was the non-probabilistic sampling method, the volunteer sampling technique.

Administration of questionnaire: Newly registered pregnant women for antenatal care visits (whose pregnancies were from the second trimester and below), were contacted on one-to-one basis and after a brief description of the study, the informed consent was handed to them. The consent form was signed by those who have read and understood the informed consent. The questionnaire was filled by those who signed the consent forms. And all those who filled the questionnaires were recruited into the study.

Laboratory diagnostic methods

All the medical laboratory diagnostic tests were carried out in the teaching laboratory of the Faculty of Health Sciences, University of Buea.

Parasitological examination: The parasitological examination was carried out once during the second trimester and once during the third trimester, for each pregnant woman. Capillay blood was collected from the finger prick and was used to prepare both the thin and the thick blood films. The blood films were air-dried and the thin blood film fixed with absolute methanol for one to two minutes. The blood films were then stained with 3% Giemsa staining solution, for 30 minutes. Buffered water was used to flush the stain from the slide, to avoid the films being covered with fine deposit of stain and the stained films were air-dried.

Examination and determination of malaria parasite density:

Thick Film: The dried slides were mounted and examined using the high power 100x objective lens. Thick blood films were used to detect the presence of *Plasmodium sp* and the level of parasitaemia, while thin blood films were examined to determine speciation. Parasite counting was done by counting the number of parasites against at least 100 leukocytes, or 200 leukocytes for the definitive count. The number of the parasites counted was calculated using the formula:

$$\text{Parasites} / \mu l \text{ of blood} = \frac{\text{Number of parasites counted} \times 8000 \text{ leukocytes}}{\text{Number of WBC Counted}}$$

For the positive cases, parasitaemia was classified as follows:

1-999 Parasites/μl of blood = Mild parasitaemia.

1,000-9,999 Parasites/μl of blood = Moderate parasitaemia.

$\geq 10,000$ Parasites/μl of blood = Severe parasitaemia [8].

Measurement of serum ferritin: The quantitative determination of serum ferritin was carried out using reagents produced by Fortress Diagnostics ISO 13485 accredited company, United Kingdom. The spectrophotometric method of measurement was employed (Batch number: BXCO441A). The calibration curve was drawn by preparing serial dilutions of the calibrator using NaCl 9 g/L as diluents. The concentration of the calibrator was multiplied by the corresponding factor, as indicated on the manufacturer's guide (Fortress Diagnostics ISO 13485 Accredited Company), to obtain the ferritin concentration of each point on the curve.

The reagents for this measurement were allowed to come to room temperature and then pipette into test tubes following the manufacturer's guide (Fortress Diagnostics ISO 13485 Accredited Company).

The contents in the test tubes were well mixed and the absorbance read and recorded immediately as A1. The absorbance was read again after 8 minutes of incubation at 37°C and recorded as A2. The absorbance difference (A2-A1) at each point of the curve was calculated and the values obtained were plotted against the ferritin concentration for each calibrator dilution. The ferritin concentration in the sample was then read from the intercept point (A2-A1) on the calibration curve.

Measurement of serum transferrin: The quantitative determination of serum transferrin was carried out using reagents produced by Fortress Diagnostics Company ISO 13485 Accredited Company. The spectrophotometric method of measurement was employed. (Batch number: BXCO741A)

Six levels of standards which accompanied the test kit had their calibrator values or concentrations labelled on it. After bringing them to room temperature, calibrators/samples, alongside with the reagents were pipetted into test tubes, following the manufacturer's guide (Fortress Diagnostics ISO 13485 Accredited Company).

The change of absorbance (A_2-A_1) was calculated. A graph using the concentrations of the six levels of standards against its absorbance (A_2-A_1) was drawn. The concentration of transferrin in patient sera was read from the graph using its change of absorbance (A_2-A_1) values.

Measurement of serum iron: The quantitative determination of serum iron was carried out using reagents produced by Fortress Diagnostics ISO 13485 Accredited Company, United Kingdom and the spectrophotometric method of measurement was employed. (Batch number: BXCO236A)

The reagents were pipette into test tubes following the manufacturer's guide (Fortress Diagnostics ISO 13485 Accredited Company).

The contents in the pipettes were mixed and incubated for 10 minutes at 37°C. The absorbance of the samples and the standards were read against the reagent blank. The iron concentrations in μmol/L were then calculated as follows:

$$\frac{\text{Absorbance of Sample} \times \text{Standard concentration}}{\text{Absorbance of Calibrator}} = \text{Sample Concentrations} (\mu mol / L)$$

Data analysis

Descriptive statistics (mean, median and mode), with the use of tables were employed in the presentation of results on age, marital status, occupation, gravidity and iron supplementation. The multiple regression analysis was used to justify a strong goodness of fit for the effect of malaria on serum ferritin, transferrin and iron in the study subjects, for the five centres of the study area.

Results

The status of malaria infection in the study area by centers is shown in Figure 1. Malaria endemicity in the study area by trimester is shown on Figure 2. The levels of parasitaemia in the entire study area by trimesters are shown on Table 1. The status of malaria infection in the study area by age, marital status, occupation, gravidity and iron supplementation in the study area is shown on Table 2. Variation of serum ferritin, transferrin, iron and WBC among the pregnant women

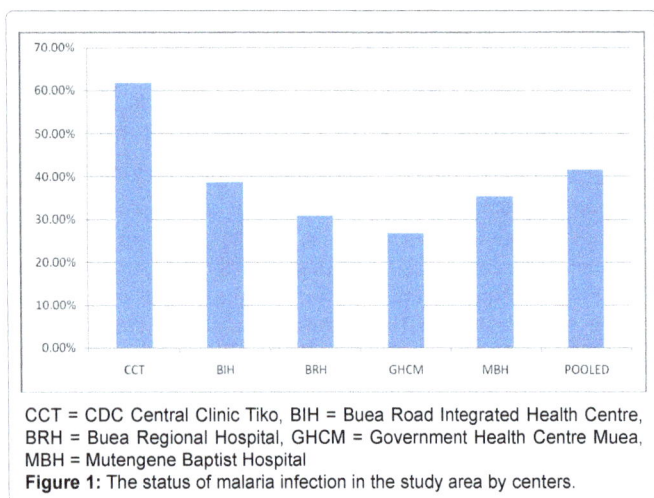

CCT = CDC Central Clinic Tiko, BIH = Buea Road Integrated Health Centre, BRH = Buea Regional Hospital, GHCM = Government Health Centre Muea, MBH = Mutengene Baptist Hospital
Figure 1: The status of malaria infection in the study area by centers.

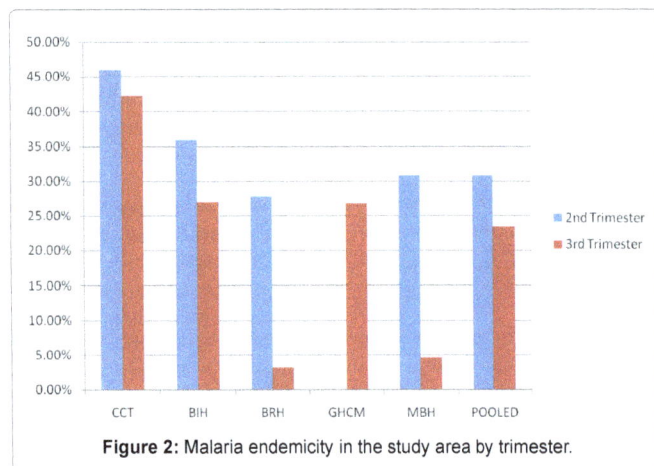

Figure 2: Malaria endemicity in the study area by trimester.

Trimester	Mild Parasitaemia (%)	Moderate Parasitaemia (%)	Severe Parasitaemia (%)	Total (%)
First	-	-	-	-
Second	57 (49.1)	54 (46.6)	05 (4.3)	116 (56.9)
Third	49 (55.7)	36 (40.9)	03 (3.1)	88 (43.1)
Total	106 (52.0)	90 (44.1)	08 (03.9)	204 (100)

Table 1: Mild Parasitaemia = 1-999 trophozoites/µL of blood; Moderate Parasitaemia = 1,000-9,999 trophozoites/µL of blood; Severe Parasitaemia = ≥10,000 trophozoites/µL of blood (WHO, 2003).

Parameters		No Examined (%)	No Infected (%)
Age	15-25yrs	165 (43.8)	63 (38.2)
	26-35yrs	190 (50.4)	83 (43.7)
	36-45yrs	22 (05.8)	10 (45.5)
Marital Status	Married	266 (70.6)	116 (43.6)
	Single	111 (29.4)	40 (36.0)
	House wives	143 (37.9)	61 (42.7)
	Public Servants	81 (21.5)	47 (58.0)
Occupation	Students	46 (12.2)	06 (13.0)
	Farmers	19 (05.0)	05 (26.3)
	Bussiness personelle	88 (23.3)	37 (42.1)
Gravidity	Multigravidae	264 (70.0)	109 (41.3)
	Primigravidae	113 (30.0)	47 (41.6)
Iron	Yes	356 (94.4)	143 (40.2)
Supplementation	No	21 (05.6)	13 (61.9)
Total for each Parameter		377	156 (41.4)

Table 2: The status of malaria infection in the study area by age, marital status, occupation, gravidity and intake of iron supplementation, in the study area.

is shown on Table 3. The variation of serum ferritin, transferrin, iron and WBC among pregnant women infected with malaria, by study centers is shown on Table 4. The quantitative regression result on the effect of malaria on serum ferritin, transferrin and iron by trimesters is shown on Table 5.

Discussion

In this study 41.4% (156/377) of the research participants were infected at least once, in their second and/or third trimester of pregnancy. This study, carried out in an area previously described as being hyper endemic for malaria reported a high percentage of malaria (41.4%) as expected. This is in agreement with the findings reported by Meeusen et al. that pregnant women in endemic areas are highly susceptible to malaria [5,9]. This is also in agreement with the work of Achidi et al. carried out in the Mutengene Maternity, in the South West Region of Cameroon, which reported a 44.7% rate of malaria infection among pregnant women, at the point of antenatal enrolment [10]. The findings agrees with that reported for Kassena-Nankana district of Ghana in which, the overall prevalence of malaria parasitaemia during pregnancy was 47%, out of 3642 pregnant women of all gravidities and gestational age of 18-32 weeks [11].

Malaria demonstrated insidious influence on SF, ST and SI stores during the period of study, as the goodness of fit value the adjusted R^2 was 88%, meaning that 88% variation in SF, ST and SI was accounted for by the presence of malaria in the study area. The value of R^2 which gives information about the inclusive and non-inclusive variables has therefore demonstrated that, the inclusive variable (malaria) had an insidious effect on SF, ST and SI. The non-inclusive variable which could be considered as control includes those variables which were not measured, which accounted for 22% variation in SF, ST and SI in the malaria positive cases. These variables could possibly include: Malaria in the first trimester, intestinal helminthic and protozoan infections associated with anaemia, variation in the physiological response to changes induced by pregnancy, variation in the nutritional content of food intake.

This results equally revealed that 1% increase in trophozoites/ul of blood in the second trimester insidiously accounted for 0.17% percent decrease in serum ferritin in CCT (P ≤ 0.01), 0.14% percent decrease in serum ferritin in BIH, 0.46% percent decrease in serum ferritin in MBH and 0.19% percent decrease in serum ferritin in BRH (P ≤ 0.01). These

Status of Infection	No Examined (%)	Low SF (%)	Normal SF (%)	High SF (%)	Low ST (%)	High ST (%)	Low SI (%)	Normal SI (%)	High SI (%)	Low WBC (%)	Normal WBC (%)	High WBC (%)
Infected	156 (41.4)	50 (32.1)	99 (63.5)	07 (04.5)	139 (89.1)	17 (10.9)	71 (45.5)	78 (50.0)	07 (04.5)	24 (15.4)	123 (78.9)	09 (05.7)
Non-infected	221 (58.62)	71 (32.1)	135 (61.1)	15 (06.8)	197 (89.1)	24 (10.9)	85 (38.5)	127 (57.5)	9 (04.1)	39 (17.7)	169 (76.5)	13 (05.9)
Total	377	121 (32.1)	234 (62.1)	22 (05.8)	336 (89.1)	41 (10.9)	156 (41.4)	205 (54.4)	16 (04.2)	63 (16.7)	292 (77.5)	22 (05.8)

Table 3: SF=Serum Ferritin, ST=Serum Transferrin and SI=Serum Iron, WBC = White blood cell count Low SF = <20 ug/), Normal SF = 20-200 ug/l, HighSF = >200 ug/l, Low ST = <200 mg/dl, Normal ST = 200-360 mg/dl, High ST = >360 mg/dl, Low SI = <9.0 umol/l, Normal SI = 9-30.4 umol/l, High SI = >30.4 umol/l, Low WBC = <4×10^9/l, Normal WBC = 4.0-10.0×10^9/l, High WBC = >10.0×10^9/l (Fortress Diagnostics ISO 13485 Accredited Company). Normal ST was not recorded.

Research Center	No Infected (%)	Low SF (%)	Normal SF (%)	High SF (%)	Low ST (%)	High ST (%)	Low SI (%)	Normal SI (%)	High SI (%)	Low WBC (%)	Normal WBC (%)	High WBC (%)
CDC Tiko	67 (61.5)	23 (34.3)	40 (59.7)	04 (06.0)	06 (91.0)	06 (09.0)	35 (52.2)	28 (41.80)	04 (06.0)	12 (17.9)	52 (77.6)	03 (04.5)
BRH	20 (30.8)	-	20 (100)	-	20 (100)	-	10 (50.0)	10 (50.0)	-	07 (35.0)	13 (65.0)	-
BIH	30 (38.5)	11 (36.7)	19 (63.3)	-	25 (83.3)	05 (16.7)	13 (43.3)	17 (56.7)	-	05 (16.7)	25 (83.3)	-
GHCM	16 (26.7)	08 (50.0)	08 (50.0)	-	13 (81.3)	03 (18.8)	03 (18.8)	13 (81.3)	-	-	13 (81.3)	03 (18.8)
MBH	23 (35.4)	08 (34.8)	12 (52.2)	03 (13.0)	20 (87.0)	03 (13.0)	10 (43.5)	10 (43.5)	03 (13.0)	-	20 (87.0)	02 (08.7)

Table 4: SF=Serum Ferritin, ST=Serum Transferrin and SI=Serum Iron, WBC = White blood cell count Low SF = <20 ug/), Normal SF = 20-200 ug/l, High SF = >200 ug/l, Low ST = <200 mg/dl, Normal ST = 200-360 mg/dl, High ST = >360 mg/dl, Low SI = <9.0 umol/l, Normal SI = 9-30.4 umol/l, High SI = >30.4 umol/l, Low WBC = <4×10^9/l, Normal WBC = 4.0-10.0×10^9/l, High WBC = >10.0×10^9/l. None was registered with Normal ST. (Fortress Diagnostics ISO 13485 Accredited Company).

	CDC Tiko	BIH	GHCM	MBH	BRH	Pooled
R²	66%	74%	78%	69%	83%	88%
F-Ratio	8.73	14.1	16.6	10.4	22.1	52.3
Degree of Freedom	4:11	0.221	0.208	0.2118	0.21	4:34
Critical Value	3.8	2.6	2.5	2.4	2.4	6.3
Judgement	s	S	S	s	S	S
Variable	PM1	PM1	PM1	PM1	PM1	PM1
SF	-0.17 (-1.99)***	-0.14 (-7.49)*	NA	-0.46 (-2.14)*	-0.19 (-2.97)*	-0.47 (-2.63)*
ST	0.04(1.78)***	0.04 (2.73)*	NA	0.05(2.45)*	0.64(6.67)*	0.38(2.20)**
SI	-0.08 (-1.78)***	-0.11 (-2.44)*	NA	-0.0(-0.58)	-0.0 (-2.21)**	-0.34 (-3.94)*
WBC	-0.13(-1.99)	0.02(1.84)	NA	-0.04(-1.63)	0.08(2.67)	0.42(3.33)
	PM2	PM2	PM2	PM2	PM2	PM2
SF	-0.03 (-1.94)***	-0.63 (-6.43)*	-0.49 (-2.21)**	-0.38 (-2.72)*	-0.33 (-1.84)***	-0.67(-4.73)*
ST	0.56(3.40)*	0.39(2.59)*	0.16(2.76)*	0.34(3.34)*	0.22(1.99)***	0.49(3.32)*
SI	-0.43(-7.31)*	-0.39(-2.79)*	-0.66 (-3.15)*	-0.39(-2.23)**	-0.84(-7.34)*	-0.34(-2.33)**
WBC	0.23(2.41)	0.06(1.79)	0.23(3.56)	0.43(3.44)	0.65(1.98)	0.56(3.03)

Table 5: The quantitative regression results of the effect of malaria on serum ferritin, transferrin and iron, by trimesters.

results are consistent with their correspondent F-ratio values, taking into consideration their degrees of freedoms which are all significant at $P \leq 0.05$.

Considering the study area as a whole, one percent increase in trophozoites/µl of blood in the second and third trimesters of pregnancy accounted for 0.47 and 0.67 percents decrease in serum ferritin respectively, at $P \leq 0.01$.

One percent increase in trophozoites/ul of blood during the third trimester of pregnancy accounted for; 0.03% decrease in serum ferritin in CCT at $P \leq 0.1$; 0.49% decrease in serum ferritin in GHCM at $P \leq 0.05$; 0.33% decrease in serum ferritin in BRH at $P \leq 0.1$; 0.38% decrease in serum ferritin in MBH and 0.63% decrease in serum ferritin in BIH, both at $P \leq 0.01$. Under steady state conditions serum ferritin level correlates with total body iron stores, therefore decrease

in ferritin levels indicates a decrease in iron storage associated with iron deficiency anaemia. But in areas of widespread infection or inflammation, defining iron deficiency using serum ferritin is difficult, as with the case of acute phase proteins, ferritin levels may be artificially high in cases of anaemia of chronic disease, where ferritin is elevated in its capacity as an acute phase protein. The expectation is therefore that serum ferritin in this study with the presence of malaria should act as an acute phase protein and therefore be elevated, with elevation persisting for several days or weeks. But this study considered the insidious effect of malaria infections in the second and third trimester, on serum ferritin levels measured at least one month after testing for malaria in the third trimester of pregnancy. Considering the fact that; parasitaemia was more endemic during the second trimester (30.8%) than the third (23.3%); 30.8% of the infected cases had consistent infections (infections in both trimesters), the decrease in serum ferritin has been statistically proven to be accounted for by an accumulated/ insidious effect of malaria over time. This effect could be supported by the fact that malaria parasites in red blood cells makes use of the available iron which is replenished from the iron stored forms, resulting to a negative effect on the iron stored forms, and more so in pregnant women with a higher demand for iron, both the development of the fetus and the mother. The result is in contrast with an assessment of iron status of 3605 school children in Zanzibar by Stoltzfus et al. [12]. In this assessment, serum ferritin concentration rose by 1.5 μg/L per 1000 parasites/uL of parasite densities greater than 1000 parasites/uL of blood. The difference might have been due to the different study groups as school children had increase in serum ferritin levels with increase parasites/uL of blood as against the pregnant women who had decrease serum ferritin levels with increase in trophozoites/μL of blood. Pregnant women have additional need for iron sources of which serum ferritin is a chief source of stored iron. The result of this study is in line with a cross-sectional study carried out by Mockenhaupt et al. in which 530 pregnant women in Ghana was studied, and ferritin levels were considerably influenced by malaria infection [13]. Unlike the study of school children, the study of pregnant women agrees with the present study.

The quantitative results on Table 5 revealed that in general, malaria acquired during the second trimester, had a positive effect on serum transferrin in all the study Centres. Considering the study area as a whole, one percent increase in trophozoites/μl of blood during the second trimester of pregnancy accounted for 0.38 percent increase in serum transferrin and 0.49 percent increase in serum transferrin was accounted for by one percent increase in trophozoites/μl of blood during the third trimester, at P ≤ 0.01. It reveals that one percent increase in trophozoites/uL of blood during the second trimester of pregnancy accounted for; 0.04 percent increase in serum transferrin in the CDC Central Clinic at P ≤ 0.1; 0.04 percent increase in serum transferrin in BIH at P ≤ 0.01; 0.05 percent increase in serum transferrin in MBH at P ≤ 0.01, and 0.64 percent increase in serum transferrin in BRH at P ≤ 0.01. In the third trimester one percent increase in trophozoites/ uL of blood accounted for; 0.56 percent increase in serum transferrin in CCT; 0.16 percent increase in serum transferrin in GHCM; 0.39 percent increase in serum transferrin in BIH; 0.34 percent increase in serum transferrin in the MBH at P ≤ 0.01 and 0.22 percent increase in serum transferrin in the BRH at P ≤ 0.1.

The normal expectation is that the concentration of transferrin increases to two or three times normal when anaemia is present, but the rise occurs only after iron stores become functionally depleted, whereas serum ferritin concentrations fall earlier, as iron stores fall [14]. As expected, while the presence of malaria had a negative impact on serum ferritin values, it had a positive impact on serum transferrin. Increase in serum transferrin during the third and second trimesters is an indicator of the body's need for iron. This study is in disagreement with the work of Rusia et al. in which serum ferritin measurements in pregnant women did not reflect the true prevalence of iron deficiency [15]. It was concluded in that study that serum transferrin receptor estimation is a more useful measure for detecting iron deficiency in pregnancy, than serum ferritin. In the same vein, Brian et al. reported that serum transferrin levels are a very sensitive means of assessing iron status, and particular in early tissue iron deficiency they reported that it reflects the adequacy of iron supply to cells in general [14]. The results therefore prove that serum ferritin as well as serum transferrin had been good indicators for iron deficiency, as a result of the presence of malaria infection.

Looking at the effects of malaria infections on serum iron, during the third trimester of pregnancy, the quantitative results reveal that one percent increase in trophozoites/uL of blood accounted for; 0.43 percent decrease in serum iron in CCT; 0.39 percent decrease in serum iron in BIH; 0.66 percent decrease in serum iron in GHCM; 0.84 percent decrease in serum iron in BRH (P ≤ 0.01) and 0.39 percent decrease in serum iron in MBH at P ≤ 0.05. It can be concluded from the quantitative regression results that, one percent increase in trophozoites/uL of blood in the second trimester of pregnancy accounted for 0.34 percent fall in serum iron in the pregnant women of the Buea and Tiko Health Districts, at P ≤ 0.01 and one percent increase in trophozoites/uL of blood during the third trimester, accounted for 0.34 percent decrease in serum iron, at P ≤ 0.05.

Considering the negative effects of malaria on iron stores and the insignificant correlation between malaria and the red blood cell indices in the study area in general, it may be inferred that, the values of the red blood cell indices, haematocrit and red blood cell counts were insignificantly affected by malaria. This is probably because iron storage forms (serum ferritin, transferrin and iron) had not been depleted, but significantly affected.

Acknowledgement

Acknowledgement goes to God Almighty, who guided this study from conception to completion. Special thanks are equally accorded to my supervisors Pr. Monday Francis, Useh and Professor A.A. Alaribe of the University of Calabar. The administration and all the workers of the four study centers who were part of this study are also appreciated. Mr. Nyingchu Robert Vuchuh, Mr. Nfor Edwin Njingti and Professor Njimanted Godfrey Forgha are appreciated for their great contributions to the success of this study.

References

1. Hastka J, Lasserre JJ, Schwarzbeck A, Strauch M, Hehlmann R (1993) Zinc protoporphyrin in anemia of chronic disorders. Blood 81: 1200-1204.

2. Brabin BJ, Hakimi M, Pelletier D (2001) An analysis of anemia and pregnancy-related maternal mortality. J Nutr 131: 604S-614S.

3. Meier PR, Nickerson HJ, Olson KA, Berg RL, Meyer JA (2003) Prevention of iron deficiency anemia in adolescent and adult pregnancies. Clin Med Res 1: 29-36.

4. Wanji S, Tanke T, Atanga SN, Ajonina C, Nicholas T, et al. (2003) Anopheles species of the Mount Cameroon Region: biting habits, feeding behavior and entomological inoculation rates. Tropical Medicine and International Health 8: 643-649.

5. Wanji S, Kimbi HK, Eyong JE, Tendongfor N, Ndamukong JL (2008) Performance and usefulness of the Hexagon rapid diagnostic test in children with asymptomatic malaria living in the Mount Cameroon region. Malar J 7: 89.

6. Uzoagulu M (1998) Fundamentals of Statistics. Churchill, United States.

7. Regional Delegation of Public Health (2010) South West Region.

8. WHO. Export Committee on Malaria (2000) Technical Report Series 892. Geneva, World Health Organisation.

9. Meeusen EN, Bischof RJ, Lee CS (2001) Comparative T-cell responses during pregnancy in large animals and humans. Am J Reprod Immunol 46: 169-179.

10. Achidi EA, Kuoh AJ, Minang JT, Ngum B, Achimbom BM, et al. (2005) Malaria infection in pregnancy and its effects on haemoglobin levels in women from a malaria endemic area of Fako Division, South West Province, Cameroon. J Obstet Gynaecol 25: 235-240.

11. Clerk CA, Bruce J, Greenwood B, Chandramohan D (2009) The epidemiology of malaria among pregnant women attending antenatal clinics in an area with intense and highly seasonal malaria transmission in northern Ghana. Tropical Medicine and International Health 1: 4-6.

12. Stoltzfus RJ, Chwaya HM, Albonico M, Schulze KJ, Savioli L, et al. (1997) Serum ferritin, erythrocyte protoporphyrin and hemoglobin are valid indicators of iron status of school children in a malaria-holoendemic population. J Nutr 127: 293-298.

13. Mockenhaupt FP, Rong B, Günther M, Beck S, Till H, et al. (2000) Anaemia in pregnant Ghanaian women: importance of malaria, iron deficiency, and haemoglobinopathies. Trans R Soc Trop Med Hyg 94: 477-483.

28

Non-alcoholic Fatty Liver Disease (NAFLD) - An Emerging Public Health Problem

Manopriya T[1], Khalid G[2], Alshaari AA[3] and Sheriff DS[3]*

[1]MAPIMS, Chennai, India
[2]Chettinad Dental College, Chennai, India
[3]Faculty of Medicine, Benghazi University, Benghazi, Libya

Abstract

NAFLD is an emerging problem in Asia, with raising prevalence and strong impact on the health care system. More and more people will suffer from not only the liver impairment of NAFLD but also the associated metabolic diseases e.g. DM and hypertension. The incidence of DM, hypertension, coronary heart diseases (CHD) and stroke will increase together with the prevalence of NAFLD and the health service expenditure will rise in coming decades. However the prevalence of and the metabolic diseases associated with NAFLD are not well studied in Asian populations. The objective of this project is to systematically review the articles related to NAFLD.

Keywords: Non-alcoholic fatty liver disease; Triglycerides; Intra peritoneal fat; Metabolic diseases

Introduction

Non-alcoholic fatty liver disease (NAFLD) represents a spectrum of medical conditions in which there is increased infiltration of fat, predominantly triglycerides, inside hepatocytes. NAFLD is defined when there is macro vesicular steatosis inside liver cells exceeding 5% of liver weight, in the absence of significant ethanol consumption or other specific causes of liver diseases [1].

Although NAFLD may occur in people with normal body weight, it is strongly associated with obesity. The prevalence among obese people (body mass index more than 30 kg/m²) in the United States has been reported as 80-90% [2]. Body mass index (BMI) of more than 35 kg/m² and an intraperitoneal fat area of more than 158 cm² are strong predictors of NAFLD [3-5]. Besides of obesity, hyperlipidemia and type 2 diabetes mellitus (DM) is associated with NAFLD [2].

Increased fat accumulation in liver or fatty liver disease can also be secondary to a number of causes, including excessive alcohol consumption, drugs (especially chemotherapeutic agents e.g. methotrexate, tamoxifen), hepatic toxins (e.g. arsenic, carbon tetrachloride), chronic viral hepatitis (e.g. hepatitis B and hepatitis C viral infection) and congenital storage diseases (e.g. Wilson disease, hemochromatosis) [6,7].

NAFLD may progress through three different stages, from hepatic steatosis to steatohepatitis and finally to cirrhosis [8,9]. Hepatic steatosis represents simple increase in accumulation of fat in liver, without evidence of inflammation or liver damage. Inflammation and liver damage is however present in steatohepatitis. Both hepatic steatosis and steatohepatitis are potentially reversible with timely intervention. Cirrhosis represents irreversible liver damage with fibrosis. NAFLD-related cirrhosis 6 may also result in liver cancer or hepatocellular carcinoma, although it is less common than in cirrhosis secondary to excessive alcohol consumption and chronic viral hepatitis.

Fatty liver disease and alcohol consumption

Excessive ethanol intake is one of the most important causes of fatty liver disease. Although there is strong and consistent evidence on ethanol induced liver damage, there is still a lack of general consensus on what should be the meaning of "excessive alcohol consumption" [10]. In the Dionysos cohort [11], it was reported that 30 g of alcohol intake per day was the threshold of alcohol induced liver damage. However, other clinical studies suggested that the individual susceptibility to ethanol induced liver toxicity was highly variable in a given population [12]. It is now generally postulated that the relationship between alcohol consumption and liver damage is probably multi-factorial. Besides of amount of ethanol intake per day, other factors such as drinking patterns, drinking habits, genetic factors and gender also determine Individual vulnerability to ethanol induced hepatic toxicity [12]. Hepatic steatosis can be induced by drinking 20-30 g of ethanol per day [13], which is now generally regarded as the upper limit in NAFLD research.

Epidemiology of non-alcoholic fatty liver disease in Western countries

NAFLD is a common problem in Western countries. It is one of the most common causes of chronic liver disease in both children and adults in the United States. The current Western diet with high saturated fat and fructose is believed to be the culprit. It had been reported that the prevalence of NAFLD was as large as 25-35% in the general population of United States [2,14]. In another study involving 31 million Americans, NAFLD has been reported to affect 31% of men and 16% of women [15]. Although the true prevalence of NAFLD in children of the United States is unknown, it has been estimated to range from 2-10% and the prevalence may even be as high as 80% in obese children [16]. Other countries report similarly high prevalence rates.

NAFLD prevalence in a Canadian autopsy study was 29% [5]. In Europe, NAFLD prevalence ranged from 16% in Italy [17] to 24% in Sweden [18-20]. In the Dionysos cohort [11] of apparently healthy subjects aged 12 to 65 years living in Northern Italy, the prevalence of NAFLD after excluding alcoholism, hepatitis B and C infection was 55%. It was more common in obese (91%) than in overweight (67%) and normal weight subjects (24.5%) (p<0.0001). The mean prevalence

*Corresponding author: Sheriff DS, PhD, Faculty of Medicine, Benghazi University, Benghazi, Libya, E-mail: drdsheriff@gmail.com

of fatty liver in Western Countries is generally accepted to range from 20-60%. It is more common in men than in women, with a ratio of 3: 1.

Inclusion and exclusion criteria

The inclusion and exclusion criteria set a priori were used to select relevant papers from those retrieved. The inclusion criteria were: a) estimated prevalence of NAFLD and/ or b) determined the metabolic risk of NAFLD in Asian countries, c) quantified the adjusted odds ratio of NAFLD risk factors (such as obesity, DM, hypertension, hyperlipidemia), d) original studies and e) human studies. The exclusion criteria were:

a) review articles/ protocols/ guidelines/ abstracts/ unpublished results/ conference presentations, b) biochemistry/ gene/ genotype/ cellular/ histology studies, c) studies only focusing on the abnormal population group such as those with smoking, DM, liver disease and obesity, d) studies which recruited the subjects with other causes of fatty liver or concurrent liver diseases, such as excessive alcohol consumption/ viral hepatitis (hepatitis B virus and hepatitis C virus) and e) studies which included non-Asian subjects. There was no

limitation or restriction on the age, gender, residency and occupations of the subjects of the studies.

Citation assessments

Based on International guidelines such as STROBE (Strengthening the Reporting of Observational studies in Epidemiology) following ten studies were analyzed [21]. Study design, sample size, representative sample size, selection bias, reliability and validity formed the bases for selecting studies that are related to the review in question and the characteristics of the studies are cited in Table 1.

Definitions of obesity, abdominal obesity, insulin resistance and metabolic syndrome

Obesity is generally defined as BMI more than 25 kg/m^2 while abdominal/ central obesity is usually defined as waist circumference more than 90 cm in men or more than 80 cm in women, following the International Diabetes Institute/ Western Pacific World Health Organization/ International Obesity Task Force [22]. Insulin resistance is estimated by homeostasis assessment (HOMA): fasting insulin (mIU/ml) × fasting glucose (mmol/l)/22.50. Individual whose HOMA

References	Sample size	Demographics	Study Design	Diagnosis of NAFLD	Prevalence of NAFLD	Significant metabolic risk factors and disease (adjusted OR and CI)
Alavian et al. [33]	996	Iran children Age-17-18 years	Cross sectional stratified multistage random sampling	US	7.10%	IR (4.4.CI=1.6-12.3).). hypertriglyceridemia (2.5 CI=1.3-4.8). Elevated TC (2.8 CI=1.5-5.1) elevated LDL-C(2.8 CI=1.5-5.3) Abdominal obesity, HT, high FPG and low HDL-C are NOT significant risk factors
Das et al. [24]	1911	Indian adults ≥ 18years of age living in rural areas	Cross sectional stratified random sampling (1 ,3 subsample i.e. every 3rd person was selected)	US and CT	8.70%	Obesity(4.3 CI=1.6-11.5)abdominal obesity(3.6 CI=1.7-7.2) high family income(2.4CI=1.2-5.0) elevated FBG(2.6 CI=1.5-4.6)
Dassanayake et al. [27]	2,985	Sri Lankan adults aged35-64 years living in urban areas	Cross sectional stratified random sampling by different age groups	US	32.60%	Obesity (3.75.CI=3.07-4.5), IR (2.16.CI=1.73-2.68) HT (1.53.CI=1.25-1.88) raised FBG (1.7.CI=1.39-2.08) Hyper triglyceridemia (1.33. CI=1.08-1.63)
Fu [29]	220	Taiwan adolescent students Aged 12-13 years	Cross sectional stratified random sampling	US	39.3% (16% in non-obese 50, 5% in over weight 63.5% in obese)	Obesity in (5.98), elevated Non HDL-C (3.8 per mg/dL)
Lee et al. [26]	13,768	Korean adults recruited from a health promotion center	Cross sectional	US	25%	Obesity (4.4-9.7) gender (0.6 women vs men)
Lee et al. [25]	589	Korea consecutive potential Liver donor, aged 21-41 years	Cross sectional	Liver biopsy	51.4	Age>30(2223,CI=1.175-4.207) obesity (5.320, CI=2.764-10.240). Hypertriglyceridemia (2.253, CI=1.140-4,450)
Li et al. [28]	8,925	Chinese adults Employee of a company attending annual checkup in 2005	Cross sectional	US	11.8% (11.6% in men and 12.1% in women)	Hyperuricaemia (1.29.CI=1.067-1.564) obesity (1.174.CI=1.120-1.231) age (1.088CI=1.080-1.096) abdominal obesity (1.09CI=1.071-1.110) Hyper triglyceridemia (1.48.CI=1.385-1.582). elevated HDL-C (0.525 CI=0.373-0.737) elevated LDL-C (1.450.CI=1.287-1.631) elevated FPG-(1.216. CI=1.131-1.308)
Mohan et al. [30]	541	Indian adults living in Urban area	Cross sectional stratified random sampling	US	325 (men 35.1% Women 29.1%)	Abdominal obesity (2.0CI=1.3-3.1), obesity (2.4CI=1.6-3.5), DM (3.4CI=2.2-5.3). IR (2.1CI=1.4-3.2) hypertriglyceridemia (1.8CI=1.2-2.7) hypercholesterolemia (1.8CI=1.2-2.6) elevated LDL-C (1.5.CI=1.0—2.3).low HDL- C (2.0.CI=1.4-3.0) MS (2.8.CI=1.9-4.2)
Shitata et al.	3,139	Japanese Male Workers of a company aged at or above 40 years	Observational cohort study	US	ND	DM (4.6.CI=3.0-6.9) (incidence of DM in NAFLD Patients 2,073 per 100,000 person years, incidence of DM in non-NAFLD group is 452 per 100,000 person-years
Zeber-Sagi et al.	326	Israel adults	Cross sectional, stratified random sampling	US	30% (38% in men and 21% in women	Male gender (2.8 CI=1.3-3.3) IR (5.8 CI=2.0-17.2) abdominal obesity (2.9 CI=1.3-6.4). hypertriglyceridemia (2.4, CI=1.3-4.5)

Table 1: Summary of the citations on the prevalence and the risk factors of NAFLD in Asia.

insulin resistance values above the third quartile for the non-diabetic population (i.e. >2.58) are classified to have insulin resistance (HOMA-IR) [23]. Metabolic syndrome, sometimes denoted as Syndrome X or dysmetabolic syndrome, is generally defined based on modified National Cholesterol Education Program and Adult Treatment Panel III (NCEP-ATPIII) guidelines [24] and International Diabetes Institute/Western Pacific World Health Organization/ International Obesity Task Force [22]. A subject is classified as having metabolic syndrome if three or more of the following criteria were fulfilled: 1) elevated triglycerides (>150 mg/dl), 2) low high-density lipoprotein (HDL)cholesterol (<40 mg/dl in men or <50 mg/dl in women), 3) high blood pressure(>130/85 mmHg), 4) elevated fasting blood glucose (>110 mg/dl) and 5) abdominal obesity (waist circumference>90 cm in men or >80 cm in women).

A number of studies in different countries documented that the prevalence of NAFLD in men was significantly higher than in women [25-45].

In India, NAFLD was more prevalent (21%) in families with high income [25] and in China NAFLD prevalence was higher in urban (20.3%) than rural areas (11.1%) [35]. The prevalence of NAFLD in children also varied by country, with 39.8% prevalence in adolescent students aged 12-13 years in Taiwan [30], 7.1% in children aged from 7 to 16 years in Iran [34], and 1.3% among children aged 7 to 18 years in China [35]. Studies focusing on the Asian elderly were very scarce. NAFLD prevalence among Israeli elderly aged 81 to 90 years was 46.2% [43]. Both obesity and abdominal obesity were independent and significant risk factors of NAFLD, with reported adjusted odds ratios 1.17-7.21 and 1.09-3.6, respectively [25,28,29,31-33,37-40,44]. Consistent with the reported impact of obesity, the insulin resistance, elevated fasting blood glucose and type 2 DM were significant risk factors for NAFLD with adjusted odds ratio of 2.1-5.8, 1.42-2.6 and 1.7-4.6, respectively [25,28,29,31,33,36,38,40,42,45].

NAFLD was associated with dysfunction of lipid metabolism or dyslipidemia with odds ratios of 1.45 - 1.8 (elevated total cholesterol), 1.45 - 1.5 (elevated low-density lipoprotein cholesterol), 1.61 - 2.0 (low high-density lipoprotein cholesterol) and 1.33-3.51 (elevated triglyceride), respectively [28,29,31,33,37-40,45]. Others have suggested an association between NAFLD and elevated blood pressure (blood pressure higher than 130/85 mmHg) with adjusted odds ratio of 1.53 - 3.7 [28,45]. Other studies reported that metabolic syndrome adjusted odds ratio between 2.37 to 2.8 [31,33] and elevated blood uric acid level (>7 mg/dl in men and >6 mg/dl in women) adjusted odds ratios ranging from 1.29 to 2.3 [26,27,29,38,46] were associated with NAFLD.

In summary, NAFLD was associated with obesity, abdominal obesity, elevated fasting blood glucose, insulin resistance, DM, elevated total cholesterol, elevated low-density lipoprotein (LDL) cholesterol, low HDL cholesterol, elevated triglyceride, hypertension, hyperuricemia and metabolic syndrome in adults. As contrast to adults, only obesity, elevated total cholesterol, elevated LDL cholesterol, elevated triglyceride and insulin resistance were associated with NAFLD in children and adolescents [30,34] but not abdominal obesity, hypertension, elevated fasting blood glucose and low HDL cholesterol [34].

Non-alcoholic fatty liver disease: why is it important?

NAFLD represents wide spectrum of liver damage, varying from simple steatosis (increase in fat accumulation), to steatohepatitis (inflammation) and liver cirrhosis (irreversible fibrosis). The natural history of NAFLD globally is currently unclear. Although it is generally believed that most patients are asymptomatic, NAFLD can potentially progress into cirrhosis and even hepatocellular carcinoma. The true incidence of chronic hepatitis, cirrhosis and hepatocellular carcinoma related to NAFLD is still unclear and the data is lacking.

According to the Queen Mary Hospital – liver clinic records, 1.5% of patients with chronic liver disease were attributed to NAFLD [47]. Among cases of chronic hepatitis of unknown etiology, the prevalence of biopsy proven non-alcoholic steatohepatitis was reported to be 16% [48]. As suggested by research elsewhere, 10-11% of these patients may progress to liver cirrhosis [49]. Some of these patients may require liver transplantation due to severe liver function impairment or may develop liver cancer [50].

However, what is much more important and crucial is the salient but high risk of NAFLD patients to develop other metabolic diseases. Like in Caucasians, studies have shown that NAFLD in Asians is strongly associated with metabolic disorders including glucose intolerance, DM, hyperlipidemia (high cholesterol and high triglyceride) and hyperuricemia. These metabolic disorders are good predictors of NAFLD.

In India, 41% (seven) patients with NAFLD developed hypertension or DM during a 6 year-follow-up [51,52] and had higher risk of CHD which reflected the findings of overseas research [36,41,51,53]. Therefore, NAFLD is not just a liver disease. Patients with NAFLD are also at risk of developing other metabolic diseases (e.g. DM, hypercholesterolemia and hypertriglyceremia), perhaps much higher than the risk of liver cirrhosis and hepatocellular carcinoma.

Non-alcoholic Fatty Liver Disease: An Emerging Public Health Problem in Asia

At present NAFLD is regarded as a liver manifestation of metabolic disorder, which more commonly affects those in affluent Western countries where the average prevalence is estimated up to 20-40%. Although a number of studies on the NAFLD of Asian countries have been published, there are some difference among these studies in terms of sample selections, population subgroup heterogeneities, study designs and diagnosis criteria. Most of these studies are city or hospital based. As a result, there is wide variation of the reported prevalence and the true nationwide prevalence of NAFLD in Asian countries is difficult to determine. However, the prevalence of NAFLD in Asia has been reported up to 51.5% [37], which is comparable to the Western countries.

Similar to results in Western world, obesity (especially central obesity), impaired glucose metabolism, DM, hyperlipidemia and metabolic syndrome are important risk factors and predictors of NAFLD in Asians. Because of the industrialization, affluence and Westernization of lifestyle, the prevalence of obesity, DM, hyperlipidemia and metabolic syndrome has rapidly increased in recent decades globally. Asia has followed suit, the prevalence of DM and obesity has risen exponentially (2- to 5- fold) over a period of 20 years in Asia-pacific region [54].

Therefore it is not surprising that the rapidly rising prevalence of obesity and DM has put a very large proportion of Asian populations at risk of developing NAFLD, and the prevalence of NAFLD is expected to increase in coming decades.

Visceral adipose mass is another important predictor of NAFLD, independent of BMI [55]. As Asians have higher proportion of visceral fat and lower proportion of lean body mass (sum of the weight of bones, muscles and organs) compared with Caucasians of similar BMI [56], the prevalence of NAFLD in normal BMI in Asians is higher than that in Caucasians. Therefore, even though only a small percentage of Asians would be classified as obesity according to Western criteria, the prevalence of NAFLD is still high.

Non-alcoholic fatty liver disease in children and adolescents

NAFLD in children was first documented in 1983 in United States [57]. The first reported pediatric case of NAFLD induced cirrhosis was an 11-year-old Japanese child who had been obese since the age of 3 [58]. Compared with adults, there is sparse published research on the epidemiology of NAFLD in Asian children and adolescents [30,34,35,59,60]. As selection bias is a feature of many of these studies, the true prevalence of NAFLD in children and adolescents is unclear. However, there is strong evidence of association between obesity and NAFLD in children. Childhood NAFLD is also more common in boys, and in children of 10 to 15 years of age.

Implications of NAFLD to India

Like other urbanized countries, DM, CHD and stroke are important contributors to the burden of healthcare in Hong Kong. The prevalence of DM was estimated up to 9.8% in India [61]. A retrospective cohort observation study estimated that the mean annual total cost of Type 2 DM in a patient was about $ 13,457, of which the government paid 78.4% [62]. In 2004, DM contributed up to 6.4% of the Authority's public sector expenditures on health and 3.9% of the total India healthcare expenditure [62]. The cost markedly increased if the diagnosis was delayed and the complications were present. Therefore early detection and treatment of DM before the appearance of complications not only improves the prognosis of the patients but also save the budgets. However, it had been estimated that up to 31.9% of DM was undiagnosed in India [63,64].

Stroke and CHD are the leading causes of death in India [64]. The average management cost of CHD was estimated to be about $85,324 India per patient per year [65]. As NAFLD is strongly associated with

metabolic disorders including hyperlipidemia, DM and hypertension – the risk factors for stroke and CHD, increasing NAFLD will increase the management cost of CHD and stroke.

However, the level of alertness of NAFLD remains low in India. A random telephone survey recruiting 521 India adults (aged>18 years), reported that up to 83% of the respondents had never heard of the term "NAFLD".

As a significant risk factor of stroke, CHD, DM and hypertension, public awareness of NAFLD should be improved. More health promotion programs and educations focusing on NAFLD by the Government should be provided. Guidelines on the management of patients with NAFLD should be designed and endorsed among the primary health care providers. People with NAFLD should be screened and regularly followed up for the associated metabolic diseases. Aggressive treatments of NALFD such as lifestyle modification and anti-obesity treatment should also be actively considered and provided (Figure 1).

Directions for Further Research

The true nationwide prevalence of NAFLD in most Asian countries still remains uncertain. Most NAFLD epidemiological studies were confined to a city, a company, a hospital or a clinic and may not represent the whole population of the country.

Therefore, it is difficult to interpret and compare these various results from different Asian countries. Countrywide cross-sectional studies with stratified random sampling would be much more representative and easier to compare.

There is strong evidence of the association between NAFLD and other metabolic disorders such as DM and hyperlipidemia, which are also the risk factors of CHD and stroke. The incidence of these metabolic disorders in NAFLD patients is however unclear. Furthermore early NAFLD (simple steatosis and steatohepatitis) is potentially reversible and can be treated by lifestyle modification and anti-obesity therapy.

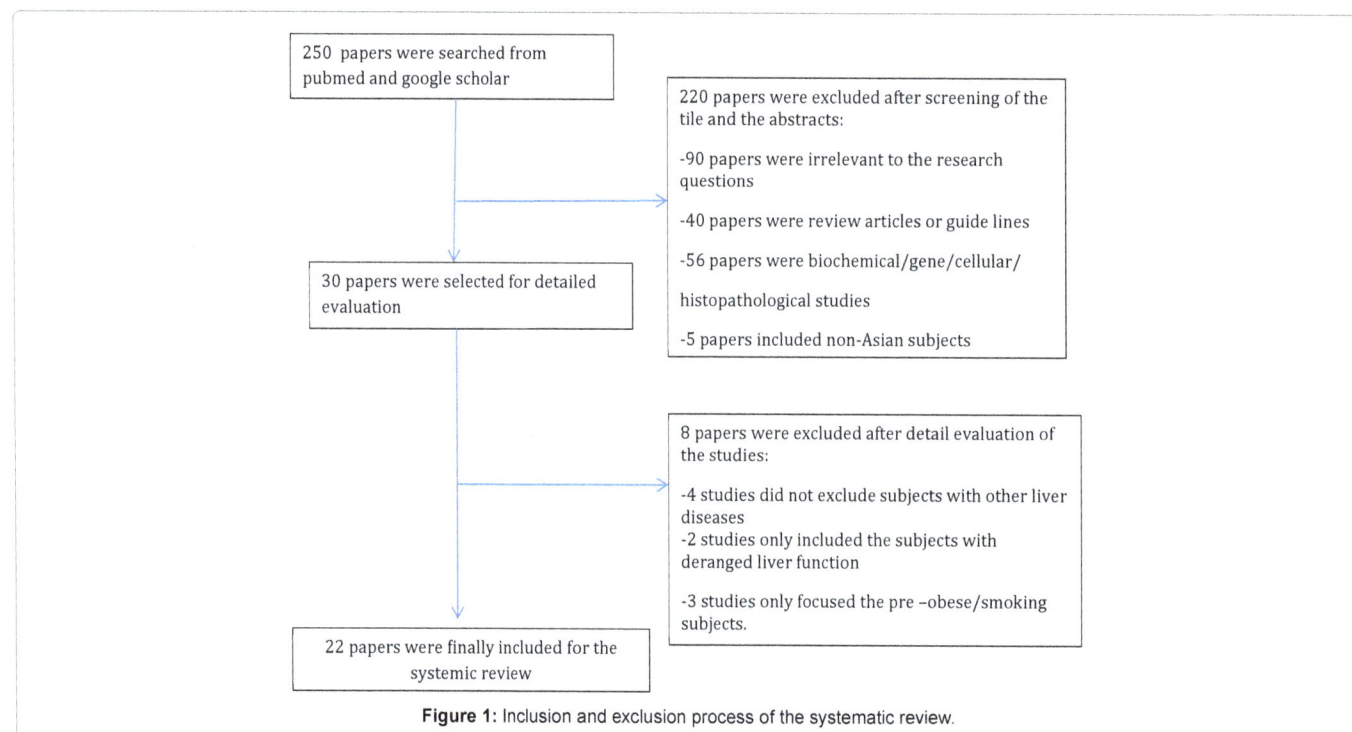

Figure 1: Inclusion and exclusion process of the systematic review.

However it is still uncertain whether the incidence of the metabolic diseases and thus the risk of cardiovascular diseases reduce after treatment of NAFLD. Prospective cohort studies would be necessary to answer these questions. The prevalence of childhood obesity and NAFLD is rising in Asia. Weight reduction is probably the only effective treatment for NAFLD in children so far, but it is still unknown how much weight should be lost to achieve the optimal outcome. .Furthermore, only few pharmacological treatments and anti-obesity drugs have been tested and investigated in children.

Limitations of this Systematic Review

As a result of industrialization, affluence, Westernization of lifestyle, lack of physical activity and over nutrition, the prevalence of NAFLD in Asian countries keeps rising and is comparable to the Western countries in recent decades. Similar to the results in Caucasian studies, obesity, glucose intolerance, DM, hyperlipidemia, hypertension and hyperuricemia are significant risk factors of NAFLD. Meanwhile, NAFLD is a strong predictor of metabolic diseases such as DM, hyperlipidemia and hypertension which are also the risk factors of cardiovascular diseases e.g. CHD and stroke. Only a small proportion of NAFLD patients may progress to liver cirrhosis and even hepatocellular carcinoma over a long period of time. However, more importantly, NAFLD patients may have much higher risks of developing diseases such as DM, hypertension, CHD and stroke.

Yet, the level of alertness of NAFLD remains low in India. As a significant risk factor of stroke, CHD, DM and hypertension, public awareness of NAFLD should be improved. More health promotion programs and educations focusing on NAFLD by the Government should be provided. Guidelines on the management of patients with NAFLD should be designed and endorsed among the primary health care providers. People with NAFLD should be screened and regularly followed up for the associated metabolic diseases. Aggressive treatments of NALFD such as lifestyle modification and anti-obesity treatment should also be actively considered and provided.

References

1. De Bruyne RM, Fitzpatrick E, Dhawan A (2010) Fatty liver disease in children: eat now pay later. Hepatol Int 4: 375-385.

2. Adams LA, Lymp JF, St Sauver J, Sanderson SO, Lindor KD, et al. (2005) The natural history of nonalcoholic fatty liver disease: a population-based cohort study. Gastroenterology 129: 113-121.

3. Sobhonslidsuk A, Jongjirasiri S, Thakkinstian A, Wisedopas N, Bunnag P, et al. (2007) Visceral fat and insulin resistance as predictors of non-alcoholic steatohepatitis. World J Gastroenterol 13: 3614-3618.

4. Duvnjak M, Lerotic I, Barsic N, Tomasic V, Jukic LV, et al. (2007) Pathogenesis and management issues for non-alcoholic fatty liver disease. World J Gastroenterol 13: 4539-4550.

5. Wanless IR, Lentz JS (1990) Fatty liver hepatitis (steatohepatitis) and obesity: an autopsy study with analysis of risk factors. Hepatology 12: 1106-1110.

6. French SW (1989) Biochemical basis for alcohol-induced liver injury. Clin Biochem 22: 41-49.

7. Hamer OW, Aguirre DA, Casola G, Lavine JE, Woenckhaus M, et al. (2006) Fatty liver: imaging patterns and pitfalls. Radiographics 26: 1637-1653.

8. Purohit V, Russo D, Coates PM (2004) Role of fatty liver, dietary fatty acid supplements, and obesity in the progression of alcoholic liver disease: introduction and summary of the symposium. Alcohol 34: 3-8.

9. El-Zayadi AR (2008) Hepatic steatosis: a benign disease or a silent killer. World J Gastroenterol 14: 4120-4126.

10. Bellentani S, Bedogni G, Miglioli L, Tiribelli C (2004) The epidemiology of fatty liver. Eur J Gastroenterol Hepatol 16: 1087-1093.

11. Bellentani S, Tiribelli C, Saccoccio G, Sodde M, Fratti N, et al. (1994) Prevalence of chronic liver disease in the general population of northern Italy: the Dionysos Study. Hepatology 20: 1442-1449.

12. List S, Gluud C (1994) A meta-analysis of HLA-antigen prevalences in alcoholics and alcoholic liver disease. Alcohol 29: 757-764.

13. Coates RA, Halliday ML, Rankin JG, Feinman SV, Fisher MM (1986) Risk of fatty infiltration or cirrhosis of the liver in relation to ethanol consumption: a case-control study. Clin Invest Med 9: 26-32.

14. Browning JD, Szczepaniak LS, Dobbins R, Nuremberg P, Horton JD, et al. (2004) Prevalence of hepatic steatosis in an urban population in the United States: impact of ethnicity. Hepatology 40: 1387-1395.

15. Crawford JM (2005) Metabolic liver disease. In Kumar V, Abbas AK, Fausto N (eds.): Robbins and Cotran, Pathologic Basis of Disease. Philadelphia: Elsevier Saunders.

16. Nobili V, Alisi A, Raponi M (2009) Pediatric non-alcoholic fatty liver disease: preventive and therapeutic value of lifestyle intervention. World J Gastroenterol 15: 6017-6022.

17. Bellentani S, Saccoccio G, Masutti F, Crocè LS, Brandi G, et al. (2000) Prevalence of and risk factors for hepatic steatosis in Northern Italy. Ann Intern Med 132: 112-117.

18. Hilden M, Christoffersen P, Juhl E, Dalgaard JB (1977) Liver histology in a 'normal' population – examinations of 503 consecutive fatal traffic casualties. Scand J Gastroenterol 12: 593-597.

19. Systematic Review (2008) Centre for Reviews and Dissemination's guidance for undertaking reviews in health care. Centre for Reviews and Dissemination, York University.

20. Elm EV, Altman DG, Egger M, Pocock SJ, Gøtzsche PC, et al. (2008) STROBE Initiative. The Strengthening the Reporting of Observational Studies in Epidemiology (STROBE) statement: guidelines for reporting observational studies. J Clin Epidemiol 61: 344-349.

21. WHO/IASO/IOTF (2000) The Asia-Pacific perspective: redefining obesity and its treatment. Health Communications Australia: Melbourne.

22. Deepa M, Farooq S, Datta M, Deepa R, Mohan V (2007) Prevalence of metabolic syndrome using WHO, ATP III and IDF definitions in Asian Indians – The Chennai Urban Rural Epidemiology Study (CURES – 34). Diabet Metab Res Rev 23: 127-134.

23. Expert Panel on Detection, Evaluation, and Treatment of High Blood Cholesterol in Adults (2001) Executive summary of the third report of the National Cholesterol Education Program (NCEP) Expert Panel on Detection, Evaluation and Treatment of High Blood Cholesterol in Adults (Adult Treatment Panel III). JAMA 285: 2486-2497.

24. Das K, Das K, Mukherjee PS, Ghosh A, Ghosh S, et al. (2010) Nonobese population in a developing country has a high prevalence of nonalcoholic fatty liver and significant liver disease. Hepatology 51: 1593-1602.

25. Lee YJ, Lee HR, Lee JH, Shin YH, Shim JY (2010) Association between serum uric acid and non-alcoholic fatty liver disease in Korean adults. Clin Chem Lab Med 48: 175-180.

26. Lee K (2009) Relationship between uric acid and hepatic steatosis among Koreans. Diabetes Metab 35: 447-451.

27. Dassanayake AS, Kasturiratne A, Rajindrajith S, Kalubowila U, Chakrawarthi S, et al. (2009) Prevalence and risk factors for non-alcoholic fatty liver disease among adults in an urban Sri Lankan population. J Gastroenterol Hepatol 24: 1284-1288.

28. Li Y, Xu C, Yu C, Xu L, Miao M (2009) Association of serum uric acid level with non-alcoholic fatty liver disease: a cross-sectional study. J Hepatol 50: 1029-1034.

29. Fu CC, Chen MC, Li YM, Liu TT, Wang LY (2009) The risk factors for ultrasound-diagnosed non-alcoholic fatty liver disease among adolescents. Ann Acad Med Singapore 38: 15-17.

30. Mohan V, Farooq S, Deepa M, Ravikumar R, Pitchumoni CS (2009) Prevalence of non-alcoholic fatty liver disease in urban south Indians in relation to different grades of glucose intolerance and metabolic syndrome. Diabetes Res Clin Pract 84: 84-91.

31. Lee K, Sung JA, Kim JS, Park TJ (2009) The roles of obesity and gender on the relationship between metabolic risk factors and non-alcoholic fatty liver disease in Koreans. Diabetes Metab Res Rev 25: 150-155.

32. Tsai CH, Li TC, Lin CC (2008) Metabolic syndrome as a risk factor for nonalcoholic fatty liver disease. South Med J 101: 900-905.

33. Alavian SM, Mohammad-Alizadeh AH, Esna-Ashari F, Ardalan G, Hajarizadeh B (2009) Non-alcoholic fatty liver disease prevalence among school-aged children and adolescents in Iran and its association with biochemical and anthropometric measures. Liver Int 29: 159-163.

34. Zhou YJ, Li YY, Nie YQ, Ma JX, Lu LG, et al. (2007) Prevalence of fatty liver disease and its risk factors in the population of South China. World J Gastroenterol 13: 6419-6424.

35. Shibata M, Kihara Y, Taguchi M, Tashiro M, Otsuki M (2007) Nonalcoholic fatty liver disease is a risk factor for type 2 diabetes in middle-aged Japanese men. Diabetes Care 30: 2940-2944.

36. Lee JY, Kim KM, Lee SG, Yu E, Lim YS, et al. (2007) Prevalence and risk factors of non-alcoholic fatty liver disease in potential living liver donors in Korea: a review of 589 consecutive liver biopsies in a single center. J Hepatol 47: 239-244.

37. Chen CH, Huang MH, Yang JC, Nien CK, Yang CC, et al. (2006) Prevalence and risk factors of nonalcoholic fatty liver disease in an adult population of Taiwan: metabolic significance of nonalcoholic fatty liver disease in non-obese adults. J Clin Gastroenterol 40: 745-752.

38. Zelber-Sagi S, Nitzan-Kaluski D, Halpern Z, Oren R (2006) Prevalence of primary non-alcoholic fatty liver disease in a population-based study and its association with biochemical and anthropometric measures. Liver Int 26: 856-863.

39. Park SH, Jeon WK, Kim SH, Kim HJ, Park DI, et al. (2006) Prevalence and risk factors of non-alcoholic fatty liver disease among Korean adults. J Gastroenterol Hepatol 21: 138-143.

40. Fan JG, Zhu J, Li XJ, Chen L, Lu YS, et al. (2005) Fatty liver and the metabolic syndrome among Shanghai adults. J Gastroenterol Hepatol 20: 1825-1832.

41. Jimba S, Nakagami T, Takahashi M, Wakamatsu T, Hirota Y, et al. (2005) Prevalence of non-alcoholic fatty liver disease and its association with impaired glucose metabolism in Japanese adults. Diabet Med 22: 1141-1145.

42. Kagansky N, Levy S, Keter D, Rimon E, Taiba Z, et al. (2004) Non-alcoholic fatty liver disease--a common and benign finding in octogenarian patients. Liver Int 24: 588-594.

43. Singh SP, Nayak S, Swain M, Rout N, Mallik RN, et al. (2004) Prevalence of nonalcoholic fatty liver disease in coastal eastern India: a preliminary ultrasonographic survey. Trop Gastroenterol 25: 76-79.

44. Shen L, Fan JG, Shao Y, Zeng MD, Wang JR, et al. (2003) Prevalence of nonalcoholic fatty liver among administrative officers in Shanghai: an epidemiological survey. World J Gastroenterol 9: 1106-1110.

45. Omagari K, Kadokawa Y, Masuda J, Egawa I, Sawa T, et al. (2002) Fatty liver in non-alcoholic non-overweight Japanese adults: incidence and clinical characteristics. J Gastroenterol Hepatol 17: 1098-1105.

46. Fung KT, Fung J, Lai CL, Yuen MF (2007) Etiologies of chronic liver diseases in Hong Kong. Eur J Gastroenterol Hepatol 19: 659-664.

47. Lang ZW, Hu ZJ, Wang SK, Zhang LJ, Meng X, et al. (2003) A clinico pathological study on nonalcoholic steatohepatitis. Zhonghua Gan Zang Bing Za Zhi 11: 81-83.

48. Sushma S (2003) Natural history and determinants of disease progression in nonalcoholic fatty liver disease: good and bad news. Hepatology 38.

49. Amarapurkar DN, Patel ND (2004) Clinical spectrum and natural history of non-alcoholic steatohepatitis with normal alanine aminotransferase values. Trop Gastroenterol 25: 130-134.

50. Fan JG, Li F, Cai XB, Peng YD, Ao QH, et al. (2007) Effects of nonalcoholic fatty liver disease on the development of metabolic disorders. J Gastroenterol Hepatol 22: 1086-1091.

51. Hui AY, Wong VW, Chan HL, Liew CT, Chan JL, et al. (2005) Histological progression of non-alcoholic fatty liver disease in Chinese patients. Aliment Pharmacol Ther 21: 407-413.

52. Targher G, Bertolini L, Poli F, Rodella S, Scala L, et al. (2005) Nonalcoholic fatty liver disease and risk of future cardiovascular events among type 2 diabetic patients. Diabetes 54: 3541-3546.

53. Yoon KH, Lee JH, Kim JW, Cho JH, Choi YH, et al. (2006) Epidemic obesity and type 2 diabetes in Asia. Lancet 368: 1681-1688.

54. Liu KH, Chan YL, Chan JC, Chan WB, Kong WL (2006) Mesenteric fat thickness as an independent determinant of fatty liver. Int J Obes (Lond) 30: 787-793.

55. Deurenberg P, Deurenberg-Yap M, Guricci S (2002) Asians are different from Caucasians and from each other in their body mass index/body fat per cent relationship. Obes Rev 3: 141-146.

56. Moran JR, Ghishan FK, Halter SA, Greene HL (1983) Steatohepatitis in obese children: a cause of chronic liver dysfunction. Am J Gastroenterol 78: 374-377.

57. Kinugasa A, Tsunamoto K, Furukawa N, Sawada T, Kusunoki T, et al. (1984) Fatty liver and its fibrous changes found in simple obesity of children. J Pediatr Gastroenterol Nutr 3: 408-414.

58. Tominaga K, Kurata JH, Chen YK, Fujimoto E, Miyagawa S, et al. (1995) Prevalence of fatty liver in Japanese children and relationship to obesity. An epidemiological ultrasonographic survey. Dig Dis Sci 40: 2002-2009.

59. Chan DF, Li AM, Chu WC, Chan MH, Wong EM, et al. (2004) Hepatic steatosis in obese Chinese children. Int J Obes Relat Metab Disord 28: 1257-1263.

60. Janus ED, Watt NMS, Lam KSL, Cockram CS, Siu STS, et al. (2000) The prevalence of diabetes, association with cardiovascular risk factors and implications of diagnostic criteria (ADA 1997 and WHO 1998) in a 1996 community based population study in Hong Kong Chinese. Diabet Med 17: 741-745.

61. Chan BS, Tsang MW, Lee VW, Lee KK (2007) Cost of Type 2 Diabetes mellitus in Hong Kong Chinese. Int J Clin Pharmacol Ther 45: 455-468.

62. Kung AWC, Janus ED, Lau C (1996) The prevalence of diabetes mellitus and its effect in elderly subjects in Hong Kong. Hong Kong Med J 2: 26-33.

63. Hospital Authority. Statistical Report 08/09. 38.

64. Lee VW, Chan WK, Lee KK (2006) A cost analysis in patients with acute coronary syndrome using clopidogrel in addition to aspirin in a Hong Kong public hospital. Int Heart J 47: 739-744.

65. Leung CM, Lai LS, Wong WH, Chan KH, Luk YW, et al. (2009) Non-alcoholic fatty liver disease: an expanding problem with low levels of awareness in Hong Kong. J Gastroenterol Hepatol 24: 1786-1790.

29

Inpatients' Outcomes Following Diabetic Myocardial Infarction: Income, Insurance, and Length of Stay in Teaching vs. Nonteaching Hospitals

Priscilla O Okunji[1]*, Johnnie Daniel[2] and Anthony Wutoh[3]

[1]Howard University College of Nursing and Allied Health Sciences, Washington, DC, USA
[2]Department of Sociology and Anthropology, Washington, DC, USA
[3]College of Pharmacy, Washington, DC, USA

Abstract

This paper assesses whether there is a significant difference in socioeconomic condition (income), insurance status, and Length of Stay (LOS) of inpatients diagnosed with diabetic myocardial infarction in teaching vs nonteaching hospitals. A retrospective data analysis of discharges was conducted from the 2008 Healthcare Cost and Utilization Project, Nationwide Inpatient Sample. Sample selection was based on the International Classification of Diseases, Ninth Revision, codes with LOS as the outcome variable. Teaching hospitals have longer LOS compared to nonteaching hospitals for patients with incomes below \$48,000 (χ^2=16.185, df=6, $P \leq 0.013$). The duration of hospital LOS is higher in teaching than in nonteaching hospitals for patient insurance (χ^2=24.975, df=6, P=0.0001). For patients with Medicare, the hospital stay of 1 day and less is lower in nonteaching hospitals. Teaching hospitals have higher rates of LOS than nonteaching hospitals for the age group, 65-74 (χ^2=37.294, df=6, P=0.0001). Especially for hospital stays of more than 6 days, the LOS is higher in teaching hospitals. The difference in LOS in teaching and nonteaching hospitals is statistically significant for males (P=0.009) vs. females (P=0.003). The results of this study indicate that the difference in LOS between teaching and nonteaching hospitals based on patient age, income, and insurance is statistically significant. When one controls for the independent variables in this study, the difference presented is large enough to affect clinical policy. These findings highlight the need for interventions to increase awareness of health care disparities that exist among inpatients with diabetic myocardial infarction, especially for low-income and older patients who do not qualify for Medicare.

Keywords: Teaching hospitals; Nonteaching hospitals; Myocardial infarction; Diabetes; Outcomes

Background

Coronary artery disease is the leading cause of premature, permanent disability in the United States, accounting for about 20% of disability allowances by the Social Security Administration (AHA) [1]. According to the 2008 National Healthcare Disparity Report, mortality from myocardial infarction (MI) in 2005 was 652,091, ranking first while diabetes ranked sixth with a mortality rate of 75,119 and total cost of \$174 billion with \$116 billion in direct medical cost. The total cost for cardiovascular diseases in 2008 was \$448.5 billion with a direct medical cost of \$296.4 billion [2]. Approximately \$86 billion, or 12%, of all US health care expenditures can be attributed to diabetes. Hospital characteristics have important effects on hospital outcomes [3]. Most, but not all, prior studies have reported lower risk-adjusted mortality in teaching hospitals as compared with nonteaching hospitals [4], perhaps because the quality and processes of care delivered in teaching hospitals are better than those in nonteaching hospitals. However, few studies have reported more mortality rates in teaching hospitals and the outcomes in minor teaching hospitals. Hence, Polanczyk et al. [5] and Dowell et al. [6] concluded that whether the outcomes observed in minor teaching hospitals were due to hospital characteristics, quality, or process of care factors still needs to undergo further investigation.

Furthermore, most studies on the hospital characteristics and their treatment outcomes have been focused on other acute and chronic diseases like AIDS [7], chronic heart failure and pneumonia [8], acute MI alone [4], and cardiovascular diseases alone [5]. Other studies concentrate on hospital characteristics and patient safety indicators [9], preventable adverse effects [10] and effects of hospital characteristics and economy on T2D [6]. No study has focused on hospital characteristics

and patients with both MI and T2D treatments with regard to patients' Length of Stay (LOS). Cook et al. [11], Dowell et al. [6], and Okunji [12] saw this need and recommended further investigation of these variables in teaching and nonteaching hospitals in the treatment of patients with T2D. Hence, the difference in teaching and nonteaching hospitals with respect to patients' LOS in MI inpatient with T2D was important for this particular population. For example, could teaching vs. nonteaching hospitals differ significantly in inpatients' LOS?

Hypothesis: Specific Aims and Hypotheses

Specific aim 1

To determine if there was a significant difference in outcome (LOS) for diabetic MI inpatients treated at teaching vs. non-teaching hospitals.

Research hypothesis 1

There was a significant difference in outcome (LOS) for diabetic MI inpatients admitted to teaching vs. nonteaching hospitals.

Specific aim 2

To determine if there was a significant difference in LOS by diabetic MI characteristics (age, gender, ethnicity, income, comorbidities, and insurance) in teaching vs. nonteaching hospitals.

*Corresponding author: Priscilla O Okunji, Howard University College of Nursing and Allied Health Sciences, Washington, DC, USA, E-mail: pokunji@aol.com

Research hypothesis 2

There was a significant difference in LOS by patient characteristics (age, gender, ethnicity, income, comorbidities, and insurance) for diabetic MI inpatients in teaching vs. nonteaching hospitals.

Theoretical Framework

The organizing framework of this study was based on the Quality of Health Model of Care. This model proposed by the American Academy of Nursing Expert Panel on Quality Health Care (1998) is useful for measuring reciprocal directions of influences of multiple variables that affect quality of care and desired health outcomes. This dynamic model applied to evaluating health care delivery systems allows researchers to utilize data bases to delineate the relevant interrelationships between patient level characteristics, the context in which care is provided, the quality of provider intervention, and, ultimately, health outcomes. This model is an expansion of the framework proposed by Donabedian [13], which posits that structure affects process and process affects outcome when patient characteristics are considered as mediating outcomes. The Quality of Health Model broadens Donebenian's framework for quality improvement and outcomes management by examining dynamic relationships with indicators that not only act on but also reciprocally affect the various components. The current study may contribute to policy decision making for organizational or system-level improvements, development of interventions and training for improved provider clinical interventions or treatment options, and descriptively address patient-level needs for self-management.

Research Design and Methodology

The study design was a secondary data analysis from the 2008 Healthcare Cost and Utilization Project (HCUP) Nationwide Inpatient Sample (NIS) [14]. HCUP is a family of health care databases and related software tools and products developed through a federal-state-industry partnership and are sponsored by the Agency for Healthcare Research and Quality (AHRQ). HCUP databases bring together the data collection efforts of state data organizations, hospital associations, private data organizations, and the federal government to create a national information resource of patient-level health care data (HCUP Partners). HCUP is the largest collection of longitudinal hospital care data in the United States and includes all-payer, encounter-level information beginning in 1988. These databases enable research on a broad range of health policy issues, including cost and quality of health services, medical practice patterns, access to health care programs, and outcomes of treatments at the national, state, and local market levels. Howard University Internal Review Board (IRB) clearance was obtained prior to the initiation of the project, along with the HIPAA certification by HCUP prior to database purchase.

Patient measures

Age (20 years and above); gender (male, female); ethnicity (white, black, Hispanic, Asian, Native American); income ($1-38,999; $39,000-$47,999; $48,000-$62,999; $63,000 and above); insurance (Medicare, Medicaid, private including HMO, self-pay, no charge).

Outcomes measures

LOS.

Study population

The HCUP NIS [14] database contains data from 5 to 8 million hospital stays from 1000 hospitals sampled to approximately a 20% stratified sample of US community hospitals. In this research,

participants' data were selected from the hospital discharge information according to patients' characteristics (age, gender, ethnicity, income, and insurance). Selection of samples was aided by the existing NIS database and ICD-9-CM (HCUP CCS) [15]. Patients aged up to 7 years were not included in this study based on the prevalence within this population of type 1 diabetes. However, among the age group 20 and above, young adults were included in this study because of the increased prevalence of type 2 diabetes in this population due to diet, lifestyle, and obesity. The NIS database samples were selected and extracted based on the following criteria: (a) inpatient diagnosed with both MI and T2D, (b) admitted in nonfederal hospitals, and (c) age 20 years and above; exclusions included (d) obstetrics-gynecologic, ear-nose-throat, orthopedic, and pediatric patients, and (e) short-term acute rehabilitation and long-term nonacute care patients, and psychiatric and alcoholism/chemical dependency treatment patients. In reviewing the statistical results of the study, we first indicated whether a finding was statistically significant. We then assessed the practical significance of the findings and indicated whether the observed differences were large enough to affect clinical policy.

Results

Nonteaching hospitals serve higher proportion of whites than do teaching hospitals Also, these patients may be transferred or die before discharge from teaching hospitals; hence other ethnic groups stay for a shorter period than the white population, with the biggest inequality among low-income patients and shorter LOS in nonteaching hospitals (Table 1).

A patient under 65 years of age was higher for teaching hospitals than for nonteaching hospitals; on the other hand the percentage of patients 75 years or older was higher for nonteaching hospitals than for teaching hospitals. The findings as it relates to Hypothesis 1 showed that teaching hospitals have longer LOS than nonteaching hospitals. Especially for a hospital stay of more than 4 days with exception of 2 days of LOS, the percentage of older patients is higher in nonteaching

	Nonteaching Hospital	Teaching Hospital
Age		
Less than 45 years	6.4	8.1
45 to 54	15.6	17.3
55 to 64	23.4	26.2
65 to 74	24.1	23.9
75 or older	**30.5**	**24.5**
Number of cases	2434	2008
$x^2 = 24$, df = 4, $P = .000$		
Gender		
Male	**56.7**	**60.3**
Female	**43.3**	**39.7**
Number of cases	2435	2008
$X^2 = 6$, df = 1, $P = .009$		
Ethnicity		
White	**75.5**	**67.5**
Black	**6.6**	**14.0**
Hispanic	8.9	9.9
Other	9.0	8.6
Number of cases	2010	1609
$X^2 = 58$, df = 3, $P = .0001$		

Table 1: Percentage Distribution of Age, Gender, and Ethnicity of Diabetic Myocardial Infarction Patients in Nonteaching and Teaching Hospitals.

hospitals. The difference in teaching and nonteaching hospitals is statistically significant because more older patients aged 65-74 years stayed longer in the hospital than their younger counterparts (χ^2=37.294, df=6, P =0.0001) (Table 2).

The percentage of males in both teaching (60.3%) and nonteaching (56.7%) hospitals was higher than the percentage of females in these hospitals. More females stayed longer days in the hospital than their male counterparts (χ^2=19.621, df=6, P=0.003) with increased length of stay of 7 to 13 days in teaching (24.9%) compared to nonteaching (21.3%) hospitals (Table 3). The difference between teaching and nonteaching hospitals is statistically significant; however, it is not large enough to affect clinical policy.

Furthermore, the results indicate that more patients with Medicare had shorter LOS (χ^2=24.975, df=6, P=0.0001) in nonteaching hospitals, but those with self-pay stayed the fewest days in both teaching and nonteaching hospitals although Medicare was the major insurance used by inpatients with MI and T2D in 2008 (Table 4).

The extent of hospital LOS for a day or less than 1 day was higher in nonteaching than in teaching hospitals for income below $48,000. Especially for the income groups of $1-$38,999 and $39,000-$47,999 the percentage was higher in nonteaching hospitals for 1 day and less and 4 days, respectively. The difference between teaching and nonteaching hospitals was statistically significant for lower-income patients and was

large enough to affect clinical policy. The results have shown that the patient's length of stay is proportional to the patient's income, which may be due to the type of insurance. Insurance type may not qualify the patient to stay longer, have quality treatment, recover, and be discharged home. The percentage of hospital length of stay for a day or less than 1 day was higher in nonteaching than in teaching hospitals for patients with insurance, especially with Medicare (Table 5).

The difference between teaching and nonteaching hospitals was statistically significant and large enough to affect clinical policy. This may be due to the aged population coupled with the fact that the government covers this insurance from age 65 years and above. Hence one policy option is that Medicaid should be expanded to cover more patients who may not be qualified for Medicare.

The hospital length of stay for a day or less than 1 day is higher in nonteaching than in teaching hospitals in terms of patients' co-morbidities. Especially for patients with hypertension, the rate is higher in nonteaching hospitals (Table 6). The percentage of longer lengths of stay (7-13 days) for congestive heart failure was also higher in nonteaching hospitals. The results correlate with the symptomatic effects of MI-high blood pressure resulting in rupture, clot, and necrotic tissues-which limit blood circulation and result in myocardial infarction. Thus, there should be a policy in place to screen all diabetic patients for hypertension and other co-morbidities to prevent complications such as MI.

	Age									
	Less than 45 years		45 to 54 years		55 to 64 years		65 to 74 years		75 years or older	
	Nonteaching Hospital	Teaching Hospital	Nonteaching Hospital	Teaching Hospital	Nonteaching Hospital	Teaching Hospital	Nonteaching Hospital	Teaching Hospital	Nonteaching Hospital	Teaching Hospital
	Length of Stay									
1 day or less than 1 day	9.0	4.9	9.8	8.6	9.0	7.2	**11.1**	**6.5**	**12.4**	**8.9**
2 days	16.0	21.0	18.7	21.0	14.6	16.3	12.8	12.9	11.3	11.6
3 days	21.2	21.0	20.3	19.5	19.7	20.5	20.3	14.0	15.7	15.7
4 days	19.2	19.8	14.2	13.2	14.2	12.5	15.5	10.6	13.6	12.0
5 to 6 days	17.3	13.0	12.9	14.1	16.9	17.5	16.7	17.5	15.2	18.3
7 to 13 days	14.7	16.0	19.3	18.1	19.5	19.8	18.1	27.5	24.0	22.6
14 days or longer	2.6	4.3	4.7	5.5	6.2	6.1	**5.6**	**11.0**	**7.8**	**11.0**
Total	100.0	100.0	100.0	100.0	100.0	100.0	100.0	100.0	100.0	100.0
Number	156	162	379	348	569	526	587	480	743	492
	χ^2 = 4.729, df = 6, P = .579		χ^2 = 1.401, df = 6, P = .966		χ^2 = 2.318, df = 6, P = .888		**χ^2 = 37.294, df = 6, P = .0001**		χ^2 = 9.025, df = 6, P = .172	

Table 2:P Percentage Distribution of the Length of Stay by Age for Diabetic Myocardial Infarction Patients in Nonteaching and Teaching Hospitals.

	Gender			
	Male		Female	
	Nonteaching Hospital	Teaching Hospital	Nonteaching Hospital	Teaching Hospital
Length of Stay				
1 day or less than 1 day	**10.6**	**7.4**	**10.6**	**7.8**
2 days	14.1	18.1	13.6	11.7
3 days	20.3	19.2	16.8	15.3
4 days	14.3	12.6	15.2	12.7
5 to 6 days	15.6	16.5	15.8	17.0
7 to 13 days	19.3	19.6	21.3	24.9
14 days or longer	5.6	6.6	**6.6**	**10.7**
Total	100.0	100.0	100.0	100.0
Number	1381	1210	1054	798
	χ^2 =17.072, df = 6, P = .009		χ^2 = 19.621, df = 6, P = .003	

Table 3: Percentage Distribution of the Length of Stay by Gender for Diabetic Myocardial Infarction Patients in Non- Teaching and Teaching Hospitals.

	Income							
	$1 to $38,999		$39,000–$47,999		$48,000–$62,999		$63,000 or Higher	
	Nonteaching Hospital	Teaching Hospital	Nonteaching Hospital	Teaching Hospital	Nonteaching Hospital	Teaching Hospital	Nonteaching Hospital	Teaching Hospital
Length of Stay								
1 day or less than 1 day	**12.1**	**6.2**	9.6	9.2	9.2	7.1	11.6	8.4
2 days	12.3	14.1	13.7	17.6	16.4	14.7	13.4	15.8
3 days	20.1	18.3	17.7	18.6	18.2	18.4	19.0	14.4
4 days	15.2	13.4	**16.4**	**9.9**	13.2	11.3	13.9	16.0
5 to 6 days	15.9	14.6	15.8	16.9	16.4	18.4	14.2	17.5
7 to 13 days	17.7	23.9	21.6	20.4	20.8	21.7	21.0	19.6
14 days or longer	6.7	9.5	5.2	7.4	6.0	8.3	6.8	8.4
Total	100.0	100.0	100.0	100.0	100.0	100.0	100.0	100.0
Number	705	568	773	544	501	434	395	418
	$\chi^2 = 23.032$, df = 6, $P = 0.001$		$\chi^2 = 16.185$, df = 6, $P = 0.013$		$\chi^2 = 4.660$, df = 6, $P = 0.588$		$\chi^2 = 8.396$, df = 6, $P = 0.211$	

Table 4: Percentage Distribution of the Length of Stay by Income for Diabetic Myocardial Infarction Patients in Nonteaching and Teaching Hospitals

	Type of Health Insurance									
	Medicare		Medicaid		Private		Self-Pay		Other	
	Nonteaching Hospital	Teaching Hospital	Nonteaching Hospital	Teaching Hospital	Nonteaching Hospital	Teaching Hospital	Nonteaching Hospital	Teaching Hospital	Nonteaching Hospital	Teaching Hospital
Length of Stay										
1 day or less than 1 day	**11.6**	**7.9**	10.0	8.6	9.1	5.5	11.1	11.8	10.2	8.7
2 days	12.0	13.0	19.4	14.1	16.4	18.0	14.8	22.1	8.0	18.5
3 days	16.3	15.0	21.9	11.7	21.0	22.0	21.6	22.8	27.3	18.5
4 days	14.3	10.8	10.6	12.3	15.9	14.4	14.2	15.4	17.0	17.4
5 to 6 days	16.4	17.5	11.9	15.3	15.1	17.6	16.7	12.5	15.9	12.0
7 to 13 days	22.2	24.9	19.4	26.4	17.5	17.9	19.8	12.5	15.9	18.5
14 days or longer	7.2	10.9	6.9	11.7	5.0	4.6	1.9	2.9	5.7	6.5
Total	100.0	100.0	100.0	100.0	100.0	100.0	100.0	100.0	100.0	100.0
Number	1298	983	160	163	569	526	162	136	88	92
	$\chi^2 = 24.975$, df = 6, $P = 0.0001$		$\chi^2 = 11.173$, df = 6, $P = 0.083$		$\chi^2 = 8.384$, df = 6, $P = 0.211$		$\chi^2 = 5.902$, df = 6, $P = 0.434$		$\chi^2 = 6.108$, df=6, $P=0.411$	

Table 5: Percentage Distribution of the Length of Stay by Type of Health Insurance for Diabetic Myocardial Infarction Patients in Nonteaching and Teaching Hospitals.

	Comorbidities					
	Congestive Heart Failure		Chronic Pulmonary Disease		Hypertension	
	Nonteaching Hospital	Teaching Hospital	Nonteaching Hospital	Teaching Hospital	Nonteaching Hospital	Teaching Hospital
Length of Stay						
1 day or less than 1 day	5.3	9.4	8.1	8.3	**10.9**	**6.9**
2 days	7.1	4.2	13.9	10.2	13.7	15.2
3 days	11.8	10.4	16.9	15.2	18.6	18.5
4 days	11.8	14.6	12.1	11.2	14.8	12.4
5 to 6 days	13.6	12.5	14.4	17.5	15.5	16.7
7 to 13 days	**34.9**	**25.0**	27.5	26.7	19.9	21.5
14 days or longer	15.4	24.0	7.1	10.9	6.5	8.8
Total	100.0	100.0	100.0	100.0	100.0	100.0
Number	169	96	396	303	1681	1457
	$\chi^2 = 7.231$, df = 6, $P = 0.300$		$\chi^2 = 6.269$, df = 6, $P = .394$		$\chi^2 = 25.236$, df = 6, $P = 0.0001$	

Table 6: Percentage Distribution of the Length of Stay by Selected Comorbidities for Diabetic Myocardial Infarction Patients in Nonteaching and Teaching Hospitals.

Discussion

The outcomes of this study are in line with those of Hogan et al. [16], who reported that although MI and T2D disorders affect all age groups, the diseases become increasingly prevalent with age and have the greatest effect on elderly people, as well as minority ethnic populations. Hogan et al. [16] estimated that more than 18% of adults older than 65 have diabetes, the majority diagnosed with type 2 diabetes. As the fifth leading cause of death in the United States, this disease has a significant effect on health, quality of life, longevity, and health care systems [16].

The result supports the observation that women usually do not exhibit classical symptoms of MI like their male counterparts, and thus they are not aggressively treated. Their conditions are usually complicated by the time they are diagnosed with MI. According to Cook et al. [11], Silent Myocardial Ischemia (SMI), a common disorder, has been studied by different research groups for the past 25 years. It is known that SMI is more common in patients with T2D than in the general population, even though the factors that contribute to the health care disparity in treatments and outcomes are unclear. Despite the fact that the number of males who were admitted far outnumbered females, the fewer females who were admitted stayed longer in the hospital than did males [11].

Between teaching and nonteaching hospitals there was a significant difference in LOS by income lower than $48,000, but this was not significant for patients with income higher than $48,000. Within the income group $1–$39,999, the difference was significant for patients with LOS of a day or less than 1 day in nonteaching hospitals (12.1%) than in teaching hospitals (6.2%). Hence the effect of income did correlate with the notion that income is proportional to the length of stay. Generally, the lower a patient's income is, the shorter his/her length of stay. This correlation may be due to the type of insurance or income that may not qualify the patient to have quality treatment procedures and enable them to stay longer. This difference is also significant among all minority ethnic groups who stayed a day or less in nonteaching hospitals compared with teaching hospitals.

Each year in the United States, the numbers of people who are underinsured and uninsured rises. As the population of the United States becomes more diverse, minorities are more likely to be uninsured because of their lack of education and cultural barriers to health care. This analysis explains why the method of health care payment is crucial to the patients' outcome. The investigators suggest that commercial insurance companies tend to focus more on profit rather than on the outcome of the patients, which explains why patients who stayed the least were not necessarily the patients most fit to be discharged. Hence, the recent proposed healthcare reform would be efficacious if one could also count on quality and affordable care. If this new reform is adopted, Medicaid will be expanded to millions of people and will increase eligibility for Medicaid to lower-income individuals. It is expected that the federal government will initially bear the entire debt or taxation burden of this expansion, with states assuming some of the burden in later years [17].

Hence, these results support the alternative hypothesis that there is a significant difference in teaching and nonteaching hospitals and LOS when one controls for patient age, gender, ethnicity, income, and insurance possession for patients admitted with both MI and T2D to US hospitals in 2008.

This study has several limitations. First, it was based on a retrospective analysis of a nationwide hospital discharge database (HCUP NIS) [14]. The variables that affected individual health status at admissions, such as duration and patterns of disease, knowledge of the disease state, adherence to therapeutic interventions, and previous lifestyle behaviors, were not included in the database [6]. Second, MI in this study includes both old MI and acute MI as classified in HCUP-NIS ICD 9 codes (41000). It is well known that the pathophysiologies of the diseases associated to this code are quite different, and the different treatment strategies may influence LOS strongly. According to Steinberg et al. [18], although ICD-9 codes have been in use for decades to classify patients with AMI in the United States, they did not allow characterization of patients with ST Elevation MI (STEMI) vs. non-ST elevation myocardial infarction (NSTEMI).

Furthermore, many factors influence people's efforts to change behavior in a way that improves and maintains health status, and the factors are not provided in the database used. These factors include life style, level of education, self-esteem, motivation, and self-image. The value placed on health, the threat of potential losses, and the perceived benefits of behavior modifications are important motivating factors. The patient-support network and availability of health-promotion programs and health care systems have influence on health care behaviors. Some people may be prevented from accessing health-promotion programs because of medical insurance, as discussed in this study.

Significance of Study

Because of the challenges involved in analyzing from secondary data the attributes that contribute to quality care, this study not only gives the data about LOS of inpatients with both MI and T2D, but it also provides the most detailed and recent data now available to compare quality of care for this population between teaching and nonteaching hospitals. There were disparities noted in the LOS outcome, most significantly in the equity area reflecting differences in patient age, gender, ethnic group, income, and insurance possession.

First, there was a significant relationship between patients' insurance and gender among patients admitted with MI and T2D. The disparity between gender and patient insurance is troubling and in line with findings. Okunji [12] reported that possession of insurance is crucial in access to health care, and these findings indicated that more men of all ethnical groups consistently had Medicare insurance (all types) than their female counterparts ($P=0.0001$). This result may explain why more males 1210 (60.3%) were admitted in teaching hospitals and more females 1054 (43.3%) were admitted in nonteaching hospitals. Older patients (65-74) had the shortest LOS. There was significant difference between the outcomes of teaching and nonteaching hospitals based on LOS. Ayanian et al. [8] reported that quality of care was consistently better in large teaching hospital than nonteaching hospitals; however, the authors confirmed the limitations of their study-documentation may have been more complete in teaching hospitals than in nonteaching hospitals because key information could be recorded by either attending or resident physicians.

Future Research

Further studies should be done to determine differences between teaching and nonteaching patient mortality rates using a more robust database that can account for all confounding variables in order to accurately predict the outcome. Results of further studies may warrant serious consideration in the formulation of national policies and programs to improve the quality of health care among inpatients with MI and T2D. Substantial overlap and inconsistency exists in ICD-9 codes for STEMI and NSTEMI patients, and the ICD-code 41000 is used for the two diseases. The new changes to future ICD-10 coding should allow a better description of quality measures and outcomes of the two different kinds of MI patients.

Implications

Acute care facilities in the United States spent $83 billion in 2008 caring for people with diabetes. One of every 5 hospitalizations involved a person with diabetes during that year. This amounts to 23% of hospital expenditures to treat all conditions in 2008. According to HCUP NIS Agency AHRQ [14], the expenditures in these hospital included costs associated with more than 540,000 hospital stays.

Hence, there is an established association between hyperglycemia, length of stay, and hospital costs in T2D inpatients. These patients are known to require longer lengths of hospitalization for any given admission diagnosis [12,19-22]. The increased LOS is probably related to the degree of hyperglycemia present during the course of hospitalization. Estrada et al. [23] found that the LOS among cardiac surgery patients with diabetes was 0.76 days longer for every 50-mg/dL increase in glucose. Further, many studies have shown that lowering the average blood glucose level of hospitalized patients has a significant benefit on important clinical outcomes such as mortality and infection rates [24,25]. According to Newton and Young [26], the decrease in the LOS for patients with diabetes has resulted in a savings of more than $2 million. This savings was calculated from the salaries of the Program Director, Program Administrative Office Assistant, as well as consultant fees for the Medical Director and the data management and product services provided by American Health ways. This added value yields a 467% return on investment [26].

Conclusions

This study has generated a new data about patient LOS with inpatient diabetic MI. The data gave a detailed and recent comparison between the quality of care in teaching and nonteaching hospitals for this population. This study has shown disparities in the LOS outcome and most significantly in the equity area in terms of differences in patient age, gender, ethnic group, comorbidities, income, and insurance possession. Hence, one notes an established association between hyperglycemia, LOS, and income in diabetic MI inpatients. However, future research should focus on more robust data and future ICD codes that would distinctively differentiate STEMI from NSTEMI for a more measurable and valid outcomes.

Acknowledgement

This grant is supported in part by National Institute of Health, National Center for Minority Health and Health Disparities, IS22 MD00241-21

References

1. Donna D. Ignatavicius , Workman ML (2009) Medical-Surgical nursing. Patient-centered collaborative care. (6thedn), Elsevier Sounders, St Loius, USA.

2. US Preventive Services Task Force (2002) Aspirin for the primary prevention of cardiovascular events: recommendation and rationale. Ann Intern Med 136: 157-160.

3. Yuan Z, Cooper GS, Einstadter D, Cebul RD, Rimm AA (2000) The association between hospital type and mortality and length of stay: a study of 16.9 million hospitalized Medicare beneficiaries. Med Care 38: 231-245.

4. Allison JJ, Kiefe CI, Weissman NW, Person SD, Rousculp M, et al. (2000) Relationship of hospital teaching status with quality of care and mortality for Medicare patients with acute MI. JAMA 284: 1256-1262.

5. Polanczyk CA, Lane A, Coburn M, Philbin EF, William, G, et al. (2002) Hospital Outcomes in Major Teaching, Minor Teaching, and Nonteaching Hospitals in New York State. Am J Med 112: 255-261.

6. Dowell MA, Rozell B, Roth D, Delugach H, Chaloux P, et al. (2004) Economic and clinical disparities in hospitalized patients with type 2 diabetes. J Nurs Scholarsh 36: 66-72.

7. Cunningham WE, Tisnado DM, Lui HH, Nakazono TT, Carlisle DM (1990) The effect of hospital experience on mortality among patients hospitalized with acquired immunodeficiency syndrome in California. Am J Medicinet 107: 137-143.

8. Ayanian JZ, Weissman JS, Chasan-Taber S, Epstein AM (1998) Quality of care for two common illnesses in teaching and nonteaching hospitals. Health Aff (Millwood) 17: 194-205.

9. Romano PS, Geppert JJ, Davies S, Miller MR, Elixhauser A, et al. (2003) A national profile of patient safety in U.S. hospitals. Health Aff (Millwood) 22: 154-166.

10. Sloan FA, Conover CJ, Provenzale D (2000) Hospital credentialing and quality of care. Soc Sci Med 50: 77-88.

11. Cook CB, Naylor DB, Hentz JG, Miller WJ, Tsui C, et al. (2006) Disparities in diabetes-related hospitalizations: relationship of age, sex, and race/ethnicity with hospital discharges, lengths of stay, and direct inpatient charges. Ethn Dis 16: 126-131.

12. Okunji PO (2010) Outcomes of patients with diabetic myocardial infarction in non federal hospitals: Effects of hospital and patient characteristics. Udini ProQuest.

13. Donabedian A (1966) Evaluating the quality of medical care. Milbank Mem Fund Q 44: 166-206.

14. Odum SM, Springer BD, Dennos AC, Fehring TK (2013) National Obesity Trends in Total Knee Arthroplasty. J Arthroplasty.

15. HCUP Clinical Classifications Software (CCS) for ICD-9-CM. Healthcare Cost and Utilization Project (HCUP) 2008. Agency for Healthcare Research and Quality, Rockville, MD.

16. Hogan P, Dall T, Nikolov P; American Diabetes Association (2003) Economic costs of diabetes in the US in 2002. Diabetes Care 26: 917-932.

17. Healthcare Reform Law (2010) Implementation Timeline for Small Business.

18. Steinberg BA, French WJ, Peterson ED, Frederick PD, Cannon CP, et al. (2006) Missed diagnosis of the diagnosis codes: comparison of International Classification of Diseases, 9th Revision coding and ST- versus non-ST-elevation myocardial infarction diagnosis in the National Registry of Myocardial Infarction. Crit Pathw Cardiol 5: 59-63.

19. Donnan PT, Leese GP, Morris AD (2000) Hospitalizations for people with type 1 and type 2 diabetes compared with the nondiabetic population of Tayside, Scotland: a retrospective cohort study of resource use. Diabetes Care 23: 1774-1779.

20. Umpierrez GE, Isaacs SD, Bazargan N, You X, Thaler LM, et al. (2002) Hyperglycemia: an independent marker of in-hospital mortality in patients with undiagnosed diabetes. J Clin Endocrinol Metab 87: 978-982.

21. Williams LS, Rotich J, Qi R, Fineberg N, Espay A, et al. (2002) Effects of admission hyperglycemia on mortality and costs in acute ischemic stroke. Neurology 59: 67-71.

22. Olveira-Fuster G, Olvera-Márquez P, Carral-Sanlaureano F, González-Romero S, Aguilar-Diosdado M, et al. (2004) Excess hospitalizations, hospital days, and inpatient costs among people with diabetes in Andalusia, Spain. Diabetes Care 27: 1904-1909.

23. Estrada CA, Young JA, Nifong LW, Chitwood WR Jr (2003) Outcomes and perioperative hyperglycemia in patients with or without diabetes mellitus undergoing coronary artery bypass grafting. Ann Thorac Surg 75: 1392-1399.

24. van den Berghe G, Wouters P, Weekers F, Verwaest C, Bruyninckx F, et al. (2001) Intensive insulin therapy in critically ill patients. N Engl J Med 345: 1359-1367.

25. Furnary AP, Gao G, Grunkemeier GL, Wu Y, Zerr KJ, et al. (2003) Continuous insulin infusion reduces mortality in patients with diabetes undergoing coronary artery bypass grafting. J Thorac Cardiovasc Surg 125: 1007-1021.

26. Newton CA, Young S (2006) Financial implications of glycemic control: results of an inpatient diabetes management program. Endocr Pract 12: 43-48.

30

Factors Associated with Metabolic Syndrome in Middle-aged Women with and without HIV

Akl LD[1,2], Valadares ALR[1,3], Gomes DC[1], Pinto-Neto AM[1] and Costa-Paiva L[1]*

[1]*State University of Campinas (UNICAMP), Campinas, SP, Brazil*
[2]*Eduardo de Menezes Hospital (HEM), Belo Horizonte, MG, Brazil*
[3]*José do Rosário Vellano University (UNIFENAS), Belo Horizonte, MG, Brazil*

Abstract

MetS is associated with an increased risk of cardiovascular disease, increases after menopause and it is probably more frequent in HIV women.

Objective: To assess MetS and associated factors in HIV seropositive and seronegative middle-aged women.

Methods: Cross-sectional study with 537 women (273 HIV seropositive and 264 HIV seronegative), between 40 and 60 years' old receiving follow-up care in two medical centers in Brazil. MetS was diagnosed based on IDF criteria. Sociodemographic, clinical, and behavioral factors were evaluated.

Results: The prevalence of MetS in the HIV group was 46.9% and 42.2% in the seronegative group (P=0.340). Multiple regression analysis showed MetS association with body mass index (BMI)>25 kg/m² (PR=2.34; 95% CI: 1.70-3.21; P<0.001), aging (PR: 0.05, 95% CI: 1.02-1.07; P<0.001), and the use of highly active retroviral therapy (HAART) (PR: 1.48; 95% CI: 1.13-1.94; P=0.005).

Conclusions: There was no association between MetS and HIV status overall. Although HAART was associated with MetS, it seems that HIV-positive women in good immunological status, after early institution of HAART and its effective use, have traditional factors associated with MetS like being overweight and having older age.

Keywords: Metabolic syndrome X; Menopause; AIDS; Overweight

Introduction

After the emergence of the human immunodeficiency virus (HIV) infection, and introduction of use of highly active antiretroviral therapy (HAART) in the 1990s, treatment of HIV patients has evolved considerably. There has been a drastic reduction in morbidity, mortality, and occurrence of opportunistic infections, and an increase in life expectancy [1].with HIV-infection acquiring the characteristics of a chronic disease [2]. With the increase in life expectancy, many HIV-infected women live to reach menopause [3], and the number of perimenopausal women with HIV infection is increasing in Brazil and elsewhere in the world [4].

Despite reducing morbidity and mortality, HAART is not without risk and is associated with some adverse effects [5-7], including metabolic abnormalities such as insulin resistance, diabetes, dyslipidemia, and body fat redistribution with increased waist circumference [8]. The natural course of HIV infection is characterized by low levels of high density lipoprotein (HDL) and low density lipoprotein (LDL), and increased levels of triglycerides (TG) [9]. With the introduction of HAART, more atherogenic changes in the lipid profile, including increased TG and LDL and decreased HDL have been observed [5-7].

The pathogenesis of dyslipidemia related to HAART is complex and involves multiple drug-induced effects, in combination with hormonal and immunological effects. Postmenopausal women who experience low estrogen levels have an increased risk of hypertension, dyslipidemia, diabetes, and cardiovascular disease (CVD) compared with premenopausal women [10]. Menopause is associated with lower energy consumption and consequent weight gain, with increased central fat deposition [10]. Thus, HIV-infected post-menopausal women have metabolic risks not only from HIV infection and HAART but also from the consequences of estrogen reduction. These metabolic changes can contribute to metabolic syndrome (MetS), defined as a complex disorder represented by a cluster of cardiovascular risk factors commonly associated with central fat deposition, insulin resistance, hypertension, and dyslipidemia [11].

There are many operational definitions for MetS [12-14]. The International Diabetes Federation (IDF) diagnostic criteria for MetS in women are: waist circumference ≥ 80 cm and two or more of the following factors: TG ≥ 150 mg/dL or treatment for this abnormality; HDL cholesterol<50 mg/dL or treatment for this abnormality; systolic blood pressure (BP) ≥ 130 mmHg or diastolic BP ≥ 85 mmHg or treatment for previously diagnosed hypertension; fasting plasma glucose (FPG) ≥ 100 mg/dL, or previously diagnosed type 2 diabetes [14].

MetS is associated with an increased risk of CVD both in HIV negative [11] and in HIV-infected individuals, [15,16] which is the main cause of death in men and women and its incidence in premenopausal women is lower than in men of the same age. This sex difference decreases with age, and women have the same risk as men after menopause [17]. Thus, ovarian failure appears to be an important cardiovascular risk factor. Hypoestrogenism leads to central adiposity and increased insulin resistance [18]. Several studies have reported a higher prevalence of MetS in postmenopausal women compared with premenopausal women [19-23]. The prevalence of MetS in postmenopausal women is 22% to 69%, varying from one country

---

*Corresponding author: Lúcia Costa-Paiva, Rua Alexander Fleming 101, Cidade State University of Campinas (UNICAMP), 13083-881 Campinas, SP, Brazil, E-mail: paivaepaiva@uol.com.br

to another and with the criteria used to diagnose MetS [21-23]. The prevalence of MetS in Brazilian postmenopausal women ranges from 34.7% to 56.9% [24-26]. World data show a higher prevalence of MetS in HIV patients than in the general population, [27,28] with increased risk of death from CVD, independent of factors such as age, sex, dyslipidemia, exercise, and smoking. This presents a major challenge to professionals involved in the care of HIV-infected individuals.

Some studies in HIV-positive patients have evaluated MetS in men and women of different age groups, [1,27-30] and many studies have evaluated MetS in climacteric women without HIV [21-26]. However, there is a lack of information specifically with regard to the impact of HIV infection on MetS in climacteric women. The study aimed to determine the prevalence and the factors associated with MetS in women in women aged between 40 and 60 years, with and without HIV infection.

Methods

Subjects

This cross-sectional study recruited women aged 40–60 years who were receiving care at the Menopause Outpatient Clinic at the University of Campinas (UNICAMP) Clinical Hospital and at the Infectious Diseases and HIV Outpatient Clinic at the UNICAMP Clinical Hospital and the Eduardo de Menezes Hospital (HEM) in Belo Horizonte, Brazil. Determination of the sample size was based on the difference in prevalence of MetS between HIV-positive and HIV-negative groups of 13 percentage points [19-26]. Considering an α error of 0.05 and a β error of 0.20, the sample size required to evaluate MetS was calculated as 242 women in each group. All women who fulfilled the inclusion criteria were invited to participate in the study. Interviews were carried out with 537 women, 273 HIV-positive and 264 HIV-negative.

HIV seropositive status was confirmed by enzyme-linked immunosorbent assay or western blotting, while women recruited to the HIV-negative group had to have a negative HIV test. Menopause status was determined by state in relation to menopause, reported by women using the definition of Jaszmann and classified as: premenopausal (women with regular menstrual cycles or menstrual pattern similar to what they had during their reproductive life), perimenopause (women with menstrual cycles in the past 12 months, but with change in menstrual pattern as the previous standards) and postmenopausal (women whose last menstrual period occurred at least 12 months before the interview). Menopausal status in women with previous hysterectomy was confirmed according to the serum levels of follicle stimulating hormone (FSH) on any day and classified as: premenopausal (<10 mIU/mL); menopausal transition (≥10 and <30 mIU/mL); and postmenopausal (≥30 mIU/mL). Bilaterally oophorectomized women, nursing mothers, pregnant women and those unable to answer the study questionnaire were excluded from the study.

Main outcome measures

A structured questionnaire was completed during an interview held in a private setting. Demographic and lifestyle data were collected, as well as information on hormone status and reproductive cycle. At the same visit, waist circumference, BP, weight and height were measured, and body mass index (BMI) was calculated. Blood samples were collected to measure fasting glucose, HDL cholesterol, TG, follicle-stimulating hormone (FSH), thyroid-stimulating (TSH), and free T4 levels. Diagnosis of MetS was based on the IDF criteria as mentioned above [14].

Independent variables

The main independent variable was HIV status. Other independent variables evaluated were age (years- continuous variable); skin color (white/other); physical activity in the previous month (none or up to twice a week/three times a week or more); schooling (<8/≥8 years); family income (≤US$ 750,00/>US$ 750,00); number of residents in the home (≤2/>2); smoking habit (none or past/current); current consumption of alcoholic beverages (yes/no or never drank); menopausal status (pre or perimenopausal/postmenopausal); weight gain (yes/no); use of hormone therapy (yes/no); self-perception of health (good or excellent/ not so good or bad); use of HAART (yes/no); other chronic diseases (yes/no); BMI (normal/abnormal); FSH (normal/abnormal); TSH (normal/abnormal); and free T4 (normal/abnormal).

Data analysis

The association between the dependent variable MetS and predictive factors was evaluated. Yates and Fisher's chi-square tests were used to compare categorical variables between groups with and without MetS. Poisson multiple regression analysis was adjusted in the various models for each of the independent variables to evaluate the factors associated with MetS. The backward manual selection method was used in which all variables were initially included, with those that were not significant being excluded, one by one, until only variables with $P<0.05$ remained in the final model. The prevalence ratio (PR) with 95% confidence interval (CI) of MetS was determined according to each factor. Data were analyzed using SPSS, version 17.0 (SPSS Inc., Chicago, IL, USA) and Stata, version 7 (Stata Corp., College Station, TX, USA).

Ethics

The study was approved by the internal review board of CAISM (Integral Care Center for Women's Health)- UNICAMP- and was conducted in compliance with the current version of the Declaration of Helsinki and with Resolution 466/12 of the Brazilian National Committee for Ethics in Research (CONEP) and its subsequent revisions. This study forms part of a larger study evaluating menopausal symptoms, bone mass, sexual function and metabolic markers. Process: Committee for Ethics in Research (CEP): 407/2010, Certificate of Presentation for Ethical Consideration (CAAE): 0313.0.146.000-10. All women gave signed informed consent for participation in the study.

Results

The mean age was 47.7 years in HIV seropositive women and 49.8 years in HIV seronegative women ($P<0.001$). Most HIV seropositive women had a body mass index<25 kg/m² (51.6%), while in the HIV seronegative women with a BMI<25 kg/m² accounted for 29.3% ($P<0.001$). Other characteristics of the groups are shown in Table 1.

The prevalence of MetS in the HIV group was 46.9% compared with 42.2% in the HIV-negative group, a non-significant difference ($P=0.340$).

In the 273 patients with HIV, 91% were taking HAART, and approximately 74% had a nadir CD4 above 200/mm³. The main risk factor for acquisition of the infection was heterosexual transmission, the mean duration of infection was 9.9 years, and the mean duration of therapy was 9.4 years (Table 1).

Table 2 shows the stratified analysis of women with MetS in relation to HIV infection. The factors significantly associated with MetS in HIV women were being postmenopausal ($P=0.032$), self-rated health considered excellent/good ($P=0.011$), and BMI>25 kg/m² ($P=0.005$).

Characteristics	Group		p-value
	HIV-seropositive (n=273)	HIV-seronegative (n=264)	
Age (years)			
40 – 44	36.60%	20.40%	
45 – 49	27.50%	28.00%	<0.01
50 – 54	19.00%	27.70%	
≥55	16.90%	23.90%	
BMI (kg/m²)			
<20.00	12.50%	1.50%	
20.00 – 24.99	39.10%	27.80%	<0.01
25.00 – 29.99	35.40%	36.90%	
≥30.00	12.90%	33.80%	
Skin color			
White	39.90%	48.10%	0.07
Non-white	60.10%	51.90%	
Schooling (years)			
≤7	58.20%	39.40%	
8-11	26.70%	37.90%	<0.01
≥12	15.10%	22.70%	
Menopausal status			
Premenopause	33.70%	22.00%	
Perimenopause	25.60%	20.00%	<0.01
Postmenopause	40.70%	58.00%	
Smoking			
Yes	28.60%	14.80%	
No	50.90%	58.00%	<0.01
Unknown	20.50%	27.20%	
Alcoholism			
Yes	29.70%	12.60%	
No	36.30%	78.60%	<0.01
Unknown	34.00%	8.80%	
Time since HIV diagnosis (years)	9.9 ± 5.4 y		
Nadir CD4 < 200 (%)	25.6		
In use of TARV (%)	91.0		
Time using TARV (years)	9.4 ± 4.8 y		
Previous or actual use of PI (%)	53.2		
Last CD4 cell count (cells/mm³)			
0-199	7.6		
≥200	92.4		
	76.9		
Quantitative viral load (copies/mL)	23.1		

Pearson's Chi-square; Yates's Chi-square; Mann-Whitney's test

Table 1: Characteristics of middle-aged women in HIV seropositive and seronegative groups (n=537).

Table 3 shows the prevalence of each of the MetS diagnostic criteria in postmenopausal women with or without HIV infection. Waist circumference ≥ 80 cm was present in all cases as it is the essential IDF criterion for MetS diagnosis. The other most prevalent factors in descending order were HDL<50 mg/dL, BP ≥ 130/85 mm Hg, TG ≥ 150 mg/dL, and blood glucose ≥ 100 mg/dL. The HIV-positive women had a worse lipid profile when compared to HIV-negative ones, with low HDL (P=0.019) and high TG (P=0.011).

In the multiple regression analysis of all women, MetS was significantly associated with BMI>25 kg/m² (PR: 2.34; 95% CI: 1.70–3.21; P<0.001), aging (PR: 1.05; 95% CI: 1.02–1.07; P<0.001), and use of HAART (PR: 1.48; 95% CI: 1.13–1.94; P=0.005) (Table 4).

Variable	Metabolic Syndrome (%)				
	HIV+ (%)	n	HIV- (%)	n	P(x)
Age (years)					
40–49	39.3	64	31.0	35	0.199
50–60	60.2	56	52.4	65	0.314
Skin color					
Other	48.0	72	45.2	56	0.728
White	45.3	48	38.9	44	0.416
Physical activity (a)					
0–2 /week	46.5	93	39.8	74	0.220
≥3 /week	47.3	26	51.0	26	0.852
Formal education (years)					
0–7	55.0	83	49.0	48	0.427
≥8	35.2	37	37.4	52	0.830
Family income (US$) (b)					
≤750.00	48.4	78	44.4	48	0.603
>750.00	43.6	41	39.8	51	0.670
House residents ©					
≤2	52.0	53	46.0	29	0.562
>2	43.8	67	41.0	68	0.691
Smoking					
No/past	45.9	84	40.4	82	0.323
Yes	49.3	36	52.9	18	0.887
Alcohol use					
No/past	47.5	87	43.1	91	0.438
Yes	45.2	33	34.6	9	0.479
Menopausal status					
Pre or peri	37.3	57	35.8	34	0.823
Postmenopausal	61.2	63	46.5	66	**0.032**
Hormone therapy (d)					
No	46.2	115	44.8	87	0.853
Yes	80.0	4	28.6	12	**0.040(y)**
Self-perception of health (d)					
Excellent/good	47.6	78	32.6	46	**0.011**
Not so good/bad	45.6	41	55.8	53	0.213
Other chronic diseases (e)					
No	44.3	74	43.7	62	>0.999
Yes	48.8	40	41.1	37	0.392
BMI (kg/m²) (b)					
≤25	28.7	39	19.7	13	0.231
>25	68.1	81	50.6	86	**0.005**
FSH (mIU/mL) (f)					
<40	37.2	51	34.8	31	0.823
≥40	58.7	61	47.2	67	0.099
TSH (mIU/mL) (g)					
≤4.5	46.0	99	41.7	86	0.429
>4.5	54.8	17	46.4	13	0.701
Free T4 (ng/dL)					
<0.90 or >1.80	51.5	17	35.7	5	0.501
0.90–1.80	46.7	99	42.5	94	0.438

(x) Yates chi-square test, (y) Fisher's exact test.
BMI: Body Mass Index; FSH: Follicle-stimulating Hormone; TSH: Thyroid-stimulating Hormone.
Missing information: (a) One in the HIV group; (b) One in each group; (c) Eight in the control group; (d) One in the control group and two in the HIV group; (e) Five in the control group and seven in the HIV group; (f) Six in the control group and 15 in the HIV group; (g) Three in the control group and 10 in the HIV group.

Table 2: Bivariate analysis of patients with metabolic syndrome according to HIV status (n=220).

VARIABLES	HIV+ (%) (n = 187)	HIV- (%) (n = 201)	P(a)	TOTAL (n = 388)
Waist circumference				
<80 cm	0	0		0
≥80 cm	100	100		100
Blood pressure			0,833	
<130/85 mm Hg	48.7	50.2		49.5
≥130/85 mm Hg	51.3	49.8		50.5
High density lipoprotein			0,019	
<50 mg/dL	56.7	44.3		50.3
≥50 mg/dL	43.3	55.7		49.7
Triglycerides			0,011	
<150 mg/dL	57.2	70.1		63.9
≥150 mg/dL	42.8	29.9		36.1
Glucose			0,470	
<100 mg/dL	75.4	71.6		73.5
≥100 mg/dL	24.6	28.4		26.5

(a) Yates chi-square

Table 3: Prevalence of each metabolic parameter according to HIV status in climacteric women with metabolic syndrome (n = 388).

VARIABLES	PR	95%CI	P
BMI (>25 kg/m²)	2.34	1.70–3.21	<0.001
Use of HAART (Yes)	1.48	1.13–1.94	0.005
Age (years)	1.05	1.02–1.07	<0.001

PR: prevalence ratio; **95% CI:** 95% confidence interval.
Missing information: (a) 46 in the whole group.
Variables considered to backward selection: age (years); skin color (white / other); physical activity (0–2 times per week / ≥3 times per week); education (0–7 years / ≥8 years); family income (≤ US$ 750.00 / >US$750.00); house residents(up to 2 / >2); smoking (yes / no); alcohol consumption (yes / no); menopausal status (pre or perimenopause / menopause); weight gain (yes / no); hormone therapy (yes / no); self-rated health (excellent or good / not so good or bad); use of HAART (yes / no); other chronic diseases (yes / no); BMI (≤25 />25 kg/m²); FSH (<40 / ≥40); TSH (≤4.5 / >4.5); free T4 (<0.90 or >1.80 / 0.90 to 1.80); group (HIV / control).

Table 4: Multiple regression analysis of the variables associated with the presence of metabolic syndrome in the total sample -HIV positive and negative women [n = 537 (a)].

Discussion

The prevalence of MetS was 46.9% and 42.2% in HIV-positive and HIV-negative women, respectively, and was similar to the rates of 22% to 69%, reported in studies that included individuals in different age groups who were HIV-positive [1,27-30].

Although there are many reports of adverse metabolic changes in HIV-positive patients in general, the effect of such changes on the development of MetS is still controversial [27,28]. No studies specifically evaluating the prevalence of MetS in HIV-infected climacteric women were found. The present study was based on the hypothesis that the prevalence of MetS would be higher in HIV-positive than in HIV-negative climacteric women. Nevertheless, in the present study HIV infection was not associated with MetS or any single parameter of MetS. The absence of an association between HIV and MetS could be related to the specific characteristics of our study population, such as good immunological status after early institution of HAART and its effective use. Krishnan et al. evaluated MetS before and after the introduction of HAART, and reported that virologic suppression and maintenance of high CD4 levels could reduce the risk of MetS [30].

There was a significant difference in the prevalence of MetS in HIV-seropositive women compared with seronegative women who perceived their health as excellent/good in the present study. The stigma of HIV infection is related to thinness and lipodystrophy, [31,32] and it

is possible that overweight could be considered a sign of health in these women rather than associated with MetS.

In the stratified analysis of factors associated with MetS according to HIV status, it was observed that HIV-positive women had a significantly higher prevalence of MetS if they were postmenopausal and had BMI>25 kg/m². This BMI association remained in the multivariate analysis, which showed that BMI>25 kg/m² was associated with a 1.34-fold increased risk of MetS.

In present study, the HIV study population was composed mostly of HAART users, and multiple regression analyses showed that the use of HAART was associated with more than twice the risk of MetS. The use of HAART has been well documented in the literature as an independent risk factor associated with MetS [1,33,34]. Signorini suggested that longer exposure (mean duration of therapy of 54 (± 36) months to HAART appeared to be associated with MetS [1]. Cahn also observed an association between long-term exposure to HAART and MetS in a study conducted in seven Latin American countries [34]. These studies included patients of both sexes aged over 18 years, in contrast to the present study, which evaluated only middle-aged women. Although MetS has been attributed to the effect of HAART, we cannot forget that aging is an important contributing factor. As HIV-seropositive patients grow older, the risk of MetS seems to increase [1,35,36]. Ramírez-Marrero conducted a study in Hispanic patients and found that older HIV patients were more likely to have MetS than younger patients, and that there was a higher prevalence in females [35]. Freitas also reported a higher prevalence of MetS in HIV patients aged older than 40 years in Portugal [36]. Signorini observed an association between MetS and aging in a study in a Brazilian HIV-infected population [1]. This study has limitations. It is a cross-sectional study, so causal relationships cannot be attributed. There were differences between the groups of HIV seropositive and seronegative women that undermined the homogeneity of the samples. Furthermore, there were some differences in the clinical characteristics of the seropositive and seronegative women. These differences could be attributed to the fact that the seronegative women were selected in outpatient clinics specialized in providing care to menopausal women, and 78% were peri or post menopause. On the other hand, in the HIV positive group 66.3% were peri or post menopause. The HIV-negative women also had greater BMI, older and had higher scholarity. However, these differences have been controlled in the multivariate analysis. In addition, the HIV-positive group had good immunological status as demonstrated by viral suppression and high CD4 levels. As these women were treated at multidisciplinary referral centers for HIV infection, the results cannot be extrapolated to the general population infected with HIV.

Conclusions

In this study, there was no association between MetS and HIV status among middle-aged women. However, HIV-positive women who were postmenopausal or had a high BMI showed a significantly higher prevalence of MetS with otherwise similar characteristics. It seems that HIV-positive women in good immunological status, after early institution of HAART and its effective use, have traditional factors associated with MetS like being overweight and having older age. There is a need for a better approach, awareness, and education of both HIV-positive and HIV-negative women to prevent and MetS. For HIV-positive middle-aged women, using effective HAART with fewer adverse effects on metabolism is an important aspect to prevent MetS.

This should be considered in clinical practice to reduce the risk of MetS in this population.

Financial Support

Funded by the São Paulo Foundation for the Support of Research (Fundação de Amparo à Pesquisa do Estado de São Paulo - FAPESP), Grant 2010/06037-5

References

1. Signorini DJ, Monteiro MC, Andrade Mde F, Signorini DH, Eyer-Silva Wde A (2012) What should we know about metabolic syndrome and lipodystrophy in AIDS? Rev Assoc Med Bras 58: 70-75.

2. Palella FJ Jr, Delaney KM, Moorman AC, Loveless MO, Fuhrer J, et al. (1998) Declining morbidity and mortality among patients with advanced human immunodeficiency virus infection. HIV Outpatient Study Investigators. N Engl J Med 338: 853-860.

3. Kojic EM, Wang CC, Cu-Uvin S (2007) HIV and menopause: a review. J Womens Health (Larchmt) 16: 1402-1411.

4. Pereira EC, Schmitt AC, Cardoso MR, Aldrighi JM (2008) Trends of AIDS incidence and mortality among women in menopause transition and post-menopause in Brazil, 1996 - 2005. Rev Assoc Med Bras 54: 422-425.

5. Carr A (2003) HIV lipodystrophy: risk factors, pathogenesis, diagnosis and management. AIDS 17 Suppl 1: S141-148.

6. Carr A, Samaras K, DJ Chisholm, Cooper DA (1998) Pathogenesis of HIV-1-protease inhibitor-associated peripheral lipodystrophy, hyperlipidaemia, and insulin resistance. The Lancet 351:1881-1883.

7. Grinspoon S, Carr A (2005) Cardiovascular risk and body-fat abnormalities in HIV-infected adults. N Engl J Med 352: 48-62.

8. Lauda LG, Mariath AB, Grillo LP (2011) Metabolic syndrome and its components in HIV-infected individuals. Rev Assoc Med Bras 57: 182-186.

9. Grunfeld C, Pang M, Doerrler W, Shigenaga JK, Jensen P, et al. (1992) Lipids, lipoproteins, triglyceride clearance, and cytokines in human immunodeficiency virus infection and the acquired immunodeficiency syndrome. JCEM 74: 1045-1052.

10. Polotsky HN, Polotsky AJ (2010) Metabolic implications of menopause. Semin Reprod Med 28: 426-434.

11. Brazilian Society of Hypertension, Brazilian Society of Cardiology, Brazilian Society of Endocrinology and Metabolism, Brazilian Society of Diabetes, Brazilian Society of Obesity Studies (2005) Brazilian guidelines on diagnosis and treatment of metabolic syndrome. Arq Bras Cardiol 84: 1-28.

12. Alberti KG, Zimmet PZ (1998) Definition, diagnosis and classification of diabetes mellitus and its complications. Part 1: diagnosis and classification of diabetes mellitus provisional report of a WHO consultation. Diabet Med 15: 539-553.

13. Grundy SM (2001) Executive Summary of the Third Report of the National Cholesterol Education Program (NCEP) Expert Panel on Detection, Evaluation, and Treatment of High Cholesterol in Adults (Adult Treatment Panel III). JAMA 285:2486-2497.

14. International Diabetes Federation (2006) The IDF consensus worldwide definition of the Metabolic Syndrome.

15. Friis-Møller N, Sabin CA, Weber R, d'Arminio Monforte A, El-Sadr WM, et al. (2003) Combination antiretroviral therapy and the risk of myocardial infarction. N Engl J Med 349: 1993-2003.

16. Triant VA, Lee H, Hadigan C, Grinspoon SK (2007) Increased acute myocardial infarction rates and cardiovascular risk factors among patients with human immunodeficiency virus disease. J Clin Endocrinol Metab 92: 2506-2512.

17. Stangl V, Baumann G, Stangl K (2002) Coronary atherogenic risk factors in women. Eur Heart J 23: 1738-1752.

18. Lobo RA (2007) Treatment of the Postmenopausal Woman: Basic and Clinical Aspects: Treatment of the postmenopausal woman: where we are today. Raven Press.

19. Deibert P, König D, Vitolins MZ, Landmann U, Frey I, et al. (2007) Effect of a weight loss intervention on anthropometric measures and metabolic risk factors in pre- versus postmenopausal women. Nutr J 6: 31.

20. Eshtiaghi R, Esteghamati A, Nakhjavani M (2010) Menopause is an independent predictor of metabolic syndrome in Iranian women. Maturitas 65: 262-266.

21. Heidari R, Sadeghi M, Talaei M, Rabiei K, Mohammadifard N, et al. (2010) Metabolic syndrome in menopausal transition: Isfahan Healthy Heart Program, a population based study. Diabetol Metab Syndr 2:59.

22. Kim HM, Park J, Ryu SY, Kim J (2007) The effect of menopause on the metabolic syndrome among Korean women: the Korean National Health and Nutrition Examination Survey, 2001. Diabetes Care 30: 701-706.

23. Pandey S, Srinivas M, Agashe S, Joshi J, Galvankar P, et al. (2010) Menopause and metabolic syndrome: A study of 498 urban women from western India. J Midlife Health 1: 63-69.

24. Neto JAF, Figuerêdo ED, Barbosa JB, Barbosa Fde F, Costa GR, et al. (2010) Metabolic syndrome and menopause: cross-sectional study in gynecology clinic. Arq Bras Cardiol 95: 339-345.

25. Nahas EAP, Padoani NP, Nahas-Neto J, Orsatti FL, Tardivo AP, et al. (2009) Metabolic syndrome and its associated risk factors in Brazilian postmenopausal women. Climacteric 12: 431-438.

26. de Oliveira EP, de Souza ML, de Lima Md (2006) Prevalence of metabolic syndrome in a semi-arid rural area in Bahia. Arq Bras Endocrinol Metabol 50: 456-465.

27. Martin Lde S, Pasquier E, Roudaut N, Vandhuick O, Vallet S, et al. (2008) Metabolic syndrome: a major risk factor for atherosclerosis in HIV-infected patients (SHIVA study). Presse Med 37: 579-584.

28. Silva EF, Bassichetto KC, Lewi DS (2009) Lipid profile, cardiovascular risk factors and metabolic syndrome in a group of AIDS patients. Arq Bras Cardiol 93: 113-118.

29. Castelo Filho A, Abrão P (2007) Metabolic changes in HIV infected patient. Arq Bras Endocrinol Metabol 51: 5-7.

30. Krishnan S, Schouten JT, Atkinson B, Brown T, Wohl D, et al. (2012) Metabolic syndrome before and after initiation of antiretroviral therapy in treatment HIV-infected individuals. J AcquirImmune Defic Syndr 61(3): 381-389.

31. Barroso CS, Peters RJ, Johnson RJ, Kelder SH, Jefferson T (2010) Beliefs and perceived norms concerning body image among African-American and Latino teenagers. J Health Psychol 15: 858-870.

32. Collins E, Wagner C, Walmsley S (2000) Psychosocial impact of the lipodystrophy syndrome in HIV infection. AIDS Read 10: 546-550.

33. Alencastro PR, Fuchs SC, Wolff FH, Ikeda ML, Brandão AB, et al. (2011) Independent predictors of metabolic syndrome in HIV-infected patients. AIDS Patient Care STDS 25: 627-634.

34. Cahn P, Leite O, Rosales A, Cabello R, Alvarez CA, et al. (2010) Metabolic profile and cardiovascular risk factors among Latin American HIV-infected patients receiving HAART. Braz J Infect Dis 14: 158-166.

35. Ramírez-Marrero FA, De Jesús E, Santana-Bagur J, Hunter R, Frontera W, et al. (2010) Prevalence of cardiometabolic risk factors in Hispanics living with HIV. Ethn Dis 20: 423-428.

36. Freitas P, Carvalho D, Souto S, Santos AC, Xerinda S, et al. (2011) Impact of Lipodystrophy on the prevalence and components of metabolic syndrome in HIV-infected patients. BMC Infect Dis 11: 246.

31

Metabolic Syndrome and Prevalent Any-site, Prostate, Breast and Colon Cancers

Thirumagal Kanagasabai[1], Jason X. Nie[1], Caitlin Mason[2] and Chris I. Ardern[1]*

[1]*School of Kinesiology and Health Science, York University, Toronto, Ontario, Canada*
[2]*University of Washington Health Promotion Research Center, Seattle, Washington, USA*

Abstract

Background: Metabolic Syndrome (MetS) is associated with elevated risk of diabetes, cardiovascular disease, and premature mortality. To date, however, the association between MetS and obesity-related cancers has not been systematically assessed within a population-based sample.

Methods: In order to quantify the association between MetS and its components on any-site, breast, prostate, and colon cancers, data from the U.S. NHANES 1999-2010 (n=15 141, 18-85 years) were used.

Results: In general, the prevalence of MetS was higher amongst those with a self-reported history of cancer. Although MetS, its individual components, and total number of components were positively related to odds of any-site, breast, prostate, and colon cancers, this effect was almost entirely eliminated after adjustment for age. In age-adjusted models, elevated blood glucose was associated with higher odds of prostate (OR: 1.67, 95% CI: 1.08-2.56) and colon cancer (OR: 1.60, 95% CI: 1.02-2.53), and a protective effect of low HDL cholesterol on prostate cancer (OR: 0.64, 95% CI: 0.43-0.94). Further adjustment for sex, ethnicity, income, education, smoking, alcohol, and recreational/leisure-time physical activity had only minimal influence on these associations. In multivariable analyses, no uniform linear trends were observed between the number of MetS components and site-specific cancers.

Conclusion: After accounting for covariates, no consistent association between MetS and any-site, breast, prostate, or colon cancer was observed. Further prospective study is necessary to confirm and extend our understanding of the role of age and other risk factors on the inter-relationship between metabolic health and cancer.

Keywords: Metabolic syndrome; Cancer; Any-site cancer; Prostate cancer; Breast cancer; Colon cancer and aging

Introduction

Metabolic syndrome (MetS) currently affects approximately one-third of U.S. adults, and is disproportionately experienced by older individuals, women, and those with excess weight [1,2]. Obesity, as a central component of MetS, is also associated with oxidative stress, which is on the causal pathway of several age-related diseases, including cardiovascular disease, diabetes and cancer [3,4]. Because aging is associated with increased oxidative stress and inflammation, free radical and immunological theories suggest a relationship between MetS and several types of cancer [5–7]. Although the relationships between MetS, obesity, and cancer survival are complex, a protective effect of physical activity and low sedentary behaviour and cancer has been demonstrated [8].

In a recent meta-analysis, men with MetS had a greater relative risk of liver (43%), colorectal (25%), and bladder (10%) cancers, but decreased prostate cancer risk (29%) compared to those without MetS. In the same study, women with MetS had increased pancreatic (58%), postmenopausal breast (56%), colorectal (34%) and endometrial (61%) cancer risk [9]. Reviews that have focused on individual MetS components (e.g. "overt diabetes", "pre-eclampsia" and obesity) have reported mixed results, and may be accounted for in part due to variation in study design, MetS criteria, and population of interest [10-16]. Similarly, a number of cohort and case-control studies have also assessed whether cancer risk varies according to the number of MetS components, yielding inconsistent results [17-22]. As with the studies of MetS overall, these investigations have largely focused on a select group of cancers, and none have explored the association within nationally representative data that allows for generalization to a geographically and demographically diverse sample of the U.S. population.

The purpose of this study was to therefore quantify the association between MetS (overall, number, and individual components), and any-site, breast, prostate and colon cancers in multiple cycles of the U.S. National Health and Nutrition Examination Survey (NHANES).

Methods

Participants

The U.S. NHANES was designed to assess the health and nutritional status of adults and children in the United States, details of which can be found elsewhere [1,8]. The initial sample included 62, 160 individuals from 1999-2010 [1999-00: n=9 965; 2001-02: n=11 039; 2003-04: n=10 122; 2005-06: n=10 348; 2007-08: n=10 149; 2009-10: n=10 537]. Subsequent exclusions were made for age (<18 y: n=26 781) and missing data for MetS components (n=20 238), for a final analytic sample of 15, 141 [age 18-85 y; 1999-00: n=2 175; 2001-02: n=2 449; 2003-04: n=2 450; 2005-06: n=2 485; 2007-08: n=2 847; 2009-10: n=2 735].

Metabolic Syndrome

MetS was defined according to the Harmonized Criteria which classifies MetS on the basis of three or more of the following: waist circumference ≥ 102 cm (men) and ≥ 88 cm (women); triglyceride ≥ 1.69

*Corresponding author: Chris I. Ardern, School of Kinesiology and Health Science, 352 Norman Bethune College, York University, 4700 Keele Street, Toronto, ON M3J1P3, Canada, E-mail: cardern@yorku.ca

mmol/L (mM); HDL-cholesterol < 1.04 nM (men), 1.29 mM (women); blood pressure (BP ≥ 130/85 mmHg of either diastolic or systolic pressures; and fasting plasma glucose ≥ 5.6 mM [23]. Participants who self-reported the use of medications for blood pressure, cholesterol, or diabetes were identified as having high blood pressure, dyslipidaemia, and high fasting glucose, respectively.

Cancer

Cancer history (yes/no) was based on a single-item self-report ('has a physician or health professional ever told you that you have a cancer or malignancy of any kind'?). Participants who responded 'yes' were then asked to report the specific type of cancer.

Covariates

On the basis of previous literature, the following were included as covariates in our analyses [24]. Total physical activity level was based on physical activity due to house/yard work, transportation and recreational/leisure-time activities. Physical activity was quantified in Metabolic Equivalent (MET) min/week from self-reported physical activity data. To calculate MET min/week, moderate and vigorous activities were assumed to have 4 MET and 8 MET energy expenditure values, respectively [25]. One MET is equivalent to the amount of oxygen consumed while in a sitting position at rest. Physical activity was then categorized as "inactive" (no reported physical activity data), "somewhat active" (<500 MET min/week) and "active" (≥500 MET min/week) [25].

Positive smoking history was defined as self-reported current smoking or having smoked ≥100 cigarettes in one's life. Body Mass Index (BMI; kg/m²) was classified as normal weight (18.5-24.9 kg/m²), overweight (25-29.9 kg/m²), or obese (≥30 kg/m²) on the basis of measured height and weight. Highest educational attainment was coded as less than high school, high school, or college; and, household income as <$20,000, $20,000-44,999, and ≥$45,000 [19]. Alcohol intake was considered high if an individual reported having ≥3 drinks per day [21].

Statistical Analyses

The prevalence of MetS and its individual components, as well as the number of MetS components present (0, 1, 2, 3, 4, or 5) was determined for the U.S. adult population. The prevalence of MetS among individuals with breast, prostate, colon, and "any" cancer group was also estimated. Mean and standard error (for continuous variables), and percentage and percent standard error (for categorical variables) were determined according to MetS status. Differences in the demographic and behavioural characteristics of participants with and without MetS were assessed by independent t-tests and χ2 analyses, as appropriate.

Logistic regression was used to estimate the crude, age, and multivariable adjusted (with and without age) odds ratios (OR) and 95% Confidence Intervals (CI) for the relationship between MetS (overall, individual components, and total number of components) and any-site, breast, prostate and colon cancers. Using a linear trend analysis, the relationship between number of MetS components and cancer history was subsequently assessed. All analyses were weighted to be representative of the U.S. adult population using SAS v9.3 (Cary, NC, U.S.A). Statistical significance was set at α <0.05.

Results

Table 1 describes characteristics of the U.S. adult population by MetS status. In general, participants with MetS were older, had lower

Characteristics	Categories	No MetS (n=9,003)	MetS (n=6,138)	P value
Age (Mean (SEM))		41.8 (0.3)	53.9 (0.3)	<0.05
Age categories (% (SE))	≤ 50 years	72.1 (0.9)	41.3 (1.0)	<0.05
	> 50 years	27.9 (0.9)	58.7 (1.0)	
Sex (% (SE))	Males	48.7 (0.6)	49.0 (0.8)	NS
	Females	51.3 (0.6)	51.0 (0.8)	
Ethnicity (% (SE))	White	69.7 (1.2)	72.7 (1.6)	<0.05
	Non-white	30.3 (1.2)	27.3 (1.6)	
Education (% (SE))	Less than high school	17.3 (0.7)	24.3 (0.8)	<0.05
	High school	23.1 (0.7)	28.5 (1.0)	
	College	59.6 (1.1)	47.2 (1.2)	
Income (% (SE))	<$20,000	17.9 (0.8)	23.3 (0.9)	<0.05
	$20,000-44,999	29.5 (0.8)	33.7 (1.1)	
	≥ $45,000	52.6 (1.0)	43.0 (1.3)	
Total Physical Activity (% (SE))	Inactive	14.2 (0.5)	23.8 (1.0)	<0.05
	Somewhat active	24.2 (0.7)	26.3 (0.9)	
	Active	61.6 (0.8)	49.9 (1.1)	
Transportation related Physical Activity (% (SE))	Inactive	73.1 (0.9)	79.7 (0.8)	<0.05
	Somewhat active	17.8 (0.7)	13.7 (0.7)	
	Active	9.1 (0.5)	6.6 (0.4)	
House/Yard Word Physical Activity (% (SE))	Inactive	40.0 (0.9)	43.4 (1.1)	<0.05
	Somewhat active	28.1 (0.7)	27.4 (1.0)	
	Active	32.0 (0.8)	29.2 (1.0)	
Recreational/Leisure-time Physical Activity (% (SE))	Inactive	33.6 (0.8)	49.5 (1.1)	<0.05
	Somewhat active	30.3 (0.7)	25.9 (0.9)	
	Active	36.1 (0.8)	24.6 (0.9)	
Smoking (% (SE))	Past or current	24.2 (0.8)	20.3 (0.7)	<0.05
Alcohol (% (SE))	≥ 3 drinks per day	36.7 (0.9)	32.7 (1.1)	<0.05
BMI (% (SE))	Normal weight	46.5 (0.7)	9.1 (0.5)	<0.05
	Overweight	35.6 (0.7)	32.3 (0.8)	
	Obese	17.9 (0.6)	58.6 (1.0)	
Doctor diagnosed cancer or malignancy (% (SE))	Any-site	7.0 (0.4)	12.0 (0.5)	<0.05
	Breast	0.9 (0.1)	1.7 (0.2)	<0.05
	Prostate	0.6 (0.1)	1.4 (0.2)	<0.05
	Colon	0.2 (0.1)	0.8 (0.1)	<0.05

Table 1: Characteristics of the U.S. adult population with and without metabolic syndrome. p<0.05, two-sided t-test or Chi-square, as appropriate. Mean (SEM) for continuous and frequency (SE) for categorical variables. Physical Activity: Inactive is no reported physical activity data; somewhat active is >0 to <500 MET min/week; Active is ≥500 MET min/week (meeting physical activity guidelines). Metabolic Syndrome (MetS) is having ≥ 3 of WC ≥ 102 cm (men) and, ≥ 88 cm (women), Triglyceride ≥ 1.69 mmol/L (mM), HDL-Cholesterol < 1.04 (men), 1.29 mM (women), blood pressure ≥ 130/85 mmHg of either diastolic or systolic pressures, and fasting plasma glucose ≥5.6 mM, based on the Harmonized Criteria. No MetS is <3 of these components. WC is waist circumference, "or medication use for hypertension, diabetes, cholesterol" before ", based on the Harmonized..." HDL is high density lipid, and NS is not significant. Weighted N= 96, 318, 456.

educational attainment and income, and were more likely to be non-Hispanic white. The frequency of any-site, breast, prostate and colon cancers were also higher in the MetS vs. non-MetS groups (740 vs. 556, 109 vs. 72, 124 vs. 80, and 65 vs. 30, respectively). On the other hand, adults without MetS were more likely to engage in "recreational/" to be consistent 'recreational/leisure-time', house/yard work-, and transport-related physical activity. Prevalence's of past or current smoking, ≥3 alcohols drinks/day, normal weight and overweight individuals were also significantly higher in the non-MetS group.

Figure 1 shows the distribution of the number of MetS components and MetS in the U.S. adult population. Overall, the prevalence of MetS was 38.1 ± 0.7% [≤ 50 years: 26.0 ± 0.7% vs. > 50 years: 56.4 ± 0.9%, p <0.0001], with no significant sex difference [M: 38.2 ± 0.8%; F: 37.9 ± 0.9%].

The distributions of MetS and the number of MetS components in adults with a history of any-site, breast, prostate, and colon cancers are shown in Figure 2. More than half the men and women with any-site cancer had MetS (Figure 2a), with higher prevalences in older (vs. younger) adults (Figure 2b). In persons with a history of any-site and site-specific cancers, generally those with 2 or 3 MetS components had the highest prevalence of any-site, prostate, post-menopausal and total breast cancers (Figure 2c, 2d). Due to a small sample size, only pooled analyses were presented for colon cancer, prostate cancer was limited to men, and breast cancer was limited to women. Consequently, the prevalences of MetS were 57.5 ± 3.0% and 68.1 ± 4.1% in those with prostate and colon cancers, respectively.

In the >50 y age group, the prevalence of any-site cancer in the subpopulation with MetS was 17.6 ± 0.8%. This prevalence ranged between 15.7-19.6%, depending on the number of MetS components and was highest in those with all 5 criteria (12.1% for men, 17.3% for women, and 4.7% for ≤ 50 years old) (data not shown).

Table 2 contains the crude, age-adjusted and multivariable logistic regression models for the association between each cancer and individual MetS components, number of MetS components, and MetS overall. Once adjusted for age, all but the association between high blood glucose and low HDL for prostate cancer, and high blood glucose and colon cancer were abolished. These associations were further attenuated after multivariable adjustment (age, sex, ethnicity, income, education,

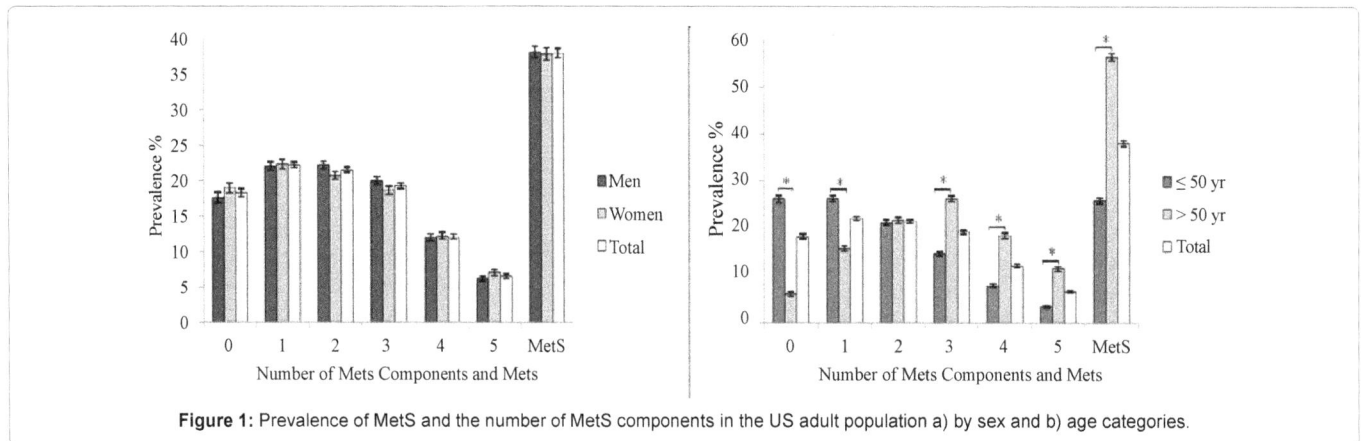

Figure 1: Prevalence of MetS and the number of MetS components in the US adult population a) by sex and b) age categories.

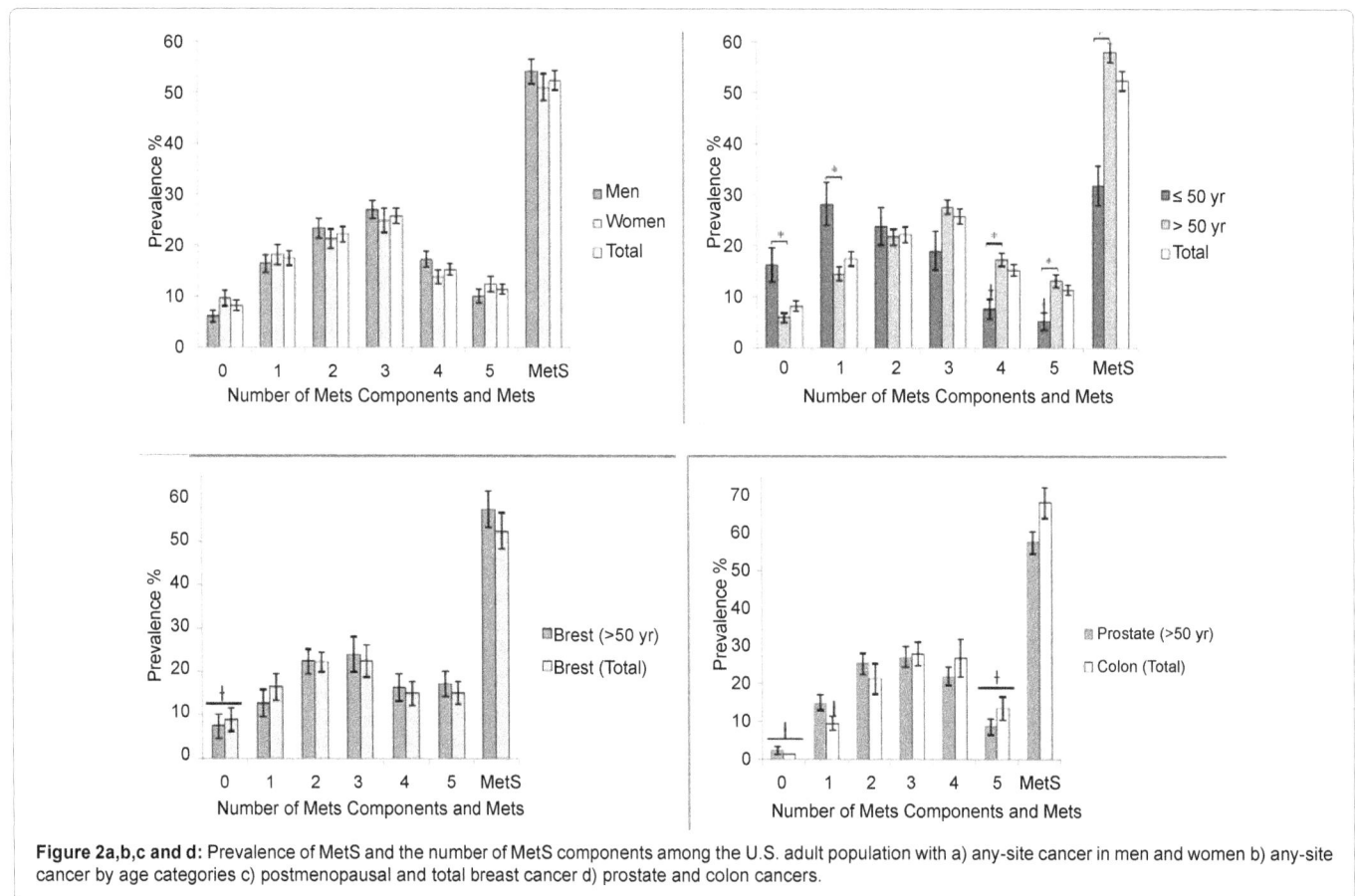

Figure 2a,b,c and d: Prevalence of MetS and the number of MetS components among the U.S. adult population with a) any-site cancer in men and women b) any-site cancer by age categories c) postmenopausal and total breast cancer d) prostate and colon cancers.

		Any-site (n=1,296)			
		ORc (95% CI)	ORage (95% CI)	ORadj (95% CI)	ORadj2 (95% CI)
Individual MetS components	High Blood Pressure	2.57 (2.24, 2.94)*	0.97 (0.83, 1.14)	1.01 (0.84, 1.22)	2.20 (1.87, 2.60)*
	High Glucose	1.87 (1.60, 2.19)*	0.99 (0.83, 1.18)	1.02 (0.81, 1.29)	1.77 (1.44, 2.17)*
	Low HDL	0.85 (0.74, 0.99)*	0.94 (0.80, 1.11)	0.94 (0.76, 1.16)	0.78 (0.64, 0.95)*
	High Triglyceride	1.38 (1.21, 1.58)*	1.01 (0.88, 1.16)	0.94 (0.78, 1.13)	1.19 (0.98, 1.43)
	High Waist Circumference	1.56 (1.32, 1.84)*	1.10 (0.92, 1.30)	1.05 (0.83, 1.32)	1.37 (1.09, 1.71)*
Number of MetS components§	1	1.76 (1.29, 2.40)*	1.08 (0.78, 1.50)	1.39 (0.91, 2.11)	2.07 (1.39, 3.09)*
	2	2.30 (1.67, 3.16)*	1.01 (0.72, 1.43)	1.23 (0.80, 1.89)	2.39 (1.60, 3.57)*
	3	3.03 (2.24, 4.10)*	1.11 (0.80, 1.55)	1.42 (0.95, 2.14)	3.27 (2.24, 4.79)*
	4	2.81 (2.06, 3.85)*	0.91 (0.65, 1.27)	0.97 (0.69, 1.37)	2.29 (1.64, 3.20)*
	5	4.02 (2.91, 5.56)*	1.16 (0.81, 1.65)	1.23 (0.76, 1.98)	3.06 (1.94, 4.81)*
p for linear trend		<0.0001	0.0311	0.123	<0.0001
MetS§§		1.82 (1.56, 2.11)*	1.02 (0.86, 1.20)	1.01 (0.82, 1.24)	1.58 (1.29, 1.94)*
		Breast (n=181)			
		ORc (95% CI)	ORage (95% CI)	ORadj (95% CI)	ORadj2 (95% CI)
Individual MetS components	High Blood Pressure	3.15 (2.05, 4.84)*	0.81 (0.49, 1.33)	0.76 (0.41, 1.42)	2.26 (1.30, 3.91)*
	High Glucose	2.25 (1.64, 3.10)*	1.04 (0.73, 1.46)	0.68 (0.42, 1.10)	1.26 (0.79, 2.02)*
	Low HDL	0.91 (0.59, 1.41)	0.94 (0.62, 1.43)	0.92 (0.53, 1.59)	0.76 (0.44, 1.32)
	High Triglyceride	1.87 (1.34, 2.63)*	1.13 (0.80, 1.58)	0.96 (0.57, 1.62)	1.34 (0.80, 2.23)
	High Waist Circumference	1.11 (0.73, 1.71)	0.75 (0.47, 1.18)	0.58 (0.32, 1.05)	0.76 (0.42, 1.35)
Number of MetS components§	1	1.57 (0.67, 3.67)ǂ	0.81 (0.32, 2.05)ǂ	0.82 (0.28, 2.36)ǂ	1.51 (0.59, 3.81)ǂ
	2	2.30 (1.03, 5.12)*ǂ	0.81 (0.33, 2.00)ǂ	0.58 (0.21, 1.63)ǂ	1.43 (0.58, 3.49)ǂ
	3	2.60 (1.17, 5.74)*ǂ	0.70 (0.28, 1.73)ǂ	0.60 (0.20, 1.86)ǂ	1.88 (0.74, 4.81)ǂ
	4	2.64 (1.27, 5.50)*ǂ	0.61 (0.26, 1.41)ǂ	0.32 (0.11, 0.92)*ǂ	1.04 (0.40, 2.69)ǂ
	5	4.68 (2.01, 10.90)*ǂ	0.91 (0.34, 2.41)ǂ	0.66 (0.17, 2.48)ǂ	2.19 (0.66, 7.35)ǂ
p for linear trend		0.0011	0.0134	0.0011	0.7349
MetS§§		1.83 (1.26, 2.65)*	0.86 (0.58, 1.27)	0.71 (0.41, 1.21)	1.25 (0.75, 2.07)
		Prostate (n=204)			
		ORc (95% CI)	ORage (95% CI)	ORadj (95% CI)	ORadj2 (95% CI)
Individual MetS components	High Blood Pressure	3.64 (1.97, 6.72)*	0.96 (0.51, 1.80)	0.92 (0.44, 1.90)	3.00 (1.45, 6.22)*
	High Glucose	3.89 (2.62, 5.79)*	1.67 (1.08, 2.56)*	1.69 (1.00, 2.85)	3.42 (2.10, 5.57)*
	Low HDL	0.52 (0.35, 0.76)*	0.64 (0.43, 0.94)*	0.80 (0.45, 1.43)	0.55 (0.32, 0.96)*
	High Triglyceride	1.39 (1.01, 1.92)*	1.16 (0.83, 1.63)	0.82 (0.50, 1.32)	0.87 (0.54, 1.38)
	High Waist Circumference	2.10 (1.51, 2.91)*	1.39 (0.98, 1.96)	1.37 (0.82, 2.26)	1.80 (1.10, 2.95)*
Number of MetS components§	1	5.46 (1.72, 17.32)*ǂ	2.04 (0.62, 6.77)ǂ	1.62 (0.33, 8.02)ǂ	4.17 (0.92, 18.97)ǂ
	2	9.21 (2.89, 29.35)*ǂ	2.04 (0.61, 6.82)ǂ	1.84 (0.37, 8.99)ǂ	7.16 (1.55, 32.96)*ǂ
	3	11.00 (3.89, 31.13)*ǂ	2.21 (0.74, 6.59)ǂ	1.69 (0.44, 6.50)ǂ	7.25 (2.05, 25.64)*ǂ
	4	14.95 (5.21, 42.91)*ǂ	2.68 (0.88, 8.18)ǂ	2.04 (0.43, 9.71)ǂ	8.05 (1.91, 33.92)*ǂ
	5	11.38 (3.46, 37.46)*ǂ	1.93 (0.57, 6.49)ǂ	1.57 (0.30, 8.18)ǂ	6.66 (1.40, 31.68)*ǂ
p for linear trend		<.0001	0.9543	0.9257	0.0002
MetS§§		2.23 (1.61, 3.08)*	1.20 (0.86, 1.66)	1.06 (0.67, 1.68)	1.67 (1.06, 2.61)*
		Colon (n=95)			
		ORc (95% CI)	ORage (95% CI)	ORadj (95% CI)	ORadj2 (95% CI)
Individual MetS components	High Blood Pressure	11.19 (4.18, 29.97)*ǂ	2.43 (0.92, 6.42)ǂ	1.53 (0.51, 4.56)ǂ	6.01 (1.87, 19.27)*ǂ
	High Glucose	3.82 (2.39, 6.11)*	1.60 (1.02, 2.53)*	1.57 (0.74, 3.36)ǂ	3.21 (1.45, 7.07)*ǂ
	Low HDL	0.82 (0.48, 1.40)	0.97 (0.56, 1.67)	1.05 (0.45, 2.43)ǂ	0.74 (0.31, 1.68)ǂ
	High Triglyceride	2.03 (1.38, 2.98)*	1.36 (0.92, 2.02)	1.39 (0.74, 2.63)	1.67 (0.86, 3.21)
	High Waist Circumference	2.05 (1.26, 3.32)*	1.31 (0.80, 2.16)	1.21 (0.65, 2.25)ǂ	1.45 (0.75, 2.82)ǂ
Number of MetS components§	1	6.28 (0.78, 50.69)ǂ	2.20 (0.26, 18.46)ǂ	1.39 (0.15, 13.16)ǂ	4.15 (0.49, 34.95)ǂ
	2	14.67 (1.92, 112.04)*ǂ	3.08 (0.36, 26.18)ǂ	1.55 (0.15, 16.54)ǂ	6.97 (0.83, 58.49)ǂ
	3	21.42 (2.91, 157.89)*ǂ	3.77 (0.49, 29.28)ǂ	2.36 (0.27, 20.63)ǂ	11.18 (1.55, 88.86)*ǂ
	4	32.88 (4.28, 252.89)*ǂ	4.95 (0.61, 40.44)ǂ	1.63 (0.17, 15.47)ǂ	8.10 (0.93, 70.73)ǂ
	5	30.19 (3.89, 234.64)*ǂ	3.83 (0.47, 31.26)ǂ	3.01 (0.29, 31.50)ǂ	13.84 (1.29, 148.17)*ǂ
p for linear trend		<.0001	0.3145	0.5796	0.0538
MetS§§		3.49 (2.09, 5.84)*	1.62 (0.98, .69)	1.56 (0.79, 3.08)	2.57 (1.29, 5.13)*

Table 2: Odds ratios for any-site, breast, prostate and colon cancers by individual MetS components, number of MetS components and MetS for the U.S. adult population. ORc is odds ratio crude, ORage is odds ratio adjusted for age, ORadj is odds ratio adjusted for age, sex, ethnicity, income, education, smoking, alcohol, and recreational/leisure-time physical activity (for breast and prostate cancers, sex was not included in the model), and ORadj2 is odds ratio adjusted for sex, ethnicity, income, education, smoke, alcohol, and recreational/leisure-time physical activity (for breast and prostate cancers, sex was not included in the model). Metabolic Syndrome (MetS) is having ≥ 3 of Waist Circumference ≥ 102 cm (men) and, ≥ 88 cm (women), Triglyceride ≥ 1.69 mmol/L (mM), HDL-Cholesterol < 1.04 (men), 1.29 mM (women), blood pressure ≥ 130/85 mmHg of either diastolic or systolic pressures, and fasting plasma glucose ≥5.6 mM, "or medication use for hypertension, diabetes, cholesterol" before ", based on the Harmonized...". §compared to 0 MetS components, §§compared to no MetS, ǂinterpret with caution as n < 20 in reference or response group; * p <0.05.General linear model was used to determine the p for trend analysis. Note: those with missing data were excluded from logistic analyses, and all data have been weighted to represent the U.S. adult population.

smoking, alcohol, and recreational/leisure-time physical activity). Although there was a linear-dose response relationship between the number of MetS components and cancer, the relationship was no longer significant after adjusting for covariates. The only remaining linear trend was for breast cancer, which must be interpreted with caution due to a small sample across the number of MetS components.

To explore age-differences in the above relationships, analyses were stratified by age (18-50 y vs. > 50 y). After stratification, the only remaining significant associations were for number of MetS components with prostate and colon cancer (Table 3).

Discussion

Our aim was to quantify the associations between the number and composition of MetS clusters and any-site, breast, prostate and colon cancers. In general, we found that individuals with MetS had higher prevalences of any-site, breast, prostate, and colon cancers. However, after adjustment for confounders, these relationships were no longer significant. Similarly, despite a graded dose-response relationship for the number of MetS components and prevalence of site-specific cancers, no consistent associations remained after multivariable adjustment.

Our estimation of MetS prevalence is slightly higher than other studies (38% vs. 34%) using similar data and definition, a finding that may be attributed in part to our exclusion of participants with any missing MetS components, and variation in NHANES data cycles

[1,2]. MetS prevalence increases gradually with time, and since we used newer data, this may further explain our modestly higher prevalence [26]. Nonetheless, cancer prevalence in our study (any-site: 8.96%; breast: 1.22%; prostate: 0.94%; and colon: 0.43%) is similar to previous estimates, with slight variation owing to differences in sample selection criteria [27].

MetS Components and Site-Specific Cancer

The above notwithstanding, our finding of no association between MetS and site-specific cancers is at odds with some, but not all previous work. For breast cancer, our finding of no significant association with further stratification by age and menopausal status (i.e., >50 y) is in contrast to the finding of elevated risk amongst those with MetS (1.58, 1.07-2.33) or its individual components (1.67, 1.06-2.63) reported elsewhere. On the other hand, null associations between diabetes, hypertension and dyslipidemia and breast cancer are not entirely unexpected, and have been found in other studies [10,18,21,28]. Variations in the multivariable model, selection criteria, innate characteristics of the study population and study design may account for some of the observed inconsistencies.

The relationship between MetS and prostate cancer also yielded inconsistent results. In our study, low HDL was associated with 36% lower odds of prostate cancer. By contrast, a hospital-based case control by Magura et al. found that men with low HDL cholesterol (<1.03 mM)

			OR (95% CI)	
			Any-site (n=1296)	
			≤50 years (n=195)	> 50 years (n=1101)
Individual MetS component		High Blood Pressure	1.42 (1.04, 1.95)*	1.30 (1.08, 1.56)*
		High Glucose	1.11 (0.74, 1.66)	1.15 (0.96, 1.38)
		Low HDL	0.94 (0.66, 1.35)	0.93 (0.79, 1.08)
		High Triglyceride	1.20 (0.89, 1.61)	1.01 (0.85, 1.20)
		High Waist Circumference	1.62 (1.17, 2.26)*	0.98 (0.82, 1.17)
Number of MetS components§		1	1.71 (0.97, 2.99)	0.94 (0.62, 1.43)
		2	1.74 (0.99, 3.04)	1.04 (0.70, 1.53)
		3	2.00 (1.07, 3.76)	1.10 (0.75, 1.62)
		4	1.46 (0.76, 2.79)ƚ	0.96 (0.63, 1.46)
		5	2.28 (0.99, 5.24)ƚ	1.23 (0.81, 1.86)
p for linear trend			0.1808	0.8029
MetS§§			1.27 (0.90, 1.81)	1.08 (0.92, 1.28)
			Breast	Prostate	Colon
			> 50 years (n=166)	> 50 years (n=204)	> 50 years (n=90)
Individual MetS component		High Blood Pressure	1.35 (0.81, 2.26)	1.38 (0.76, 2.50)	6.78 (2.34, 19.60)*
		High Glucose	1.20 (0.85, 1.69)	1.76 (1.17, 2.64)*	2.01 (1.25, 3.25)*
		Low HDL	0.91 (0.59, 1.41)	0.61 (0.42, 0.89)	0.95 (0.55, 1.66)
		High Triglyceride	1.19 (0.84, 1.68)	1.06 (0.76, 1.46)	1.23 (0.78, 1.93)
		High Waist Circumference	0.73 (0.47, 1.13)	1.19 (0.86, 1.66)	1.21 (0.70, 2.08)
Number of MetS components§		1	0.63 (0.23, 1.67)ƚ	2.79 (0.88, 8.81)ƚ	2.59 (0.31, 21.71)ƚ
		2	0.92 (0.36, 2.36)ƚ	3.00 (0.94, 9.58)ƚ	3.81 (0.50, 29.23)ƚ
		3	0.77 (0.31, 1.89)ƚ	2.76 (0.96, 7.92)ƚ	5.25 (0.70, 39.20)ƚ
		4	0.68 (0.29, 1.61)ƚ	3.52 (1.20, 10.27)*ƚ	6.94 (0.88, 54.56)ƚ
		5	1.06 (0.37, 3.08)ƚ	2.62 (0.80, 8.56)ƚ	5.50 (0.69, 43.96)ƚ
p for linear trend			0.4133	0.0254*	0.0078*
MetS§§			0.99 (0.66, 1.49)	1.12 (0.82, 1.55)	1.97 (1.21, 3.19)*

Table 3: Age-stratified association between individual MetS components, number of MetS components and MetS and any-site, breast and colon cancers, OR is crude odds ratio. Metabolic Syndrome (MetS) is having ≥ 3 of WC ≥ 102 cm (men) and, ≥ 88 cm (women), Triglyceride ≥ 1.69 mmol/L (mM), HDL-Cholesterol < 1.04 (men), 1.29 mM (women), blood pressure ≥ 130/85 mmHg of either diastolic or systolic pressures, and fasting plasma glucose ≥5.6 mM, "or medication use for hypertension, diabetes, cholesterol" before ", based on the Harmonized...". §compared to 0 MetS components, §§compared to no MetS, ƚinterpret with caution as n < 20 in reference or response group; * p <0.05. Due to small number of site-specific cancers among ≤50 year, only results for >50 years are shown for age stratification. Note: those with missing data were excluded from logistic analyses, and all data have been weighted to represent the U.S. adult population but n of samples used in weighing are given.

had a 57% (1.04-2.36) greater likelihood of prostate cancer compared to those with high HDL [29]. Two other studies using cohort designs have produced null associations [20,30]. Although we report a positive association between high blood glucose and prostate cancer, null and negative associations amongst older men and certain ethnic groups (RR: 0.65 [95% CI: 0.50-0.84] for European Americans, RR: 0.89 [95% CI: 0.77-1.03] for African Americans) have also been found [12,20,31]. Differences in blood glucose level (i.e., high glucose (≥5.6 mM) vs. diabetes (≥11.1 mM)) may have exaggerated these differences, as only 22 of 204 prostate cancer cases had physician diagnosed diabetes in our study. Given the central role of obesity in MetS and its high prevalence in the US population, it is also possible that duration of obesity (or elevated blood glucose) may be an important factor in prostate cancer development through oxidative stress induced cell proliferation, reduced adiponectin levels, and hyperinsulinemia induced prostate/colon cancer cell proliferation [3,4,32,33]. When taken together, the discrepancy between the findings may be due to variation in: i) confounding variables and sample (i.e. hospital-based vs. nationally representative); ii) classification of past and current smokers; and iii) multivariable adjustment.

Number of MetS Components and Cancer

Studies evaluating the linear dose-response relationship between the number of MetS components and colorectal, colon, prostate, and postmenopausal breast cancers have found mixed results [17-22]. Contrary to some but not all studies, our linear trends were generally insignificant. Despite pooling multiple cycles of NHANES, the sample size available to explore the dose-response relationship between site-specific cancers and number of MetS components was small, and results must be interpreted with caution [17,18,20,21].

Once more, while the general pattern crude analyses was suggestive of a relationship between number of MetS clusters and any-site cancer, these associations were almost entirely reversed by age, a phenomenon known as Simpson's paradox [34-36]. Cancer risk progressively increases with age and may be linked to age-related increases in susceptibility to carcinogens, hormonal imbalance, immunologic dysfunction, and decreased capacity for cell repair/apoptosis [37]. Although several experimental studies have reported the Simpson's paradox of age, we are not aware of any population-based study that has reported the Simpson's paradox of age between cancer and MetS or its composition. Furthermore, since our results suggest that age is on the causal pathway between metabolic dysfunction and cancer, it is not a genuine confounder [34,38]. Taken together, these findings reinforce therapeutic and preventive strategies targeting age-related causal mechanisms such as immunological decline [39].

Limitations

First, given that our analysis is limited to cross-sectional data, cause and effect cannot be inferred. Second, because only cancer survivors are included, results may be an underestimate of the true association between MetS and cancer [40]. Finally, it is possible that changes in behaviour (consequent to cancer diagnosis) and the self-reported nature of lifestyle factors and cancer history may have also contributed to a lack of observed associations.

Conclusions

Significant crude association between the number (or composition) of MetS clusters and any-site, breast, prostate, and colon cancers are present, but accounting for age alone attenuated most of the associations. In light of the strong effect of age on these associations,

additional prospective studies are needed to explore the effects of MetS components on the development and prognosis of obesity-related cancers.

Reference

1. Mozumdar A, Liguori G (2011) Persistent Increase of Prevalence of Metabolic Syndrome Among U.S. Adults: NHANES III to NHANES 1999–2006. Diabetes Care 34: 216–219.

2. Ford ES, Li C, Zhao G (2010) Prevalence and correlates of metabolic syndrome based on a harmonious definition among adults in the US. J Diabetes 2: 180–193.

3. Khandekar MJ, Cohen P, Spiegelman BM (2011) Molecular mechanisms of cancer development in obesity. Nat Rev Cancer 11: 886–895.

4. Wolin KY, Carson K, Colditz GA (2010) Obesity and Cancer. The Oncologist 15: 556–565.

5. Cowey S, Hardy RW (2006) The metabolic syndrome: A high-risk state for cancer? Am J Pathol 169: 1505-1522.

6. Calle EE, Kaaks R (2004) Overweight, obesity and cancer: epidemiological evidence and proposed mechanisms. Nat Rev Cancer 4: 579-591.

7. Jin K (2010) Modern Biological Theories of Aging. Aging Dis 1: 72-74.

8. Kim RB, Phillips A, Herrick K, Helou M, Rafie C, et al. (2013) Physical activity and sedentary behavior of cancer survivors and non-cancer individuals: results from a national survey. PLoS One 8: e57598.

9. Esposito K, Chiodini P, Colao A, Lenzi A, Giugliano D (2012) Metabolic syndrome and risk of cancer: a systematic review and meta-analysis. Diabetes Care 35: 2402-2411.

10. Larsson SC, Mantzoros CS, Wolk A (2007) Diabetes mellitus and risk of breast cancer: a meta-analysis. Int J Cancer 121: 856-862.

11. Larsson SC, Orsini N, Wolk A (2005) Diabetes mellitus and risk of colorectal cancer: a meta-analysis. J Nat Cancer Inst 97: 1679-1687.

12. Kasper JS, Giovannucci E (2006) A meta-analysis of diabetes mellitus and the risk of prostate cancer. Cancer Epidemiol Biomarkers Prev 15: 2056-2062.

13. Bellamy L, Casas JP, Hingorani AD, Williams DJ (2007) Pre-eclampsia and risk of cardiovascular disease and cancer in later life: systematic review and meta-analysis. BMJ 335: 974.

14. Larsson SC, Wolk A (2007) Obesity and colon and rectal cancer risk: a meta-analysis of prospective studies. Am J Clin Nutr 86: 556-565.

15. Berrington de Gonzalez A, Sweetland S, Spencer E (2003) A meta-analysis of obesity and the risk of pancreatic cancer. Br J Cancer 89: 519-523.

16. Guh DP, Zhang W, Bansback N, Amarsi Z, Birmingham CL, et al. (2009) The incidence of co-morbidities related to obesity and overweight: a systematic review and meta-analysis. BMC Public Health 9: 88.

17. Ahmed RL, Schmitz KH, Anderson KE, Rosamond WD, Folsom AR (2006) The metabolic syndrome and risk of incident colorectal cancer. Cancer 107: 28-36.

18. Agnoli C, Berrino F, Abagnato CA, Muti P, Panico S, et al. (2010) Metabolic syndrome and postmenopausal breast cancer in the ORDET cohort: a nested case-control study. Nutr Metab Cardiovasc Dis 20: 41-48.

19. Tsilidis KK, Brancati FL, Pollak MN, Rifai N, Clipp SL, et al. (2010) Metabolic syndrome components and colorectal adenoma in the CLUE II cohort. Cancer Causes Control 21: 1-10.

20. Tande AJ, Platz EA, Folsom AR (2006) The metabolic syndrome is associated with reduced risk of prostate cancer. Am J Epidemiol 164: 1094-1102.

21. Rosato V, Bosetti C, Talamini R, Levi F, Montella M, et al. (2011) Metabolic syndrome and the risk of breast cancer in postmenopausal women. Ann Oncol 22: 2687-2692.

22. Pelucchi C, Negri E, Talamini R, Levi F, Giacosa A, et al. (2010) Metabolic syndrome is associated with colorectal cancer in men. Eur J Cancer 46: 1866-1872.

23. Alberti KGMM, Eckel RH, Grundy SM, Zimmet PZ, Cleeman JI, et al. (2009) Harmonizing the Metabolic Syndrome A Joint Interim Statement of the International Diabetes Federation Task Force on Epidemiology and Prevention; National Heart, Lung, and Blood Institute; American Heart Association; World Heart Federation; International Atherosclerosis Society; and International Association for the Study of Obesity. Circulation 120: 1640–1645.

24. Penaranda EK, Shokar N, Ortiz M (2013) Relationship between Metabolic Syndrome and History of Cervical Cancer among a US National Population. ISRN Oncol 2013: 840964.

25. Janssen I, Carson V, Lee IM, Katzmarzyk PT, Blair SN (2013) Years of life gained due to leisure-time physical activity in the U.S. Am J Prev Med 44: 23-29.

26. Ford ES, Giles WH, Mokdad AH (2004) Increasing prevalence of the metabolic syndrome among u.s. Adults. Diabetes Care 27: 2444-2449.

27. Howlader N, Noone AM, Krapcho M, Garshell J, Neyman N, et al. (2013) SEER Cancer Statistics Review, 1975-2010, National Cancer Institute. Bethesda, MD.

28. Kucharska-Newton AM, Rosamond WD, Mink PJ, Alberg AJ, Shahar E, et al. (2008) HDL-cholesterol and incidence of breast cancer in the ARIC cohort study. Ann Epidemiol 18: 671-677.

29. Magura L, Blanchard R, Hope B, Beal JR, Schwartz GG, et al. (2008) Hypercholesterolemia and prostate cancer: a hospital-based case-control study. Cancer Causes Control 19: 1259-1266.

30. Mondul AM, Weinstein SJ, Virtamo J, Albanes D (2011) Serum total and HDL cholesterol and risk of prostate cancer. Cancer Causes Control 22: 1545-1552.

31. Waters KM, Henderson BE, Stram DO, Wan P, Kolonel LN, et al. (2009) Association of diabetes with prostate cancer risk in the multiethnic cohort. Am J Epidemiol 169: 937-945.

32. Doyle SL, Donohoe CL, Lysaght J, Reynolds JV (2012) Visceral obesity, metabolic syndrome, insulin resistance and cancer. Proc Nutr Soc 71: 181-189.

33. Su LJ, Arab L, Steck SE, Fontham ET, Schroeder JC, et al. (2011) Obesity and prostate cancer aggressiveness among African and Caucasian Americans in a population-based study. Cancer Epidemiol Biomarkers Prev 20: 844-853.

34. Julious SA, Mullee MA (1994) Confounding and Simpson's paradox. BMJ 309: 1480-1481.

35. Tu YK, Gunnell D, Gilthorpe MS (2008) Simpson's Paradox, Lord's Paradox, and Suppression Effects are the same phenomenon--the reversal paradox. Emerg Themes Epidemiol 5: 2.

36. Yancik R, Ries LA (1994) Cancer in older persons. Magnitude of the problem--how do we apply what we know? Cancer 74: 1995-2003.

37. Ukraintseva S, Yashin AI. (2003) Individual Aging and Cancer Risk: How are They Related? Demogr Res 9: 163–196.

38. Ameringer S, Serlin RC, Ward S (2009) Simpson's paradox and experimental research. Nurs Res 58: 123-127.

39. DePinho RA (2000) The age of cancer. Nature 408: 248-254.

40. Courneya KS, Katzmarzyk PT, Bacon E (2008) Physical activity and obesity in Canadian cancer survivors: population-based estimates from the 2005 Canadian Community Health Survey. Cancer 112: 2475-2482.

32

H$_2$O$_2$ Treatment of HUVECs Facilitates PKC Mediated Thr495 Phosphorylation on eNOS when Pre-treated with High Glucose Levels

Thomas J Guterbaum[1,2,6*], **Thomas H Braunstein**[1,2], **Anna Fossum**[3], **Niels-Henrik Holstein-Rathlou**[1,2], **Christian Torp-Pedersen**[4] and **Helena Domínguez**[1,2,5]

[1]The National Research Foundation Center for Cardiac Arrhythmia, Denmark
[2]Department of Biomedical Sciences, Faculty of Health Sciences, University of Copenhagen, Denmark
[3]Biotech Research and Innovation Center, FACS Facility, University of Copenhagen, Copenhagen, Denmark
[4]Department of Health Science and Technology, Aalborg University, Aalborg, Denmark
[5]Department of Cardiology Y, Bispebjerg Hospital, Frederiksberg Section, Frederiksberg, Denmark
[6]Department of Cardiology MK, Odense University Hospital, Svendborg Section, Svendborg, Denmark

Abstract

Objective: Metabolic syndrome entails hypertension, hyperglycemia, obesity and hypercholesterolemia. This syndrome increases the risk of cardiovascular disease and diabetes. Hyperglycemia during coronary reperfusion is associated with a poor prognosis. Contrastingly, targeting correction of hyperglycemia in clinical trials has not improved clinical outcome or has even been detrimental. H$_2$O$_2$ is produced under hyperglycemic conditions and under reperfusion. This study aims to provide a mechanistic approach evaluating the impact of high glucose on the endothelial nitric oxide pathway in a H$_2$O$_2$-rich environment.

Methods and results: HUVECs (human umbilical vein endothelial cells) were exposed to high glucose (20 mM) for either 20 or 72 hours co-incubated with or without H$_2$O$_2$ (400 µM) for 30 minutes as models of increased oxidative stress during acute and prolonged hyperglycemia, respectively. The presence of reactive oxygen species (ROS) in both mitochondria and cytoplasm was measured by fluorescence activated cell sorting (FACS). Phosphorylation of endothelial nitric oxide synthase (eNOS) on threonine 495 (Thr495) and serine 1177 (Ser1177) was assessed by western blotting. Short-term (20 hours) high concentration of glucose alone increased ROS in mitochondria to 133.5% ($p<0.05$), whereas prolonged (72 hours) did not increase mitochondrial ROS. The increase in mitochondrial ROS could be attenuated by the anti-oxidant N-acetyl-L-cysteine (NAC). Incubation with H$_2$O$_2$ for 30 minutes resulted in an increase in Thr495 phosphorylation (to 425%, $p<0.01$) and a decrease in Ser1177 phosphorylation (to 50.6%, $p<0.01$). Pre-incubation for 20 hours with 10 and 20 mM glucose did not affect phosphorylation of Thr495 and Ser1177. Stimulating HUVECs that were pre-incubated with 20 mM glucose for 72 hours with H$_2$O$_2$ increased Thr495 phosphorylation to 146.6% ($p<0.05$). PKC inhibition attenuated the H$_2$O$_2$-induced Thr495 phosphorylation in cells incubated with high glucose levels for 72 hours.

Conclusion: Acute exposure to high glucose induces oxidative stress. H$_2$O$_2$ leads to phosphorylation of eNOS at Thr495 and dephosphorylation of Ser1177. After prolonged exposure to high glucose levels, the addition of H$_2$O$_2$ yields phosphorylation of Thr495 through the PKC pathway.

Keywords: Endothelial nitric oxide synthase; Thr495 phosphorylation; Ser1177 phosphorylation; High glucose levels; Mitochondrial radical oxygen species

Introduction

The present study aims to provide information on how chronic and acute high glucose affect the activation of endothelial nitric oxide (NO) in an oxidative-stress rich environment. An important manifestation of endothelial dysfunction is the decrease in endothelial derived nitric oxide bioavailability [1]. The production of NO by vascular endothelial cells is central in maintaining normal endothelial function and preventing the development of atherosclerosis. In clinical settings, decreased endothelium-derived NO is an independent predictor of cardiovascular events [2], which probably is related to the ability of NO to inhibit platelet aggregation, attachment of neutrophils to endothelial cells and proliferation of smooth muscle cells [3]. Diabetes is characterized by hyperglycemia and endothelial dysfunction [4,5]. Two interdependent mechanisms seem to contribute to endothelial dysfunction in diabetes: Hyperglycemia and reactive oxygen species (ROS). The experiments conducted in humans by Calver et al. and McVeigh et al. showed that forearm blood flow in diabetic patients was impaired due to decreased availability of NO [6,7]. Studies in healthy subjects during hyperglycemic clamps suggest an important role of hyperglycemia as the response of forearm vessels to methacholine,

as it is attenuated during the clamps [8]. The reperfusion that follows prolonged ischemia provides oxidative stress which may contribute to an impairment of NO production [9,10]. Thus, a combination of hyperglycemia and reperfusion following myocardial ischemia has been regarded as a possible explanation for a poorer outcome in patients with diabetes who suffer from myocardial infarction [11-18]. The results of the DIGAMI-1 study seemed to support this notion, as correcting glycaemia in diabetic patients with high glucose levels (blood glucose >11 mM) at admission for acute myocardial infarction seemed to reduce mortality in these patients [19,20], even though subsequent studies do not support the use of insulin to achieve glycemic control [21]. Since phosphorylation of eNOS at Ser1177 is necessary for eNOS to synthesize NO [22]. While phosphorylation at Thr495 hinders its enzymatic activity [23,24], it is expectable, that conditions where

---

*Corresponding author: Thomas Jeremy Guterbaum, Department of Cardiology MK, Odense University Hospital, Svendborg Section, Valdemarsgade 53, 5700 Svendborg, Denmark; E-mail: guterbaum_thomas@hotmail.com

increased phosphorylation of eNOS-Thr495 occur, lead to a decreased eNOS enzymatic activity and, consequently, to decreased NO production. Indeed, prolonged periods (2-3 days) of exposure of high glucose levels in rat aortic endothelial cells, smooth muscle cells and bovine retina endothelial cells increase the total diacylglycerol (DAG) levels, leading to the activation of the DAG-PKC pathway, and eNOS Thr495 phosphorylation [25].

During the reperfusion that follows acute target organ ischemia, there is a substantial increase of the presence of H_2O_2 [26], which may induce specific phosphorylation of eNOS regulating the synthesis of NO. This effect may also be mediated by increases in the endothelial calcium concentrations or changes in membrane potential [27-29]. In regard to ROS, it has been shown that high glucose levels lead to increased superoxide production by inducing NADPH oxidase [30], which will decrease eNOS expression in endothelial cells [31]. Furthermore, uncoupling of eNOS results in production of superoxide, which reacts rapidly with NO producing peroxynitrite ultimately leading to decreased NO bioavailability [32]. In some studies H_2O_2 appears to be have bidirectional effects, with an early promotion of NO production though eNOS phosphorylation at Ser1177 [33,34] and later inhibition of NO production [35] while only an inhibitory effect is apparent in other [36]. Hence, it is still obscure to what extent eNOS expression, eNOS cofactor availability or oxidative stress contribute to a decreased NO activity in diabetes.

Our study aims to investigate the effects of glucose and ROS on phosphorylation of eNOS Thr495 and Ser1177 in HUVECs. We hypothesized that the presence of high glucose levels in an environment rich in H_2O_2 would lead to eNOS Thr495 phosphorylation and Ser1177 dephosphorylation. Based on previous results, in which we observed increased mitochondrial ROS after H_2O_2 incubation [36], we expected to see an increase in mitochondrial ROS generation with high glucose alone and with H_2O_2 incubation. By extension, we anticipated phosphorylation changes of eNOS after high glucose levels alone and with H_2O_2 and an additive effect by combining the two. We have previously shown that incubating HUVECs with H_2O_2 led to an ERK and ROCK mediated phosphorylation of eNOS at Thr495 [36]. We hypothesized that incubating HUVECs for longer duration (72 hours) with high glucose levels would lead to a facilitation of the PKC pathway and therefore expected to see an increase in Thr495 phosphorylation with high glucose levels alone or combined with H_2O_2 and that the phosphorylation could be hindered by inhibition of PKC.

Materials and Methods

Cell culture and medium

Pooled HUVECs (human umbilical vein endothelial cells) from 15 women were obtained from Lonza (CC-2519, Lonza, Basel, Switzerland) and were grown to confluency in EBM-2 medium (CC-3156) with growth factor and additional supplements (CC-4176, both Lonza, Basel, Switzerland) and 5% Bovine Serum (10270-106, Invitrogen, Carlsbad, CA, USA). According to vendor supplements contained ascorbic acid. Final concentration of ascorbic acid or whether it was in stable form is not stated. Cells were not serum deprived prior to experiments and only cells in passage 3 and 4 were used. The cells were grown to confluency and co-incubated with relevant chemicals in 6 well plates (92006, Techno Plastic Products AG, TPP, Trasdingen, Switzerland) coated with 10.5 µg/cm² gelatin (214340, Difco Laboratories, Beckton, USA). Cells were grown at 20% O_2 (ambient air). HUVECs exposed to glucose were incubated in concentrations of 5, 10 or 20 mM for either 20 hours or 72 hours. It has been shown that HUVECs grown in high glucose levels (19 or 33 mM) for at least 36 hours undergo apoptosis, which

could be reverted by ascorbic acid (100 µM) [37]. Because HUVECs were grown in and treated with high glucose levels with ascorbic acid, we did not expect to induce apoptosis. In concurrent experiments, HUVECs were exposed to 400 µM H_2O_2 for 30 minutes to simulate ischemia/reperfusion. Suppressible oxidative stress was assessed by pre-incubating the relevant subset of HUVECs with 10 mM N-acetyl-L-cysteine ((NAC), A9165, Sigma-Aldrich, Steinheim, Germany) for 20 hours before stimulation with H_2O_2.

The pan-PKC-inhibitor (3-(N-[Dimethylamino]propyl-3-indolyl)-4-(3-indolyl)maleimide, Bisindolylmaleimide I,3-[1-[3-(Dimethylamino) propyl]1H-indol-3-yl]-4-(1Hindol-3-yl)1H-pyrrole-2,5dione) GF109203X (GFX) in a concentration of 1 µM, (G2911, Sigma-Aldrich, Inc., Steinheim, Germany) was used to investigate the role of Protein kinase C (PKC) in Thr495-eNOS phosphorylation and was added 1 hour before harvest.

Western blot procedure

HUVECs were washed twice in ice-cold PBS and harvested with RIPA buffer (R0278), which contained protease (P8340) and phosphatase inhibitor cocktails I and II (P2850, P5726). Additional 1 mM sodium orthovanadate (S6508) and 1 mM phenylmethanesulfonyl fluoride (PMSF, 78830) was added to robustly preserve the phosphorylation of eNOS and inhibit serine proteases, respectively (all compounds from Sigma-Aldrich, Steinheim, Germany). The cell lysate was ultrasonicated and centrifuged for 30 minutes at 20,000 g. After discarding the pellet the solubilized protein concentration was determined with Bradford Protein Assay, according to the producer's recommendations (500-0006, Bio-Rad Laboratories, Hercules, California, USA). After obtaining the protein concentration of each lysate, the concentration was corrected with RIPA buffer to attain equivalent protein amounts. The samples were run on a 7% Novex Tris-Acetate gel (EA03585BOX, Invitrogen Corporation, Carlsbad, CA, USA). After transfer to a nitrocellulose membrane, the equal loading of the gel lanes was confirmed with protein detection Ponceau S staining. The nitrocellulose membrane was blocked by submerging it in a blocking buffer containing 5% (w/v) Skim milk in Tris Buffered Saline (TBS) with 0.05% Tween-20 (TBS-T) for 1 hour at room temperature. Then the membrane was washed 3 times in TBS-T followed by overnight incubation at 4°C with relevant primary antibodies in 5% BSA in TBS-T, which consisted of 1:1000 anti-phospho-eNOS (Thr495) mouse antibody (612707, BD Transduction Laboratories, Franklin Lakes, NJ, USA), 1:1000 anti-phospho-eNOS (Ser1177) mouse antibody (612393, BD Transduction Laboratories, Franklin Lakes, NJ, USA) and rabbit polyclonal anti-eNOS (07-520, Upstate, Lake Placid, NY, USA), followed by washing of the nitrocellulose membrane three times with TBS-T. Thereafter we applied blocking buffer containing a secondary HRP-conjugated anti-rabbit antibody (1858415, Pierce Biotechnology, Rockford, IL, USA) or a HRP-conjugated anti-mouse antibody (1858413, Pierce Biotechnology, Rockford, IL, USA) for 1h at room temperature (1:5000). After washing the nitrocellulose membrane three times it was incubated in SuperSignal West Femto Maximum Sensitivity Substrate (34095, Pierce Biotechnology, Rockford, IL, USA) for 1 minute followed by densitometric quantification (LabWorks, Ultra-Violet Products Ltd, Cambridge, UK). The membranes were also analyzed for equal loading with beta-tubulin. We used the ratio between Thr495 and total eNOS for comparison of eNOS phosphorylation in all western blotting experiments.

Fluorescent activated cell sorting (FACS)

HUVECs were analyzed in separate wells for intracellular and intramitochondrial ROS by incubating cells in medium with 5 µM

5-(and-6)-chloromethyl-2´,7´-dichlorodihydrofluorescein diacetate (CM-H2DCFDA) (C6827, Invitrogen, Eugene, Oregon, USA) or MitoSOX Red mitochondrial superoxide indicator (M36008, Invitrogen, Eugene, Oregon, USA), respectively for 15 minutes at 37°C in the dark. HUVECs were suspended in cold PBS with 1% BSA and analyzed by flow cytometry on a FACS-Aria from BD Biosciences (New Jersey, USA), armed with a blue (488 nm), red (633 nm) and violet (405 nm) laser. CM-H2DCFDA was measured with a 525/50 bandpass filter and MitoSOX Red with a 585/42 bandpass filter. Ten thousand data points were accumulated for each round of analysis.

Statistical analysis

As the absolute signal value from each round of experiment displayed variation we normalized to the control situation in each western gel, thus reflecting the variation in the control level of phosphorylation in an increased variation in the treatment groups. Data are expressed in arbitrary units as percent changes compared to Control (unstimulated cells) and are expressed as average +SEM unless otherwise stated. Groups of data were analyzed by ANOVA followed by the Scheffé post hoc analysis (Statistica, Statsoft, Tulsa, OK, USA). To maintain variance homogeneity relevant data sets underwent logarithmic transformation. Paired comparisons were analyzed by Student's T-test for unequal variance. A p-value <0.05 was considered statistically significant. The letter "n" refers to the number of times an experiment was repeated.

Results

To assess the capability of high glucose levels to induce ROS we exposed HUVECs to a glucose concentration of 20 mM for 20 hours and analyzed the level of ROS in mitochondria as described above. Figure 1a shows that this increased the amount of ROS in mitochondria to 133.5%, p<0.05. This effect could be abolished by simultaneous treatment of cells with 10 mM NAC for 20 hours (Figure 1b). We also investigated the effect of glucose on the cytoplasmic levels of ROS. FACS analysis showed that there was no difference in these levels (data not shown).

We wished to investigate combinations of high glucose and ROS to model the short and long term ischemic conditions and to find additive or synergistic effects between the two. We therefore analyzed Thr495 phosphorylation levels in response to increasing concentrations of glucose in combination with a high amount of H_2O_2. Figure 2 show that H_2O_2 increased Thr495 phosphorylation (to 425% (5 mM), 370% (10 mM), 308% (20 mM)). As these increases after H_2O_2 addition in Thr495 phosphorylation were not significantly different from each other, there was no combined effect of glucose and H_2O_2 on Thr495 phosphorylation. Regarding phosphorylation of Ser1177 in response to glucose and H_2O_2, Fig. 3 shows that H_2O_2 decreased Ser1177 phosphorylation (to 50.6% (5 mM), 31.2% (10 mM), 29.4% (20 mM), p<0.01). As these decreases in Ser1177 phosphorylation were not significantly different from each other, there was no combined effect of glucose and H_2O_2 on Ser1177 dephosphorylation (Figure 3).

Studies have shown that the production of diacylglycerol (DAG) is significant after prolonged exposure to of high glucose concentrations (72 hours). [see Rask-Madsen and King(Rask-Madsen and King 2005) for a review]. DAG stimulates PKC which in turn is capable of phosphorylating Thr495. We therefore hypothesized that although the short term effect of H_2O_2 is not mediated by PKC, prolonged incubation with glucose concentrations in the range of hyperglycemia could facilitate the PKC pathway. We therefore stimulated cells with 20 mM glucose for 72 hours and added 400 μM H_2O_2 for the last 30 minutes, which increased Thr495 phosphorylation with 146.4% (from 112.9% to 165.4%) compared to 20 mM (p<0.05) (Figure 4). This effect was significantly reduced by the pan-PKC inhibitor GFX indicating an enhanced role of PKC by the combined effects of glucose and H_2O_2.

Stimulation with H_2O_2 induced phosphorylation of eNOS Thr495 after 72 hours of incubation with high levels of glucose and was paralleled by an accumulation of ROS in the mitochondria to 235% (5 mM) and 267% (20 mM) (p<0.05) (Figure 5). No significant difference of mitochondrial ROS accumulation was observed between control (5 mM) and 20 mM without H_2O_2 stimulation.

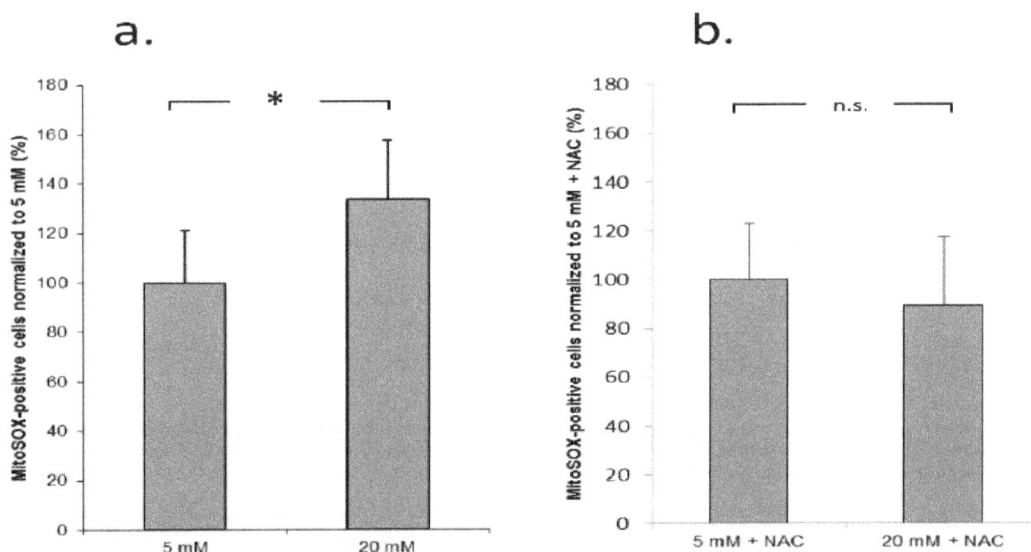

a. The results are presented as normalized means + SEM. N=5. (*p < 0.05: 20 mM glucose treatment for 20 hours vs. control (5 mM))
b. The results are presented as normalized means + SEM. N=4. (n.s. p>0.05; 5 mM + NAC: Control (5 mM glucose) co-incubated with 10 mM NAC for 20 hours. 20 mM + NAC: Cells incubated with 20 mM glucose and 10 mM NAC for 20 hours.

Figure 1: FACS analysis of the ROS formation assessed by application of MitoSOX red mitochondrial superoxide indicator.

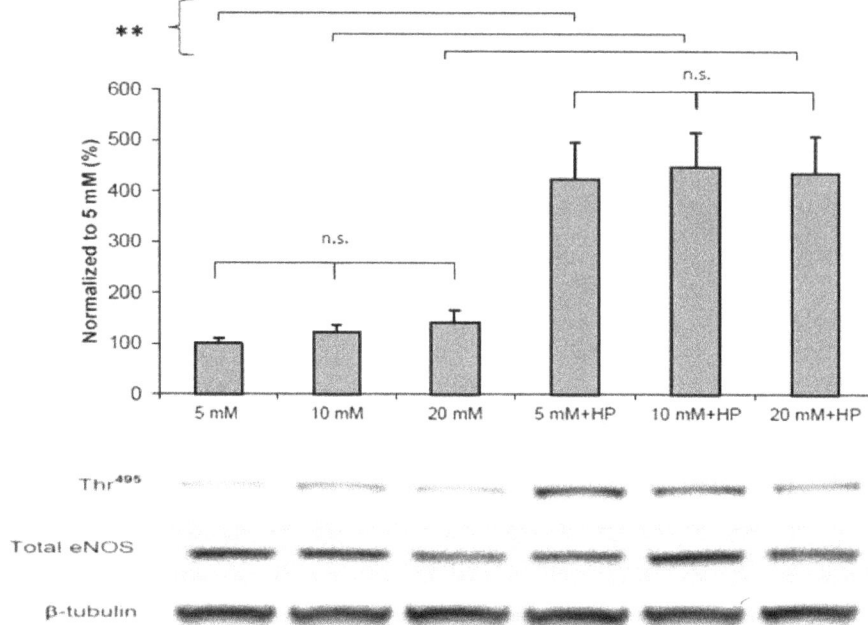

30 minutes of H$_2$O$_2$ stimulation (400 µM) increased phosphorylation of Thr495 significantly. Incubating cells with increasing amounts of glucose (5, 10, 20 mM) did not significantly alter the Thr495 phosphorylation level. No combined effect of H$_2$O$_2$ and glucose was observed. The results are presented as densitometric means of ratios between Thr495 and Total eNOS signals (+/- SEM). Below the graph is shown Thr495, total eNOS and Beta tubulin. (HP: H$_2$O$_2$; n.s.: p>0.05; ** p<0.01).

Figure 2: Western blotting analysis of the role of H$_2$O$_2$ and glucose on phosphorylated threonine 495 residue on eNOS (p -Thr495) (n=8).

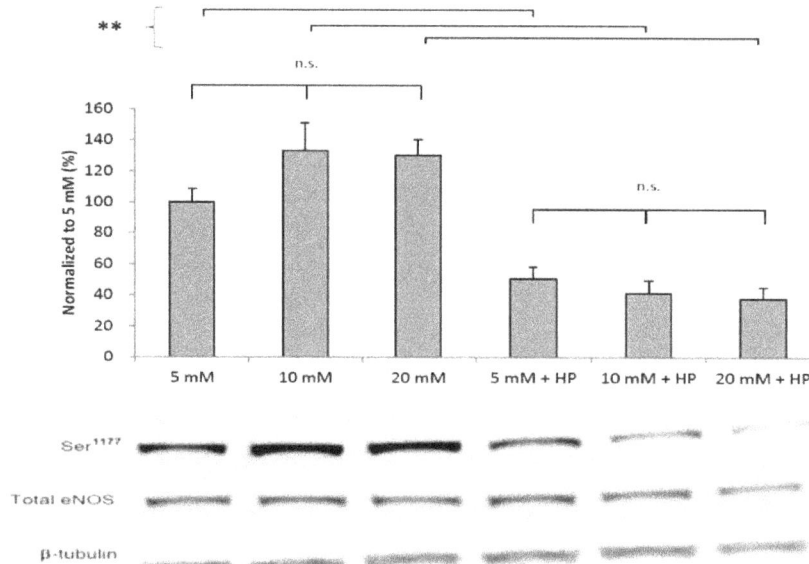

30 minutes of H$_2$O$_2$ stimulation (400 µM) decreased Ser1177 phosphorylation 30 minutes of H$_2$O$_2$ stimulation (400 µM) decreased phosphorylation of Ser1177 significantly. Incubating cells with increasing amounts of glucose (5, 10, 20 mM) did not significantly alter the Ser1177 phosphorylation level. No combined effects of H$_2$O$_2$ and glucose was observed. The results are presented as densitometric means of ratios between Thr495 and Total eNOS signals (+/- SEM). Below the graph is shown Ser1177 as a representative blot as well as the same blot reprobed with total eNOS. Beta tubulin is shown below. (HP: H$_2$O$_2$; n.s.: p>0.05; ** p<0.01).

Figure 3: Western blotting analysis of Ser1177 phosphorylation in HUVECs stimulated with H$_2$O$_2$ and glucose (n=8).

Discussion

The main findings in our study is that 72 hours after exposure of HUVECs to 20 mM glucose followed by addition of 400 µM H$_2$O$_2$ for 30 minutes induced Thr495 phosphorylation mediated by PKC.

These findings support earlier reports from other groups. Inoguchi et al. observed increased DAG content and PKC activation in aortas of streptozotocin induced diabetic rats and BAECs grown in 22.2 mM glucose for four days also displayed the same characteristics [38]. The

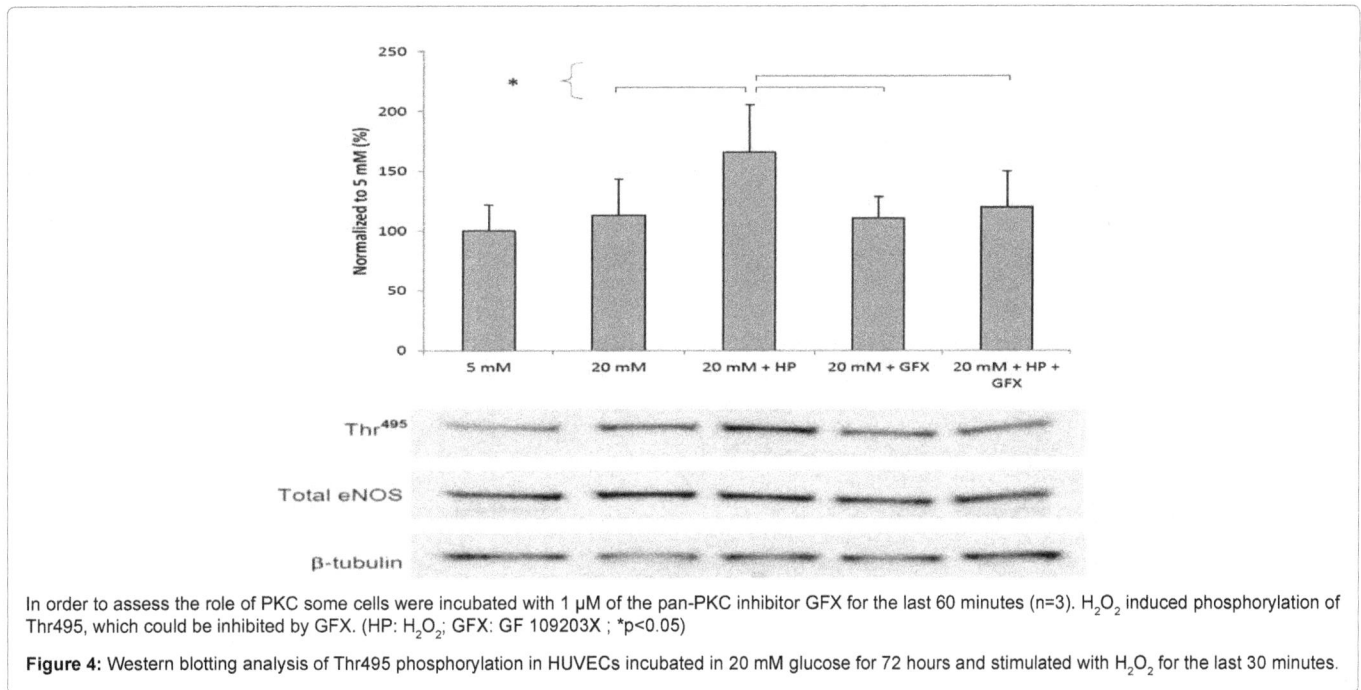

In order to assess the role of PKC some cells were incubated with 1 µM of the pan-PKC inhibitor GFX for the last 60 minutes (n=3). H_2O_2 induced phosphorylation of Thr495, which could be inhibited by GFX. (HP: H_2O_2; GFX: GF 109203X ; *p<0.05)

Figure 4: Western blotting analysis of Thr495 phosphorylation in HUVECs incubated in 20 mM glucose for 72 hours and stimulated with H_2O_2 for the last 30 minutes.

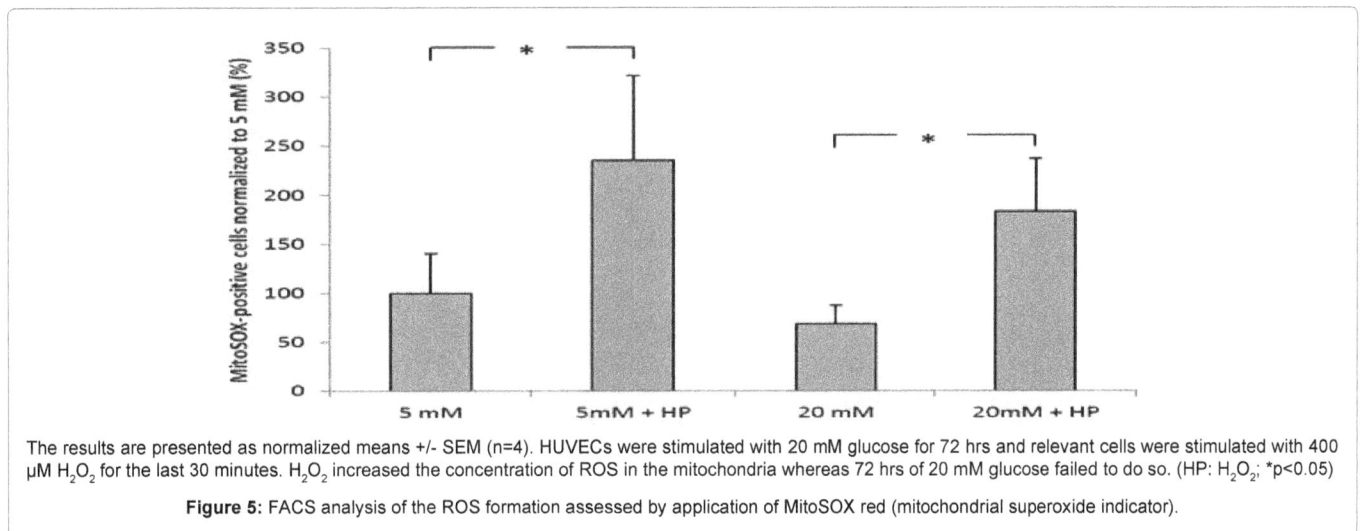

The results are presented as normalized means +/- SEM (n=4). HUVECs were stimulated with 20 mM glucose for 72 hrs and relevant cells were stimulated with 400 µM H_2O_2 for the last 30 minutes. H_2O_2 increased the concentration of ROS in the mitochondria whereas 72 hrs of 20 mM glucose failed to do so. (HP: H_2O_2; *p<0.05)

Figure 5: FACS analysis of the ROS formation assessed by application of MitoSOX red (mitochondrial superoxide indicator).

source of the increased DAG has in bovine or rat aortic endothelial and smooth muscle cells grown under the same circumstances for three days been shown to derive from *de novo* synthesis [39]. Xia et al. also demonstrated that endothelial and smooth muscle cells grown in 22 mM glucose for two to three days increased DAG levels which originated from *de novo* synthesis [25]. This increase in DAG levels and activity has the pivotal effect of activating PKC [25,38] Similarly, Craven et al. detected an increased PKC activity which correlated with increased DAG content in non-diabetic rat glomeruli incubated in 30 mM glucose [40]. Consequentially an increased PKC activity leads to phosphorylation of eNOS Thr495 [41]. Our study failed to show that elevated glucose *per se* would lead to increased phosphorylation of eNOS Thr495. We have previously shown [36] that incubation of HUVECs with H_2O_2 increased phosphorylation of Thr495 not through PKC activation but ROCK and MEKK/ERK activation. In the current study, however, stimulation with H_2O_2 in cells incubated 72 hours after exposure to high glucose levels demonstrated that this phosphorylation

can be inhibited by application of the pan-PKC inhibitor GFX. As DAG production is increased after high glucose exposure for 72 hours [3] we therefore expected phosphorylation of Thr495 after glucose exposure alone. Although we failed to observe this, we obtained results that suggest that elevated glucose concentrations for 72 hours facilitate signaling via the DAG-PKC pathway when cells are exposed to H_2O_2, something we failed to see previously [36]. The applied concentration of the pan-PKC inhibitor GFX of 1 µM exceeds the IC_{50} value of around 20 nM [42], which should completely inhibit PKC with the applied concentration. In pilot experiments we observed that pre-incubation with 1 µM GFX inhibited Thr495 phosphorylation in both HUVECs and BAECs stimulated with PMA. We do recognize that GF109203X may have off-target effects with the applied concentration of 1µM as it has been shown that GF109203X is not a selective inhibitor of PKC isoforms α,β and γ. Both MAPKAP-K1β and p70 S6 kinase are inhibited by similar potency of GF109203X with MAPKAP-K1β having IC_{50}=50 nM and p70 S6 kinase IC_{50}=100 nM [43]. This is crucial because these kinases are involved in signaling pathways activating PKC. In conducting research applying GFX one should ensure that the effects obtained are not due to MAPKAP-K1β and p70 S6 kinase inhibition conducting control experiments with specific inhibitors PD 98059 and rapamycin, respectively. The medium was not changed during the 72 hours of incubation. Studies have shown that HUVECs consume approximately 0.1 mM glucose per hour regardless of outset glucose concentration, yielding a concentration of about 18 mM after 20 hours and 13 mM after 72 hours, without affecting the morphology of the cells [44,45]. This relationship is well established and robust among other cell types also. Altamirano et al. measured consumption rates of glucose in CHO cells. If grown initially at 20 mM the glucose concentration after 20 hours was approximately 17-19 mM, whereas after 72 hours the concentration dropped to around 13 mM [46]. Rheinwald et al. observed in V79 cells grown with complex carbohydrates, when these complex carbohydrates were depleted the concentration of glucose would decline from around 20 mM to approximately 11 mM after 3 days [47]. In all cases the 72 hour time point was still hyperglycemic. Cells incubated with normoglycemic medium would on the other hand experience a slight hypoglycemic environment after 72 hours [45]. It is possible that the used glucose concentration was insufficient to elicit a phosphorylation response without concomitant H_2O_2 stimulation. To convey this, cells could be incubated with higher glucose concentrations, and assess whether it is possible to obtain a dose dependent relationship in both mitochondrial ROS generation and Thr495 phosphorylation. Higher mortality has been shown in patients with myocardial infarction with an admission glucose levels above 8.44 [48], 9-10 [49,50], 11 [51-53] and 11.7 [54]. mM. Based on these values we incubated HUVECs with high glucose levels with an outset concentration of 20 mM reaching calculated concentrations of 18 mM and 13 mM after 20 and 72 hours, respectively. We thus calculate that the cells remained within the concentration range that is associated with higher mortality in clinical trials. Williams et al. showed that the minimum concentration of glucose to activate PKC is 15 mM [55]. Based on the calculations exposed above, such a concentration is reached after 50 hours. This may explain why we observe mitochondrial increase in ROS after 20 hours, but not after 72 hours. Furthermore, we found in preliminary studies, that HUVECs that have been either serum deprived or have not had changed medium (5 mM glucose) for several days could not elicit a phosphorylation response upon stimulation with H_2O_2 (data not shown). The rationale behind starvation is poorly defined and it induces an artificial condition where most of the cells are in an arrested state. The effects of serum starvation seem grave as it induces phosphorylation of many signaling molecules, such as a more than tenfold change in ERK phosphorylation in different cell lines [56]. Therefore, we chose not to starve our cells prior to the studies.

In the micromolar concentration range, H_2O_2 induces changes in membrane potential [57] and intra-cellular calcium in human endothelial cells [57,58], which is not the case at higher concentrations [58]. Thus, intracellular calcium changes are probably not part of the changes that we have observed in our studies.

The applied concentration (400 μM) of H_2O_2 is enough to cause apoptosis in HUVECs [59] and PKC inhibition could inhibit PKC-dependent cell apoptosis [60]. It is in our model not elucidated whether apoptotic pathways play a role in eNOS phosphorylation on Thr495.

Activation of eNOS by phosphorylation at Ser1177 is accompanied by a decrease in the dependence of eNOS for Ca^{2+}/calmodulin [61]. The role of high glucose levels on NO production and the effect on Ser1177 phosphorylation are somewhat unclear. Carneiro et al. showed that

diabetic rats had decreased eNOS phosphorylation levels at Ser1177 in corpora cavernosa [62] and Schnyder et al. showed that high glucose levels in HUVECs (15-30 min; 25 mM) inhibited NO production [63]. Salt et al., however, showed in Human Aortic Endothelial Cells (HAECs) that 25 mM glucose for 48 hours inhibited insulin stimulated NO production although phosphorylation at Ser1177 was not reduced [64]. Furthermore even shorter periods (5 hours) of high glucose levels inhibits Thr495 dephosphorylation and phosphorylation of Ser1177 in bradykinin-stimulated PAECs (porcine aortic endothelial cells) [65]. A recent study on adult cardiac myocytes showed that 10 μM hydrogen peroxide stimulation increased phosphorylation of eNOS at Ser1177 [66]. Likewise, Thomas et al. incubated PAECs with 130-300 μM H_2O_2 for 30 minutes yielding the same result [34]. Also Urao et al. showed that endogenous H_2O_2 increases Ser1177 phosphorylation in a mouse hind limb ischemia model [67]. Our experiments did not show an effect of increased ROS generated by high glucose concentrations on the phosphorylation of Ser1177. In fact, high concentrations of hydrogen peroxide had the opposite effect with a decrease in Ser1177 phosphorylation regardless of the concomitant glucose concentration. The explanation for these apparently contradictory results is suggested by a study by Hu et al. who described a dose-dependent biphasic response to H_2O_2 in which 500 μM initially increased Ser1179 phosphorylation in eNOS transfected HEK 293 cells and BAECs grown in serum-containing medium followed by a drastic decline in phosphorylation after 30 minutes [35]. It is possible that the same mechanism has taken place in our cells, even though this remains speculative as we only have assessed the phosphorylation response after 30 minutes of H_2O_2 stimulation. A clinical trial showed that infusion of a peptide inhibitor of PKCδ (delcasertib) given at reperfusion reduced infarct size when given to STEMI patients [68]. IC_{50} of GFX on PKCδ inhibition is 0.21 μM. Thus a substantial suppression of PKCδ to about 10% activity is achieved with 1 μM used in our study [69]. The findings, however, could not be replicated in the PROTECTION-MI trial, which was a multicenter, double-blind trial was performed in patients presenting within 6 hours undergoing primary PCI for STEMI [70]. We confirm here in an *in vitro* model of reperfusion that PKC is involved in Thr495 phosphorylation giving an indication that inhibition of PKC could prevent endothelial dysfunction which is seen in conjunction to reperfusion damage and high glucose levels. Oxidative stress leads to mitochondrial dysfunction [9,71,72] and H_2O_2 has been suggested as a retrograde signaling molecule deriving from the cytoplasm, as it seems to be supported by the finding that neuronal mitochondria release H_2O_2 in response to incubation with H_2O_2 [73]. Nevertheless, our previous studies failed to confirm this hypothesis [36]. Here we also found no clear indication of a possible retrograde signaling from the mitochondrion to eNOS, since 20 mM of glucose elicited ROS accumulation in the mitochondrion that was not paralleled by phosphorylation or dephosphorylation of eNOS, while externally applied H_2O_2, both accumulated eNOS and induced phosphorylation changes of eNOS. We cannot conclude whether 72 hours of high glucose levels have an effect on mitochondrial ROS accumulation since the final glucose concentrations probably were insufficient to provoke this response. To amend this problem, future studies with higher glucose levels are warranted.

Because a decrease in eNOS-derived NO bioavailability is an important manifestation of endothelial dysfunction, it could be argued that we should have attempted to measure the available NO after HUVECs had been exposed to high glucose levels or H_2O_2. However, we have previously described [36] a decrease in NO production (DAF-2DA chemiluminescence) in acetylcholine stimulated HUVECs pre-incubated with H_2O_2 and thus showed a correlation between an increase in Thr495 phosphorylation and a decrease in NO production.

Conclusion

Incubation of HUVECs with 20 mM glucose for 20 hours increased mitochondrial ROS but did not induce phosphorylation of Thr495 or dephosphorylation of Ser1177, and did not act synergistically with H_2O_2. Exposure to 400 μM of H_2O_2 for 30 minutes in a physiologic glucose concentration phosphorylates Thr495 and dephosphorylates Ser1177 along with increased ROS in mitochondria. High glucose levels were neither able to increase mitochondrial ROS after 72 hours nor did it induce phosphorylation of Thr495. Addition of H_2O_2 elicited phosphorylation of this residue, which could be prevented by PKC inhibition. This suggests that 72 hours exposure to high glucose levels facilitates the PKC pathway in opposition to our previous studies where HUVECs naïve to high glucose levels phosphorylated Thr495 through MEK/ERK and ROCK in response to H_2O_2. Thus, this model points toward two different pathways being involved in eNOS phosphorylation in response to acute ROS as a model of ischemia and reperfusion in the normoglycemic and hyperglycemic state. Our findings support that high glucose levels induce changes in eNOS phosphorylation which leads to decrease in enzymatic activity and thus NO production. These findings have clinical implications with respect to metabolic syndrome underscoring the importance of optimizing glycemic control in these patients thus minimizing development of endothelial dysfunction and by extension the incidence of cardiovascular events.

Acknowledgements

We acknowledge Ninna Buch Petersen for her laboratory skills as well as Christian Rask-Madsen at the Joslin Diabetes Center, Harvard University, Boston, Mass., USA for guidance on techniques. Laboratory expenses were covered by McKinney Møller og hustrus fond til almene formal.

References

1. Napoli C, de Nigris F, Williams-Ignarro S, Pignalosa O, Sica V, et al. (2006) Nitric oxide and atherosclerosis: an update. Nitric Oxide 15: 265-279.

2. Suwaidi JA, Hamasaki S, Higano ST, Nishimura RA, Holmes DR Jr, et al. (2000) Long-term follow-up of patients with mild coronary artery disease and endothelial dysfunction. Circulation 101: 948-954.

3. Rask-Madsen C, and King GL (2005) Proatherosclerotic Mechanisms Involving Protein Kinase C in Diabetes and Insulin Resistance. Arterioscler Thromb Vasc Biol 25: 487-496.

4. Koya D, King GL (1998) Protein kinase C activation and the development of diabetic complications. Diabetes 47: 859-866.

5. Naruse K, Rask-Madsen C, Takahara N, Ha SW, Suzuma K, et al. (2006) Activation of Vascular Protein Kinase C-Beta Inhibits Akt-Dependent Endothelial Nitric Oxide Synthase Function in Obesity-Associated Insulin Resistance. Diabetes 55: 691-698.

6. Calver A, Collier J, Vallance P (1992) Inhibition and stimulation of nitric oxide synthesis in the human forearm arterial bed of patients with insulin-dependent diabetes. J Clin Invest 90: 2548-2554.

7. McVeigh GE, Brennan GM, Johnston GD, McDermott BJ, McGrath LT, et al. (1992) Impaired endothelium-dependent and independent vasodilation in patients with type 2 (non-insulin-dependent) diabetes mellitus. Diabetologia 35: 771-776.

8. Beckman JA, Goldfine AB, Gordon MB, Garrett LA, Creager MA (2002) Inhibition of Protein Kinase Cbeta Prevents Impaired Endothelium-Dependent Vasodilation Caused by Hyperglycemia in Humans. Circ Res 90:107-111.

9. Davidson SM, Duchen MR (2007) Endothelial mitochondria: contributing to vascular function and disease. Circ Res 100: 1128-1141.

10. Jugdutt BI (2002) Nitric oxide and cardioprotection during ischemia-reperfusion. Heart Fail Rev 7: 391-405.

11. Barbash GI, White HD, Modan M, Van de Werf F (1993) Significance of Diabetes Mellitus in Patients with Acute Myocardial Infarction Receiving Thrombolytic Therapy. Investigators of the International Tissue Plasminogen Activator/Streptokinase Mortality Trial. J Am Coll Cardiol 22: 707-713.

12. Behar S, Boyko V, Reicher-Reiss H, Goldbourt U (1997) Ten-Year Survival after Acute Myocardial Infarction: Comparison of Patients with and without Diabetes. SPRINT Study Group. Secondary Prevention Reinfarction Israeli Nifedipine Trial. Am Heart J 133: 290-296.

13. Berger AK, Breall JA, Gersh BJ, Johnson AE, Oetgen WJ, et al. (2001) Effect of diabetes mellitus and insulin use on survival after acute myocardial infarction in the elderly (the Cooperative Cardiovascular Project). Am J Cardiol 87: 272-277.

14. Löwel H, Koenig W, Engel S, Hörmann A, Keil U (2000) The Impact of Diabetes Mellitus on Survival after Myocardial Infarction: Can It Be Modified by Drug Treatment? Results of a Population-Based Myocardial Infarction Register Follow-up Study. Diabetologia 43: 218-226.

15. Mak KH, Moliterno DJ, Granger CB, Miller DP, White HD, et al. (1997) Influence of Diabetes Mellitus on Clinical Outcome in the Thrombolytic Era of Acute Myocardial Infarction. GUSTO-I Investigators. Global Utilization of Streptokinase and Tissue Plasminogen Activator for Occluded Coronary Arteries. J Am Coll Cardiol 30: 171-179.

16. Miettinen H, Lehto S, Salomaa V, Mähönen M, Niemelä M, et al. (1998) Impact of diabetes on mortality after the first myocardial infarction. The FINMONICA Myocardial Infarction Register Study Group. Diabetes Care 21: 69-75.

17. Mukamal KJ, Nesto RW, Cohen MC, Muller JE, Maclure M, et al. (2001) Impact of diabetes on long-term survival after acute myocardial infarction: comparability of risk with prior myocardial infarction. Diabetes Care 24: 1422-1427.

18. Zuanetti G, Latini R, Maggioni AP, Santoro L, Franzosi MG (1993) Influence of diabetes on mortality in acute myocardial infarction: data from the GISSI-2 study. J Am Coll Cardiol 22: 1788-1794.

19. Malmberg K (1997) Prospective Randomised Study of Intensive Insulin Treatment on Long Term Survival after Acute Myocardial Infarction in Patients with Diabetes Mellitus. DIGAMI (Diabetes Mellitus, Insulin Glucose Infusion in Acute Myocardial Infarction) Study Group. BMJ 314: 1512-1515.

20. Malmberg K, Rydén L, Efendic S, Herlitz J, Nicol P, et al. (1995) Randomized Trial of Insulin-Glucose Infusion Followed by Subcutaneous Insulin Treatment in Diabetic Patients with Acute Myocardial Infarction (DIGAMI Study): Effects on Mortality at 1 Year. J Am Coll Cardiol 26: 57-65.

21. Mellbin LG, Malmberg K, Norhammar A, Wedel H, Rydén L, et.al. (2008) The Impact of Glucose Lowering Treatment on Long-Term Prognosis in Patients with Type 2 Diabetes and Myocardial Infarction: A Report from the DIGAMI 2 Trial. Eur Heart J 29: 166-176.

22. Dimmeler S, Fleming I, Fissithaler B, Hermann C, Busse R, et al. (1999) Activation of nitric oxide synthase in endothelial cells by Akt-dependent phosphorylation. Nature 399: 601-605.

23. Fleming I, Busse R (1999) Signal Transduction of eNOS Activation. Cardiovascular research 43: 532-541.

24. Michell BJ, Chen Zp, Tiganis T, Stapleton D, Katsis F, et al. (2001) Coordinated control of endothelial nitric-oxide synthase phosphorylation by protein kinase C and the cAMP-dependent protein kinase. J Biol Chem 276: 17625-17628.

25. Xia P, Inoguchi T, Kern TS, Engerman RL, Oates PJ, et al. (1994) Characterization of the mechanism for the chronic activation of diacylglycerol-protein kinase C pathway in diabetes and hypergalactosemia. Diabetes 43: 1122-1129.

26. Kelley EE, Khoo NK, Hundley NJ, Malik UZ, Freeman BA, et al. (2010) Hydrogen peroxide is the major oxidant product of xanthine oxidase. Free Radic Biol Med 48: 493-498.

27. Jornot L, Maechler P, Wollheim CB, Junod AF (1999) Reactive oxygen metabolites increase mitochondrial calcium in endothelial cells: implication of the Ca2+/Na+ exchanger. J Cell Sci 112 : 1013-1022.

28. Lückhoff A, Busse R (1990) Calcium influx into endothelial cells and formation of endothelium-derived relaxing factor is controlled by the membrane potential. Pflugers Arch 416: 305-311.

29. Mülsch A, Bassenge E, Busse R (1989) Nitric oxide synthesis in endothelial cytosol: evidence for a calcium-dependent and a calcium-independent mechanism. Naunyn Schmiedebergs Arch Pharmacol 340: 767-770.

30. Inoguchi T, Li P, Umeda F, Yu HY, Kakimoto M, et al. (2000) High Glucose Level and Free Fatty Acid Stimulate Reactive Oxygen Species Production through Protein Kinase C--Dependent Activation of NAD(P)H Oxidase in Cultured Vascular Cells. Diabetes 49: 1939-1945.

31. Srinivasan S, Hatley ME, Bolick DT, Palmer LA, Edelstein D, et al. (2004) Hyperglycaemia-Induced Superoxide Production Decreases eNOS Expression via AP-1 Activation in Aortic Endothelial Cells. Diabetologia 47: 1727-1734.

32. Cai H, Harrison DG (2000) Endothelial dysfunction in cardiovascular diseases: the role of oxidant stress. Circ Res 87: 840-844.

33. Cai H, Li Z, Davis ME, Kanner W, Harrison DG, et al. (2003) Akt-Dependent Phosphorylation of Serine 1179 and Mitogen-Activated Protein Kinase Kinase/extracellular Signal-Regulated Kinase 1/2 Cooperatively Mediate Activation of the Endothelial Nitric-Oxide Synthase by Hydrogen Peroxide. Mol Pharmacol 63: 325-331.

34. Thomas SR, Chen K, Keaney JF Jr (2002) Hydrogen Peroxide Activates Endothelial Nitric-Oxide Synthase through Coordinated Phosphorylation and Dephosphorylation via a Phosphoinositide 3-Kinase-Dependent Signaling Pathway. J Biol Chem 277: 6017-6024.

35. Hu Z, Chen J, Wei Q, Xia Y (2008) Bidirectional actions of hydrogen peroxide on endothelial nitric-oxide synthase phosphorylation and function: co-commitment and interplay of Akt and AMPK. J Biol Chem 283: 25256-25263.

36. Guterbaum TJ, Braunstein TH, Fossum A, Holstein-Rathlou NH, Torp-Pedersen CT, et.al. (2013) Endothelial Nitric Oxide Synthase Phosphorylation at Threonine 495 and Mitochondrial Reactive Oxygen Species Formation in Response to a High H2O2 Concentration. J Vasc Res 50: 410-420.

37. Ho FM, Liu SH, Liau CS, Huang PJ, Lin-Shiau SY (2000) High glucose-induced apoptosis in human endothelial cells is mediated by sequential activations of c-Jun NH(2)-terminal kinase and caspase-3. Circulation 101: 2618-2624.

38. Inoguchi T, Battan R, Handler E, Sportsman JR, Heath W, et al. (1992) Preferential elevation of protein kinase C isoform beta II and diacylglycerol levels in the aorta and heart of diabetic rats: differential reversibility to glycemic control by islet cell transplantation. Proc Natl Acad Sci U S A 89: 11059-11063.

39. Inoguchi T, Xia P, Kunisaki M, Higashi S, Feener EP, et al. (1994) Insulin's effect on protein kinase C and diacylglycerol induced by diabetes and glucose in vascular tissues. Am J Physiol 267: E369-379.

40. Craven PA, Davidson CM, DeRubertis FR (1990) Increase in diacylglycerol mass in isolated glomeruli by glucose from de novo synthesis of glycerolipids. Diabetes 39: 667-674.

41. Payne GA, Bohlen HG, Dincer UD, Borbouse L, Tune JD (2009) Periadventitial Adipose Tissue Impairs Coronary Endothelial Function via PKC-Beta-Dependent Phosphorylation of Nitric Oxide Synthase. Am J Physiol Heart Circ Physiol 297: H460-65.

42. Toullec D, Pianetti P, Coste H, Bellevergue P, Grand-Perret T, et al. (1991) The bisindolylmaleimide GF 109203X is a potent and selective inhibitor of protein kinase C. J Biol Chem 266: 15771-15781.

43. Alessi DR (1997) The protein kinase C inhibitors Ro 318220 and GF 109203X are equally potent inhibitors of MAPKAP kinase-1beta (Rsk-2) and p70 S6 kinase. FEBS Lett 402: 121-123.

44. Gong Y, Fan Y, Liu L, Wu D, Chang Z, et al. (2004) Erianin induces a JNK/SAPK-dependent metabolic inhibition in human umbilical vein endothelial cells. In Vivo 18: 223-228.

45. Watanabe K, Fairclough GF Jr, Jaffe EA (1992) Hypoglycemia rapidly develops in cultures of human endothelial cells. In Vitro Cell Dev Biol 28A: 73-74.

46. Altamirano C, Paredes C, Cairó JJ, Gòdia F (2000) Improvement of CHO cell culture medium formulation: simultaneous substitution of glucose and glutamine. Biotechnol Prog 16: 69-75.

47. Rheinwald JG, Green H (1974) Growth of cultured mammalian cells on secondary glucose sources. Cell 2: 287-293.

48. Beck JA, Meisinger C, Heier M, Kuch B, Hörmann A, et al. (2009) Effect of Blood Glucose Concentrations on Admission in Non-Diabetic versus Diabetic Patients with First Acute Myocardial Infarction on Short- and Long-Term Mortality (from the MONICA/KORA Augsburg Myocardial Infarction Registry). Am J Cardiol 104: 1607-1612.

49. Bellodi G, Manicardi V, Malavasi V, Veneri L, Bernini G, et al. (1989) Hyperglycemia and prognosis of acute myocardial infarction in patients without diabetes mellitus. Am J Cardiol 64: 885-888.

50. Leor J, Goldbourt U, Reicher-Reiss H, Kaplinsky E, Behar S (1993) Cardiogenic Shock Complicating Acute Myocardial Infarction in Patients without Heart Failure on Admission: Incidence, Risk Factors, and Outcome. SPRINT Study Group. Am J Med 94: 265-273.

51. Sewdarsen M, Vythilingum S, Jialal I, Becker PJ (1989) Prognostic importance of admission plasma glucose in diabetic and non-diabetic patients with acute myocardial infarction. Q J Med 71: 461-466.

52. Stranders I, Diamant M, van Gelder RE, Spruijt HJ, Twisk JW, et al. (2004) Admission blood glucose level as risk indicator of death after myocardial infarction in patients with and without diabetes mellitus. Arch Intern Med 164: 982-988.

53. Wahab NN, Cowden EA, Pearce NJ, Gardner MJ, Merry H, et al. (2002) Is blood glucose an independent predictor of mortality in acute myocardial infarction in the thrombolytic era? J Am Coll Cardiol 40: 1748-1754.

54. Hadjadj S, Coisne D, Mauco G, Ragot S, Duengler F, et al. (2004) Prognostic value of admission plasma glucose and HbA in acute myocardial infarction. Diabet Med 21: 305-310.

55. Williams B, Schrier RW (1992) Characterization of glucose-induced in situ protein kinase C activity in cultured vascular smooth muscle cells. Diabetes 41: 1464-1472.

56. Pirkmajer S, Chibalin AV (2011) Serum starvation: caveat emptor. Am J Physiol Cell Physiol 301: C272-279.

57. Bychkov R, Pieper K, Ried C, Milosheva M, Bychkov E, et al. (1999) Hydrogen peroxide, potassium currents, and membrane potential in human endothelial cells. Circulation 99: 1719-1725.

58. Hu Q, Corda S, Zweier JL, Capogrossi MC, Ziegelstein RC (1998) Hydrogen peroxide induces intracellular calcium oscillations in human aortic endothelial cells. Circulation 97: 268-275.

59. Park WH (2013) The effects of exogenous H2O2 on cell death, reactive oxygen species and glutathione levels in calf pulmonary artery and human umbilical vein endothelial cells. Int J Mol Med 31: 471-476.

60. Wang SS, Xu YH, Feng L, Zhu Q, He B (2011) A PKC-beta inhibitor prompts the HUVECs apoptosis-induced by advanced glycation end products. Pharmazie 66: 881-887.

61. Fleming I, Fisslthaler B, Dimmeler S, Kemp BE, Busse R (2001) Phosphorylation of Thr(495) regulates Ca(2+)/calmodulin-dependent endothelial nitric oxide synthase activity. Circ Res 88: E68-75.

62. Carneiro FS, Giachini FR, Carneiro ZN, Lima VV, Ergul A, et al. (2010) Erectile dysfunction in young non-obese type II diabetic Goto-Kakizaki rats is associated with decreased eNOS phosphorylation at Ser1177. J Sex Med 7: 3620-3634.

63. Schnyder B, Pittet M, Durand J, Schnyder-Candrian S (2002) Rapid Effects of Glucose on the Insulin Signaling of Endothelial NO Generation and Epithelial Na Transport. Am J Physiol Endocrinol Metab 282: E87–94.

64. Salt IP, Morrow VA, Brandie FM, Connell JM, Petrie JR (2003) High Glucose Inhibits Insulin-Stimulated Nitric Oxide Production without Reducing Endothelial Nitric-Oxide Synthase Ser1177 Phosphorylation in Human Aortic Endothelial Cells. J Biol Chem 278: 18791-18797.

65. Zhang XH, Yokoo H, Nishioka H, Fujii H, Matsuda N, et al. (2010) Beneficial effect of the oligomerized polyphenol oligonol on high glucose-induced changes in eNOS phosphorylation and dephosphorylation in endothelial cells. See co Br J Pharmacol 159: 928-938.

66. Sartoretto JL, Kalwa H, Pluth MD, Lippard SJ, Michel T (2011) Hydrogen Peroxide Differentially Modulates Cardiac Myocyte Nitric Oxide Synthesis Proc Natl Acad Sci U S A 108: 15792-15797.

67. Urao N, Sudhahar V, Kim SJ, Chen GF, McKinney RD, et al. (2013) Critical role of endothelial hydrogen peroxide in post-ischemic neovascularization. PLoS One 8: e57618.

68. Bates E, Bode C, Costa M, Gibson CM, Granger C, et al. (2008) Intracoronary KAI-9803 as an Adjunct to Primary Percutaneous Coronary Intervention for Acute ST-Segment Elevation Myocardial Infarction. Direct Inhibition of Delta-Protein Kinase C Enzyme to Limit Total Infarct Size in Acute Myocardial Infarction. Circulation 117: 886-896.

69. Martiny-Baron G, Kazanietz MG, Mischak H, Blumberg PM, Kochs G, et al. (1993) Selective inhibition of protein kinase C isozymes by the indolocarbazole Gö 6976. J Biol Chem 268: 9194-9197.

70. Lincoff AM, Roe M, Aylward P, Galla J, Rynkiewicz A, et al. (2014) Inhibition of Delta-Protein Kinase C by Delcasertib as an Adjunct to Primary Percutaneous Coronary Intervention for Acute Anterior ST-Segment Elevation Myocardial Infarction: Results of the PROTECTION AMI Randomized Controlled Trial. Eur Heart J 35:2516-2523.

71. Dröge W (2002) Free radicals in the physiological control of cell function. Physiol Rev 82: 47-95.

72. Zhuang S, Kinsey GR, Yan Y, Han J, Schnellmann RG (2008) Extracellular Signal-Regulated Kinase Activation Mediates Mitochondrial Dysfunction and Necrosis Induced by Hydrogen Peroxide in Renal Proximal Tubular Cells. J Pharmacol Exp Ther 325: 732-740.

73. Kudin AP, Bimpong-Buta NY, Vielhaber S, Elger CE, Kunz WS (2004) Characterization of Superoxide-Producing Sites in Isolated Brain Mitochondria J Biol Chem 279: 4127-4135.

33

Non-Alcoholic Fatty Liver Disease and the Left Ventricle Mass Index in Obese Children

Beray Selver[1], Enver Simsek[2]*, Ugur Kocabas[3] and Yildiz Dallar[1]

[1]Department of Pediatrics, Ankara Research and Training Hospital, Ankara, Turkey
[2]Department of Pediatrics, Division of Endocrinology, Eskisehir Osmangazi University, School of Medicine, Eskisehir, Turkey
[3]Department of Cardiology, Ankara Research and Training Hospital, Ankara, Turkey

Abstract

Objective: To investigate Nonalcoholic Fatty Liver Disease (NAFLD), the Left Ventricle Mass Index (LVMI), and the relationship between NAFLD and LVMI in obese children.

Material and methods: Systolic (SBP) and Diastolic (DBP) Blood Pressure and waist and hip circumferences were measured. Fasting blood glucose and insulin concentrations, total cholesterol, and Triglycerides (TG) were assayed. The diagnosis of NAFLD was based on sonographic evidence of a fatty liver. The Left Ventricle Mass (LVM) was calculated from two-dimensionally guided M-mode echocardiographic measurements of the left ventricle. LVMI was calculated as LVM (g)/height (m)$^{2.7}$ and Left Ventricular Hypertrophy (LVH) was defined as LVMI ≥ 95th percentile for age and gender

Results: Forty-three obese children with NAFLD, 55 obese children without NAFLD, and 48 non-obese controls were studied. Fasting insulin, homeostasis model assessment-estimated insulin resistance (HOMA-IR) index, TG, and total cholesterol levels in the obese children were significantly higher than in the controls (all $p < 0.001$); SBP and DBP in the obese children were also higher than in the controls. LVMI was higher in the obese children ($p < 0.001$), although the mean LVMI did not differ significantly between obese children with and without NAFLD ($p > 0.05$). The prevalence of LVH differed significantly between the obese groups and controls (all $p < 0.001$), while there was no significant difference between the obese subjects with and without NAFLD. LVH was present in 5 of 48 (10.4%) control subjects, 25 of 79 (31.6%) obese subjects with normotensive subjects, and 6 of 19 (36.8%) obese subjects with hypertension. The prevalence of LVH differed significantly between the obese groups and controls (all $p < 0.001$), whereas no significant difference was observed between obese subjects with or without hypertension ($p > 0.05$). In a multiple linear regression analysis, NAFLD, SBP, and DBP were not correlated with LVMI. The LVMI was closely related to the Body Mass Index-Standard Deviation Score (BMI-SDS), and Liver Longitudinal Dimension (LLD) percentile. The BMI-SDS was the only independent predictor of NAFLD and LVMI.

Conclusions: LVH and NAFLD are two important and independent covariates in obese children. Obese children with or without hypertension have significant LVH as compared with non-obese control subjects. NAFLD and casual blood pressure measurements are not predictors of LVMI in obese children.

Keywords: Children; Obesity; Left ventricle mass index; Non-alcoholic fatty liver disease

Introduction

The prevalence of childhood obesity is increasing, not only in developed countries, but also in some developing countries [1]. It is associated with several risk factors for later heart disease and other chronic diseases, including hyperlipidemia, hyperinsulinemia, hypertension, and early atherosclerosis [2]. Children who are overweight and obese are more likely to become overweight and obese adults [3].

Non-Alcoholic Fatty Liver Disease (NAFLD) describes a spectrum of liver damage, ranging from simple steatosis to steatohepatitis, advanced fibrosis, and cirrhosis in persons who have not consumed alcohol so as to cause liver damage, and in whom no other etiology for fatty liver is present. An increased prevalence of NAFLD has been observed along with a dramatic rise in obesity in children during the past three decades. Obesity and insulin resistance are hallmarks of NAFLD. The exact prevalence of NAFLD is unclear. Pooling data from studies performed primarily in tertiary medical centers, the reported prevalence of NAFLD in obese children ranges from 20 to 77% [1,4-6].

Left Ventricular Hypertrophy (LVH) has prognostic importance in adults and is generally considered to have a similar prognostic value in children. Numerous population-based and hypertensive cohort studies investigating the impact of adiposity on left ventricle structure have shown that LVH is more prevalent in obese individuals than in their lean counterparts [7,8]. No reported study has analyzed the relationship between NAFLD and the Left Ventricle Mass Index (LVMI) in obese children. Thus, this study investigated the risk factors for left ventricle hypertrophy and determined the relationship between NAFLD and the LVMI in obese children.

Material and Methods

This was a cross-sectional study that included 98 obese children and 48 age- and gender-matched non-obese children as a control group. Subjects were enrolled randomly from among the obese children admitted to the Pediatric Endocrinology Department of Ankara Research and Training Hospital. To compare variables that differed significantly between the obese children and controls, the obese children were subdivided into two groups according to the presence of NAFLD.

*Corresponding author: Prof. Dr. Enver Simsek, Department of Pediatrics, Division of Pediatric Endocrinology, Eskisehir Osmangazi University, School of Medicine, Eskisehir, Turkey; E-mail: enversimsek06@hotmail.com

Inclusion criteria included a Body Mass Index (BMI) ≥ 95th percentile for age and gender. Children were excluded if they had any condition known to influence body composition, insulin action, or insulin secretion (e.g., glucocorticoid therapy, hypothyroidism, Cushing's syndrome), or a history of medication use that could affect body mass or lipid profile. Children were also excluded if they had a history of medication use that causes liver inflammation, diabetes mellitus, or tested positive for hepatitis B or C.

At enrollment, the subjects all underwent physical examinations that included weight, standing height, BMI, and blood pressure measurements. Height was measured to the nearest 0.1 cm without shoes using a Harpenden stadiometer (Harpenden, Holtain, UK). Weight was measured to the nearest 0.1 kg on a standard beam scale with the subject dressed only in light underwear and without shoes. All measurements were repeated twice.

The weight status was recorded as the BMI, which was calculated as weight (kg)/height^2 (m). Because the BMI changes rapidly with normal growth, and varies with age and gender, it was standardized for age and gender by converting to a "z score" [9]. Data were expressed as the Body Mass Index-Standard Deviation Score (BMI-SDS), which was calculated as [individual measurement-population mean]/population SD. Obesity was defined as a BMI ≥ 95th percentile according to reference curves for Turkish children [10]. The waist circumference was measured at the smallest point between the iliac crest and rib cage, and the hip circumference was measured at the largest width over the greater trochanter.

The resting Systolic (SBP) and Diastolic (DBP) Blood Pressures were measured twice in the right arm after a 10-min rest in a supine position by one investigator using a standard mercury sphygmomanometer and a validated protocol [11]. All subjects were considered hypertensive when the SBP or DBP was ≥ 95th percentile for age, gender, and height according to a percentiles chart for Turkish children [12]. Patients with evidence of secondary hypertension and those already on antihypertensive medication were excluded. Secondary hypertension was excluded by history, physical examination, serum chemistry, urinalysis, renal ultrasound, and other tests as indicated. Obese subjects were divided into four groups (with or without NAFLD and with or without hypertension) to compare the frequency of LVMI and LVH.

Biochemical analysis

After an overnight fast, blood samples were taken for the analysis of serum glucose, plasma insulin, Total Cholesterol (TC), Triglycerides (TG), Alanine Aminotransferase (ALT), Aspartate Aminotransferase (AST), Hepatitis B surface Antigen (HBsAg), and anti-Hepatitis C Virus antibody (anti-HCV). Glucose was measured using the glucose-oxidase colorimetric method using an automated analyzer (Hitachi, Roche Diagnostics, Mannheim, Germany). Fasting insulin was analyzed with a radio-immunochemical method (Pharmacia & Upjohn Diagnostics AB, Uppsala, Sweden). The detection limit was 0.5 μU/mL, and the intra- and interassay coefficients of variation were 6.5 and 9.1%, respectively. The homeostasis model assessment of insulin resistance (HOMA-IR) was used to evaluate insulin sensitivity [13]. The HOMA-IR was calculated as HOMA-IR = [fasting insulin (μU/mL) × fasting glucose (mmol/L)] / 22.5. A HOMA-IR > 3.16 was taken as a surrogate measure of insulin resistance [14].

The ALT, AST, fasting TC, and TG were measured using enzymatic colorimetric methods on an automated analyzer (Hitachi 904, Roche Diagnostics). Elevated liver enzymes were defined an ALT or AST ≥ 40 units/L. Cut-off points ≥ 95th percentile of healthy children were used to define dyslipidemia in accordance with international recommendations.

These cut-off points were 200 mg/dL (5.1 mmol/L) for cholesterol and 150 mg/dL (1.7 mmol/L) for triglycerides [15]. HBsAg and anti-HCV were measured using microparticle enzyme immunoassays (Abbott Laboratories, Abbott Park, IL, USA).

Liver ultrasound and echocardiographic examination

An ultrasound examination was performed to identify NAFLD and to measure the Liver Longitudinal Dimension (LLD). The procedure was carried out by an experienced radiologist who was unaware of both the study aims and the participants' biochemical profiles. An ultrasound device (GE LOGIQa 100 MP, GE Medical System, Milwaukie, WI, USA) with a 5-mHz probe in younger children and a 3.5-mHz probe in larger or markedly obese children was used. Fatty liver was diagnosed based on the ultrasonographic pattern and graded as absent, mild, moderate, and severe, according to the criteria of Needleman et al. [16]. In this study, the diagnosis of NAFLD was based on sonographic evidence of a fatty liver and negative test results for HBsAg and anti-HCV antibody. No participant had a history of liver disease, hypertension, or diabetes.

Echocardiograms were performed in all study subjects to evaluate LVH. All echocardiography was conducted by a single cardiologist. To determine the Left Ventricular Mass (LVM), two-dimensional echocardiography was performed in M-mode (General Electric Vivid 3, Norway) according to the guidelines of the American Society of Echocardiography [17]. All measurements were made at end-diastole, which was defined as the time of the maximum left ventricle dimension. Electronic calipers were used to measure the left ventricle internal diameter, interventricular septal thickness, and left ventricle posterior wall thickness from the M-mode images. The measurements were repeated over three consecutive cardiac cycles and averaged. The Devereux formula was used to estimate the LVM [18]. Because the LVM increases during growth and normal must be defined in the context of body size, the Left Ventricular Mass Index (LVMI) was calculated for all children as the LVM in grams divided by height in meters to the 2.7th power [19,20]. Using pediatric criteria, Left Ventricle Hypertrophy (LVH) was defined as LVMI ≥ 95th percentile for gender, which was 39.36 g/m$^{2.7}$ for boys and 36.88 g/m$^{2.7}$ for girls [21].

The study was conducted in accordance with the guidelines proposed in the Declaration of Helsinki and was approved by the Ethics Committee of Ankara Research and Training Hospital. Written informed consent was obtained from all participants over 12 years of age, and informed parental consent was obtained for all children regardless of age.

Statistical Analysis

Statistical analyses were performed using the Statistical Package for the Social Sciences (SPSS/PC+, ver. 13.0, Chicago, IL, USA). The following variables were included in the analysis: clinical data [Weight Standard Deviation Score (WSDS), Height Standard Deviation Score (HSDS), BMI-SDS, SBP, DBP, and pubertal status], biochemical parameters (fasting serum insulin and glucose concentrations, and HOMA-IR), LLD, NAFLD, LVM, and LVMI. The data are expressed as the mean ± standard deviation (SD) or median (min-max) where appropriate. Test selection was based on evaluating the variables for a normal distribution using the Shapiro–Wilk test. If the variables were distributed normally, a Student's t-test was used; otherwise, the Mann-Whitney U-test was used. Categorical data were evaluated using Pearson's chi-squared or Fisher's exact test where applicable. Statistical correlations were calculated using Spearman's correlation. Multiple linear regression analysis was performed with LVMI and NAFLD as dependent variables, and age, BMI-SDS, HOMA-IR, AST, ALT, and LLD

	Obese children n=98 (%)	Non-obese controls n=48 (%)	p
Age (year)	12.4 ± 2.4	11.6 ± 2.2	0.385[a]
Boy/Girl	41/57	27/21	0.101[b]
Pubertal/Prepubertal	67/31	31/17	0.648[b]
BMI-SDS	2.6 (0.55-5.14)	0.42 (-1.71 – 1.94)	< 0.001[c]
Waist circumference (WC)(cm)	86 (63-117)	62 (49-79)	< 0.001[c]
Hip circumference (HC) (cm)	99.9 ± 11.9	78.8 ± 9.1	< 0.001[a]
WC/HC ratio	0.88 ± 0.087	0.80 ± 0.082	< 0.001[a]
SBP > 95th percentile	19 (19.4%)	none	< 0.001[b]
DBP > 95th percentile	14 (14.3%)	none	0.005[d]
Glucose (mg/dl)	82 (53-225)	84 (67-98)	0.154[c]
Insulin (µU/ml)	17.8 (2.3-113.6)	9.2 (3.4-22.7)	< 0.001[c]
HOMA-IR	3.6 (0.5-21.3)	1.9 (0.7-4.4)	< 0.001[c]
Triglyceride (mg/dl)	124 (38-432)	82 (33-207)	< 0.001[c]
Total cholesterol (mg/dl)	165 ±27	141 ±24	< 0.001[a]
AST (U/L)	23 (11-96)	24 (15-40)	0.742[c]
ALT (U/L)	19 (7-199)	17 (9-35)	< 0.001[c]
NAFLD	43 (43.9%)	1 (2.1%)	< 0.001[b]
LVM (g)	119.8 (63.3-243.5)	82.0 (32.3-128.7)	< 0.001[c]
LVMI (g/m2.7)	40.1 (26.4-98.2)	29.7 (15.6-42.0)	< 0.001[c]

SBP: Systolic Blood Pressure; DBP: Diastolic Blood Pressure; HOMA-IR: Homeostasis Model Assessment Of Insulin Resistance; AST: Aspartate Aminotransferase; ALT: Alanine Aminotransferase; NAFLD: Non-Alcoholic Fatty Liver Disease; LLD: Liver Longitudinal Dimension; LVM: Left Ventricle Mass; LVMI: Left Ventricle Mass Index.
[a]Student's t-test
[b]Pearson's chi-squared test
[c]Mann Whitney U test
[d]Fisher's exact test

Table 1: Clinical characteristics, laboratory data, LLD percentile, LVM, and LVMI in obese children and non-obese controls.

	Obese children with NAFLD (N=43)	Obese children without NAFLD (N=55)	Control subjects (N=48)	p1	p2	p3
BMI-SDS	2.55 (2.27-2.84)	2.66 (2.37-2.95)	0.41 (-0.42-1.01)	< 0.001	< 0.001	0.18
LLD percentile	90 (75-95)	75 (50-90)	50 (25-75)	< 0.001	< 0.001	0.65
Triglyceride (mg/dl)	125 (88-149)	123 (92-158)	82 (63-117)	< 0.001	< 0.001	0.46
Total cholesterol (mg/dl)	167 (± 29)	164 (± 27)	141 (± 25)	< 0.001	< 0.001	0.84
ALT (U/L)	19 (16-26)	19 (15-23)	17 (12-21)	<0.001	<0.001	0.99
Fasting insulin (µU/ml)	17.6 (13.2-22.88)	17.9 (12.6-23.4)	9.24 (7.3-11.6)	< 0.001	< 0.001	0.96
HOMA-IR	3.57 (2.92-5.10)	3.56 (2.47-4.60)	1.94 (1.47-2.60)	< 0.001	< 0.001	0.98
LVMI (g/m$^{2.7}$)	40.4 (35.8-46.1)	39.6 (34.6-45.6)	29.7 (25.2-33.6)	< 0.001	< 0.001	0.92

*The data are expressed as the mean ± SD or median (25%-75%) where appropriate; BMI-SDS: Body Mass Index – Standard Deviation Score; LLD: Liver Longitudinal Dimension Percentile; ALT: Alanine Aminotransferase; HOMA-IR: Homeostasis Model Assessment of Insulin Resistance; NAFLD: Non-Alcoholic Fatty Liver Disease; LVMI: Left Ventricle Mass Index; LVH: Left Ventricle Hypertrophy; NAFLD: Non-Alcoholic Fatty Liver Disease
p1: obese children with NAFLD vs. control; p2: obese children without NAFLD vs. control; p3: obese children with NAFLD vs. obese without NAFLD

Table 2: Obesity related risk factors in obese children with NAFLD, obese children without NAFLD, and control subjects*.

percentile as independent variables. Logarithmic transformed data for LVM and LVMI were used because of their non-normal distributions. Multiple linear regression analysis was performed with LVMI as a dependent variable, NAFLD as a main predictor variable, and BMI-SDS as a covariate (model I). In model II, LVMI was the dependent variable, NAFLD was the main predictor variable, and BMI-SDS, SBP, and DBP were covariates. P-values < 0.05 were considered statistically significant.

Results

Of the participants, six were excluded because they tested positive for HBsAg (n = 5) or anti-HCV (n = 1). The study included 98 obese children and 48 non-obese control children. Of the obese subjects, 43 had NAFLD and 55 did not. The physical characteristics, laboratory results, LLD, LVM, and LVMI of the obese children and controls are summarized in Table 1. Compared with the controls, the obese children had significant differences in several clinical risk factors, including body weight, BMI, BMI-SDS, SBP, DBP, waist circumference, hip circumference, and waist/hip ratio (all p < 0.001). Nineteen (19.4%)

of the 98 obese children had systolic or diastolic hypertension; none of the control subjects did. Insulin resistance was seen in 66 (67%) of the obese children and only two (4%) of the controls. The median LLD percentile in obese children and control subjects was the 82.5 (5–95) and 50 (10–95) percentile, respectively (p < 0.001). Forty-three (44%) of the obese children had NAFLD, while only one (2%) control subject did. The median LVMI in obese and control subjects was 40.1 (26.4–68.2) and 29.7 (15.6–42.0) g/m$^{2.7}$, respectively (p < 0.001). Comparisons of obesity-related risk factors between obese children with and without NAFLD and control subjects are presented in Table 2. All obesity-related risk factors differed significantly between the controls and obese children with or without NAFLD (all p < 0.001; Table 2). However, the same variables did not differ between obese children with and without NAFLD (Figure 1). LVH was present in 5 of 48 (10.4%) control subjects and 30 of 98 (30.6%) obese subjects. When obese children were grouped according to whether or not they had hypertension, LVH was present in 24 of 79 (30.3%) obese subjects without hypertension and 6 of 19 (36.8%) obese subjects with hypertension. The frequency of LVH differed significantly between the obese children and controls

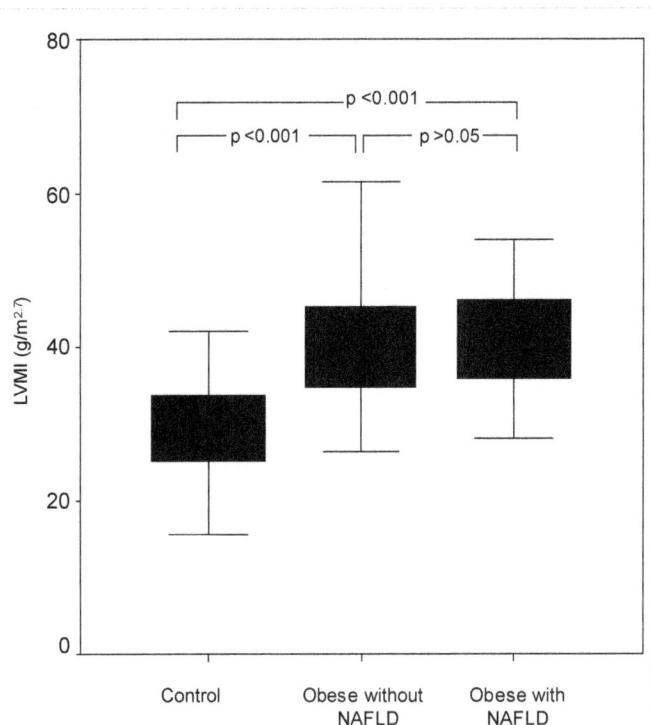

Figure 1: Adjusted pair-wise comparison of the left ventricle mass index (LVMI) of obese children with non-alcoholic fatty liver disease (NAFLD), obese children without NAFLD, and control subjects.

Models		β	95% Confidence Interval		P
			Lower Limit	Upper Limit	
Model I	(Constant)	3.378	3.316	3.440	<0.001
	NAFLD	0.042	-0.044	0.128	0.333
	Obesity	0.308	0.225	0.392	<0.001
Model II	(Constant)	3.357	3.282	3.431	<0.001
	NAFLD	0.040	-0.046	0.126	0.358
	Obesity	0.305	0.217	0.392	<0.001
	SBP Percentile	0.007	-0.021	0.035	0.627
	DBP Percentile	0.004	-0.002	0.010	0.218

NAFLD: Non-Alcoholic Fatty Liver Disease; SBP: Systolic Blood Pressure; DBP: Diastolic Blood Pressure
Table 5: Multiple linear regression analysis for predictors of left-ventricle mass index (LVMI)

	BMI-SDS	
	r	p
Glucose	- 0.075	0.369
Insulin	0.470	< 0.001
HOMA-IR	0.436	< 0.001
Triglyceride	0.362	< 0.001
Total cholesterol	0.446	< 0.001
AST	0.033	0.694
ALT	0.270	< 0.001

HOMA-IR: Homeostasis Model Assessment of Insulin Resistance; AST: Aspartate Aminotransferase; ALT: Alanine Aminotransferase
Table 3: Univariate Spearman's correlation coefficients between the study variables and body mass index-standart deviation scores (BMI-SDS).

	LVM		LVMI	
	r	p	r	p
Age	0.526	<0.001	0.094	0.259
BMI-SDS	0.561	<0.001	0.675	<0.001
HOMA-IR	0.490	<0.001	0.250	0.002
AST	0.221	0.007	0.007	0.935
ALT	0.060	0.473	0.155	0.062
LLD percentile	0.540	<0.001	0.331	<0.001

BMI-SDS: Body Mass Index-Standart Deviation Scores; HOMA-IR: Homeostasis Model Assessment of Insulin Resistance; AST: Aspartate Aminotransferase; ALT: Alanine Aminotransferase; LLD: Liver Longitudinal Dimension; LVM: Left Ventricle Mass
Table 4: Univariate Spearman's correlation coefficients between the study variables and left ventricle mass (LVM) and LVMI index.

(p < 0.001), whereas no significant difference was observed between the obese children with and without hypertension. The serum ALT differed significantly between obese children with or without NAFLD and control subjects (all p < 0.001). Eight (18.6%) of 43 obese children with NAFLD had an abnormal ALT.

In the univariate Spearman's correlation analysis, BMI-SDS was directly related to the fasting insulin level, HOMA-IR, TG, TC, and ALT levels (Table 3), whereas, LVMI was positively correlated with BMI-SDS, HOMA-IR, and LLD percentile (Table 4). In the multiple linear regression analysis, LVMI (β = 0.119; p < 0.001) and NAFLD (β = 0.213; p < 0.001) remained independent correlates of BMI-SDS. The Spearman's correlation analysis indicated no significant correlation between blood pressure and LVMI. In multiple linear regression models with NAFLD, BMI-SDS, SBP, and DBP as covariates, NAFLD was a significant predictor of LVMI (β = 3.4, p < 0.001). When BMI-SDS was added to the model, NAFLD as a predictor of LVMI was strongly attenuated and no longer statistically significant (β = 0.4). BMI-SDS remained a significant predictor of LVMI (β = 0.3, p < 0.001). When SBP and DBP were added to the model, the NAFLD association was also attenuated (β =0.4). BMI-SDS remained a significant predictor of LVMI (β = 0.3, p < 0.001). SBP and DBP were not significant predictors of LVMI (β= 0.007) (Table 5).

Discussion

In addition to the current rise in obesity, NAFLD is becoming responsible for a large percentage of liver disease in children [1]. The actual prevalence of NAFLD remains unknown largely because of the lack of population-based studies and reliable noninvasive screening tools. The reported frequency of NAFLD is 20% of obese children and adolescents from the US [22], 44% from Italy [23], and 74% from China [24]. In the present study, the frequency of NAFLD was 44% in obese subjects.

NAFLD encompasses a spectrum of diseases, from asymptomatic steatohepatitis to cirrhosis. The pathogenesis of NAFLD has remained poorly understood since the earliest description of the disease. Studies have reported the pathophysiology of NAFLD in obese patients in detail [1,25,26]. Insulin resistance and oxidative stress have critical roles in NAFLD pathogenesis. The molecular basis of the association between insulin resistance and hepatic steatosis is unclear. In this study, fasting insulin level, HOMA-IR ALT (as a parameter of insulin resistance), TG, TC, and ALT did not differ between obese children with and without NAFLD. In multiple regression analyses, insulin resistance itself was not an independent predictor of NAFLD, whereas the severity of obesity (as BMI-SDS) showed a significant correlation with NAFLD. In contrast, some studies have reported that insulin resistance is associated with the development of NAFLD in obese subjects [27,28]. Taken together, previous results and our current findings suggest that the molecular pathogenesis of insulin resistance is multifactorial. Mildly to moderately elevated serum ALT or AST levels are the most common and often the only laboratory abnormalities in NAFLD. In previous studies, the frequency of an elevated ALT level was between 10 and 30% in subjects with NAFLD [29,30]. In our study, the ALT levels differed significantly between obese children and controls, whereas no significant difference was observed between obese children with and without NAFLD. Only 8 of 43 (18.6%) obese children with NAFLD had abnormal ALT levels. A large portion of obese children may be missed at screening based only on serum aminotransferases. Fishbein et al. [31] reported that enzymatic abnormalities in fatty livers occur only in severe cases. Furthermore, Mofrad et al. [32] reported that the entire spectrum of NAFLD could be seen in subjects with normal ALT values. An ultrasound examination is preferred for identifying a fatty liver due to its noninvasiveness, availability, and high sensitivity and specificity. Joseph et al. [33] reported a sensitivity of 89% and specificity of 93% for detecting steatosis in the liver. Furthermore, we found that no subject with a normal liver ultrasound had an elevated ALT, and ultrasound revealed liver steatosis in all patients with elevated ALT levels. These findings suggest that an elevated ALT, higher BMI-SDS, and echogenic liver parenchyma, revealed by ultrasonography, are predictors of NAFLD.

The other obesity-related cardiovascular risk factor includes an increased LVMI or LVH. A number of studies have examined the relationship between LVM, BP, and obesity (as BMI or BMI-SDS) with conflicting results. A high BP (i.e., BP > 95th percentile) of between 18 and 35% has been reported in overweight and obese children [34,35]. In this study, 19 of 98 (19.4%) obese children were hypertensive. The frequency of LVH differed significantly between the obese children and controls, whereas no significant difference was observed between the obese children with and without hypertension. In a multiple linear regression analysis of the obesity-related risk factors (BMI-SDS, glucose, fasting insulin levels, HOMA-IR, TC, and TGs) that may be responsible for the pathogenesis of increased LVMI, BMI-SDS was the only significant predictor of increased LVMI. Furthermore, in a multiple linear regression analysis, BP and NAFLD were not significant predictors of LVMI. Our findings are supported by previous studies [2,36-39]. The Bogalusa Heart Study showed a strong association between LVM in childhood and the degree of obesity, but childhood BMI was the only independent predictor for adult LVMI [2]. Dhuper et al. [40] reported that obesity is a major predictor of concentric remodeling (CR) of the left ventricle, and the prevalence of CR of the left ventricle was similar in both the hypertensive and normotensive obese groups. Daniels et al. [41] showed a strong association between BMI and increased LVMI, independent of SBP. Finally, adult studies also reported that LVM is increased in normotensive obese adults, and that it is more closely associated with BMI and insulin resistance rather than BP [42,43]. Obesity affects cardiac muscle through multiple mechanisms. Factors other than BP, such as increased sympathetic activity, insulin resistance, vascular remodeling, neurohumoral modulation, volume overload, endothelial dysfunction, oxidative stress, and inflammation, which were not evaluated in the present study, may play a role in the pathogenesis of increasing LVMI in obese subjects. In contrast, some studies have shown that LVMI is positively associated with elevated BP [44-46]. Sorof et al. [47] found that LVMI is strongly correlated with 24-hour ambulatory measurements of the SBP index, whereas LVMI did not correlate with casual BP. Maggio et al. [48] reported a similar observation. In contrast, de Simone et al. [46] reported that the risk of LVH was significantly higher in children with a high casual BP as compared with children with normal BP, independent of the effects of obesity. These contradictory findings may be explained by different BP measurement methods and masked hypertension, which is defined as elevated ambulatory BP measurement without concomitant elevation of casual BP measurement.

Although NAFLD and increased LVMI or LVH are two important

obesity-related covariates, this is the first study to identify a relationship between NAFLD and LVMI in obese children. Components of Metabolic Syndrome (MS, i.e., hypertension, hyperinsulinism, dyslipidemia, impaired glucose tolerance, and obesity) are strongly associated with NAFLD [49,50]. Children with NAFLD often have multiple cardiovascular risk factors, including abnormal waist circumference, dyslipidemia, hypertension, insulin resistance [51], and increased carotid intima media thickness [52]. In a case control study comparing 150 pediatric patients with biopsy-proven NAFLD versus 150 overweight controls, children with MS had a five-fold increased risk of NAFLD [51]. Considering these studies, it can be concluded that NAFLD represents a liver manifestation of MS. It is well known that a major risk factor for mortality from MS is cardiovascular disease. Studies have shown that mortality among patients with NAFLD is higher than that in the general population, mainly due to concomitant cardiovascular diseases [53-56]. The natural history of NAFLD in the pediatric population is not clearly understood due to a lack of prospective studies evaluating children over time [57,58]. In our study, LVMI was significantly higher in obese children with or without NAFLD as compared with non-obese children. However, LVMI was not significantly different between obese subjects with or without NAFLD. Furthermore, the multiple linear regression analysis revealed that NAFLD was not a significant predictor for LVMI and that BMI-SDS was the only main predictor of LVMI. The findings of this study highlight that there is no relationship between NAFLD and LVMI. This finding may be explained by the different pathophysiology of NAFLD and increased LVMI in obese children. The higher mortality rate secondary to cardiovascular diseases in NAFLD may be explained because NAFLD is a significant predictor of liver damage in MS.

Our study had two limitations. The current study was cross-sectional in design; therefore, temporal associations between obesity, BP elevation, LVMI, and NAFLD could not been evaluated. We used the method of casual BP measurement to screen for hypertension. Casual BP may not reflect the most comprehensive view of BP and may miss a diagnosis of hypertension.

In conclusion, this study has demonstrated that LVH and NAFLD are two important and independent obesity-related covariates in obese children. Obese children with or without hypertension have a higher frequency of LVH compared to non-obese control subjects. In addition, LVMI may be influenced by fat mass rather than casual BP. The 24-hour ambulatory BP measurement may be a potential tool to improve risk stratification in obesity studies. NAFLD and casual BP measurements are not predictors of LVMI in obese children. Collectively, NAFLD is an obesity-related risk factor for chronic liver disease and is expected to become one of the most common causes of end-stage liver disease in children.

References

1. Pacifico L, Nobili V, Anania C, Verdecchia P, Chiesa C (2011) Pediatric nonalcoholic fatty liver disease, metabolic syndrome and cardiovascular risk. World J Gastroenterol 17: 3082-3091.

2. Li X, Li S, Ulusoy E, Chen W, Srinivasan SR, et al. (2004) Childhood adiposity as a predictor of cardiac mass in adulthood: the Bogalusa Heart Study. Circulation 110: 3488-3492.

3. Serdual MK, Ivery D, Coates RJ, Freedman DS, Williamson DF, et al. (1993) Do obese children become obese adults? A review of the literature. Prev Med 22: 167-177.

4. Chan DF, Li AM, Chu WC, Chan MH, Wong EM, et al. (2004) Hepatic steatosis in obese Chinese children. Int J Obes Relat Metab Disord 28: 1257-1263.

5. Tominaga K, Kurata JH, Chen YK, Fujimoto E, Miyagawa S, et al. (1995) Prevalence of fatty liver in Japanese children and relationship to obesity. An epidemiological ultrasonographic survey. Dig Dis Sci 40: 2002-2009.

6. Franzese A, Vajro P, Argenziano A, Puzziello A, Iannucci MP, et al. (1997) Liver involvement in obese children. Ultrasonography and liver enzyme levels at diagnosis and during follow-up in an Italian population. Dig Dis Sci 42: 1428-1432.

7. Hanevold C, Waller J, Daniels S, Portman R, Sorof J, et al. (2004) The effects of obesity, gender, and ethnic group on left ventricular hypertrophy and geometry in hypertensive children: a collaborative study of the International Pediatric Hypertension Association. Pediatrics 113: 328-333.

8. Galvan AQ, Galetta F, Natali A, Muscelli E, Sironi AM, et al. (2000) Insulin resistance and hyperinsulinemia: No independent relation to left ventricular mass in humans. Circulation 102: 2233-2238.

9. Cole TJ, Bellizzi MC, Flegal KM, Dietz WH (2000) Establishing a standard definition for child overweight and obesity worldwide: international survey. BMJ 320: 1240-1243.

10. Bundak R, Furman A, Gunoz H, Darendeliler F, Bas F, et al. (2006) Body mass index references for Turkish children. Acta Paediatr 95: 194-198.

11. Soergel M, Kirschstein M, Busch C, Danne T, Gellermann J, et al. (1997) Oscillometric twenty-four-hour ambulatory blood pressure values in healthy children and adolescents: a multicenter trial including 1141 subjects. J Pediatr 130: 178-184.

12. Tümer N, Yalçinkaya F, Ince E, Ekim M, Köse K, et al. (1999) Blood pressure nomograms for children and adolescents in Turkey. Pediatr Nephrol 13: 438-443.

13. Matthews DR, Hosker JP, Rudenski AS, Naylor BA, Treacher DF, et al. (1985) Homeostasis model assessment: insulin resistance and beta-cell function from fasting plasma glucose and insulin concentrations in man. Diabetologia 28: 412-419.

14. Keskin M, Kurtoglu S, Kendirci M, Atabek ME, Yazici C (2005) Homeostasis model assessment is more reliable than the fasting glucose/insulin ratio and quantitative insulin sensitivity check index for assessing insulin resistance among obese children and adolescents. Pediatrics 115: e500-e503.

15. (1992) American Academy of Pediatrics. National Cholesterol Education Program: Report of the Expert Panel on Blood Cholesterol Levels in Children and Adolescents. Pediatrics 89: 525–584.

16. Needleman L, Kurtz AB, Rifkin MD, Cooper HS, Pasto ME, et al. (1986) Sonography of diffuse benign liver disease: accuracy of pattern recognition and grading. AJR Am J Roentgenol 146: 1011-1015.

17. Schiller NB, Shah PM, Crawford M, DeMaria A, Devereux R, et al. (1989) Recommendations for quantitation of the left ventricle by two-dimensional echocardiography. American Society of Echocardiography Committee on Standards, Subcommittee on Quantitation of Two-Dimensional Echocardiograms. J Am Soc Echocardiogr 2: 358-367.

18. Devereux RB, Alonso DR, Lutas EM, Gottlieb GJ, Campo E, et al. (1986) Echocardiographic assessment of left ventricular hypertrophy: comparison to necropsy findings. Am J Cardiol 57: 450-458.

19. de Simone G, Daniels SR, Devereux RB, Meyer RA, Roman MJ, et al. (1992) Left ventricular mass and body size in normotensive children and adults: assessment of allometric relations and impact of overweight. J Am Coll Cardiol 20: 1251-1260.

20. de Simone G, Devereux RB, Daniels SR, Koren MJ, Meyer RA, et al. (1995) Effect of growth on variability of left ventricular mass: assessment of allometric signals in adults and children and their capacity to predict cardiovascular risk. J Am Coll Cardiol 25: 1056-1062.

21. Daniels SR (1999) Hypertension-induced cardiac damage in children and adolescents. Blood Press Monit 4: 165-170.

22. Strauss RS, Barlow SE, Dietz WH (2000) Prevalence of abnormal serum aminotransferase values in overweight and obese adolescents. J Pediatr 136: 727-733.

23. Sartorio A, Del Col A, Agosti F, Mazzilli G, Bellentani S, et al. (2007) Predictors of non-alcoholic fatty liver disease in obese children. Eur J Clin Nutr 61: 877-883.

24. Chan DF, Li AM, Chu WC, Chan MH, Wong EM, et al. (2004) Hepatic steatosis in obese Chinese children. Int J Obes Relat Metab Disord 28: 1257-1263.

25. Alisi A, Manco M, Vania A, Nobili V (2009) Pediatric nonalcoholic fatty liver disease in 2009. J Pediatr 155: 469-474.

26. Feldstein AE, Charatcharoenwitthaya P, Treeprasertsuk S, Benson JT, Enders FB, et al. (2009) The natural history of non-alcoholic fatty liver disease in children: a follow-up study for up to 20 years. Gut 58: 1538-1544.

27. Feldstein AE (2010) Novel insights into the pathophysiology of nonalcoholic fatty liver disease. Semin Liver Dis 30: 391-401.

28. Fabbrini E, Sullivan S, Klein S (2010) Obesity and nonalcoholic fatty liver disease: biochemical, metabolic, and clinical implications. Hepatology 51: 679-689.

29. Tazawa Y, Noguchi H, Nishinomiya F, Takada G (1997) Serum alanine aminotransferase activity in obese children. Acta Paediatr 86: 238-241.

30. Vajro P, Fontanella A, Perna C, Orso G, Tedesco M, et al. (1994) Persistent hyperaminotransferasemia resolving after weight reduction in obese children. J Pediatr 25: 239-241.

31. Fishbein MH, Miner M, Mogren C, Chalekson J (2003) The spectrum of fatty liver in obese children and the relationship of serum aminotransferases to severity of steatosis. J Pediatr Gastroenterol Nutr 36: 54-61.

32. Mofrad P, Contos MJ, Haque M, Sargeant C, Fisher RA, et al. (2003) Clinical and histologic spectrum of nonalcoholic fatty liver disease associated with normal ALT values. Hepatology 37: 1286-1292.

33. Joseph AE, Saverymuttu SH, al-Sam S, Cook MG, Maxwell JD (1991) Comparison of liver histology with ultrasonography in assessing diffuse parenchymal liver disease. Clin Radiol 43: 26-31.

34. Raj M, Sundaram KR, Paul M, Deepa AS, Kumar RK (2007) Obesity in Indian children: time trends and relationship with hypertension. Natl Med J India 20: 288-293.

35. l'Allemand D, Wiegand S, Reinehr T, Müller J, Wabitsch M, et al. (2008) Cardiovascular risk in 26,008 European overweight children as established by a multicenter database. Obesity (Silver Spring) 16: 1672-1679.

36. Friberg P, Allansdotter-Johnsson A, Ambring A, Ahl R, Arheden H, et al. (2004) Increased left ventricular mass in obese adolescents. Eur Heart J 25: 987-992.

37. Kinik ST, Varan B, Yildirim SV, Tokel K (2006) The effect of obesity on echocardiographic and metabolic parameters in childhood. J Pediatr Endocrinol Metab 19: 1007-1014.

38. Van Putte-Katier N, Rooman RP, Haas L, Verhulst SL, Desager KN, et al. (2008) Early cardiac abnormalities in obese children: importance of obesity per se versus associated cardiovascular risk factors. Pediatr Res 64: 205-209.

39. Chinali M, de Simone G, Roman MJ, Lee ET, Best LG, et al. (2006) Impact of obesity on cardiac geometry and function in a population of adolescents: the Strong Heart Study. J Am Coll Cardiol 47: 2267-2273.

40. Dhuper S, Abdullah RA, Weichbrod L, Mahdi E, Cohen HW (2011) Association of obesity and hypertension with left ventricular geometry and function in children and adolescents. Obesity (Silver Spring) 19: 128-133.

41. Daniels SR, Witt SA Glascock B, Khoury PR, Kimball TR (2002) Left atrial size in children with hypertension: the influence of obesity, blood pressure, and left ventricular mass. J Pediatr 141: 186-190.

42. Wong CY, O'Moore-Sullivan T, Leano R, Byrne N, Beller E, et al. (2004) Alterations of left ventricular myocardial characteristics associated with obesity. Circulation 110: 3081-3087.

43. Iacobellis G, Ribaudo MC, Zappaterreno A, Vecci E, Tiberti C, et al. (2003) Relationship of insulin sensitivity and left ventricular mass in uncomplicated obesity. Obes Res 11: 518-524.

44. Daniels SR, Kimball TR, Morrison JA, Khoury P, Witt S, et al. (1995) Effect of lean body mass, fat mass, blood pressure, and sexual maturation on left ventricular mass in children and adolescents. Statistical, biological, and clinical significance. Circulation 92: 3249-3254.

45. Malcolm DD, Burns TL, Mahoney LT, Lauer RM (1993) Factors affecting left ventricular mass in childhood: The Muscatine Study. Pediatrics 92: 703-709.

46. de Simone G, Mureddu GF, Greco R, Scalfi L, Del Puente AE, et al. (1997) Relations of left ventricular geometry and function to body composition in children with high casual blood pressure. Hypertension 30: 377-382.

47. Sorof JM, Cardwell G, Franco K, Portman RJ (2002) Ambulatory blood pressure and left ventricular mass index in hypertensive children. Hypertension 39: 903-908.

48. Maggio AB, Aggoun Y, Marchand LM, Martin XE, Herrmann F, et al. (2008) Associations among obesity, blood pressure, and left ventricular mass. J Pediatr 152: 489-493.

49. Loria P, Lonardo A, Carulli L, Verrone AM, Ricchi M, et al. (2005) Review article: the metabolic syndrome and non-alcoholic fatty liver disease. Aliment Pharmacol Ther 22: 31-36.

50. Mencin AA, Lavine JE (2011) Nonalcoholic fatty liver disease in children. Curr Opin Clin Nutr Metab Care 14: 151-157.

51. Schwimmer JB, Pardee PE, Lavine JE, Blumkin AK, Cook S (2008) Cardiovascular risk factors and the metabolic syndrome in pediatric nonalcoholic fatty liver disease. Circulation 118: 277-283.

52. Demircioğlu F, Koçyiğit A, Arslan N, Cakmakçi H, Hizli S, et al. (2008) Intima-media thickness of carotid artery and susceptibility to atherosclerosis in obese children with nonalcoholic fatty liver disease. J Pediatr Gastroenterol Nutr 47: 68-75.

53. Adams LA, Lymp JF, St Sauver J, Sanderson SO, Lindor KD, et al. (2005) The natural history of nonalcoholic fatty liver disease: a population-based cohort study. Gastroenterology 129: 113-121.

54. Ekstedt M, Franzén LE, Mathiesen UL, Thorelius L, Holmqvist M, et al. (2006) Long-term follow-up of patients with NAFLD and elevated liver enzymes. Hepatology 44: 865-873.

55. Rafiq N, Bai C, Fang Y, Srishord M, McCullough A, et al. (2009) Long-term follow-up of patients with nonalcoholic fatty liver. Clin Gastroenterol Hepatol 7: 234-238.

56. Söderberg C, Stål P, Askling J, Glaumann H, Lindberg G, et al. (2010) Decreased survival of subjects with elevated liver function tests during a 28-year follow-up. Hepatology 51: 595-602.

57. Loomba R, Sirlin CB, Schwimmer JB, Lavine JE (2009) Advances in pediatric nonalcoholic fatty liver disease. Hepatology 50: 1282-1293.

58. Argo CK, Northup PG, Al-Osaimi AM, Caldwell SH (2009) Systematic review of risk factors for fibrosis progression in non-alcoholic steatohepatitis. J Hepatol 51: 371-379.

34

The Changes of the Expression of PGC-1α and the Level of Oxidative Stress in NAFLD as well as the Effects of Metformin on NAFLD

Jian-hua Jiang*, Jing Cheng, Bao Zhang, Shi-xia Guan and Li-li Hou

Department of Clinical Nutriology, the FirstAffiliated Hospital ofAnhui Medical University, Hefei, China

Abstract

Purpose: The objective of this study was to determine how metformin regulates the major activator of hepatic gluconeogenesis, peroxisome proliferator-activated receptor γ coactivator 1α (PGC-1α) and the PGC-1α controlled liver functions.

Methods: In population study, we selected 40-69 years old patients with NAFLD, 77, and 102 healthy subjects as a control group. We detect the levels of serum PGC-1α, MDA and the activity of SOD of the two groups. In vitro study, L-02 cells were treated by 20 μg/ml oleic acid to induce the NAFLD cells model. The control group added ordinary 1640 culture medium. The model group cells were cultured in the medium containing 2.5, 5, 7.5mmol/l concentrations of metformin. Used RT-PCR analysis of PGC-1α mRNA, detected the level of triglycerides in cells, measured the content of MDA and the activity of SOD.

Results: In population study, the level of MDA in the case group were increased obviously and the activity of SOD was decreased compared with the control group. There had no difference of the level of PGC-1α between the two groups. In vitro study, compared with the control groups, the level of triglyceride and the concentration of MDA in the model groups were increased and the activity of SOD as well as the expression of PGC-1α mRNA were decreased; When the final concentration of metformin is 7.5 mmol/l, the level of triglyceride and MDA were decreased as well as the activity of SOD and the expression of PGC-1α mRNA were increased compared with the model group.

Conclusion: Metformin can adjust the expression of PGC-1α and the level of oxidative stress which can decrease the fat accumulation, Our results thus identify selective modulation of hepatic PGC-1α functions as a novel mechanism involved in the therapeutic action of metformin.

Keywords: Nonalcoholic fatty liver; PGC-1α; MDA; SOD; Metformin

Introduction

With the improvement of people's living standard and the change of lifestyle as well as population aging, the incidence of non-alcoholic fatty liver disease (NAFLD) in China is increasing gradually [1-3]. Nonalcoholic steatohepatitis (NASH) is the main stage in the progression of NAFLD, which can also lead to liver cirrhosis [4] even hepatocellular carcinoma [5]. In addition, NAFLD is associated with increased risk of inflammation, cardiovascular disease [6,7] as well as insulin resistance (IR) and type 2 diabetes [8]. Although the pathogenesis of NAFLD is not clearly understood, it is known that insulin resistance assumes a pivotal role and it is generally regarded as the hepatic component of the metabolic syndrome (MetS) [9]. However, there is no accepted standard medication in the treatment of NAFLD. But drugs which can improve insulin sensitivity are widely used because insulin resistance play an important role in the pathophysiology of NAFLD [10]. A open label trial in well-characterized patients with NASH, metformin therapy was associated with improvements in insulin sensitivity in most patients and with weight loss, decreases in serum aminotransferase levels and improvements in liver histology in approximately 30% of patients [11]. Metformin is a biguanide drug that improves insulin sensitivity in the liver and skeletal muscle [12]. Metformin is known to stimulate AMP-activated protein kinase (AMPK) activity in primary hepatocytes, a hepatoma cell line and in whole liver [13-15]. Researchers describing the possible mechanisms by which metformin or other AMPK activators regulate the expression of genes for gluconeogenesis through AMPK [16]. The exact mechanisms of action are not fully understood, but probably involve the activation of AMPK, which results in the suppression of the production of glucose [17], cholesterol, and triglycerides, and stimulation of fatty acid oxidation [18].

Peroxisome proliferator activated receptor γ coactivator 1α (PGC-1α) is a regulator of myocardial energy metabolism and mitochondrial biogenesis [19,20]. PGC-1α can regulate mitochondrial antioxidant enzyme's activity and expression in brain tissues [21] and cultured vascular endothelial cells [22]. The expression of mitochondrial antioxidants including superoxide dismutase 2 (SOD2) and uncoupling protein 2 (UCP2) were reduced and had a increased vulnerability to oxidative injury of the dopaminergic neurons in the brain tissue of PGC-1α null mice [21]. Overexpression of PGC-1α in vascular endothelial cells increased mitochondrial antioxidant enzyme expression, and decreased oxidative stress and cell death [22]. In liver, PGC-1α stimulates gluconeogenesis, fatty acid oxidation and heme biosynthesis [23]. Because PGC-1α has been shown to play an important role in regulation of gluconeogenesis, it has also been suggested to be involved in the hepatic action of metformin [24]. Although PGC-1α is a key regulator of energy metabolism, the effects of metformin on hepatic PGC-1α expression and function have not been specifically studied. Thus, it appears timely to intensify research on metformin in the context of NAFLD and to begin delineating cellular and molecular events that may be activated beneficially in liver. Therefore, the aim of this study was to evaluate the effects of metformin on important phenotypic modifiers in NAFLD.

---

*Corresponding author: JIANG Jian-hua, Department of Clinical Nutriology, the First Affiliated Hospital of Anhui Medical University, No.218 Jixi Road, Hefei, Anhui Province 230032, China; E-mail: jhua@yeah.net

Materials and Methods

Population study

Subjects: All patients with clinical and evidence of NAFLD were selected from July to November 2012 at the medical center of the First Affiliated Hospital of Anhui Medical University. 77 patients and 102 normal population aged 40-69 years old were selected, there had no statistically significant differences in the constitute of age and gender between the two groups. Health questionnaires including general demographic characteristics, lifestyle, disease history were performed in all objects. Inclusion criteria were: patients without alcohol use or occasional use (< 30gr alcohol per day in men, and <20 grains in women). Results of liver ultrasound study meet the diagnostic criteria of mild diffuse fatty liver and cannot be explained by other reasons. Exclusion criteria were: chronic hepatic disease (hepatitis B and C, hemochromatosis), systemic comorbidities and neoplasm, hepatotoxic drugs during the past 6 months [25]. Subjects had to keep on an empty stomach more than 12 hours, and not taking lipid-lowering drugs, high-fat foods and alcohol within the 24 hours. This study was approved by the ethics committees. Informed consent was obtained from all patients.

Methods

Ultrasonic testing: All subjects were received the examination of liver ultrasound (by Toshiba 660, Japan) in the same condition. To avoid inter-operator discordance, we used an expert radiologist performed ultrasonic evaluations for all the subjects and repeated the suspicious ultrasonographies.

The determination of biochemical indicators: peripheral venous blood were collected on an empty stomach, we used automatic biochemical analyzer (by Hitachi - 7600, Japan) test fasting blood glucose (FBG), total cholesterol (TC), triglyceride (TG), very low density lipoprotein (VLDL -c), high-density lipoprotein (HDL - C), low density lipoprotein (LDL - C) and uric acid (UA), biochemical reagents bought from Roche Co., Ltd.

Determination of PGC-1α level in serum: Using ELISA method (PGC-1α ELISA kit was purchased from beijing biotechnology research institute, China), first to join the standard and sample to be tested, set up the negative control, under the condition of 37°C reacting 30 min, washing board for four times, adding enzyme reagent, under the condition of 37°C reacting 30 min, washing board for four times, adding color reagent A and B, under the condition of 37°C coloring 15 min, then join the terminated reagent, the absorbance (A) values were measured at 450 nm, finally, draw the standard curve and calculate the concentration of PGC-1α.

The determination of the level of MDA and the activity of SOD in serum: All subjects were not take antioxidants within a month, all subjects were collected 4 ml venous blood on an empty stomach, centrifuged the blood at a room temperature (2500 r / min, 8min), serum was separated and placed in a 20°C cryopreservation. The level of MDA in the serum were measured by thiobarbituric acid method (TBA), the determination of SOD was by xanthine oxidation method (XTO) (the kits above were purchased from Nanjing Jiancheng biological reagent company, China). One unit SOD is defined as the amount of the protein that inhibitis the rate of NBT reduction by 50% (U/ml)

Vitro study

Materials and cells: The human normal hepatocyte cell line L-02 was purchased from the cell bank of the Institute of Biochemistry and Cell Biology (Shanghai, China). RPMI 1640 medium without sugar and phenol (were purchased from Gibco BRL Co. Ltd. USA); fetal calf serum (HyClone, Logan, UT, USA); 1:125 trypsin (Gibco, USA); streptomycin, penicillin(China Pharmaceutical Husheng Co. Ltd.); metformin (Sigma, USA); TG test kit, Malonyldialdehyde (MDA) and superoxide dismutase (SOD) assay kits were obtained from Nanjing Jiancheng biological reagent company, China. BCA protein assay kit (Biocolor Bioscience & Technology Com-pany). TRIzol PrimeScript RT reagent kit and T SYBR Premix Ex Taq kit (Takara Biotechnology Co., Ltd.).

Experimental protocols: The L-02 cells were cultured in RPMI 1640 medium supplemented with 10% heat-inactivated fetal calf serum and 1% v/v penicillin/streptomycin in a 5% CO2 humidified atmosphere at 37°C. According to the methods from literatures [26], the L02 cells were grown to 80% confluence added 20μg/ml oleic acid (dissolved by 0.5% DMSO) into the medium for 24h to induce the cell model of nonalcoholic fatty liver disease. The control group added ordinary 1640 culture medium containing 10% fetal calf serum. The cells of the model group were cultured in the medium containing 2.5, 5, 7.5 mmol/l concentrations of metformin which were marked group 1, 2, 3 and continue to cultivate 24 hour then collected cells. There were five replicates in each group.

The evaluation of the non-alcoholic fatty liver cells model: Cells were treated by oleic acid for 24 hours, collected cells by the digestion of trypsin and then observed under the electron microscope. Have a biochemical detection of intracellular triglyceride of each groups.

Determination of intracellular triglyceride: About 1×105 cells were implanted in each hole of the 6 hole plate. The supernatant was discarded after packet processing, then collected the cells in each cell culture plate and frozen- thawed the cells repeatedly, After centrifugation for 5 min at 3,000 rpm the decanted supernatant was saved as the TG extract. Using TG test kit(Nanjing Jincheng Corp, China)to detect the contents of TG. Take the remaining liquid for the quantitation of proteins, the protein content was measured using a BCA protein assay.

Assay for intracellular contents of SOD and MDA: The culture medium was collected, then cells were washed with D-Hanks, scraped from the plates into 1 ml of icecold PBS (0.1 M, containing 0.05 mM of EDTA), and homogenized. The homogenate was centrifuged at 4000 r/min for 10 minutes at 4 °C, the MDA contents and SOD activities in the supernatant were measured by the assay kit (Nanjing Jincheng Corp, China) according to its provider's instructions. The activities of SOD were expressed as units per milligram protein. MDA was measured at a wavelength of 532 nm by reacting with thiobarbituric acid to form a stable chromophoric production. Values of MDA level were expressed as nanomoles per milligram protein.

The measurement of the expression of PGC-1α mRNA by RT-PCR: The total RNA of cells was extracted using TRIzol reagent and cDNA was synthesized according to the instructions from the PrimeScript RT reagent kit. RT-PCR primers were as follows: Upstream of PGC-1α: CAGCAAGTCCTCAGTCCTCAC; downstream of PGC-1α: TGCCTCCAAAGTCTCTCTCAG; product size:247bp. Upstream of β-action: GAAATGGAGGCACCCCTTC; downstream of β-action:TTGCCGACAGGATGCAGAA; product size:100bp.The reaction system was prepared according to the instructions of the SYBR Premix Ex Taq kit and then DNA was amplified as follows: 95°C for 10 minutes; then 95°C for 15 sec, 61°C for 15 sec and 72°C for 15 sec for 40 cycles; and finally 95°C for 1 minutes, 55°C for 30 secponds and 95°C for 30 sec. PCR products were electrophoresed in agarose gel, to determine the expression of target and reference gene.

Observed under the electron microscope: The fixation and treating of cells as well as sections were made by professionals from Electron Microscopy Room in Anhui Provincial Hospital (In Anhui province of China). Observing organelles structures, mitochondria and lipid droplet under the electron microscope.

Statistical analysis:

The continuous variables were summarized by the mean and range. Other categorical variables were summarized by count and percentage. The SPSS Statistics 15.0 package was utilized to analyze the data. Spearman rank correlation coefficients were used to summarize monotonic relationships between PGC-1α and triglyceride, MDA, SOD in cells. Differences among groups were analyzed using the one-way analysis of variance (ANOVA), followed by multiple comparisons by LSD test. The $p < 0.05$ was considered statistically significant.

Results

Population study

Baseline characteristics: There had no difference of the age, sex and blood pressure between the two groups; Compared with the control group, BMI in the case group was increased obviously, and the difference was statistically significant ($p < 0.05$) (Table 1).

The comparison of biochemical indicators: Compared with the control group, the level of TC, TG, VLDL-C , LDL-C , FBG, UA and ALT in the case group were increased obviously, and the level of HDL in the case group was decreased, the differences were statistically significant ($p < 0.05$). There had no difference of the level of AST between the two groups (Table 2).

The comparison of the level of PGC-1α MDA and the activity of SOD in serum: Compared with the control group, the level of MDA in the case group were increased obviously, and the vitality of SOD in the case group was decreased, the differences were statistically significant ($p < 0.05$). There had no difference of the level of PGC-1α between the two groups (Table 3).

In vitro study

The structure of organelles under the electron microscope: Many mitochondria can be seen in cells of control group, their shape is elliptical or round, and the membrane and carinulae of mitochondria were clear. In the model group, the number of mitochondria was decreased apparently. The membrane and inner carinulae in deformed mitochondria were absent, most of mitochondrions changed to vacuole after the cells exposed to oleic acid (the level of intracellular triglyceride by biochemical detection showed that an increasing level in model group, it indicated that we successfully built up NAFLD cells model). In the cells of Group1 (metformin 2.5 mmol/l) and Group 2 (metformin 5 mmol/l), the vacuolation of mitochondria decreased. In the cells of Group3 (metformin 7.5 mmol/l), the mitochondria were a little swelling, but the membrane and carinulae of mitochondria were clear and with an obvious reduction of vacuolation (Figure 1).

The effect of metformin on the level of triglyceride in L-02 cells

Compared with the control group, the level of triglyceride in the cells of the model group increased obviously, and the difference was statistically significant ($p < 0.05$). When the final concentration of metformin is 7.5 mmol/l, the level of triglyceride decreased compared with the model group and the difference was statistically significant ($p < 0.05$). The level of triglyceride in the Group3 (metformin 7.5mmol/l) decreased compared with Group1 (metformin 2.5 mmol/l), the difference was statistically significant ($p < 0.05$) (Figure 2).

The effect of metformin on the level of MDA and the activity of SOD in cells

Compared with the control group, the concentration of MDA was increased apparently with a difference of statistical significance ($p < 0.05$), and the vitality of SOD is reduced significantly, the difference was statistically significant ($p < 0.05$). Compared with the model group, when the final concentration of metformin is 5 mmol/l, 7.5 mmol/l, the concentration of MDA was decreased apparently with a difference of statistical significance ($p < 0.05$), and the activity of SOD is increased significantly, the difference was statistically significant ($p < 0.05$).

Variable	Case group (n=77)	Control group (n=102)	p value
Age (years)	47.40 ± 6.79	49.13 ± 7.83	>0.05
Male, n (%)	47(61.0)	62(60.8)	>0.05
SBP (mmHg)	121.63 ± 10.67	119.42 ± 9.21	>0.05
DBP (mmHg)	75.54 ± 8.16	73.26 ± 7.89	>0.05
BMI (kg/m²)	25.52 ± 4.59	22.0 ± 2.36	<0.001

Table 1: Baseline characteristics (age 40–69) of the NAFLD case and control populations.

Variable	Case group (n=77)	Control group (n=102)	p value
TC (mmol/L)	5.10 ± 1.02	4.48 ± 0.69	<0.001
TG (mmol/L)	2.03 ± 1.09	1.16 ± 0.52	<0.001
HDL-C (mmol/L)	1.15 ± 0.27	1.36 ± 0.31	<0.001
VLDL-C (mmol/L)	0.75 ± 0.40	0.43 ± 0.19	<0.001
LDL-C (mmol/L)	3.19 ± 0.97	2.69 ± 0.65	<0.001
FBG (mmol/L)	5.18 ± 0.40	4.63 ± 1.10	<0.001
UA (μmol/L)	356.34 ± 70.34	305.37 ± 76.91	<0.001
ALT(IU/L)	28.08 ± 14.13	18.64 ± 8.10	<0.001
AST(IU/L)	20.51 ± 5.95	19.23 ± 5.03	>0.05

Table 2: Biochemical indicators.

Variable	Case group (n=77)	Control group (n=102)	p value
PGC-1α (nmol/L)	25.76 ± 8.00	24.28 ± 6.14	>0.05
SOD (U/ml)	75.65 ± 6.35	98.19 ± 7.03	<0.001
MDA (μmol/L)	5.08 ± 0.42	3.85 ± 0.36	>0.001

Table 3: The level of PGC-1α MDA and the vitality of SOD in serum.

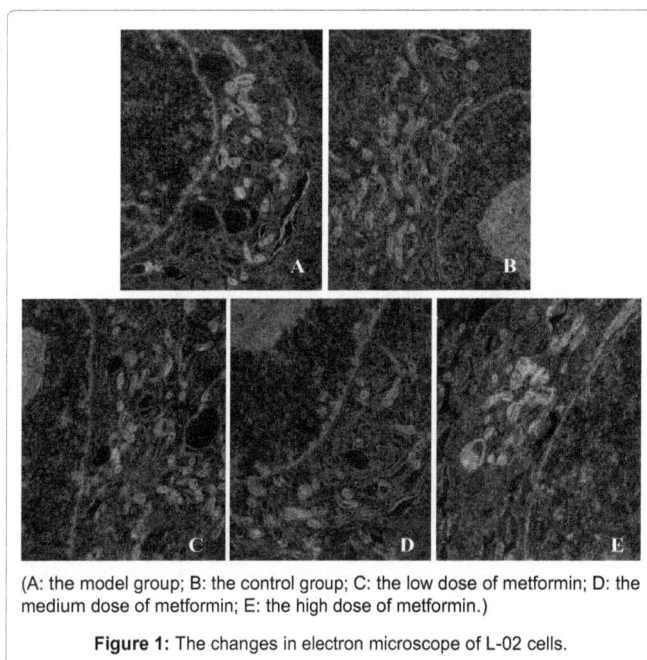

(A: the model group; B: the control group; C: the low dose of metformin; D: the medium dose of metformin; E: the high dose of metformin.)

Figure 1: The changes in electron microscope of L-02 cells.

Compared with the final concentration of metformin was 2.5 mmol/l group, when the final concentration of metformin was respectively 5 mmol/l, 7.5 mmol/l, the concentration of MDA was reduced apparently with a difference of statistical significance (p<0.05), and the vitality of SOD is increased significantly, the difference was statistically significant (p<0.05) (Figures 3 and 4).

The effect of metformin on the expression of PGC-1α mRNA in L-02 cells

Compared with the control group, the expression of PGC-1α mRNA in L-02 cells in model group decreased apparently with a difference of statistical significance (p<0.05). Compared with the model group, when the final concentration of metformin was respectively 2.5 mmol/l,Group1), 5 mmol/l, Group2), 7.5 mmol/l, Group3), the expression of PGC-1α mRNA in L-02 cells were increased obviously and with a differences of statistical significance (p<0.05). The expression of PGC-1α mRNA in Group3 was higher than that in Group1 with a difference of statistical significance (p<0.05) (Figures 5 and 6).

Correlation

The expression of PGC-1α mRNA showed a negative correlation with the levels of triglyceride and the concentration of MDA in L-02

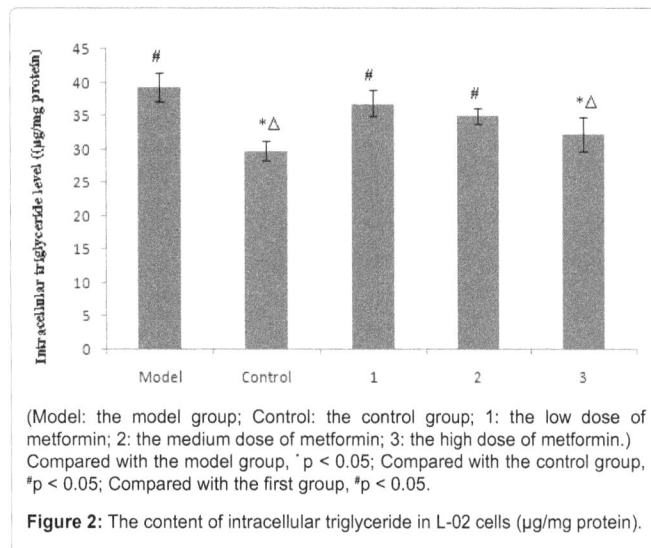

(Model: the model group; Control: the control group; 1: the low dose of metformin; 2: the medium dose of metformin; 3: the high dose of metformin.) Compared with the model group, ˙ p < 0.05; Compared with the control group, #p < 0.05; Compared with the first group, #p < 0.05.

Figure 2: The content of intracellular triglyceride in L-02 cells (μg/mg protein).

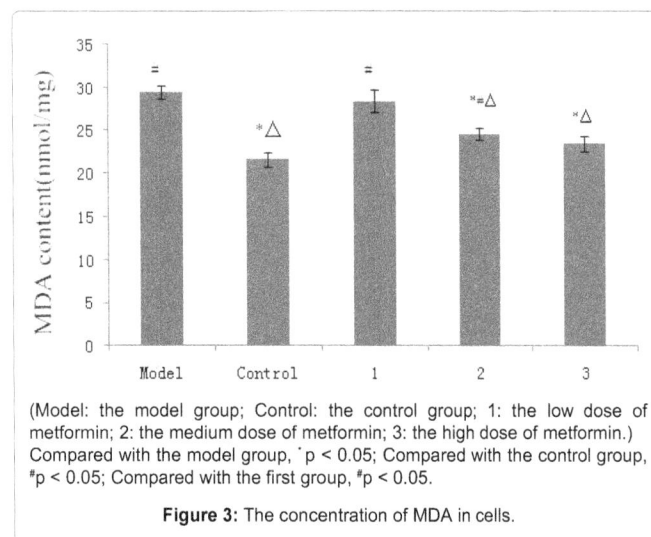

(Model: the model group; Control: the control group; 1: the low dose of metformin; 2: the medium dose of metformin; 3: the high dose of metformin.) Compared with the model group, ˙ p < 0.05; Compared with the control group, #p < 0.05; Compared with the first group, #p < 0.05.

Figure 3: The concentration of MDA in cells.

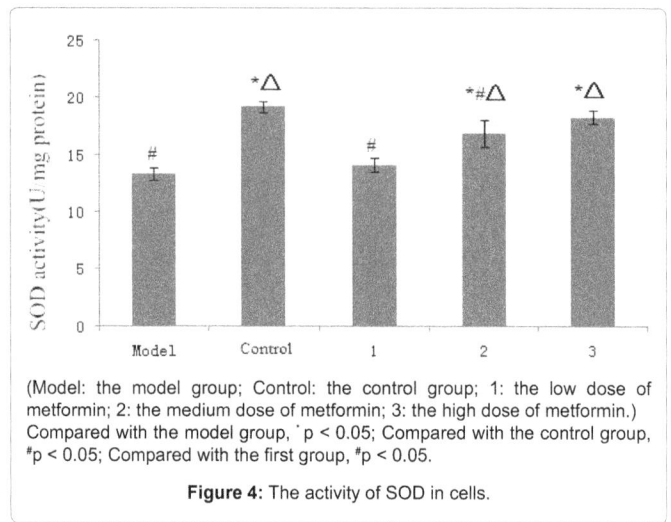

(Model: the model group; Control: the control group; 1: the low dose of metformin; 2: the medium dose of metformin; 3: the high dose of metformin.) Compared with the model group, ˙ p < 0.05; Compared with the control group, #p < 0.05; Compared with the first group, #p < 0.05.

Figure 4: The activity of SOD in cells.

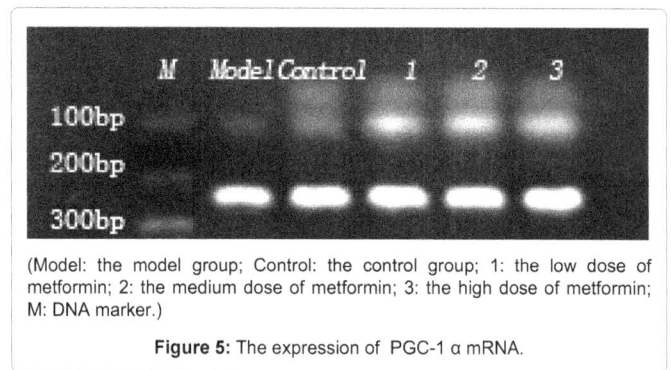

(Model: the model group; Control: the control group; 1: the low dose of metformin; 2: the medium dose of metformin; 3: the high dose of metformin; M: DNA marker.)

Figure 5: The expression of PGC-1 α mRNA.

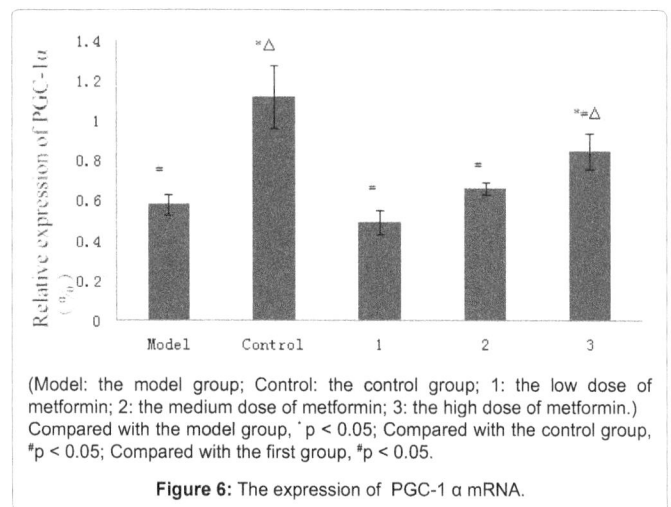

(Model: the model group; Control: the control group; 1: the low dose of metformin; 2: the medium dose of metformin; 3: the high dose of metformin.) Compared with the model group, ˙ p < 0.05; Compared with the control group, #p < 0.05; Compared with the first group, #p < 0.05.

Figure 6: The expression of PGC-1 α mRNA.

cells (r=-0.581, -0.629, p<0.05); the expression of PGC-1α mRNA showed a positive correlation with the activity of SOD in L-02 cells (r=0.746, p<0.05).

Discussion

PGC-1α regulates mitochondrial biogenesis and function, oxidative stress, gluconeogenesis, and lipogenesis, all of which are key factors in the development of NAFLD [27]. PGC-1α interacts with different transcription factors and activates distinct biological programs in different tissues, including gluconeogenesis in the liver, thermogenesis in brown fat, and angiogenesis in skeletal muscles [28]. In hepatocytes, PGC-1α orchestrates broad energy programs, including gluconeogenesis and mitochondrial fatty acid β-oxidation [29]. As IR is closely related to the pathogenesis of NAFLD, there had a study founded that mild and long-term decreased expression of PGC-1α is one of the reasons causing IR in mice liver [30]. However, Koo et al. [31] demonstrated that a sharp, adenoviral-mediated reduction of hepatic PGC-1α increased insulin sensitivity *in vivo*. In our population study, there had no difference of the level of PGC-1α between the case group and control group. However, the expression of PGC-1α mRNA in the cells of the model group was decreased apparently compared with the control group in our vitro study. The reason of this result may be due to the complexity of human body system and the difference of the detection method, but by vitro experiments we concluded that the decrease of the expression of PGC-1α may play an important role in the pathogenesis of NAFLD.

Oxidative stress damages multiple cellular components including DNA, lipids, and proteins and has been linked to pathological alterations in NAFLD. Reactive oxygen species (ROS) attack polyunsaturated fatty acids and initiate lipid peroxidation within the cell, which results in the formation of aldehyde by-products such as MDA. Thus, MDA is widely used as a marker of lipid oxidation that reflects the level of oxidative stress. Study have found that the content of MDA which was increased obviously in NAFLD patients was positively related to the degree of inflammatory necrosis and fibrosis in liver tissue [32]. In our study we founded that the content of MDA both in NAFLD patients and cells model were increased as well as and the activity of SOD were decreased, it prompt that the imbalance of the level of oxidation and antioxidant play a important role in the formation of NAFLD. PGC-1α not only can regulate the induction of antioxidant defenses including SODs, catalase and GPx [33] but also can increase the expression of the metabolic sensor NAD^+-dependent deacetylase sirtuin 3 (Sirt3), a key regulator of the mitochondrial antioxidant system [34]. We founded that the expression of PGC-1α mRNA showed a negative correlation with the levels of triglyceride and the concentration of MDA as well as showed a positive correlation with the activity of SOD in L-02 cells, it means that PGC-1α is closely related to the level of oxidative stress.

In view of the fact that insulin resistance plays a key role in the pathogenesis of NAFLD, improving insulin resistance and increasing insulin sensitivity may be a target in the treatment of NAFLD. Metformin and insulin sensitizing agents are the drugs that commonly used. Metformin appears to be both an anti-hyperglycemic drug and a therapeutic tool for the treatment of insulin resistance, in which it plays a pivotal role in depressing of fatty acid oxidation and treating the metabolic syndrome [35]. The activation of AMP-activated protein kinase (AMPK) may play a central role in metformin's actions [15]. AMPK is an important regulatory factor of energy metabolism in cells, it can not only regulates the oxidation of fatty acid and was also involved in the regulation of the insulin sensitivity. However, a recent study showed that AMPK deficiency did not abolish the effects of metformin on hepatic glucose production, indicating that the role of AMPK is dispensable [36]. The liver-protective mechanisms of metformin in NAFLD may be attributed to the down regulation of the inflammatory response and protection of mitochondrial function [37]. In this experiment, after the intervention of metformin, the level of triglyceride in the cells of drug group was lower than the cells in the model group. But the specific molecular mechanism that the metformin decreases the level of triglyceride in hepatocyte is unclear, We speculate that it is relate to the PGC-1α which is involved in mitochondrial damage and the disorder of lipid metabolic.

In this experiment, undering the action of oleic acid the expression of PGC-1α and the activity of SOD in the cells of model group is decreased compared with the control group. We found that after the intervention of metformin, the expression of PGC-1α and the activity of SOD was increased significantly in the cells of model groups. Through the experiment we come to the conclusion that Metformin can adjust the expression of PGC-1α and the level of oxidative stress which can decrease the fat accumulation. Consistent with the results of our research, it had demonstrated that the expression of PGC-1α is reduced in skeletal muscle in vivo and also in the failing heart [38], and metformin increases the expression of PGC-1α protein [39]. Severeness of steatosis is associated with impaired PGC-1α expression and reduced mitochondrial gene expression [40].

In conclusion, Metformin can adjust the expression of PGC-1α and the level of oxidative stress. The increment of mitochondria aftering the treatment of metformin would at least partially be expected to be due to the increased expression of PGC-1α. A previous study [22] demonstrated the expression of PGC-1α can stimulate mitochondrial proliferation and increase the mtDNA copy number, Such a role of PGC-1α for improving the mitochondrial capacity is one of the possible mechanisms for the metformin action.

References

1. Leng SX, Tian XP, Durso S, Lazarus G, Lu C, et al. (2008) The aging population and development of geriatrics in China. J Am Geriatr Soc 56: 571-573.

2. Adams LA, Lymp JF, St Sauver J, Sanderson SO, Lindor KD, et al. (2005) The natural history of nonalcoholic fatty liver disease: a population-based cohort study. Gastroenterology 129: 113-121.

3. Kawada N, Imanaka K, Kawaguchi T, Tamai C, Ishihara R, et al. (2009) Hepatocellular carcinoma arising from non-cirrhotic nonalcoholic steatohepatitis. J Gastroenterol 44: 1190-1194.

4. Jansen PL (2004) Non-alcoholic steatohepatitis. Eur J Gastroenterol Hepatol 16: 1079-1085.

5. Bugianesi E, Leone N, Vanni E, Marchesini G, Brunello F, et al. (2002) Expanding the natural history of nonalcoholic steatohepatitis: from cryptogenic cirrhosis to hepatocellular carcinoma. Gastroenterology 123: 134-140.

6. Arslan N, Makay B (2010) Mean platelet volume in obese adolescents with nonalcoholic fatty liver disease. J Pediatr Endocrinol Metab 23: 807-813.

7. Aygun C, Kocaman O, Sahin T, Uraz S, Eminler AT, et al. (2008) Evaluation of metabolic syndrome frequency and carotid artery intima-media thickness as risk factors for atherosclerosis in patients with nonalcoholic fatty liver disease. Dig Dis Sci 53: 1352-1357.

8. Shoelson SE, Herrero L, Naaz A (2007) Obesity, inflammation, and insulin resistance. Gastroenterology 132: 2169-2180.

9. Martín-Domínguez V, González-Casas R, Mendoza-Jiménez-Ridruejo J, García-Buey L, Moreno-Otero R (2013) Pathogenesis, diagnosis and treatment of non-alcoholic fatty liver disease. Rev Esp Enferm Dig 105: 409-420.

10. Loomba R, Lutchman G, Kleiner DE, Ricks M, Feld JJ, et al. (2009) Clinical trial: pilot study of metformin for the treatment of non-alcoholic steatohepatitis. Aliment Pharmacol Ther 29: 172-182.

11. Loomba R, Lutchman G, Kleiner DE, Ricks M, Feld JJ, et al. (2009) Clinical trial: pilot study of metformin for the treatment of non-alcoholic steatohepatitis. Aliment Pharmacol Ther 29: 172-182.

12. Scarpello JH, Howlett HC (2008) Metformin therapy and clinical uses. Diab Vasc Dis Res 5: 157-167.

13. Zang M, Zuccollo A, Hou X, Nagata D, Walsh K, et al. (2004) AMP-activated protein kinase is required for the lipid-lowering effect of metformin in insulin-resistant human HepG2 cells. J Biol Chem 279: 47898-47905.

14. Yin W, Mu J, Birnbaum MJ (2003) Role of AMP-activated protein kinase in cyclic AMP-dependent lipolysis In 3T3-L1 adipocytes. J Biol Chem 278: 43074-43080.

15. Zhou G, Myers R, Li Y, Chen Y, Shen X, et al. (2001) Role of AMP-activated protein kinase in mechanism of metformin action. J Clin Invest 108: 1167-1174.

16. Miller RA, Birnbaum MJ (2010) An energetic tale of AMPK-independent effects of metformin. J Clin Invest 120: 2267-2270.

17. Grisouard J, Timper K, Radimerski TM, Frey DM, Peterli R, et al. (2010) Mechanisms of metformin action on glucose transport and metabolism in human adipocytes. Biochem Pharmacol 80: 1736-1745.

18. Kaser S, Ebenbichler CF, Tilg H (2010) Pharmacological and non-pharmacological treatment of non-alcoholic fatty liver disease. Int J Clin Pract 64: 968-983.

19. Arany Z, He H, Lin J, Hoyer K, Handschin C, et al. (2005) Transcriptional coactivator PGC-1 alpha controls the energy state and contractile function of cardiac muscle. Cell Metab 1: 259-271.

20. Finck BN, Kelly DP (2006) PGC-1 coactivators: inducible regulators of energy metabolism in health and disease. J Clin Invest 116: 615-622.

21. St-Pierre J, Drori S, Uldry M, Silvaggi JM, Rhee J, et al. (2006) Suppression of reactive oxygen species and neurodegeneration by the PGC-1 transcriptional coactivators. Cell 127: 397-408.

22. Valle I, Alvarez-Barrientos A, Arza E, Lamas S, Monsalve M (2005) PGC-1alpha regulates the mitochondrial antioxidant defense system in vascular endothelial cells. Cardiovasc Res 66: 562-573.

23. Handschin C (2009) The biology of PGC-1Î± and its therapeutic potential. Trends Pharmacol Sci 30: 322-329.

24. Viollet B, Guigas B, Leclerc J, Hébrard S, Lantier L, et al. (2009) AMP-activated protein kinase in the regulation of hepatic energy metabolism: from physiology to therapeutic perspectives. Acta Physiol (Oxf) 196: 81-98.

25. Razavizade M, Jamali R, Arj A, Talari H (2012) Serum parameters predict the severity of ultrasonographic findings in non-alcoholic fatty liver disease. Hepatobiliary Pancreat Dis Int 11: 513-520.

26. Okamoto Y, Tanaka S, Haga Y (2002) Enhanced GLUT2 gene expression in an oleic acid-induced in vitro fatty liver model. Hepatol Res 23: 138-144.

27. Soyal S, Krempler F, Oberkofler H, Patsch W (2006) PGC-1alpha: a potent transcriptional cofactor involved in the pathogenesis of type 2 diabetes. Diabetologia 49: 1477-1488.

28. Handschin C, Spiegelman BM (2006) Peroxisome proliferator-activated receptor gamma coactivator 1 coactivators, energy homeostasis, and metabolism. Endocr Rev 27: 728-735.

29. Lin J, Handschin C, Spiegelman BM (2005) Metabolic control through the PGC-1 family of transcription coactivators. Cell Metab 1: 361-370.

30. Estall J L, KahnM, CooperM P, Fisher FM, Wu MK, et al. (2009) Sensitivity of lipid metabolism and insulin signaling to genetic alterations in hepatic peroxisome proliferator-activated receptor-gamma coac-tivator-1 alpha expression. Diabetes 58: 1499-1508.

31. Koo SH, Satoh H, Herzig S, Lee CH, Hedrick S, et al. (2004) PGC-1 promotes insulin resistance in liver through PPAR-alpha-dependent induction of TRB-3. Nat Med 10: 530-534.

32. Yesilova Z, Yaman H, Oktenli C, Ozcan A, Uygun A, et al. (2005) Systemic markers of lipid peroxidation and antioxidants in patients with nonalcoholic Fatty liver disease. Am J Gastroenterol 100: 850-855.

33. St-Pierre J, Drori S, Uldry M, Silvaggi JM, Rhee J, et al. (2006) Suppression of reactive oxygen species and neurodegeneration by the PGC-1 transcriptional coactivators. Cell 127: 397-408.

34. Kong X, Wang R, Xue Y, Liu X, Zhang H, et al. (2010) Sirtuin 3, a new target of PGC-1alpha, plays an important role in the suppression of ROS and mitochondrial biogenesis. PLoS One 5: e11707.

35. Muntoni S (1999) Metformin and fatty acids. Diabetes Care 22: 179-180.

36. Foretz M, Hébrard S, Leclerc J, Zarrinpashneh E, Soty M, et al. (2010) Metformin inhibit s hepatic gluconeogenesis in mice independently of the LKB1/AMPK pathway via a decrease in hepatic energy state. J Clin Invest 120: 2355-2369.

37. Huang Y, Fu JF, Shi HB, Liu LR (2011) [Metformin prevents non-alcoholic fatty liver disease in rats: role of phospholipase A2/lysophosphatidylcholine lipoapoptosis pathway in hepatocytes]. Zhonghua Er Ke Za Zhi 49: 139-145.

38. Huss JM, Kelly DP (2005) Mitochondrial energy metabolism in heart failure: a question of balance. J Clin Invest 115: 547-555.

39. Suwa M, Egashira T, Nakano H, Sasaki H, Kumagai S (2006) Metformin increases the PGC-1alpha protein and oxidative enzyme activities possibly via AMPK phosphorylation in skeletal muscle in vivo. J Appl Physiol (1985) 101: 1685-1692.

40. Lin J, Handschin C, Spiegelman BM (2005) Metabolic control through the PGC-1 family of transcription coactivators. Cell Metab 1: 361-370.

35

Prevalence of Metabolic Syndrome Diagnosed by Three Different Criteria in School-Aged Children from Rural and Urban Areas

Cecilia Ramírez-Murillo, Elizabeth Guillot-Sánchez, Elizabeth Artalejo-Ochoa Q B, Alma E. Robles-Sardin, José A. Ponce-Martínez, María I Grijalva-Haro, Graciela Caire-Juvera, María I. Ortega-Vélez and Martha N. Ballesteros-Vásquez*

Centro de Investigación en Alimentación y Desarrollo, A.C. Carretera a la Victoria km 0.6, Hermosillo, Sonora México

Abstract

The International Diabetes Federation (IDF) does not justify the evaluation of metabolic syndrome (MetS) in children aged less than 10 years, unless they have a family history of risk factors. The prevalence of overweight and obesity in the Northwest of Mexico has increased in recent decades, making it possible to consider that MetS is already present in this group of population.

Objective: The primary objective of this study was to determine the prevalence of metabolic syndrome in children aged 6 to 9 years living in rural (RA) or urban (UA) areas of Northwest of Mexico. A secondary objective was to find adequate criteria to diagnose the prevalence of MS in children.

Methods: Participated 268 school-aged children in a random-selected cross sectional study. Anthropometric and blood pressure measurement were performed, and biochemical indicators were analyzed. MetS was defined as the presence of three or more risk factors and diagnosed using three different criteria. One of them according to what was proposed by the International Diabetes Federation (IDF) for children and two additional criteria proposed by this study considering suitable cutoffs for age for lipids and blood pressure.

Results: The general prevalence of MetS according to the three different criteria used was as follows.1) IDF criteria, 4.1%; 2) using cutoffs suggested for age for lipids and blood pressure and taking into account waist circumference as a criterion for MetS, 6.3%; and 3) cutoffs suggested for age, lipids and blood pressure without considering waist circumference as a criterion for MetS, 10.4%. Children living in the RA with a history of obesity and cardiovascular disease had higher waist circumference, triglycerides, and very low-density lipoprotein-C, and children from the UA had higher systolic and diastolic blood pressure, and higher levels of glucose and insulin.

Conclusion: MetS is present in children aged 6 to 9 years in the northwest region of Mexico, with higher proportions of the syndrome observed in overweight and obese children. The second criteria used in this study could be the most suitable for diagnosis of MetS, and the third criteria, for children at higher risk for cardiovascular disease and type 2 diabetes mellitus associated to heredity factors.

Keywords: Metabolic syndrome; Obesity; School-Aged Mexican children; Cardiovascular disease; Type 2 diabetes mellitus

Introduction

Overweight and obesity are highly associated with metabolic syndrome (MetS). This is defined as a clustering of metabolic abnormalities characterized by risk factors that are associated with cardiovascular disease and type 2 diabetes mellitus (T2DM). These factors are abdominal obesity, lipid profile alterations, glucose intolerance, and hypertension [1]. The presence of MetS increases the risk of developing cardiovascular disease and T2DM [2]. For adolescents, the evaluation criteria are not well defined and there is no accepted definition to diagnose MetS [3]. The International Diabetes Federation (IDF) [4]. does not justify the evaluation of MetS in children less than 10 years old, suggesting that the presence of MetS is out that its presence is unlikely in this population. Nevertheless, IDF states that more studies are needed to corroborate this statement.

One of the difficulties in evaluating MetS in children is the constant change in the level of insulin during childhood and the presence of physiological insulin resistance during puberty [5]. However, evidence indicates that people who develop diabetes in adulthood had higher body mass index (BMI) and subscapular skin fold as well as higher levels of glucose, triglycerides, and insulin, higher blood pressure, and lower levels of HDL-cholesterol (HDL-C) during childhood than those who do not develop diabetes [6]. Additionally, the American Pediatric Association suggests that cardiovascular risk factors be evaluated in

children between 2 and 10 years of age when they have family history of cardiovascular diseases [7].

Currently, research on MetS focuses on identifying its components in different populations and at different ages as well as developing a useful definition for clinical and epidemiological practices. In addition to the traditional components of MetS, researchers are considering other indicators that could be helpful in identifying people at higher risk, such as acanthosis nigricans (AN) and inflammatory markers [8,9].

In Mexico, T2DM and cardiovascular diseases are the main causes of mortality in the adult population [10]. Risk factors leading to these pathologies could be present during childhood mainly due to heredity or life style factors such as inadequate diets higher in carbohydrates or fat, together with low levels of physical activity [11,12].

In this context and according to data from the National Health and Nutrition Survey in Mexico in 2012, the state of Sonora, located in the

*Corresponding author: Martha N. Ballesteros Vásquez, Centro de Investigación en Alimentación y Desarrollo, A.C. Carretera a la Victoria km 0.6, Hermosillo, Sonora México; E-mail: nydia@ciad.mx

northwest region of Mexico, is one of the states in the country with a higher prevalence of childhood overweight and obesity (36.9%). Both rural and urban areas are affected, although in different ways; there are more overweight (24.8%) than obese (6.4%) children in rural areas, whereas the urban areas have more obese (19.4%) than overweight (18.3%) children [13]. Among the complications associated with excess body fat are insulin resistance [14], non-alcoholic fatty liver disease, hypertension, dyslipidemias, sleep disorders, orthopedic problems, and psychological and social issues [15].

The evaluation of MetS in children and adolescents is important for timely prevention and control of non-communicable disease development such as heart disease and T2DM. Therefore, the primary objective of this study was to determine the prevalence of metabolic syndrome in children aged 6 to 9 years living in rural and urban areas of Northwest of Mexico. A secondary objective was to compare MetS prevalence differences based on three criteria in a sample of children from Sonora, Mexico and determine the most appropriate criterion to diagnose it in a pediatric population.

Materials and Methods

Study design and sample selection

For this study, a cross-sectional sample of school-aged children aged 6 to 9 years was assessed. Eighteen public elementary schools located in two different areas (rural and urban) in the state of Sonora in northwest Mexico participated in the study. In the rural area, 7 schools from different towns were involved. In the urban area, 11 schools located in the city of Hermosillo (the capital) participated in the study. The rural and urban areas were defined according to the criteria established by Villalvazo [16], who defined a rural area as having less than 15,000 inhabitants. A total of 295 children participated in the study.

Study protocol

The experimental protocol was approved by the Ethical Review Board of Centro de Investigación en Alimentación y Desarrollo A.C. We used simple random sampling for the selection of the schools. Forty invitations were left in each school, inviting parents who had children between 6 and 9 years old to participate in the study. Parents and children who attended the invitation, received a detailed explanation of the protocol and provided informed consent. The parents answered a clinical questionnaire about family history of diabetes or cardiovascular risks, current medical conditions, and medication use.

A standard questionnaire was used to collect information about socio-demographic characteristics, and patient´s medical and family history during face-to-face interviews conducted by trained staff. Family history of obesity, diabetes, and cardiovascular disease were defined as the existence of these conditions in at least one first-degree relative.

Anthropometric measurements were performed according to standard procedures. Body weight was measured using an electronic scale with a capacity of 0 to 150 ± 0.05 kg (AND FV-150 KA1; A&D Co. Japan), and height was measured using a portable stadiometer (Holtain Limited Dyfed, Britain, UK). BMI was calculated using weight and height (kg/m^2) and BMI for age z score, height for age z score, and weight for age z score were calculated using the Anthro Plus software [17]. Obesity was defined following World Health Organization (WHO) criteria for children of the same age. Waist circumference (WC), was measured with non-elastic tape (Lafayette Instruments, USA) at the midpoint between the lower rib margin and the iliac crest, perpendicular to the long axis of the body, with the subject

standing balanced on both feet. Body composition was measured using bioelectrical impedance analysis (Impedimed IMP5™). Since we could not assess a hydration status of the children before measurement, we applied a brief clinical questionnaire to the parents in order to know if their children presented illness or diarrhea episodes 5 days before the evaluation. If the answer was positive, the child was not included in the study. Total body fat and lean mass were obtained using the Ramirez-López formula developed for the population of school children living in Sonora [18]. Body fat percentage was classified according to Freedman´s values for age and gender [19].

Blood pressure was measured according to the technique proposed by the National High Blood Pressure Education Program (NHBPEP) for children and adolescents [20] after 5 minutes of rest in a sitting position with the child's feet on the floor and their arms supported at heart level. Two measurements were performed at 10-minute intervals using mercurial sphygmomanometers (Desk Model Mercurial Sphygmomanometer, Model 100, China Meheco Medical instrument, RPC) with an appropriate cuff for the arm diameter. Hypertension was defined as the average systolic (SBP) or diastolic (DBP) blood pressure level greater than or equal to the 95th percentile for the child's sex, age, and height. AN was defined as a skin darkening and thickening at the neck [21]. The determination of AN child was assessed by a trained individual.

Biochemical analyses

Plasma obtained after overnight fasting was used to determine plasma glucose, total cholesterol (TC), HDL-C, triglycerides, and insulin. Two fasting (12-h) blood samples were collected from each subject on 2 different days. Blood was collected in tubes containing 0.15 g/100 g EDTA to determine plasma lipids. Plasma was separated by centrifugation at 1500 g for 20 min at 4°C then placed into vials containing phenyl methyl sulfonyl fluoride (0.015 g/100 g), sodium azide (0.01 g/100 g), and aprotinin (0.01 g/100 g).

TC was determined using an enzymatic method (CHOD-PAO) with Roche-Diagnostic standards and kits [22]. HDL-C was measured in supernatant after precipitation of apo B-containing lipoproteins [23], and low density lipoprotein (LDL)-C was determined using the Friedwald equation [24]. Triglycerides were measured using an enzymatic method (GPO-PAP) with Roche-Diagnostics standards and kits [25]. Means of two blood draws were used.

Plasma glucose was determined using an enzymatic method (GOD-PAO) with Roche Diagnostic kits [26]. Fasting plasma insulin concentration was determined by enzyme-linked immunosorbent assay (ELISA) using a sandwich type immunoassay (ALPCO Diagnostics, NH, USA). The homeostasis model assessment (HOMA) [27] was used to calculate insulin resistance (IR) according to the following equation: IR (HOMA IR) – fasting insulin (µU/mL) fasting glucose (mmol/L) ÷22.5. The HOMA model has been shown to be a reliable method for measuring insulin resistance in various populations when other more invasive methods are not feasible [28]. The HOMA-IR value of 3.4 was chosen as the reference value to define IR [28] and the insulin blood concentration was classified as normal, borderline, or high [29].

Definition of metabolic syndrome

Because there is no single accepted criteria for the diagnosis of MetS in children aged 6 to 9 years, the presence of MetS in this population was determined using three different criteria as follows: 1) according to the definition proposed by IDF [4] for children aged 10 years, considering the presence of central obesity as a mandatory condition for diagnosis coupled with the presence of two or more additional risk factors; 2) considering the presence of central obesity according to the provisions of the IDF [4], but using predefined cutoffs for lipids specific for children [30] and blood pressure [20]; 3) establishing the presence of three or more risk factors regardless of central obesity as a mandatory condition and using predefined cutoffs determined by the IDF [4] for waist circumference and glucose, the National Cholesterol Education Program (NCEP) criteria [30] for lipids, and the NHBPEP criteria [20] for blood pressure (Table 1).

Central obesity was defined as a waist circumference value at or above the 90th percentile for sex, age, and ethnicity from the IDF definition [4]. For the lipid profile, we considered the cut off values from the National Cholesterol Education Program [30]. Triglycerides, LDL-C, and TC were considered elevated when values were at or above the 95th percentile for age and sex, and HDL-C was considered low when the values were at or under the 5th percentile [30]. Elevated SBP or DBP were defined as values at or above the 95th percentile for age, sex, and height [20]. The reference value for impaired fasting glucose was taken from the IDF and considered as 100 mg/dL or higher.

Statistical analysis

Normality of the data was verified and descriptive statistics were performed to show the study population characteristics by rural/urban area. Data are presented as means ± standard deviations and as medians and interquartile ranges accordingly. Normality and equality of variances were evaluated and the tests were used accordingly. Two-sample Student's t-test was used to compare both areas of study. For non-normal variables, we used the Mann Whitney U Test. For non-equal variances, the Aspin Welch p value was selected. The Chi-squared test for Independence was used to compare frequencies. Differences with p<0.05 were considered significant. The kappa coefficient was used to test the level of agreement for the three definitions. All data were analyzed using NCSS 2007 (Number Cruncher Statistical System for Windows, Kaysville, Utah, USA) Software.

Results

Children's anthropometric characteristics by area (rural and urban) are presented in Table 2. The mean age of the children was 7.4 ± 1.03

Indicator	Total (n=268)	Rural area (n=119)	Urban area (n=149)	p¹
Age (years)*	7.5 (1.4-3.9)	7.6 (1.3-3.7)	7.3 (1.45-3.9)	0.54
Weight (Kg)*	24.59 (8.86-44.65)	25.29 (7.8-44.65)	24.14 (10.17-31.05)	0.25
Height (cm) †	124.05 ± 7.30 (105.2-144.4)	124.76 ± 7.13 (105.2-144.4)	123.48 ± 7.40 (108.5-140.9)	0.15
z-BMI/A*	0.015 (2.07-8.33)	0.12 (2.02-7.49)	-0.06 (2.27-7.87)	0.15
z-H/A†	0.006 ± 0.99 (-2.54-2.56)	0.093 ± 0.99 (-2.54-2.54)	-0.06 ± 0.99 (-2.33-2.56)	0.20
z-W/A*	0.21 (2.06-8.11)	0.28 (1.81-7.72)	0.14 (2.19-7.04)	0.38
WC (cm) *	55.4 (10.57-55.5)	56.4 (10.1-50.6)	55.0 (10.5-45.3)	0.21
% fat mass (BIA) †	28.06 ± 8.93 (8.49-50.22)	27.49 ± 8.78 (11.46-49.70)	28.52 ± 9.05 (8.49-50.22)	0.35
Triglycerides (mg/dL) *	88.29 (44.38-341.0)	92.04 (40.75-174.95)	84.55 (45.67-341.0)	0.01
TC (mg/dL) †	170.82 ± 33.40 (86.07-304.92)	172.23 ± 33.79 (86.78-304.92)	169.69 ± 33.15 (86.07-277.15)	0.53
HDL-C (mg/dL) *	48.71 (11.89-96.68)	51.27 (13.07-96.68)	47.01 (11.59-60.3)	0.01
LDL-C (mg/dL) *	101.12 (43.54-194.01)	103.06 (39.32-189.08)	99.8 (48.40-169.95)	0.61
VLDL (mg/dL) *	17.66 (8.87-68.2)	18.41 (8.15-34.99)	16.91 (9.13-68.2)	0.01
SBP (mmHg) *	90 (20-70)	90 (20-70)	90 (15-60)	0.30
DBP (mmHg) *	60 (17.5-67.5)	60 (17.5-52.5)	60 (18.75-65)	0.60
Fasting glucose (mg/dL) †	93.29 ± 13.99 (44.82-130.21)	89.86 ± 14.40 (44.82-126.64)	96.04 ± 13.05 (61.65-130.21)	<0.01
Insulin (mU/L) *	6.24 (6.21-62.51)	5.32 (5.41-38.95)	7.27 (6.97-62.51)	0.03
HOMA*	1.4 (1.53-15.02)	1.22 (1.17-10.21)	1.70 (1.83-15.02)	<0.01
AN, n (%)**	15 (5.6)	9 (7.6)	6 (4)	0.21

†Mean ± standard deviation (minimum - maximum).
*Median (interquartile range [p25-p75]).
¹Difference between groups by two sample Student's t-test and Mann Whitney U Test for non-normal data (p<0.05). **Chi-squared test.
Abbreviations: z-BMI/A z: score of body mass index for age, z-H/A z: score height for age, z-W/A z: score weight for age, SBP: systolic blood pressure, DBP: diastolic blood pressure, AN: acanthosis nigricans, WC: waist circumference, HDL-C: high density lipoprotein cholesterol, TC: total cholesterol, LDL-C: low density lipoprotein, VLDL: very low density lipoprotein, HOMA: Homeostasis Model Assessment.

Table 2: Anthropometric characteristics and metabolic profile of the total population and by rural or urban area.

years, ranging from 5 to 10 years. No statistically significant differences were observed between rural and urban areas in the anthropometric variables, blood pressure and the AN indicator (p>0.05). According to the z BMI/A, the prevalence of overweight and obesity was 31.1% in rural areas and 32.9% in urban areas. Waist circumference was at or above the 90th percentile in 10.1% of children in rural areas and 12% in urban areas. Likewise, children with moderate and high body fat percentage were observed in both study areas: 26% and 33% in rural and 27% and 36% in urban areas, respectively.

There were statistically significant differences between the urban and rural areas in some metabolic variables. Fasting blood glucose, insulin, and the HOMA index were higher in the urban area, whereas concentrations of triglycerides, HDL-C, and very low density lipoprotein (VLDL)-C were higher in the rural area (Table 2).

Risk factor	IDF, 2007	IDF (2007), NCEP (1991), NHBPEP (2005) (proposed in this study)	Three or more risk factors NCEP (1991), NHBPEP (2005) without WC as a condition. (proposed in this study)
Obesity	Obligatory presence of waist circumference ≥ 90th percentile for age and sex + 2 risk factors	Obligatory presence of waist circumference ≥ 90th percentile for age and sex [4] + 2 risk factors	Waist circumference in ≥90th percentile for age and sex [4]
Triglycerides (mg/dL)	≥150	≥ 95th percentile for age and sex [28]	≥ 95th percentile for age and sex [28]
Glucose (mg/dL)	≥ 100	≥ 100 mg/dL [4]	≥ 100 mg/dL [4]
HDL-C (mg/dL)	<40	≤ 5th percentile for age and sex [28]	≤ 5th percentile for age and sex [28]
SBP and/or DBP (mm Hg)	Systolic ≥130 Diastolic ≥ 85	≥ 95th percentile for age, sex and height [18]	≥ 95th percentile for age, sex and height [18]

Abbreviations: HDL-C: High Density Lipoprotein Cholesterol, IDF: International Diabetes Federation, NCEP: National Cholesterol Education Program, NHBPEP: National High Blood Pressure Education Program, SBP: Systolic Blood Pressure, DBP: Diastolic Blood Pressure.

Table 1: Criteria used to diagnose metabolic syndrome.

According to the American Diabetes Association [31], fasting glucose values in children with normal, impaired, and probable diagnosis of diabetes are 86.1 mg/dL, 108.5 mg/dL, and 128.4 mg/dL (p<0.01), respectively. Figure 1a shows the classification of the study population according to their blood glucose concentration.

Glucose data were divided according to normal, borderline, and high insulin blood levels. There were no differences in concentrations of glucose (p=0.99) relative to insulin levels, even when we found borderline and high values of insulin (Figure 1b).

According to the HOMA index, insulin resistance was present in 9 children from the rural area (7.5%) and 22 from the urban area (14.8%). There were no statistically significant differences between study groups (p=0.06). AN, which is associated with high levels of insulin, was found in 15 children including 9 from the rural and 6 from the urban areas (Table 2). This indicator was observed only in children with a high body fat mass.

Results of the anthropometric and metabolic characteristics in the population stratified by family history of obesity, diabetes, and cardiovascular disease are shown in Table 3. Children with a history of obesity had a significantly higher weight/age (W/A) and percentage of fat mass compared to children with no familiar history of obesity. Those with a history of diabetes had higher BMI/A and waist circumference, and children from families with a history of cardiovascular disease had higher systolic blood pressure, DBP, TC, and LDL-C compared with children without a family history of cardiovascular disease. Particularly in the rural area, a family history of obesity and cardiovascular diseases was present in children with a higher waist circumference (58.5 vs. 53.8 cm, p<0.02; 59 vs. 54.2 cm, p<0.01). In contrast, urban children had higher SBP (94.46 ± 11.97 vs. 88.17 ± 10.98 mmHg, p<0.001) and DBP (63.36 ± 12.92 vs 57.60 ± 10.08 mmHg; p<0.001) when a family history of obesity and cardiovascular diseases was present.

Table 4 shows the proportion of children with MetS according to the different definitions used in the present study. For the first criteria suggested by the IDF [4], MetS was present in 11 children (4.1%). In the rural and urban areas, 2.5% and 5.4% of the children had MetS,

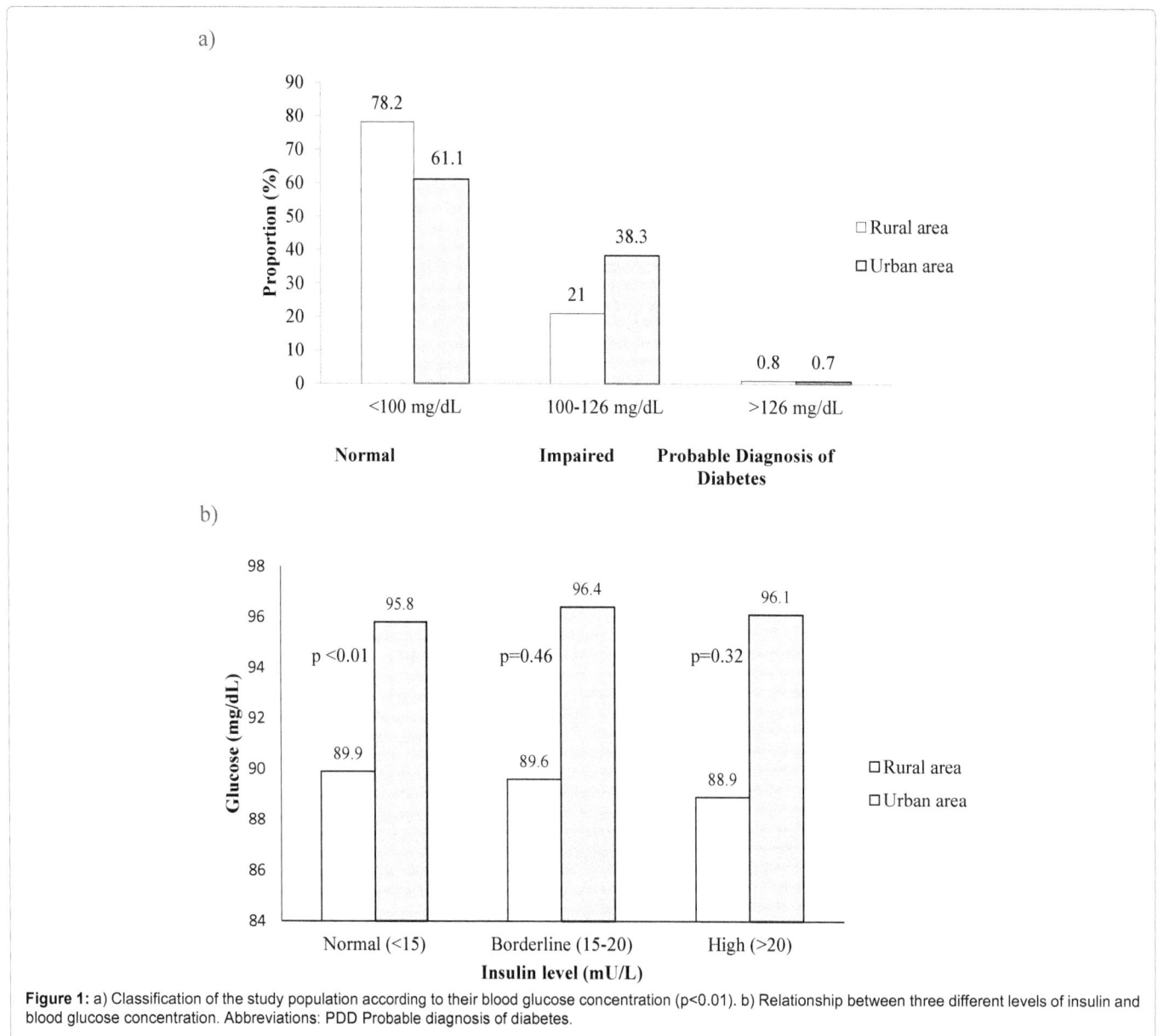

Figure 1: a) Classification of the study population according to their blood glucose concentration (p<0.01). b) Relationship between three different levels of insulin and blood glucose concentration. Abbreviations: PDD Probable diagnosis of diabetes.

Indicator	Without obesity (n =44)	Obesity (n=90)	p¹	Without diabetes (n=93)	Diabetes (n=18)	p¹	Without CVD (n = 63)	CVD (n= 25)	p¹
Age (years)	7.5 ± 0.7† (6.1-9)	7.4 ± 0.9 (6-9.7)	0.58	7.3 ± 0.9† (6-9.7)	7.5 ± 0.7 (6.1-8.4)	0.47	7.33 ± 0.73† (6.1-8.8)	7.46 ± 0.94 (6.1-9.7)	0.49
Weight (Kg)	25.9 ± 7.1† (16.1-43)	28.36 ± 8.1 (16.3-60.7)	0.10	24.9* (10.6-44.6)	28.1 (10.6-32)	0.04	25.4* (9.3-30.2)	27.9 (11.4-34.2)	0.34
Height (cm)	123.75 ± 7.2† (108.8-136.9)	125.14 ± 7.3 (108.5-144.4)	0.29	123.7 ± 7.9† (108.5-144.4)	126.7 ± 5.7 (116.1-134.4)	0.16	124.24 ± 5.9† (111.8-134.4)	124.45 ± 7.9 (108.9-144.4)	0.89
z-BMI/A	0.34 ± 1.7† (-1.8-4.7)	0.86 ± 1.6 (-2.8-5.5)	0.08	0.48 ± 1.5† (-2.8-4.2)	1.31 ± 1.7 (-0.9-5.5)	0.04	0.60 ± 1.44† (-1.9-3.7)	1.1 ± 1.83 (-1.4-5.5)	0.17
z-H/A	0.03 ± 1.0† (-2.0-2.0)	0.3 ± 0.9 (-2.2-2.56)	0.06	0.13 ± 0.9† (-2.0-2.5)	0.45 ± 0.7 (-0.96-1.8)	0.23	0.2 ± 0.85† (-1.9-2.5)	0.08 ± 1.07 (-2.0-2.0)	0.60
z-W/A	0.3 ± 1.6† (-2.3-4.1)	0.9 ± 1.5 (-2.3-5.3)	0.03	0.46 ± 1.5† (-2.3-4.8)	1.32 ± 1.5 (-0.7-5.3)	0.04	0.59 ± 1.3† (-2.1-3.8)	0.88 ± 1.7 (-2.3-5.3)	0.39
WC (cm)	57.2 ± 9.1† (44.5-80)	60.5 ± 10.3 (45.5-96.6)	0.08	55.6* (11.2-50.6)	59.7 (15.9-36.1)	0.02	56.6* (9.8-39.6)	58.5 (14.6-39.3)	0.35
% fat mass (BIA)	26.9 ± 9.1† (13-48.3)	30.5 ± 9.5 (11.5-50.2)	0.03	28.1 ± 9.0† (11.5-50.2)	31.2 ± 10.1 (13-49.3)	0.32	28.47 ± 9.2† (11.5-49.5)	30.8 ± 2.0 (15.8-49.3)	0.29
Triglycerides (mg/dL)	98.6 ± 57.3† (47.8-378.5)	99.9 ± 34.4 (37.5-193)	0.86	89.2* (42.6-225.5)	123.4 (56.7-310.3)	0.19	86.9* (41.2-341)	102.3 (58.4-129.5)	0.37
TC (mg/dL)	175 ± 33.3† (86.8-277.1)	173.8 ± 37.2 (86.1-304.9)	0.86	179.43 ± 32.6† (86.8-304.9)	159.6 ± 21.7 (129.3-76.8)	0.01	168.79 ± 35.6† (86.1-251.7)	185.36 ± 33.9 (142.4-277.1)	0.04
HDL-C (mg/dL)	47.14 ± 10.7† (19.2-70.1)	51.3 ± 12.1 (8-104.7)	0.05	50.6* (11.7-81)	46.3 (10.7-71.5)	0.36	51.3* (12.5-96.7)	50.2 (14.6-48.4)	0.64
LDL-C (mg/dL)	108.1 ± 31.3† (37.4-200.2)	102.5 ± 34.0 (30.2-224.2)	0.36	108.9 ± 30.5 (37.4-186.9)	87.6 ± 20.8 (47.9-126.3)	0.00	98.18 ± 33.0† (30.2-179.3)	114.22 ± 30.7 (78.8-200.2)	0.03
VLDL (mg/dL)	19.7 ± 11.5† (9.6-75.7)	19.9 ± 6.9 (7.5-38.6)	0.86	17.8* (8.5-45.1)	24.7 (11.3-62)	0.19	17.4* (8.2-68.2)	20.5 (11.7-25.9)	0.37
SBP (mmHg)	90* (10-55)	90 (15-55)	0.82	92.3 ± 11.3† (70-130)	98.7 ± 15.8 (75-127.5)	0.03	90* (15-50)	90 (20-55)	0.03
DBP (mmHg)	59.3* (18.7-42.4)	61.9 (20-65)	0.30	59.3 ± 11.9† (37.5-90)	65.4 ± 15.4 (40-105)	0.05	59.72 ± 10.9† (37.5-80)	67.7 ± 15.0 (45-105)	0.02
Fasting glucose (mg/dL)	96.5 ± 15.0† (61.9-126.4)	92.2 ± 14.4 (49.8-119)	0.11	93.70 ± 14.0† (49.8-120.7)	96.6 ± 14.1 (79.3-122.8)	0.32	94.53 ± 14.3† (52.6-122.8)	97.0 ± 17.0 (24.4-71.9)	0.47
Insulin (mU/L)	7.56 ± 5.4† (0-24.4)	7.74 ± 6.33 (0-38.9)	0.87	7.2* (6.3-38.9)	6.2 (8-25.4)	0.31	7.02* (5.3-25.4)	7.5 (6.4-17.2)	0.37
HOMA	1.5 (1.8-6.8)	1.5 (1.8-10.2)	0.59	1.61* (1.6-10.2)	1.57 (1.8-6.6)	0.60	1.56 (1.32-6.6)	1.79 (2.2-4.4)	0.24
AN, n (%) **	0 (0)	8 (8.9)	0.04	6(6.4)	2(11.7)	0.48	3 (4.7)	3 (12)	0.22

†Mean ± standard deviation (minimum - maximum). *Median (interquartile range [p25-p75]). *Abbreviations*: z-BMI/A z: score of body mass index for age, z-H/A z: score height for age, z-W/A z: score weight for age, SBP: systolic blood pressure, DBP: diastolic blood pressure, AN: acanthosis nigricans, WC: waist circumference, HDL-C: high density lipoprotein cholesterol, SBP: systolic blood pressure, DBP: diastolic blood pressure, TC: total cholesterol, LDL-C: low density lipoprotein, VLDL: very low density lipoprotein, HOMA: Homeostasis Model Assessment. ¹Difference between groups by two sample Student's t-test and Mann Whitney U Test for non-normal data (p<0.05). **Chi-squared test.

Table 3: Anthropometric characteristics and metabolic profile of the total population and categorized by family history of obesity, diabetes, and cardiovascular disease.

Criteria	IDF (2007) for children over 10 years old (%)	IDF (2007), NCEP (1991), NHBPEP (2005) (this study analysis) (%)	Three or more risk factors NCEP (1991), NHBPEP (2005) without WC as a condition. (this study analysis) (%)
Total	4.1	6.3	10.4
Area			
Rural	2.5	5.0	10.1
Urban	5.4	7.4	10.7
Sex			
Girls	5.7	7.9	11.4
Boys	2.3	4.7	9.4

Abbreviations: IDF: International Diabetes Federation, NCEP: National Cholesterol Education Program, NHBPEP: National High Blood Pressure Education Program.

Table 4: Proportion (%) of children with metabolic syndrome according to the different criteria used in this study.

and the differences between groups was not significant (p=0.24). The second criteria for MetS (Table 5) considered abdominal obesity plus two other risk factors according to the NCEP [30] and NHBPEP [20] percentiles. MetS was found in 17 children (6.3%), 5.0% from the rural and 7.4% from the urban areas, with no significant differences between groups. The third criteria for MetS diagnosis considered children with three or more risk factors for MetS and the presence of abdominal obesity was not obligatory. Of the total population, 10.4% had MetS,

and the same percentage of children with MetS was present in both areas of study (rural 10.1% vs. urban 10.7%, p=0.86). The reliability analysis using the kappa coefficient (0.6487, p=0.000) showed that the agreement was substantial in the total population.

Discussion

This study demonstrates that MetS is present in children aged 6 to 9 years living in urban and rural areas of northwest Mexico. In this study

Indicator	Without MS (n=251)	With MS (n=17)	p[1]
Age (years)*	7.5 (1.3-3.9)	7.3 (1.45-2.7)	0.45
Weight (Kg)*	24.14 (8.1-31.85)	42.69 (9.87-28.8)	<0.01
Height (cm)[†]	123.67 ± 7.24 (123-124.8)	129.58 ± 5.97 (122.7-129.2)	<0.01
WC (cm)*	55 (8.8-45.3)	78.5 (8.15-27.5)	<0.01
z-BMI/A*	-0.06 (1.81-6.52)	3.37 (1.73-3.52)	<0.01
Body fat (%)*	26.37 (9.92-41.73)	44.13 (5.12-9.85)	<0.01
Triglycerides (mg/ dL)*	85.95 (41.93-225.54)	138.88 (65.57-301.42)	<0.01
TC (mg/dL)*	169.38 (46.26-191.08)	178.31 (43.30-162.1)	0.05
HDL-C (mg/dL)*	49.75 (11.84-96.68)	42.35 (10.98-35.57)	<0.01
LDL-C (mg/dL)[†]	100.76 ± 30.49 (30.2-200.1)	117.88 ± 38.30 (47.9-224.2)	0.07
VLDL (mg/dL)*	17.19 (8.39-45.11)	27.78 (13.11-60.28)	<0.01
SBP (mmHg)*	90 (20-70)	115 (20-40)	<0.01
DBP (mmHg)*	60 (15-52.5)	80 (11.25-55)	<0.01
Glucose (mg/dL)*	92.98 (19.51-85.39)	100.78 (14.2-55.9)	0.27
Insulin (mU/L)*	5.7 (5.72-33.79)	13.74 (10.89-57.09)	<0.01
HOMA*	1.34 (1.38-7.18)	3.21 (2.27-14.31)	<0.01
AN, n (%)**	7(2.8)	8(47.1)	<0.01

[†]Mean ± standard deviation (minimum - maximum). *Median (interquartile range [p25-p75]).
[1]Difference between groups by two sample Student's t-test and Mann Whitney U Test for non-normal data (p<0.05). **Chi-squared test.
Abbreviations: z-BMI/A z: score of body mass index for age, z-H/A z: score height for age, z-W/A z: score weight for age, SBP: systolic blood pressure, DBP: diastolic blood pressure, AN: acanthosis nigricans, WC: waist circumference, HDL-C: high density lipoprotein cholesterol, SBP: systolic blood pressure, DBP: diastolic blood pressure, TC: total cholesterol, LDL-C: low density lipoprotein, VLDL: very low density lipoprotein, HOMA: Homeostasis Model Assessment.

Table 5: Anthropometric characteristics and metabolic profile according to the presences of metabolic syndrome (MS) with abdominal obesity as an obligatory factor (second criteria used in this study).

population, overweight and obesity represented one of the risk factors for MetS. In both the rural and urban areas, the prevalence of obesity was elevated (31.1% and 37%, respectively). The percentage of urban children with obesity was higher than that reported by the Nutrition and Health National Survey 2012 [32].

Towards the end of the first year of life, a physiological loss of fat mass takes place, so that in normal conditions a child between 5 and 6 years should be physiologically thinner. When a 6-year old is an obese child, the probability of persistent obesity increases by 50% [33]. Obesity in parents influenced the development of obesity in their children and this influence seemed higher when the child was aged less than 10 years [33,34]. In this study, the results from the family history questionnaire on chronic diseases showed that children from the rural area with a family history of cardiovascular diseases and obesity had higher waist circumference. In contrast, children from the urban area with the same family history had higher systolic and diastolic blood pressure (data not shown). We do not have a clear idea of the differences between urban and rural children, as they have similar family history. A possible

explanation is that in the urban areas, there is a greater tendency to consume fast foods that typically have a high sodium content, which probably could be affecting the gene expression associated with blood pressure. Kuschnir and Mendoça mentioned that the risk of developing hypertension is higher when both parents have the disease [35].

Beside heredity, other factors that may contribute to the growing prevalence of obesity and its complications in this population are low physical activity and an inadequate diet. Although data on dietary habits and physical activity were not collected. Results from others studies [36-38] in urban locations of the same region showed that children consumed a hypercaloric diet, with adequate quantities of protein and fiber but excessive amounts of simple carbohydrates and saturated fat and a low quantity of polyunsaturated fat. Those studies also showed that most of the children were sedentary [36,38]. The development of obesity secondary to genetic or excessive consumption of food has been proposed as a risk factor for developing metabolic alterations including insulin resistance and diabetes mellitus [39]. Transnational food chains have made energy-dense, low-cost food available and accessible to Mexican children in a community environment where food regulation is still scarce [40].

The analysis of the metabolic profile showed that children from the rural area had more alterations in their lipid profile, with higher triglyceride and VLDL-C values than children from the urban area. In contrast, children from the urban area had more alterations in glucose metabolism, with higher concentrations of glucose and insulin and higher HOMA than children from the rural area. These results suggest that children from the urban area at greater risk for developing heart disease or diabetes, possibly due to risk factors related to lifestyle. Studies on the migration of people from rural to urban areas have reported similar changes in body composition and clinical markers associated with their new lifestyle, which involve higher consumption of energy-dense foods and less physical activity [41,42].

A simple analysis of fasting blood glucose does not determine the diagnosis of diabetes, but it may be the first step in its detection. In this study, we classified fasting blood glucose concentrations according to the American Diabetes Association [31]. Of the total population of the study, 31.3% (21% rural, 38.3% urban) of children had impaired fasting blood glucose. These children are probably producing more insulin to compensate for the elevated glucose, but the two are not balancing each other out [43]. We could assume that this situation has progressed for some time and could turn into T2DM in the future.

T2DM begins with reduced insulin action due to an impairment in the ability of the target cells to respond to this hormone, which leads to insulin resistance. During this process, there is a decrease in the peripheral consumption of glucose and also in hepatic glycogenesis, and an increase in glyconeogenesis with results in hyperglycemia. Also, β cells from the pancreatic islet cells hypersecrete insulin to compensate for the excess glucose, producing hyperinsulinemia and normoglycemia. When the cycle is exhausted, it leads to glucose intolerance and, in later stages to T2DM [43,44].

We found children with insulin resistance in both areas (7.5% rural, 14.8% urban, p=0.06). Even when we did not detect significant differences between groups, the proportion of children with insulin resistance was higher in the urban area. Secondary to obesity, insulin resistance may be a common etiopathogenic mechanism for hypertension and dyslipidemia. Generally, children with obesity have a higher prevalence of hypertriglyceridemia and low levels of HDL-C [45]. In adipose tissue, hyperinsulinemia increases lipolysis, leading to more availability of free fatty acids, an increase in the hepatic synthesis of VLDL, and a decrease in HDL-C [46].

AN was found only in children with high body fat mass, and this coincided with insulin resistance being present only in children with high fat mass. The prevalence of high SBP and/or DBP was 16% rural vs 11.4% urban, the presence of hypertension at an early age is might be an early sign of glucose intolerance [47] and a risk factor for coronary disease [48].

Another risk factor for coronary disease is dyslipidemia. In this study, 32.1% of children had hypertriglyceridemia and 19% had low HDL-C. Other studies in Sonoran children reported low levels of HDL-C and the predominant subfraction was HDL$_3$, which is associated with higher cardiovascular risk [38]. Obesity, hypertension, hypertriglyceridemia, low HDL-C, and impaired glucose are components of MetS.

One of the most important goals of this study was to evaluate the prevalence of MetS in children using three different diagnostic criteria and determine which of them might be more appropriate for the diagnosis of MetS in a pediatric population. The first criteria used for the diagnosis of MetS in this study were the one according to the IDF [4] for 10-year-old children. These criteria use cutoffs for adults for the biochemical indicators and account for the presence of waist circumference $\geq$ 90th percentile for the diagnosis of MetS. The general prevalence of MetS using these criteria was 4.1% (2.5% rural; 5.4% urban). The IDF does not consider the presence of MetS in children aged < 10 years and does not recommend its diagnosis unless the children have a family history of risk factors [4]. This study demonstrates that even when criteria for adults is used, there are children with MetS in the region of Sonora. A study by Elizondo-Montemayor et al. [49] using the IDF criteria [4] in overweight children age 6 to 12 years from Mexico City reported a prevalence of MetS of 6.7%. When they observed age groups of 6-9 years and 10-12 years, the prevalence of MetS was 7.3% and 5.9% (p=0.91), respectively. These authors mentioned that there were more children with MetS in the younger age group, and this may be due to the fact that the percentage of children with waist circumference above the 90th percentile [4] was significantly higher (p<0.001) in the group of children aged 6-9 years compared with the older age group .

Another study done in Campeche, México, used the same IDF criteria [4] and reported a prevalence of 20% MetS in adolescents aged 11 to 13 years. Nevertheless, only obese participants (BMI $\geq$ 95th percentile) were included [3].

The second way in which we determined the prevalence of MetS also considered the IDF criteria [4] using a waist circumference $\geq$ 90th percentile as a condition for the diagnosis, but also employed adequate cutoffs for metabolic measurements in children aged 6 to 9 years provided by the NCEP [30] for the lipid profile, and by the NHBPEP [20] for blood pressure. Thus, the observed prevalence of MetS in the total study population was 6.3% (5.0% rural vs. 7.4% urban, p=0.43). Thus, the ratio obtained was similar to that reported by Elizondo-Montemayor et al. (7.3%) in obese children aged 6-9 years [49]. However, they used the IDF definition [4] without adjusting the cutoffs for children. Differences in physical and metabolic characteristics between children with and without the presence of MetS were evident (Table 5). Children with MetS had higher values in all the body composition variables and metabolic risk factors, and approximately 50% of children diagnosed with MetS presented AN. The consideration of central obesity plus the appropriate clinical cutoffs for children, could be a better criterion for evaluating MetS in a pediatric population

The third way to diagnose MetS did not take into account the presence of a waist circumference $\geq$90th percentile as a condition for evaluating MetS and used lipid profile metabolic indicator cutoffs for children aged 6 to 9 years from the NCEP and blood pressure criteria from the NHBPEP. Thus, the prevalence of MetS using these criteria was 10.4% (10.1% rural vs. 10.7% urban), and 32.1% of the children presented with AN. When we diagnosed MetS this way, children with a normal body composition met this criterion because other risk factors like impaired fasting glucose, hypertension, hypertriglyceridemia, or low HDL-C were present. Even without considering obesity, some children may have altered metabolic factors, possibly due to genetic factors that put children at risk. High levels of TC, LDL-C, plasma glucose, and high blood pressure are risk factors that could be influenced by family history due to shared genetic and environmental factors [5].

Considering central obesity as the major factor for the diagnosis of MetS may underestimate the risk of developing cardiovascular diseases and T2DM because it excludes children without obesity who have other metabolic alterations.

The proportions of MetS identified in this population of children varied depending on the criteria used. We hypothesize that the IDF [4] criteria could underestimate the prevalence of MetS in children aged less than 10 years because the cutoffs for the lipid profile and blood pressure are not adequate for this age group. Instead, the second criteria included cutoffs suggested for this age from the NCEP [30] and the NHBPEP [20], which may detect more accurately children with MetS. The third criteria for evaluation of MetS included children with a normal waist circumference but who presented with three other risk factors. This third way of diagnosing MetS could be useful for identifying children at risk for cardiovascular and T2DM due to heredity factors.

We recognize that one of the limitations of this study was that we did not collect data on dietary habits and physical activity as factors related to obesity; however, data from recent studies were available for a proper discussion. The main strength of this study is that we measured MetS in children aged less than 10 years from rural and urban areas. We established three different criteria for evaluating MetS in children, and all the techniques used were applied by trained personnel.

Conclusions

This study demonstrates that MetS is present in children aged 6 to 9 years living in a community with serious problems of obesity and cardiovascular diseases. We also demonstrate that MetS is more prevalent in overweight and obese children. The second criteria used in this study could be most suitable for diagnosis of MetS in a pediatric population because it takes into account the appropriate cutoffs suggested for this age. Considering abdominal obesity as an obligatory factor for the diagnosis of MetS could underestimate the number of children at risk for cardiovascular diseases and T2DM because the criteria exclude children without abdominal obesity but who do have metabolic alterations. Therefore, MetS should be diagnosed using an age-appropriate definition. Our information suggests that metabolic problems in children from an urban area are at increased risk for heart disease and diabetes compared to the rural area.

Because obesity is associated risk factors for cardiovascular diseases and T2DM, health promotion programs should consider the combination of genetic and environmental factors. If these factors are detected and controlled in time, the development of non-communicable diseases related to MetS could be prevented.

Implications for School Health

The development of metabolic syndrome or related-conditions including obesity, hypertension, cardiovascular diseases, and type 2 diabetes mellitus in school-aged children could interfere with their adequate physical and mental development. The diagnostic criteria evaluated in this study may be useful to develop a useful definition for clinical and epidemiological practices of pediatric population in risk of chronic diseases.

Human Subjects Approval Statement

This research was approved by the Ethics Committee of the Food and Development Research Center (CIAD) (Document code CE/018/2009).

Acknowledgments

We thank the children and their parents for their participation. We also thank the School Breakfast Program of Sonora (DIF, Sonora) for supporting this study.

References

1. Alberti G, Zimmet P, Shaw J (2006) Metabolic syndrome- a new world-wide definition. A Consensus Statement from the International Diabetes Federation. Diabet Med 23: 469-480.

2. Gami A, Witt BJ, Howard D, Erwin P, Gami L, et al. (2007) Metabolic syndrome and risk of incident cardiovascular events and death: a systematic review and meta-analysis of longitudinal studies. J Am Coll Cardiol 49: 403-414.

3. Juárez-López C, Klunder-Klunder M, Medina-Bravo P, Madrigal-Azcarate A, Mass-Diaz E, et al. (2010) Insulin resistance and its association with the components of the metabolic syndrome among obese children and adolescents. BMC Public Health 10: 318.

4. Zimmet P, Alberti G, Kaufman F, Tajima N, Silink M, et al. (2007) The metabolic syndrome in children and adolescents: the IDF consensus. Diabetes Voice 52: 29-32.

5. Steinberger J, Daniels SR, Eckel RH, Hayman L, Lustig RH, et al. (2009) Progress and challenges in metabolic syndrome in children and adolescents: A scientific statement from the American Heart Association Atherosclerosis, Hypertension, and Obesity in the Young Committee of the Council on Cardiovascular Disease in the Young; Council on Cardiovascular Nursing; and Council on Nutrition, Physical Activity, and Metabolism Circulation 119: 628-647.

6. Nguyen QM, Srinivasan SR, Xu JH, Chen W, Berenson GS (2008) Changes in risk variables of metabolic syndrome since childhood in pre-diabetic and type 2 diabetic subjects. Diabetes Care 31: 2044-2049.

7. Daniels SR, Greer F (2008) Committee on Nutrition Lipid screening and cardiovascular health in childhood. Pediatrics 122: 198-208.

8. Ayaz T, Baydur Azahin S, Sahin OZ (2014) Relation of acanthosis nigricans to metabolic syndrome in overweight and obese women. Metab Syndr Relat Disord 12: 320-323.

9. Garg MK, Dutta MK, Brar KS (2012) Inflammatory markers in metabolic syndrome. Int J Diabetes Dev Ctries 32: 131-137.

10. Secretaría de Salud (2007) Programa Nacional de Salud 2007-2012 Por un México sano: construyendo alianzas para una mejor salud. Pp. 28-29.

11. Morrison J, Glueck C, Horn P, Wang P (2010) Childhood predictors of adult type 2 diabetes at 9- and 26-year follow-ups. Arch Pediatr Adolesc Med 164: 53-60.

12. Morrison JA, Friedman LA, Gray-McGuire C (2007) Metabolic syndrome in childhood predicts adult cardiovascular disease 25 years later: The Princeton lipid research clinics follow-up study. Pediatrics 120: 340-345.

13. INSP (2013) Encuesta Nacional de Salud y Nutrición 2012. Resultados por entidad federativa, Sonora. Cuernavaca, México, Instituto Nacional de Salud Pública.

14. Steinberger J, Daniels SR (2003) Obesity, Insulin Resistance, Diabetes, and Cardiovascular Risk in Children: An American Heart Association Scientific Statement From the Atherosclerosis, Hypertension, and Obesity in the Young Committee (Council on Cardiovascular Disease in the Young) and the Diabetes

Committee (Council on Nutrition, Physical Activity, and Metabolism). Circulation 107:1448-1453.

15. Barlow SE, Dietz WH (1998) Obesity evaluation and treatment: Expert Committee Recommendations. Pediatrics 102: E29.

16. Villalvazo P, Corona JP, García S (2002) Urbano-rural, constante búsqueda de fronteras conceptuales. Notas, revista de información y análisis 20: 17-24.

17. WHO (2010) Anthro for personal computers version 3.2.2, 2011: Software for assessing growth and development of the world's children Geneva, World Health Organization.

18. Ramírez-Lopez E, Grijalva-Haro MI, Valencia ME, Ponce JA, Artalejo E (2005) Impacto de un programa de desayunos escolares en la prevalencia de obesidad y factores de riesgo cardiovascular en niños sonorenses. Salud Publica Mex 47: 126-133.

19. Freedman D, Wang J, Thornton J, Mei Z, Sopher A, et al. (2009) Classification of body fatness by body mass index-for-age categories among children. Arch Pediatr Adolesc Med 163: 805-811.

20. NHBPEP (2005) National High Blood Pressure Education Program Working Group on High Blood Pressure in Children and Adolescents. The fourth report on the diagnosis, evaluation, and treatment of high blood pressure in children and adolescents. Bethesda, MD, National Insitutes of Health.

21. Higgins SP, Freemark M, Prose NS (2008) Acanthosis nigricans: a practical approach to evaluation and management. Dermatol Online J 14 :2.

22. Allain CC, Poon LS, Chan CSG, Richmond W, Fu PC (1974) Enzymatic determination of total serum cholesterol. Clin Chem 20: 470-475.

23. Warnick GR, Benderson J, Albers JJ (1982) Dextran sulfate-Mg2+ precipitation procedure for quantitation of high-density-lipoprotein cholesterol. Clin Chem 28(6): 1379-1388.

24. Friedewald WT, Levy RI, Fredrickson DS (1972) Estimation of the concentration of low-density lipoprotein cholesterol in plasma, without use of the preparative ultracentrifuge. Clin Chem 18: 499-502.

25. Siedel J, Schmuck R, Staepels J (1993) Long-term stable liquid ready-to-use monoreagent for the enzimatic assay of serum or plasma trigliceries (GPO PAP method), AACC Meeting (Abstract 34). Clin Chem 39: 1127.

26. Trinder P (1969) Determination of blood glucose using an oxidase-peroxidase system with a non-carcinogenic chromogen. J Clin Pathol 22 :158-161.

27. Matthews DR, Hosker JP, Rudenski AS, Naylor BA, Treacher DF, et al. (1985) Homeostasis model assessment: insulin resistance and beta-cell function from fasting plasma glucose and insulin concentrations in man. Diabetologia 28: 412-419.

28. Garcia-Cuartero B, Garcia-Lacalle C, Jimenez-Lobo C, Gonzalez-Vergaz A, Calvo-Rey C, et al. (2007) Indice HOMA y QUICKI, insulina y péptido C en niños sanos. Puntos de corte de riesgo cardiovascular. An Pediatr (Barc.) 66: 481-490.

29. Williams CL, Hayman LL, Daniels SR, Robinson TN, Steinberger J, et al. (2002) Cardiovascular health in childhood: A statement for health professionals from the Committee on Atherosclerosis, Hypertension, and Obesity in the Young (AHOY) of the Council on Cardiovascular Disease in the Young. American Heart Association. Circulation 106: 143-160.

30. NCEP (1991) National Cholesterol Education Panel. The Expert Panel On Blood Cholesterol Levels In Children and Adolescents. Nutrition Today 26: 36-41.

31. ADA (2012) American Diabetes Association Standards of medical care in diabetes-2012. Diabetes Care 35: S11-S63.

32. INSP (2007) Encuesta Nacional de Salud y Nutrición 2006. Resultados por entidad federativa, Sonora. Cuernavaca, México, Instituto Nacional de Salud Pública-Secretaria de Salud.

33. Moran R (1999) Evaluation and treatment of childhood obesity. Am Fam Physician 59(4):861-868.

34. Whitaker R, Wright J, Pepe M, Seidel K, Dietz W (1997) Predicting obesity in young adulthood from childhood and parental obesity. N Engl J Med 337: 869-873.

35. Kuschnir MC, Mendoça GA (2007) Risk factors associated with arterial hypertension in adolescents. J Pediatr 83: 335-342.

36. Ballesteros MN, Cabrera RM, del Socorro Saucedo M, Fernandez ML (2004)

Dietary cholesterol does not increase biomarkers for chronic disease in a pediatric population from northern Mexico. Am J Clin Nutr 80: 855-861.

37. Enríquez-Leal MC, Montano-Figueroa CA, Saucedo-Tamayo MS, Vidal Ochoa M, Rivera-Icedo BM, et al. (2010) Incidencia, características clínicas y estado nutricional en niños y adolescentes mexicanos con diabetes. Interciencia 35: 455-460.

38. Ballesteros-Vásquez MN, Amaya M, Guerrero EV, García Vedugo K, Grijalva-Haro MI, et al. (2012) Patrón de predominancia de las subfracciones de la lipoproteína HDL y su asociación con riesgo cardiovascular en niños escolares. In Congreso de la Sociedad Latinoamericana de Nutrición SLAN, Ed. Habana, Cuba, Sociedad Latinoamericana de Nutrición, pp. 251.

39. van Vliet M, Heymans M, von Rosenstiel I, Brandjes D, Beijnen J, et al. (2011) Cardiometabolic risk variables in overweight and obese children: a worldwide comparison. Cardiovasc Diabetol 10: 106.

40. Hawkes C (2006) Uneven dietary development: linking the policies and processes of globalization with the nutrition transition, obesity and diet-related chronic diseases. Global Health 2: 4.

41. Hujava Z, Lesniakova M (2011) Anthropometric risk factors of aterosclerosis: Differences between urban and rural East-Slovakian children and adolescents. Bratisl Lek Listy 112: 491-496.

42. Hernandez-Valero MA, Bustamante-Montes LP, Hernández M, Halley-Castillo E, Wilkinson AV, et al. (2012) Higher risk for obesity among Mexican-American and Mexican immigrant children and adolescents than among peers in Mexico. J Immigr Minor Health 14: 517-522.

43. Wilcox G (2005) Insulin and Insulin Resistance. Clinical Biochemist Reviews 26: 19-39.

44. Barja S, Arteaga A, Acosta A (2003) Resistencia insulínica y otras expresiones del síndrome metabólico en niños obesos chilenos. Rev Med Chil 131: 259-268.

45. Chiarelli F, Marcovecchio ML (2008) Insulin resistance and obesity in childhood. Eur J Endocrinol 159: S67-S74.

46. Cruz ML, Weigensberg MJ, Huang TTK, Ball G, Shaibi GQ, et al. (2004) The metabolic syndrome in overweight hispanic youth and the role of insulin sensitivity J Clin Endocrinol Metab 89: 108-113.

47. Yanes-Quesada M, Perich-Amador P, González-Suárez R, Yanes-Quesada M, Cruz-Hernández J, et al. (2007) Factores clínicos relacionados con la hipertensión arterial en pacientes con trastornos de tolerancia a los carbohidratos. Rev Cubana Med Gen Integ 23.

48. Luma GB, Spiotta RT (2006) Hypertension in children and adolescents. Am Fam Physician 73: 1558-1568.

49. Elizondo-Montemayor L, Serrano-Gonzalez M, Ugalde-Casas PA, Cuello-Garcia C, Borbolla-Escoboza JR (2010) Metabolic syndrome risk factors among a sample of overweight and obese Mexican children. J Clin Hypertens 12: 380-387.

36

Serum Melatonin Level Disturbance is Related to Metabolic Syndrome and Subclinical Arterial Dysfunction in Shift Working Healthy Men

Radina Eshtiaghi[1]* and Ali Reza Khoshdel[2,3]

[1]Department of Internal Medicine, Faculty of Medicine, AJA University of Medical Sciences, Tehran, Iran
[2]Department of Epidemiology, Faculty of Medicine, AJA University of Medical Sciences, Tehran, Iran
[3]Department of Nephrology, John Hunter Hospital, The University of Newcastle, NSW, Australia

Abstract

Background: NW (night work) and SW (shift work) are associated with increased risk for metabolic conditions and cardiovascular disease. This study was planned to evaluate serum melatonin level related to metabolic syndrome and subclinical vascular consequences in shift working men.

Methods: Eighty-six shift working healthy men between 30-55 years old were studied .Anthropometric parameters and fasting blood glucose, lipids, Ox-LDL, Insulin and morning melatonin were measured. Pulse wave analysis was performed via SphygmoCor® to obtain surrogate markers for arterial stiffness.

Results: Of the 86 subjects, 19 (21.1%) had metabolic syndrome .Serum melatonin level was significantly lower in subjects with metabolic syndrome compared with normal group (p = 0.014). Insulin resistance was present in 27(30.7%) of cases .In addition, Serum melatonin was higher in group with Framingham's risk score ≤ 5% versus group with scores ≥5% (p=0.02). Melatonin had inverse correlation with radial and aortic systolic pressures P= 0.005, p=0.02, radial and aortic pulse pressures (P < 0.001, p=0.0001) and cardiac end systolic pressure,(p=0.03), respectively. Odds ratio of low melatonin level (<50%) for Pulse pressure amplification ≤ 75% quartile was 3.25, P=0.02.

Conclusions: Taken together, the inverse relationship of melatonin level and metabolic syndrome and Framingham risk score as well as peripheral and central blood pressure, cardiac end systolic pressure, and its direct relation to pulse pressure amplification highlighted its potential impact on pathogenesis of metabolic syndrome and arterial stiffness.

Keywords: Arterial dysfunction; Insulin resistance syndrome; Metabolic Syndrome

Introduction

Available evidence indicates that in most developed and developing countries 20 - 30% of the adult population can be characterized as having MetS [1]. The pathophysiological mechanisms involved in the development of obesity-induced MetS, from adipose tissue dysregulation to a chronic inflammatory state, are complex and not well understood. A USA national survey showed that patients with MetS were found to have a low serum antioxidant capacity compared with those without MetS [2]. It has been suggested that occupational stress, such as shift work, may be as a risk factor for cardiovascular disease [3,4]. Apart from performance decrements and elevated vulnerability to accidents, NW(night work) and SW(shift work) are associated with increased risk for various long-term health effects, ranging from sleep disorders to metabolic conditions and Cardiovascular Disease (CVD), among others [5,6].

Melatonin or N-acetyl-5-methoxytryptamine is the hormone secreted mainly by the pineal gland that is under the control of the Suprachiasmatic Nucleus (SCN) of the hypothalamus. Convincing evidence exists for the association of circadian system derangement (chronodisruption), sleep deprivation and melatonin suppression in MetS and obesity [7]. Melatonin exerts its physiological functions through its chronobiotic, antiexcitatory, antioxidant, anti-inflammatory, immunomodulatory and vasomotor activities [8]. Besides its direct free radical scavenger and indirect antioxidant activity [9], the contribution of MT receptors in the cardioprotective properties has also been emphasized [10,11]. It was reported that melatonin enhanced glucose transport via the IRS-1/ PI-3-kinase pathway, suggesting the potential existence of signaling pathway cross-talk between melatonin and insulin in glucose homeostasis [12,13] Furthermore, Contreras-Alcantara et al. [14] have demonstrated recently that removal of the

Type 1 Melatonin receptor (MT1) significantly impairs the ability of mice to metabolize glucose and suggesting that MT1 receptors are implicated in the pathogenesis of type2DM. The purpose of this study was to investigate association of melatonin level as a surrogate of chronic sleep disturbance and metabolic syndrome parameters and their subclinical vascular consequences in SW and NWers.

Methods and Materials

A consecutive group of eighty-six healthy men between 30-55 years old were studied by analytical cross-sectional design. This group had been recruited for their job as pilots after an intense medical assessment. This group of healthy men had many unpredictable nocturnal duties over more than 20 years, but was out of shift work for a week before sampling. They experienced many unpredictable nocturnal work shifts which could disturb their usual sleep patterns.The participants did not take any medications or consumed alcohol. Coronary Heart Disease (CHD) and other health problems were excluded by periodic medical investigation in the study group. Height and weight were measured with the subjects wearing light clothes, without shoes. The Body-Mass Index (BMI) was calculated as weight in kilograms divided by height in square-meters. Blood samples for biochemical determinations were taken from an ante-cubital vein after a 12 h overnight fasting, prior to exercise and routine work programs. Biochemical measurements included FBS, lipid

---

*Corresponding author: Ali Reza Khoshdel, Department of Epidemiology, Faculty of Medicine, AJA University of Medical Sciences, Etemadzadeh Avenue, Fatemi Street, Tehran, Iran, PO Box: 16315-781
E-mail: alikhoshdel@yahoo.com

profiles, Ox-LDL and uric acid. Total serum cholesterol was analyzed by an enzymatic method. HDL-cholesterol was measured after precipitation of VLDL and LDL with phosphotungstic acid and magnesium chloride. LDL-cholesterol was measured directly. Non-HDL-cholesterol levels were calculated as total cholesterol minus HDL-cholesterol levels. Serum triglycerides were measured by an enzymatic method (Roche Diagnostics GmbH).Ox-LDL and Fasting Insulin and melatonin levels were measured by Eliza assays (Mercodia UPPSALA Sweden and USCN-Missouri,USA).HOMA-IR calculated according to Matthewset's formula: HOMA-IR = fasting insulin (μU/L)* fasting glucose (mmol/ l)] /22.5. Insulin resistance was present if HOMA-IR $\geq$ 2.5 or fasting insulin level <75% of its quartile according to WHO definitions.Beta cell function was defined via HOMA-B = 20* Fasting Insulin (μU/L) /[FBS (mmol)-3.5] with normal cut off 81.8 [15]. Framingham cardiovascular risk score was calculated for all cases using traditional calculator. The metabolic syndrome was defined according to modified IDF (normal waist circumference assumed if it was less than 90 cm according to national study in Iran) and NCEP ATPIII definition [16,17]. Pulse wave analysis was evaluated using the radial artery pressure waveform recorded over 10 seconds using a validated tonometer (Millar SPC-301B, Huston, USA), and then processed with dedicated software (SphygmoCor®, version 7.1, AtCor Medical, Sydney, Australia). Time to peak of the first, second, and reflected wave, augmentation index (AI) and pulse reflection time, as well as ejection duration and Buckberg subendocardial viability index(SEVR%) and end systolic pressure were calculated, and central arterial pressure was estimated based on a transfer function. PP amplification was the ratio of peripheral to central PP. Adjusted AI for a heart rate equal to 75 beats per minute was estimated based on an internal nomogram in the software [18].

Statistical analysis

Quantitative variables are expressed as mean ± SD unless otherwise stated. Normality was checked by Kolmogrov-Smirnov test. Log-transformed values for non-normal variables were applied. Categorical variables were compared by χ^2-tests. Comparisons of quantitative variables between groups were performed by means of two-way ANOVA with and without covariates, as appropriate. Pearson's Correlation was applied for association investigation followed by regression analysis for adjustment of co- variables. All comparisons were two-tailed. A P-value <0.05 was considered statistically significant. All statistical calculations were made by means of the statistical software package SPSS for Windows (16.0).

Results

The mean age of subjects was 41.5 years old with range of 30-55 from whom 24(30.4%) were active smoker. The characteristics of the cohort according to the components of metabolic syndrome are shown in Table 1. Of the 86 subjects, 19 (21.1%) had metabolic syndrome according to IDF and 14(16.3%) based on ATP III definitions. Insulin resistance was present in 27(30.7%) of cases. The significant correlation was found between HOMA-IR and the number of metabolic syndrome components. (p = 0.007 between groups). Insulin resistance was significantly related to waist circumference, triglycerides and uric acid, (r =0.32, P=0.003), (r =0.22, p=0.04), (r =0.24, p=0.02), respectively.

We found significant correlation between Ox-LDL and serum triglycerides and non-HDL Cholesterol (r = 0.27, P = 0.01), (r = 0.63, p=0.0001), respectively. In addition, Framingham risk score (FRS) were related to triglycerides (r = 0.29, p=0.005), Ox-LDL, (r = 0.36, P= 0.001) and Non-HDL Cholesterol (r = 0.47, p =0.0001) but not LDL cholesterol. There was no difference in Ox-LDL or uric acid between metabolic syndrome and normal subjects. Table 2 presents the comparison of

Factors	Values (mean ± SD)
Number	86
Age (years)	41.5 ± 7.1
Occupation (years)	22.3 ± 7.5
Sport (hour/week)	4.4 ± 3.7
Stress (Score)	2.9 ± 0.9
Smoking, n (%)	24 (30.4)
BMI (kg/m2) ≥ 25(%)	27.1 ± 2.8 76.1
GFR (ml/min)	148.8±49.3
Total Chol(mg/dl))	189.0 ± 36.2
LDL –C(mg/dl)	129.6 ± 35.3
NonHDL-C(mg/dl)	141.7± 37.6
Chol/HDL	4.2 ± 1.2
Ox-LDL(u/l)	68.5 ± 15.0
Uric Acid	6.4 ± 1.4
Insulin (mU/l))	9.4 ± 5.9
Melatonin(pg/dl)	114.2 ±173.9
Cortisol (µg/dl)	9.2 ± 3.8
CRP-hs (mg/l)	1.7 ± 2.3
TNF-α (pg/ml)	6.3 ± 5.3
Endothelin-1 (pg/dl)	0.6 ± 0.2
Framingham's Score (%)	5.0 ± 3.3
Components of Metabolic Syndrome:	
Waist circumference(cm) ≥90 cm (%)	91.9 ± 6.2 50
SBP (mmHg) ≥130 mmHg (%)	117 ± 12 23.9
DBP (mmHg) ≥85 mmHg (%)	76 ± 8 47.7
TG (mg/dl) ≥150 mg/dl (%)	162.7 ± 93.1 44.3
HDL-C (mg/dl) <40mg/dl (%)	47.3 ± 9.3 27.3
FBS (mg/dl) ≥100 mg/dl (%)	91.2 ± 13.0 19.3

Table 1: Baseline characteristics of the cohort and frequencies of components of metabolic syndrome in a group of healthy men.

Factors	MetS - ve	MetS + ve	p-value
No(%)	66(75%)	19(22.1%)	-
Age (year)	40.6 ± 6.7	43.3 ± 7.8	ns
Waist circumference	90.4 ± 5.5	97.6 ± 4.9	0.000
BMI	26.4 ± 2.5	29.3 ± 2.3	0.001
physical activity	4.3 ± 2.9	4.6 ± 5.4	ns
GFR(ml/min)	84.2 ± 23.3	106.3 ± 35.9	0.019
Uric Acid	6.4 ± 1.3	6.5 ± 1.8	ns
LDL-C(mg/dl)	131.0 ± 34.7	124.7 ± 38.3	ns
Non-HDL(mg/dl)	137.2 ± 37.8	153.9 ± 36.4	ns
Chol/HDL	3.9 ± 1.1	4.9 ± 1.5	0.003
Ox-LDL(u/l)	67.5 ± 15.2	70.6 ± 14.9	ns
IRI(mU/l)	7.9 ± 4.4	13.6 ± 7.7	0.002
Cortisol (µg/dl)	9.2 ± 4.2	8.9 ± 2.6	ns
CRP-hs (mg/l)	1.7 ± 2.5	1.7 ± 1.7	ns
TNF-α (pg/ml)	6.5 ± 4.7	6.0 ± 6.9	ns
Endothelin-1 (pg/dl)	0.61 ± 0.2	0.63 ± 0.2	0.08
HOMA-IR	1.7 ± 1.1	3.4 ± 2.2	0.001
HOMA-B	142.6 ± 92.2	135.6 ± 94.7	ns
Melatonin (pg/dl)	131.6 ± 197.6	61.2 ± 58.9	0.014
Framingham's Risk Score (5%)	4.5 ± 2.7	6.6 ± 4.2	0.013

Table 2: Comparison of metabolic risk factors and melatonin level between cases with /without metabolic syndrome.

cardiovascular risk factors and melatonin level in cases with/without metabolic syndrome. Serum melatonin level was significantly lower in subjects with metabolic syndrome than normal cases (62.3 ± 61.3 pg/dl vs.131.6 ± 193.7 pg/dl, p = 0.014). Hypertension is a dominant factor in this difference (63.7 ± 66.5 pg/dl vs. 134.4 ± 198.3 pg/dl, p=0.01). A significant difference of insulin level and HOMA-IR index were found between quartiles of serum melatonin. (P=0.018 and P=0.027 between groups, respectively)

Figure 1 showed that serum melatonin was significantly different between categorized Framingham's risk scores <5% vs. ≥ 5% (194.6 ± 23.9 pg/dl vs. 70.8 ±15.1 pg/dl, p=0.02). We could not found any relation between melatonin and uric acid, Ox-LDL, CRP (hs), Endothelin-1, TNF (α) or cortisol levels.

Characteristics of pulse wave analysis parameters compared with cases with/out metabolic syndrome were defined in Table 3. As Figure 2 shows, Melatonin had inverse correlation with radial and aortic systolic pressures (r =-0.34, P= 0.005), (r = -0.30, p=0.02), radial and aortic pulse pressures (r =-0.47, P < 0.0001), (r =-0.45, p=0.0001) and end systolic pressure, (r =-0.25, p=0.03), respectively. In multivariate analysis, melatonin level remained as a significant determinant of aortic pulse pressure after adjustment for age, BMI, smoking, renal function (β=-0.25, P=0.04). We found that low melatonin level for pulse pressure amplification less than 75% quartiles had odds ratio equals to 3.7 (95% CI: 1.14 - 12.17, p= 0.024). Figure 3 could illustrate that melatonin level had inversely correlation with augmentation pressure and directly related to pulse pressure amplification.

Discussion

In humans, melatonin production significantly lowers in age-related diseases such as metabolic syndrome [19]. Chronic sleep deficit is now known to be an independent risk factor for obesity [20]. New emerging data show that melatonin may play an important role in body weight regulation and energy metabolism focusing on its effects in obesity, insulin resistance and leptin resistance [21]. There are solid grounds to postulate that melatonin may act peripherally by regulating insulin secretion and insulin action on sensitive tissues [22-24]. Moreover, the relationship between night-time melatonin level and insulin concentration is more pronounced in patients with

Factors	Total	MetS -ve	MetS +ve	p-value
Number	68	66	19	-
Redial parameters:				
Systolic pressure	119.0 ± 12.0	117.0 ± 11.8	127.4 ± 9.4	0.004
Diastolic pressure	77.2 ± 8.5	76.0 ± 8.8	82.2 ± 4.1	0.001
Pulse pressure	41.8 ± 7.9	41.1 ± 7.8	44.2 ± 8.1	ns
Mean pressure	91.3 ± 9.2	89.7 ± 9.4	97.5 ± 4.7	0.006
Aortic Parameters:				
Systolic pressure	105.6 ± 10.7	103.8 ± 10.7	113.1 ± 7.1	0.005
Diastolic pressure	78.2 ± 8.6	71.0 ± 8.9	83.5 ± 4.5	0.014
Pulse pressure	27.4 ± 5.8	26.8 ± 5.1	29.1 ± 6.2	ns
Central Hemodynamic Parameters:				
Heart Rate	87.0 ± 9.9	77.2 ± 9.3	81.8± 11.7	ns
Ejection Duration%	37.3 ± 3.0	36.9 ± 2.8	38.8 ± 3.5	0.04
Aortic T1	112.9 ± 2.3	112.4 ± 9.4	114.7 ± 9.2	ns
Aortic T2	201.1 ± 18.4	201.1 ± 19.2	201.2 ± 16.1	ns
Aortic Tr	150.4 ± 10.4	149.9 ± 9.9	151.7 ± 11.6	ns
Aortic Augmentation (AP)	3.2 ± 2.8	3.1 ± 2.6	3.4 ± 3.7	ns
Aortic AIx(AP/PP)%	10.7 ± 9.4	10.8 ± 8.5	10.5 ± 12.3	ns
Aortic AIx(P2/P1)%	111.7 ± 18.8	113.2 ± 11.6	107.2 ± 32.1	ns
AIx(AP/PP)@HR75%	12.2 ± 7.9	12.1 ± 17.4	12.7 ± 9.4	ns
Buckberg SEVR%	148.7 ± 18.0	150.9 ± 17.9	139.8 ± 17.2	0.045
End Systolic Pressure	98.6 ± 9.9	97.2 ± 10.0	105.1 ± 6.5	0.008
PP amplification%	153.6 ± 15.7	153.7 ± 14.8	153.4 ± 18.6	ns

Table 3: Characteristic of pulse wave analysis parameters and comparison between cases +/- metabolic syndrome.

metabolic syndrome [25]. In our study, Morning melatonin was considerably lower in cases with metabolic syndrome compared with normal subjects. These findings can emphasize the association between chronic sleep deficit in NW and SWers and metabolic syndrome. We found a significant difference of insulin level / HOMA-IR index between quartiles of serum melatonin. Theses evidences implied that melatonin and insulin concentration must have some interaction with each other.

Melatonin administered for 2 months significantly improved antioxidative defense and lipid profile (decrease in LDL-C), and lowered blood pressure [26]. Pechanova et al. demonstrated that melatonin reduces blood pressure significantly and that this treatment enhanced nitric oxide synthase activity reduced oxidative stress and decreased NF-kb [27]. Several reports have indicated a direct effect of melatonin on blood pressure through its anti-adrenergic effects and nitric oxide availability [28]. A meta-analysis of randomized controlled trials by Grossman et al. [29] indicated that melatonin administration was effective to reduce nocturnal systolic and diastolic blood pressure in patients with nocturnal hypertension. Melatonin was reported to reduce Systolic Blood Pressure (SBP) along with aortic pulse wave velocity, which is regarded as an important indicator of total cardiovascular risk estimation [30]. We found that low serum melatonin was associated with higher Framingham's cardiovascular risk scores. This evidence introduces that inadequate melatonin level could be as risk factor of atherosclerosis in human being. Oxidized-LDL is a critical factor in progression of atherosclerosis and it contributes to endothelial dysfunction and plaque destabilization through multiple mechanisms [31]. Because of lipophilic nature, melatonin readily enters the lipid phase of the low-density lipoprotein particles and prevents lipid peroxidation [32]. Dominguez-Rodriguez et al. [33] showed an association between nocturnal elevated Ox-LDL and reduced

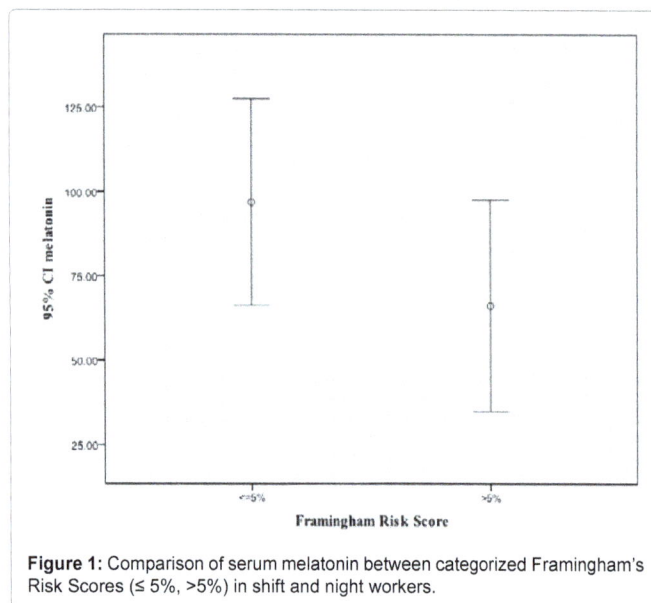

Figure 1: Comparison of serum melatonin between categorized Framingham's Risk Scores (≤ 5%, >5%) in shift and night workers.

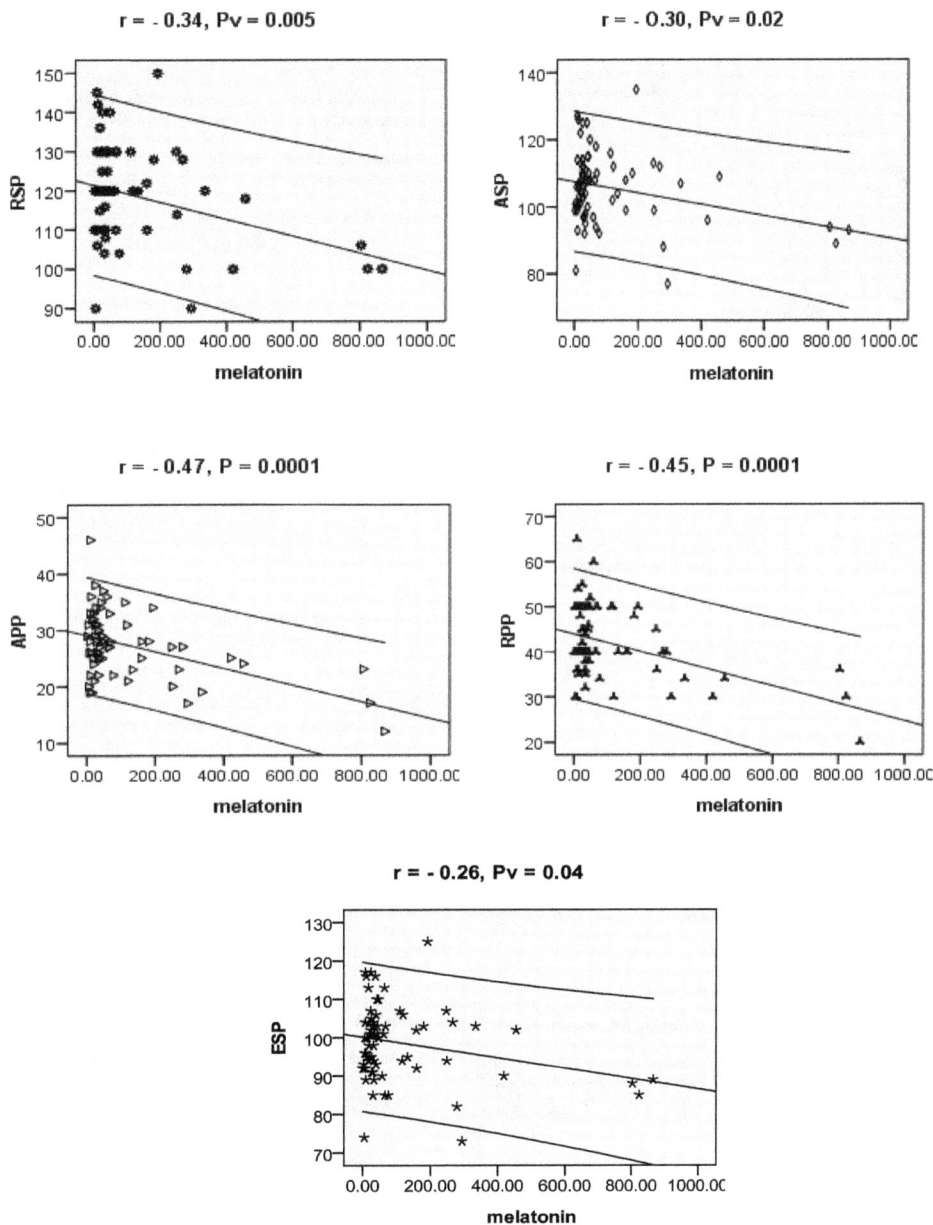

Figure 2: The Correlation between serum melatonin and pulse wave analysis parameters: radial systolic pressure (RSP), aortic systolic pressure (ASP), end systolic pressure (ESP), radial pulse pressure (RPP), aortic pulse pressure (APP) in shift and night workers.

melatonin levels in patients with acute myocardial infarction. But, we did not found any correlation between morning melatonin and Ox-LDL or pro-inflammatory factors in our cohort.

In addition to not well-characterized central regulatory mechanisms, MEL can modulate directly vascular tone [28]. However, the data testing the influence of MEL on vascular reactivity appear diverse, vessel-specific, and sometimes conflicting. Melatonin administration, as compared with placebo, decreases carotid-femoral PWV and systolic blood pressure in healthy young men [34]. Our results from pulse wave analysis, especially confirmed the inverse relationship between morning melatonin level and systolic peripheral and aortic pressures as well as pulse pressure and heart End systolic pressure which can partially explain vascular damages in chronic sleep disturbance. Amplification of the central-to-brachial PP is inversely related to large artery stiffness,

as assessed by carotid-femoral Pulse Wave Velocity (PWV) or total arterial compliance, peripheral arterial resistance, and characteristics of the reflected waves, such as the AI, the Time to reflection (Tr), and the reflection coefficient [35]. Serum melatonin had direct correlation with pulse pressure amplification and inversely with augmentation pressure which confirmed above evidences in our study.

This study had some limitations such as few numbers of cases with metabolic syndrome in homogenous population with limited age range and no comparable group. We measured melatonin level in morning in men worked in unpredictable nocturnal work shifts. Also, the study was constrained by cost-effectiveness to repeat measurement of melatonin in night or during subjects' vacation times. This report can be a preliminary study and should be followed by further researches in areas of interaction between low melatonin level and metabolic syndrome

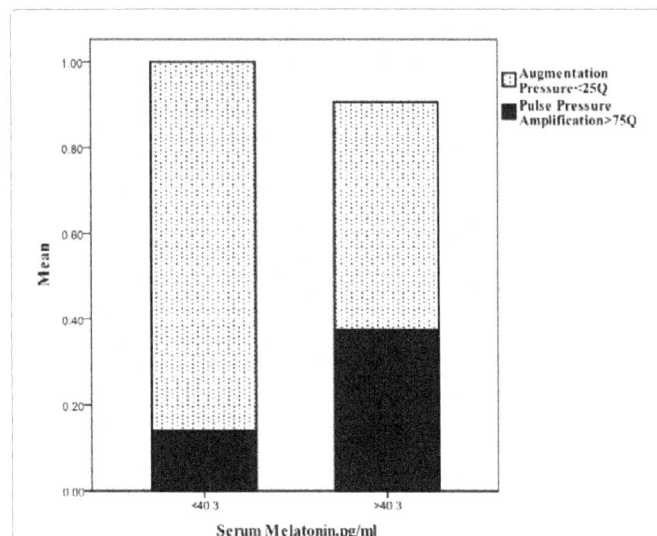

Figure 3: Comparison of Trends of means of pulse pressure amplification and augmentation pressure with changes in melatonin levels (lower /higher than 50% of quartiles).

and their potential impacts on emergence of subclinical atherosclerosis in larger cohorts.

Conclusion

The inverse relationship of melatonin level with metabolic syndrome, cardiovascular risk score as well as peripheral and central blood pressure, pulse pressure, End systolic pressure, and its direct relation to pulse pressure amplification highlighted its potential impact on pathogenesis of metabolic syndrome and arterial stiffness and possible effectiveness of melatonin therapy on prevention of cardiovascular disease in shift and night workers.

References

1. Grundy SM (2008) Metabolic syndrome pandemic. Arterioscler Thromb Vasc Biol 28: 629-636.

2. Beydoun MA, Shroff MR, Chen X, Beydoun HA, Wang Y, et al. (2011) Serum antioxidant status is associated with metabolic syndrome among U.S. adults in recent national surveys. J Nutr 141: 903-913.

3. Rajaratnam SM, Arendt J (2001) Health in a 24-h society. Lancet 358: 999-1005.

4. Erren TC, Reiter RJ (2009) Defining chronodisruption. J Pineal Res 46: 245-247.

5. Karlsson B, Knutsson A, Lindahl B (2001) Is there an association between shift work and having a metabolic syndrome? Results from a population based study of 27,485 people. Occup Environ Med 58: 747-752.

6. Knutsson A, Hammar N, Karlsson B (2004) Shift workers' mortality scrutinized. Chronobiol Int 21: 1049-1053.

7. Reiter RJ, Tan DX, Korkmaz A, Ma S (2012) Obesity and metabolic syndrome: association with chronodisruption, sleep deprivation, and melatonin suppression. Ann Med 44: 564-577.

8. Pandi-Perumal SR, Srinivasan V, Maestroni GJ, Cardinali DP, Poeggeler B, et al. (2006) Melatonin: Nature's most versatile biological signal? FEBS J 273: 2813-2838.

9. Tengattini S, Reiter RJ, Tan DX, Terron MP, Rodella LF, et al. (2008) Cardiovascular diseases: protective effects of melatonin. J Pineal Res 44: 16-25.

10. Grossini E, Molinari C, Uberti F, Mary DA, Vacca G, et al. (2011) Intracoronary melatonin increases coronary blood flow and cardiac function through β²-adrenoreceptors, MT1/MT2 receptors, and nitric oxide in anesthetized pigs. J Pineal Res 51: 246-257.

11. Lamont KT, Somers S, Lacerda L, Opie LH, Lecour S (2011) Is red wine a SAFE sip away from cardioprotection? Mechanisms involved in resveratrol- and melatonin-induced cardioprotection. J Pineal Res 50: 374-380.

12. Ha E, Yim SV, Chung JH, Yoon KS, Kang I, et al. (2006) Melatonin stimulates glucose transport via insulin receptor substrate-1/phosphatidylinositol 3-kinase pathway in C2C12 murine skeletal muscle cells. J Pineal Res 41: 67-72.

13. Nishida S (2005) Metabolic effects of melatonin on oxidative stress and diabetes mellitus. Endocrine 27: 131-136.

14. Contreras-Alcantara S, Baba K, Tosini G (2010) Removal of melatonin receptor type 1 induces insulin resistance in the mouse. Obesity (Silver Spring) 18: 1861-1863.

15. Matthews DR, Hosker JP, Rudenski AS, Naylor BA, Treacher DF, et al. (1985) Homeostasis model assessment: insulin resistance and beta- cell function from fasting plasma glucose and insulin concentrations in man. Diabetologia 28: 412-419.

16. Song Y, Manson JE, Tinker L, Howard BV, Kuller LH, et al. (2007) Insulin sensitivity and insulin secretion determined by homeostasis model assessment and risk of diabetes in a multiethnic cohort of women: the Women's Health Initiative Observational Study. Diabetes Care 30: 1747-1752.

17. Esteghamati A, Ashraf H, Rashidi A, Meysamie A (2009) Waist circumference cut-off points for the diagnosis of metabolic syndrome in Iranian adults. Dia Res Clin Pract 84: 279-287.

18. Khoshdel AR, Carney SL, Trevillian P, Gillies A (2010) Evaluation of arterial stiffness and pulse wave reflection for cardiovascular risk assessment in diabetic and nondiabetic kidney transplant recipients. Iran J Kidney Dis 4: 237-243.

19. Altun A, Yaprak M, Aktoz M, Vardar A, Betul UA, et al. (2002) Impaired nocturnal synthesis of melatonin in patients with cardiac syndrome X. Neurosci Lett 327: 143-145.

20. Taheri S, Lin L, Austin D, Young T, Mignot E (2004) Short sleep duration is associated with reduced leptin, elevated ghrelin, and increased body mass index. PLoS Med 1: e62.

21. Nduhirabandi F, du Toit EF, Lochner A (2012) Melatonin and the metabolic syndrome: a tool for effective therapy in obesity-associated abnormalities? Acta Physiol (Oxf) 205: 209-223.

22. Peschke E, Fauteck JD, Musshoff U, Schmidt F, Beckmann A, et al. (2000) Evidence for a melatonin receptor within pancreatic islets of neonate rats: functional, autoradiographic, and molecular investigations. J Pineal Res 28: 156-164.

23. Poon AM, Choy EH, Pang SF (2001) Modulation of blood glucose by melatonin: a direct action on melatonin receptors in mouse hepatocytes. Biol Signals Recept 10: 367-379.

24. Kosa E, Maurel D, Siaud P (2001) Effects of pinealectomy on glucagon responsiveness to hypoglycaemia induced by insulin injections in fed rats. Exp Physiol 86: 617-620.

25. Robeva R, Kirilov G, Tomova A, Kumanov P (2008) Melatonin-insulin interactions in patients with metabolic syndrome. J Pineal Res 44: 52-56.

26. Koziróg M, Poliwczak AR, Duchnowicz P, Koter-Michalak M, Sikora J, et al. (2011) Melatonin treatment improves blood pressure, lipid profile, and parameters of oxidative stress in patients with metabolic syndrome. J Pineal Res. 50: 261-266.

27. Pechánová O, Zicha J, Paulis L, Zenebe W, Dobesová Z, et al. (2007) The effect of N-acetylcysteine and melatonin in adult spontaneously hypertensive rats with established hypertension. Eur J Pharmacol 561: 129-136.

28. Paulis L, Simko F (2007) Blood pressure modulation and cardiovascular protection by melatonin: potential mechanisms behind. Physiol Res 56: 671-684.

29. Grossman E, Laudon M, Zisapel N (2011) Effect of melatonin on nocturnal blood pressure: meta-analysis of randomized controlled trials. Vasc Health Risk Manag 7: 577-584.

30. Yildiz M, Akdemir O (2009) Assessment of the effects of physiological release of melatonin on arterial distensibility and blood pressure. Cardiol Young 19: 198-203.

31. Landmesser U, Harrison DG (2001) Oxidant stress as a marker for cardiovascular events: Ox marks the spot. Circulation 104: 2638-2640.

32. Wakatsuki A, Okatani Y, Ikenoue N, Shinohara K, Watanabe K, et al. (2001) Melatonin protects against oxidized low-density lipoprotein-induced inhibition of nitric oxide production in human umbilical artery. J Pineal Res 31: 281-288.

33. Dominguez-Rodriguez A, Abreu-Gonzalez P, Garcia-Gonzalez M, Ferrer-Hita J, Vargas M, et al. (2005) Elevated levels of oxidized low-density lipoprotein and impaired nocturnal synthesis of melatonin in patients with myocardial infarction. Atherosclerosis 180: 101-105.

34. Yildiz M, Sahin B, Sahin A (2006) Acute effects of oral melatonin administration on arterial distensibility, as determined by carotid-femoral pulse wave velocity, in healthy young men. Exp Clin Cardiol 11: 311-313.

35. Avolio AP, Van Bortel LM, Boutouyrie P, Cockcroft JR, McEniery CM, et al. (2009) Role of pulse pressure amplification in arterial hypertension: experts' opinion and review of the data. Hypertension 54: 375-383.

37

The Brain Adenylyl Cyclase Signaling System and Cognitive Functions in Rats with Neonatal Diabetes under the Influence of Intranasal Serotonin

Alexander O Shpakov[1]*, Kira V Derkach[1], Oksana V Chistyakova[1], Ivan B Sukhov[1], Valery N Shipilov[1] and Vera M Bondareva[1]

Sechenov Institute of Evolutionary Physiology and Biochemistry, Russian Academy of Sciences, Thorez av. 44, 194223 St. Petersburg, Russia

Abstract

Type 2 diabetes mellitus is often associated with the neurodegenerative changes, and this is regarded as being the cause of cognitive deficit and other brain dysfunctions. The data obtained by us and the other authors showed that alterations in the brain signaling systems regulated by different hormones and neurotransmitters contribute to triggering and development of neurodegenerative processes in diabetes. However, the activity of brain adenylyl cyclase system and the cognitive functions, their interrelation, and the influence of intranasal serotonin on them in type 2 diabetes are poorly understood yet. We investigated the hormonal sensitivity of adenylyl cyclase system in the brain of female rats with the neonatal model of type 2 diabetes and the influence of 8-weeks treatment with intranasal serotonin (20 µg/rat daily) on the brain adenylyl cyclase system and cognition in diabetes. It was shown that in the diabetic brain the regulatory effects of hormones (relaxin, adrenergic agonists, dopamine, serotonin) activating adenylyl cyclase via Gs proteins changed in a receptor-specific manner and were restored by intranasal serotonin. The effects of hormones inhibiting adenylyl cyclase via Gi proteins were significantly decreased, especially in the case of agonists of type 1 serotonin receptors. The intranasal serotonin treatment led to their partial or complete restoration. Using Morris water maze test we showed that intranasal serotonin improves diabetes-associated impaired learning and spatial memory. Summing up, in the brain of diabetic rats the functional activity of hormone-sensitive adenylyl cyclase signaling system was altered, most dramatically in the G_i-coupled cascades. The intranasal serotonin treatment improved both the signal transduction via the brain adenylyl cyclase system and cognitive functions in type 2 diabetes.

Keywords: Adenylyl cyclase; Brain; Cognition; Diabetes mellitus; Dopamine; 5-hydroxytryptamine receptor; Intranasal serotonin; Morris water maze test; Somatostatin; Spatial memory

Abbreviations: AC: Adenylyl Cyclase; AR: Adrenergic Receptor; DAR: Dopamine Receptor; DM: Diabetes Mellitus; EMD-386088: 5-chloro-2-methyl-3-(1,2,3,6-tetrahydro-4-pyridinyl)-1H-indole; G_s and G_i proteins: Heterotrimeric G proteins of the stimulating and inhibitory types, respectively; GppNHp, β,γ-imidoguanosine-5'-triphosphate; 5-HT, 5-hydroxytryptamine (serotonin); 5-HTR, 5-Hydroxytryptamine Receptor; IS: Intranasal Serotonin; 5-MeO-DMT: 5-Methoxy-N,N-Dimethyltryptamine; MWM test: Morris Water Maze Test; PACAP-38: Pituitary Adenylyl Cyclase-Activating Polypeptide-38; STZ: Streptozotocin; T1DM and T2DM: Types 1 and 2 Diabetes Mellitus.

Introduction

Diabetes mellitus (DM) is one of the most severe metabolic disorders in humans characterized by hyperglycemia due to a relative or an absolute lack of insulin or its action on the target tissue or both. Many neurodegenerative disorders, such as diabetic encephalopathy and Alzheimer's disease, are associated with the types 1 and 2 diabetes mellitus (T1DM and T2DM) [1]. Manifestation of these disorders in diabetic patients includes alterations in neurotransmission, electrophysiological abnormalities, structural changes and cognitive deficit [2]. In the case of T2DM it is generally accepted that the main factors responsible for the neurodegenerative changes are the resistance of the peripheral tissues to insulin action, which leads to moderate hyperglycemia, and the recurrent hypoglycemia induced by inadequate insulin therapy and glycemic control [3]. Recently, many evidences have been obtained to the effect that the alterations and abnormalities of hormonal signaling systems regulated by insulin, insulin-like growth factor-1, leptin, biogenic amines, and peptide hormones controlling fundamental processes in the neuronal and glial cells contribute to

triggering and development of neurodegenerative changes in the diabetic brain [4,5]. In our view, the changes in the brain signaling systems, on the one hand, may be due to formation of a compensatory response to physiological and biochemical dysfunctions occurring in DM, and, on the other hand, may themselves be the cause of these dysfunctions.

Earlier we and the other authors showed that in human DM and animal models of this disease the functioning of hormone-sensitive adenylyl cyclase (AC) signaling system undergoes changes in tissue- and hormone-specific manner [6-11]. In both types of DM the most pronounced alterations were found in the regulation of AC activity by hormones inhibiting the enzyme via heterotrimeric G proteins of the inhibitory type (G_i) [6,7,10,11]. At the same time, the functional state of AC signaling system in the brain of rats with experimental models of T2DM and the regulation of AC activity by hormones interacting with G proteins of the stimulatory type (G_s) or G_i proteins, or activating simultaneously both G protein types, have not been investigated. The study of AC signaling in the diabetic brain may throw light on the molecular mechanisms of neurodegeneration in human T2DM; it may also be helpful in finding new approaches for the treatment of T2DM-induced cognitive deficit and neurological disorders.

Now insulin is commonly accepted as drug to be used in treatment of T1DM as well as T2DM, especially when β cell function falls [12]. Usually, insulin is injected subcutaneously, but recently the other ways of delivery of hormone and its analogues, such as oral and intranasal,

Corresponding author: Alexander O. Shpakov, Sechenov Institute of Evolutionary Physiology and Biochemistry, Russian Academy of Sciences, Thorez av. 44, 194223 St. Petersburg, Russia, E-mail: alex_shpakov@list.ru

have been used. Intranasal insulin allows successful glycemic control, improves learning and memory and prevents cognitive decline in diabetic patients [13]. This is confirmed by our findings that the therapy of rats with T2DM by intranasal insulin normalizes the functioning of insulin signaling system, restores cAMP-dependent signaling cascades and improves their cognitive functions [11,14]. However, in the recent years, along with insulin in the treatment of T2DM and pre-diabetic state and, first of all, to correct DM-associated neurodegenerative diseases, have been widely used bromocriptine, a selective agonist of type 2 dopamine receptor (DA$_2$R) [15], and the selective serotonin (5-HT) reuptake inhibitors [16]. It was found that both bromocriptine and 5-HT reuptake inhibitors increase the brain serotonin level markedly decreased in DM [15,17]. The data is available suggesting that abnormalities in the serotonergic system in the diabetic brain provoke disturbances in neuronal processing, induce alteration of the plasticity of neurotransmission and, thus, play an important role in DM-induced behavioral abnormalities, therefore there are all reasons to expect that the increased level of brain serotonin will lead to restoration of the serotonin signaling in the brain and improve the impaired cognitive functions [17]. With this in mind, we made an attempt to examine the influence of intranasal route of serotonin delivery on the functioning of the brain in rats with T2DM.

The aim of this work was to study the functional state and hormonal sensitivity of AC signaling system in the brain of female rats with the neonatal model of T2DM and to investigate the influence of 8-weeks intranasal serotonin (IS) on this system and cognitive functions in diabetic animals. To determine the specificity of alterations in brain AC system, we studied AC and β,γ-imidoguanosine-5'-triphosphate (GppNHp) binding effects of hormones and their analogues activating receptors of the serpentine type coupled with G$_s$ or G$_i$ proteins. To do this, were chosen the hormones activating G$_s$-coupled receptors, such as isoproterenol, agonist of β-adrenergic receptors (β-AR), 5-HT$_6$R-agonist 5-chloro-2-methyl-3-(1,2,3,6-tetrahydro-4-pyridinyl)-1H-indole (EMD-386088), pituitary AC-activating polypeptide-38 (PACAP-38) and relaxin-2, and the hormones activating G$_i$-coupled receptors, such as DA$_2$R-agonist bromocriptine, 5-HT$_{1B/1D}$R-agonist 5-nonyloxytryptamine, 5-HT$_{1/2}$R-agonist 5-methoxy-N,N-

dimethyltryptamine (5-MeO-DMT) and somatostatin-14, as well as the hormones activating both G$_s$- and G$_i$-coupled receptors, i.e. serotonin, norepinephrine and dopamine (Figure 1). Being involved in the regulation of synaptic plasticity and metabolic and growth processes in neuronal and glial cells, these hormones are very important for the functioning of the central nervous system (CNS). They are also responsible for cellular processes in the peripheral organs and tissues involved in the insulin synthesis and secretion, and thus controlling the glucose homeostasis in the brain and in the whole organism. To detect cognitive deficit in DM and the influence of IS on formation of the long-term spatial memory and learning, a spatial version of the Morris water maze (MWM) test was used.

Materials and Methods

Animals

The female Wistar rats were housed in plastic sawdust-covered cages with a normal light–dark cycle and free access to food and water. The experiments were carried out under the Institutional Guidelines (the Bioethics Committee, December 23, 2010) and "Guidelines for the treatment of animals in behavior research and teaching" [18]. All efforts were made to minimize animal suffering and reduce the number of animals used.

Four groups of animals were investigated: control animals (n = 9, Group C), IS-treated control animals (n = 8, Group C-S), animals with the neonatal model of T2DM (n = 7, Group D), and IS-treated diabetic animals (n = 7, Group D-S).

Neonatal model of T2DM

Neonatal DM was provoked by intraperitoneal administration of streptozotocin (STZ) dissolved in citrate-acidified solution containing 0.9% NaCl, pH 4.5, at the dose of 80 mg/kg of body weight in newborn (5 days) rats using 26 gauge (5/8 in. long) needle [19,20]. The injection site was the dorsal midpoint between pelvis and ribs close to the right side of the spine. Control animals received citrate-acidified physiological solution injected in a similar manner. Typically treatment with STZ induces destruction of β-cells and the insulin production is almost

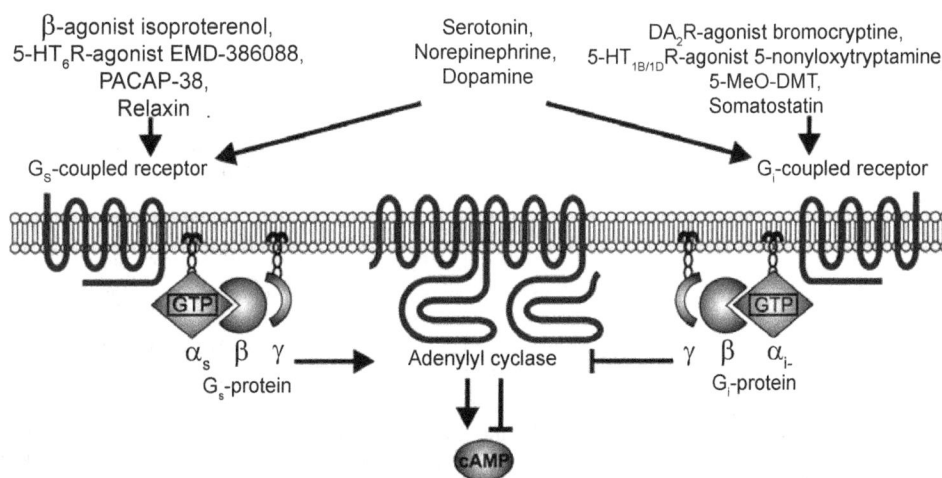

Figure 1: Transduction of hormonal signals generated by biogenic amines, polypeptide hormones and their synthetic analogues via AC signaling system. Isoproterenol, EMD-386088, PACAP-38 and relaxin interact with Gs protein-coupled receptors, stimulate AC activity, increase the intracellular level of second messenger cAMP and trigger cAMP-dependent signaling cascades involved in the regulation of growth, differentiation and metabolism of the neuronal and glial cells. Bromocriptine, 5-nonyloxytryptamine, 5-MeO-DMT and somatostatin interact with Gi protein-coupled receptors, inhibit AC activity and block cAMP-dependent pathways. Serotonin, norepinephrine and dopamine are capable of interacting with both Gs protein- and Gi protein-coupled receptors.

completely blocked. However, at the early stages of development of rats (the first week after birth), a partial restoration of insulin-producing function of β-cells can occur due to their regeneration [21,22]. As a rule, 50–70 % of STZ treatment infant rats show signs of T2DM on reaching the age of 2.5–3 months [23]. In our experiments 70 % of 3 month-old STZ-treated rats had glucose tolerance, as was assessed in the glucose tolerance test (GTT), and these animals were used for experiments (Groups D and D-S). Alongside, we observed moderate hyperglycemia (the fasting glucose concentration was no higher than 7 mM), moderate hypoinsulinemia and the increased plasma levels of triglycerides and HDL-cholesterol. This is in good agreement with the corresponding parameters of the rats with neonatal model of T2DM obtained by the other authors [19,20,23]. In our case impaired glucose tolerance can be associated with moderate hypoinsulinemia, which was due to damage of β-cells in the neonatal period of development and with insulin resistance, which was due to decrease of insulin signaling in the tissues of rats with STZ-induced neonatal DM [14,24]. Earlier, we showed that the insulin binding capacity of insulin receptors in the liver membranes of rats with neonatal model of T2DM was lower compared with healthy animals due to a smaller number of insulin receptors with high and low affinity [14].

Plasma glucose, insulin, triglycerides and HDL-cholesterol measurements

The glucose in the whole blood from the tail vein was measured using test strips One Touch Ultra (USA) and a glucometer (Life Scan Johnson & Johnson, Denmark). The insulin concentration in rat serum was determined using Rat Insulin ELISA (Mercodia AB, Sweden). Triglycerides was determined by Trinder-based GPO-PAP colorimetric end-point method and high density lipoproteins(HDL)-cholesterol by direct clearance method using kits of Randox Laboratories Ltd. (UK) and Sapphire 400 automated clinical chemistry analyzer (Niigata Mechatronics Co., Ltd., Japan). The whole blood was obtained from the tail vein under local (sc) anesthesia with 2 % Lidocaine per 2-4 mg/kg of body weight.

Intranasal delivery of serotonin

Intranasal delivery of serotonin to 6-months old healthy rats (Group C-S) and to diabetic rats of the same age with 3-months neonatal DM (Group D-S) was carried out according to Thorne and coworkers [25]. Serotonin at final concentration of 1 mg/ml was dissolved in saline, pH 4.5. Each rat was placed in a supine position and then an average of 20 μl of serotonin solution containing 20 μg of hormone was administrated by Eppendorf pipette as 5 μl drops in each nostril, in turn, every 1–2 min. Control animals were given the equal volume of saline, pH 4.5. All in all, the IS treatment covered 8 weeks (one week prior to physiological experiments and 7 weeks in the course of experiments).

Chemicals and radiochemicals

The chemicals used in the study were purchased from Sigma-Aldrich (St. Louis, MO, USA) and Calbiochem (San Diego, CA, USA). STZ, GppNHp, somatostatin-14, PACAP-38, serotonin, norepinephrine, dopamine, isoproterenol, bromocryptine, and 5-MeO-DMT were purchased from Sigma-Aldrich (St. Louis, MO, USA). 5-Nonyloxytryptamine and EMD-386088 were purchased from Tocris Cookson Ltd. (United Kingdom). Human relaxin-2 was kindly provided by Prof. J. Wade (Howard Florey Institute, University of Melbourne, Australia). [α-32P]-ATP (4 Ci/mmol) was purchased from Isotope Company (St. Petersburg, Russia), β,γ-imido[8-^{3}H]-guanosine-5'-triphosphate ([8-^{3}H]-GppNHp) (5 Ci/mmol) was from Amersham

(UK); the type HA 0.45 μm nitrocellulose filters were from Sigma-Aldrich Chemie GmbH (Germany).

Synaptosomal membrane preparation

The 8-months old diabetic and non-diabetic animals were decapitated under anesthetics (a mixture of Ketamine and Xylazine at the doses of 90 and 10 mg/kg of body weight, respectively) 24 hours after the last intranasal administration of serotonin or saline, and the brain was rapidly removed and frozen to prepare synaptosomal membrane fractions. The preparation of the rat brain membranes was obtained as described earlier [26]. The brain tissues were dissected on ice and homogenized with a Polytron in 30 volumes of ice-cold 50 mM Tris-HCl buffer (pH 7.4) containing 10 mM $MgCl_2$, 2 mM EGTA, 10% (w/v) sucrose and a cocktail of protease inhibitors (Buffer A). The obtained material underwent centrifugation at 4°C. The crude homogenate was centrifuged at 1000 × g for 10 min; the resulting pellet was discarded and the supernatant was centrifuged at 9000 × g for 20 min. The pellet was resuspended in Buffer A (without sucrose) and centrifuged at 35000 × g for 10 min. The final pellet was resuspended in 50 mM Tris-HCl buffer (pH 7.4) to produce the membrane fraction with a protein concentration range 1–3 mg/ml and stored at -70°C. The protein concentration of each membrane preparation in all experiments was measured by the method of Lowry and colleagues, using BSA as a standard.

Adenylyl cyclase assay

The AC (EC 4.6.1.1) activity was measured as described earlier [26]. The reaction mixture (final volume 50 μl) contained 50 mM Tris-HCl (pH 7.5), 5 mM $MgCl_2$, 1 mM ATP, 1 μCi [α-^{32}P]-ATP, 0.1 mM cAMP, 20 mM creatine phosphate, 0.2 mg/ml creatine phosphokinase, and 15–45 μg of the membrane protein. Incubation was carried out at 37°C for 10 min. The reaction was initiated by the addition of membrane protein and terminated by the addition of 100 μl of 0.5 M HCl, followed by immersing the tubes with mixture in a boiling water bath for 6 min. 100 μl of 1.5 M imidazole was added to each tube. In these conditions the AC activity was linear. [^{32}P]-cAMP formed as a result of the enzyme reaction was separated using column chromatography. The samples were placed on neutral alumina columns and cAMP was eluted with 8 ml of 10 mM imidazole-HCl buffer (pH 7.4). The eluates were collected in scintillation vials and counted using a LS 6500 scintillation counter (Beckman Instruments Inc., USA). Each assay was carried out in triplicate at least three times, and the results were expressed as pmol cAMP/min per mg of membrane protein. The basal activity was measured in the absence of hormones, GppNHp and forskolin. To measure the AC inhibitory effect of hormone, the enzyme was pre-activated by diterpene forskolin (10^{-5} M).

GppNHp binding assay

[8-^{3}H]-GppNHp binding to heterotrimeric G proteins was determined as described earlier [27]. The reaction mixture (final volume 50 μl) contained 25 mM HEPES-Na buffer (pH 7.4), 1 mM EDTA, 5 mM $MgCl_2$, 100 mM NaCl, 1 mM dithiothreitol, 1 μM GppNHp, 0.1% BSA, 0.5–1 μCi [8-^{3}H]-GppNHp. The reaction was started by the addition of 50–100μg of membrane protein and carried out at 30°C for 45 min. The reaction mixture was incubated and rapidly diluted with 100 μl of the washing buffer (20 mM K$^+$-Na$^+$ phosphate buffer, pH 8.0) containing 0.1% Lubrol-PX and the samples were filtered under vacuum through 0.45 μm nitrocellulose filters (type HA). In each case the filter was washed three times with 2 ml of washing buffer and dried. The filter-bound radioactivity was estimated in a toluene scintillator using a LKB 1209/1215 RackBeta scintillation counter. Unlabeled 10 mM

GppNHp was added to the reaction mixture to estimate non-specific binding. The specific GppNHp binding was assessed as the difference between a total and non-specific binding. Each assay was carried out in triplicate at least three times and the results were expressed as pmol [8-^{3}H]-GppNHp per mg of membrane protein.

Morris water-maze test

Throughout the behavioral experiments the groups of 6–8 months old diabetic and non-diabetic rats, IS-treated and untreated, were investigated. Prior to the experiments the animals were acclimated to handling over a week. A spatial training of rats was performed in MWM test [28]. The test efficiency was estimated by how long it took the animals swimming in a circular pool (120 cm in diameter and 30 cm in height filled with turbid water with chalk at 24 ± 1 °C) to find a 13 cm diameter hidden platform located 2 cm below the water level.

In the first series of experiments the animals swam daily for five days. Each rat had four attempts of 120 seconds for search of the hidden platform from four starting points. The animals were allowed to swim until either they located the platform, climbing upon it, or when 120 seconds elapsed. If the rats did not find the platform, they were compulsorily placed on it. Between the attempts the animals remained on the platform for 30 seconds rest. Post-testing, rats were placed under a heating lamp to get warm. The escape latency, the length of search path, and search speed during each trial were taken as indicators of successful formation and consolidation of spatial memory and learning.

A month later the testing was repeated (the second series) and the rats were given the trials similar to those of the first series. In addition, on the fifth day of the first and second series 40 minutes after the basic testing the rats were placed for 60 seconds in the pool where the hidden platform was removed and the number of annulus crossings over the previous platform location was recorded. This parameter provides replicates of the experiment for estimation of the strength and accuracy of the memory of the previous platform location. The swimming path and the escape latency were recorded by video camera for each rat during the trial. The obtained data were processed using Real Timer software 1.2 (Open Science Ltd., Russia) and Smart Junior (Panlab, S.L.U., Harvard Apparatus, USA).

Statistical analysis

The data was presented as the mean ± SD. Testing the assumption of normality was performed by using Shapiro-Wilk test. The results of the test confirmed that the obtained data is a sample from a normal distribution at $\alpha = 0.05$. The difference in the basal activity of AC or the basal level of GppNHp binding in the tissue membrane fractions of control and diabetic animals as well as the difference in the AC activity or GppNHp binding in the membrane fractions treated by hormones and non-hormonal AC regulators in each case was statistically assessed using one-way analysis of variance (ANOVA) and considered significant at $P < 0.05$. The analysis of the data obtained in MWM test

was carried out using one-way analysis of variance (ANOVA) followed by Student's Newman-Keuls post hoc test or unpaired t-test as required, and the difference was considered significant at $P < 0.05$.

Results

Neonatal model of T2DM and IS treatment

In our biochemical and physiological experiments were used 6–8-months old diabetic rats with neonatal DM duration of 3–5 months. Prior to IS treatment the body weight of 6-months old diabetic rats was higher as compared with control animals of the same age and following 8-weeks treatment with IS the difference in the body weight between IS-treated diabetic (D-S) and healthy (C-S) animals decreased (Table 1). In diabetic rats the level of fasting blood glucose was no higher than 7 mM (moderate hyperglycemia) and the level of plasma insulin was slightly decreased (moderate hypoinsulinemia). The level of triglycerides in the blood of the diabetic rats was significantly increased compared with control animals (1.50 ± 0.19 vs. 0.88 ± 0.12 nM, $P < 0.001$), while the increase of the level of HDL-cholesterol in DM was not significant (0.55 ± 0.08 vs. 0.46 ± 0.07 mM). These data is in good agreement with characteristics of the rat neonatal DM obtained by the other authors [19,23]. In our case, the IS treatment had a weak influence on glucose, insulin, triglycerides and HDL-cholesterol concentrations both in diabetic and control rats. In glucose tolerance test 2 hours after glucose load the concentration of plasma glucose in control rats reached normal level, while in diabetic rats remained much higher compared with control (13.5 ± 2.6 vs. 5.3 ± 1.0 mM) (Figure 2). In the IS-treated diabetic rats the concentration of glucose in glucose tolerance test also did not decrease to normal level and was higher than in Group C-S (11.1 ± 2.0 vs. 5.7 ± 1.5 mM). At the same time,

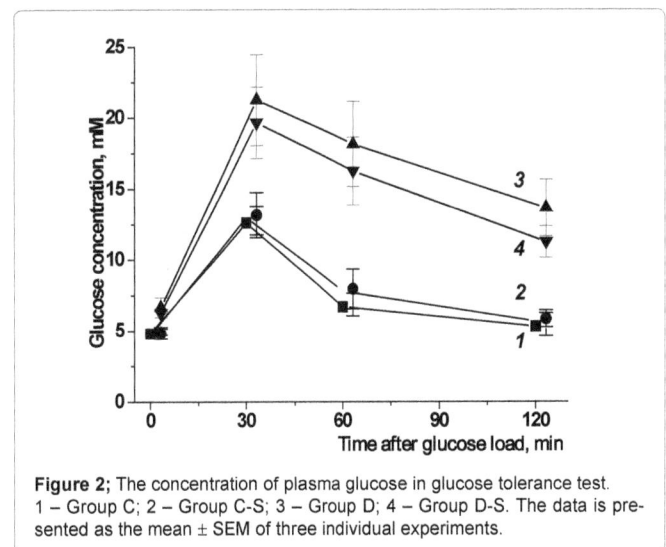

Figure 2; The concentration of plasma glucose in glucose tolerance test. 1 – Group C; 2 – Group C-S; 3 – Group D; 4 – Group D-S. The data is presented as the mean ± SEM of three individual experiments.

	Body weight, g		Plasma glucose, mM		Plasma insulin, ng/mL	
	6 months	8 months	6 months	8 months	6 months	8 months
C (n = 9)	226 ± 19	259 ± 1&&	5.0 ± 0.7	4.7 ± 0.9&	2.4 ± 0.3	2.3 ± 0.3&
C-S (n = 8)	219 ± 17	256 ± 15&&	5.1 ± 0.6	4.5 ± 0.5&&	2.4 ± 0.4	2.1 ± 0.2&&
D (n = 7)	261 ± 22	296 ± 26&	6.9 ± 1.1*	6.5 ± 1.2**&	1.4 ± 0.3*	1.6 ± 0.4&
D-S (n = 7)	268 ± 12++	278 ± 16&&	6.9 ± 1.4+	6.0 ± 1.2+&&	1.5 ± 0.4+	1.8 ± 0.3&&

C – control animals, C-S – IS-treated healthy animals, D – diabetic animals; D-S – IS-treated diabetic animals. & - control and diabetic rats after 8-weeks intranasal administration of saline instead of serotonin; && - healthy and diabetic rats after 8-weeks IS treatment (20 μg/rat every day). Values are the mean ± SD of three individual experiments. *, ** - the statistically significant difference between Groups D and C at $P < 0.05$ and $P < 0.01$; +, ++ - the statistically significant difference between Groups D-S and C-S at $P < 0.05$ and $P < 0.01$, respectively.

Table 1: The body weight, fasting glucose and insulin levels in 6- and 8-months healthy and diabetic rats.

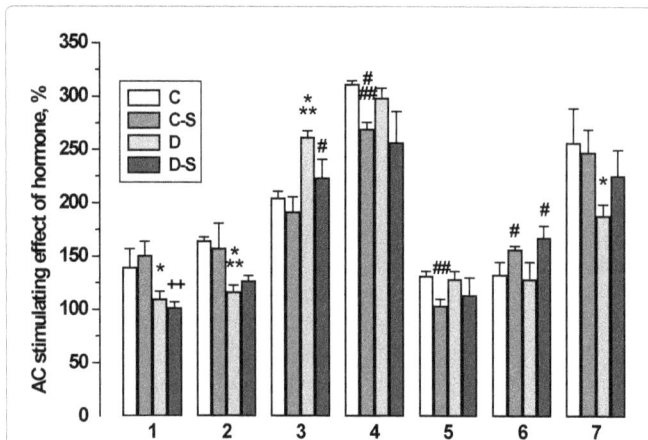

Figure 3: The stimulating effects of hormones on AC activity in the brain of untreated and IS-treated diabetic and control rats.
1 – norepinephrine; 2 – isoproterenol; 3 – dopamine; 4 – serotonin; 5 – EMD-386088 (10^{-5} M each); 6 – PACAP-38, 10^{-7} M; 7 – relaxin, 10^{-8} M.
C – control animals, C-S – IS-treated healthy animals, D – diabetic animals; D-S – IS-treated diabetic animals. Values are the mean ± SD of three individual experiments, each performed in triplicate.
*, *** - the statistically significant difference between Groups D and C at $P <$ 0.05 and $P < 0.001$; #, ##, ### - the statistically significant difference between Groups D-S and D or Groups C-S and C at $P < 0.05$, $P < 0.01$ and $P < 0.001$, respectively; ++ - the statistically significant difference between Groups D-S and C-S at $P < 0.01$.

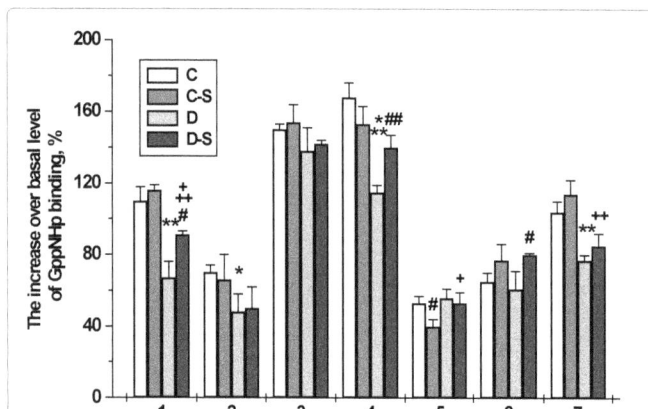

Figure 4: The hormone-induced increase of GppNHp binding in the brain of untreated and IS-treated diabetic and control rats.
1 – norepinephrine; 2 – isoproterenol; 3 – dopamine; 4 – serotonin; 5 – EMD-386088 (10^{-5} M each); 6 – PACAP-38, 10^{-7} M; 7 – relaxin, 10^{-8} M.
The basal level of GppNHp binding is taken as 100 %. Values are the mean ± SD of three individual experiments, each performed in triplicate.
*, **, *** - the statistically significant difference between Groups D and C at $P < 0.05$, $P < 0.01$ and $P < 0.001$; #, ## - the statistically significant difference between Groups D-S and D or Groups C-S and C at $P < 0.05$ and $P < 0.01$; +, ++, +++ - the statistically significant difference between Groups D-S and C-S at $P < 0.05$, $P < 0.01$ and $P < 0.001$, respectively.

in Group D-S the plasma glucose level was 18 % lower compared with Group D, which indicates a rather moderate IS-induced improvement in sensitivity of the peripheral tissues to insulin.

The influence of IS on the basal and GppNHp- and forskolin-stimulated adenylyl cyclase activities and on GppNHp binding in the brain of diabetic and control rats

The basal AC activity in the brain of diabetic rats did not differ significantly from control (23.0 ±1.7 vs. 24.4 ± 1.5 pmol cAMP/min per mg of membrane protein). Non-hydrolysable analog of GTP, GppNHp

(10^{-5} M), activator of G_s proteins, stimulated AC activity in control and diabetic rats by 188 and 197 %, and forskolin (10^{-5} M) acting directly on the catalytic site of the enzyme stimulated AC activity by 281 and 273 %, respectively. The basal AC activity in the brain of IS-treated diabetic and control rats was 21.3 ± 2.0 and 20.9 ± 1.3 pmol cAMP/min per mg of membrane protein, which did not differ significantly from the basal activity of the enzyme in the untreated animals. The IS treatment did not influence the stimulating effects of GppNHp and forskolin on AC activity.

The basal level of GppNHp binding in the brain of diabetic animals did not differ significantly from control (4.25 ± 0.28 vs. 4.51 ± 0.26 pmol [8-^{3}H]-GppNHp/mg of membrane protein), and 8-weeks IS treatment increased, but not significantly, it in Groups D-S and C-S, which was now 4.55 ± 0.19 and 4.73 ± 0.22 pmol [8-^{3}H]-GppNHp/mg of membrane protein, respectively. This prompts a suggestion that in the brain of rats with neonatal model of T2DM the functional activity of AC system in the basal state and/or under stimulation by non-hormonal agents does not undergo significant alterations, and IS did not significantly affect AC and G_s protein, the catalytic and the transducing components of this system.

The regulation of AC system by hormones acting via G_s-coupled receptors in DM under the influence of IS

In our experiments the biogenic amines and their analogues, such as norepinephrine, β-AR-agonist isoproterenol, dopamine, serotonin and 5-HT$_6$R-agonist EMD-386088, as well as the polypeptide hormones PACAP-38 and relaxin stimulated AC activity and GppNHp binding in the brain of both diabetic and control animals (Figures 3,4). In the diabetic brain AC stimulating effects of relaxin and AR-agonists isoproterenol and norepinephrine were decreased, the corresponding effect of dopamine was on the contrary increased, and AC effects of 5-HTR-agonists and PACAP-38 remained unchanged. The stimulating effects of relaxin, AR-agonists and serotonin on GppNHp binding were decreased in the diabetic brain, and the corresponding effects of the other hormones were close to control.

The IS treatment of control and diabetic rats led to a decrease of AC stimulating effects of serotonin and EMD-386088 and to an increase of the corresponding effect of PACAP-38. In the diabetic brain the stimulating effects of serotonin and PACAP-38 on GppNHp binding were increased, whereas the corresponding effect induced by EMD-386088 did not change significantly. IS led to partial restoration of both AC effect of relaxin decreased in the diabetic brain and the corresponding effect of dopamine increased in DM. IS did not significantly affect AC stimulating effects of AR ligands that in DM are decreased, but increased norepinephrine-induced stimulation of GppNHp binding (Figures 3,4). Thus, in the brain of rats with neonatal T2DM the functional activity of some signaling pathways mediating AC stimulation by hormones of different nature is changed. The changes we identified were hormone-specific, being as a rule associated with pathways regulated by AR ligands and relaxin. IS restored the transduction of AC stimulating signals in the diabetic brain and also affected AC stimulating effects of 5-HTR agonists and PACAP-38 in the healthy rats treated by IS.

The regulation of AC system by hormones acting via G_i-coupled receptors in DM under the influence of IS

The hormonal regulators acting via G_i-coupled receptors – the biogenic amines and their synthetic analogues, such as norepinephrine, dopamine, serotonin, selective 5-HT$_{1B/1D}$R agonist 5-nonyloxytryptamine, 5-HT$_{1/2}$R agonist 5-methoxy-

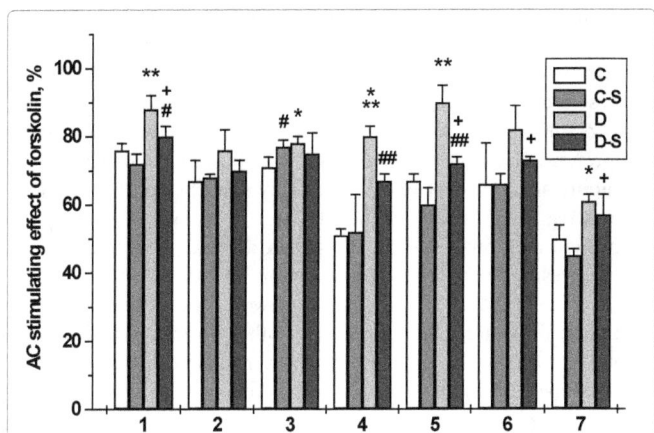

Figure 5: The inhibitory effects of hormones on forskolin-stimulated AC activity in the brain of untreated and IS-treated diabetic and control rats.
1 – norepinephrine; 2 – dopamine; 3 – bromocriptine; 4 – serotonin; 5 – 5-nonyloxytryptamine; 6 – 5-MeO-DMT (10^{-5} M each); 7 – somatostatin, 10^{-6} M.
The stimulating effect of forskolin (10^{-5} M) on the basal AC activity is taken as 100 %. Values are the mean ± SD of three individual experiments, each performed in triplicate.
*, **, *** - the statistically significant difference between Groups D and C at $P < 0.05$, $P < 0.01$ and $P < 0.001$; #, ## - the statistically significant difference between Groups D-S and D or Groups C-S and C at $P < 0.05$ and $P < 0.01$, respectively; + - the statistically significant difference between Groups D-S and C-S at $P < 0.05$.

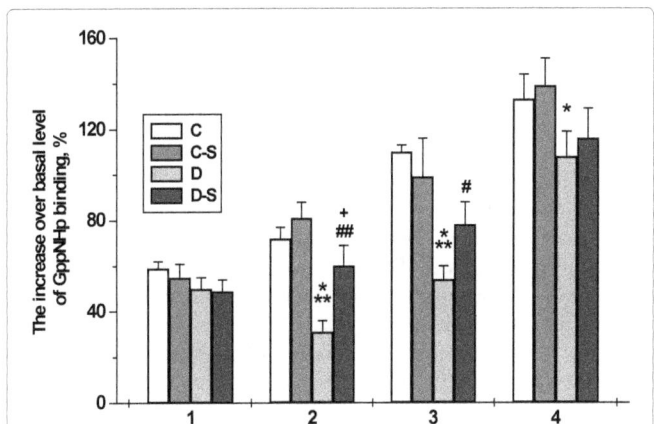

Figure 6: The increase of basal GppNHp binding by hormones activating preferably G_i proteins.
1 – bromocriptine; 2 – 5-nonyloxytryptamine; 3 – 5-MeO-DMT (10^{-5} M each); 4 – somatostatin, 10^{-6} M.
The basal level of GppNHp binding is taken as 100 %. Values are the mean ± SD of three individual experiments, each performed in triplicate.
*, *** - the statistically significant difference between Groups D and C at $P < 0.05$ and $P < 0.001$, respectively; #, ## - the statistically significant difference between Groups D-S and D or Groups C-S and C at $P < 0.05$ and $P < 0.01$, respectively; + - the statistically significant difference between Groups D-S and C-S at $P < 0.05$.

N,N-dimethyltryptamine, DA_2R agonist bromocriptine, and the neuropeptide somatostatin – all decreased forskolin-stimulated AC activity in the synaptosomal membranes in control rats (Figure 5). Besides, these hormones increased basal GppNHp binding (Figures 4,6). In Group D the inhibiting effects of hormones on AC activity and their stimulating effects on GppNHp binding were markedly decreased, especially in the case of serotonin and 5-HT_1R agonists. In the diabetic brain the stimulating effects of norepinephrine, serotonin, 5-nonyloxytryptamine, 5-methoxy-N,N-dimethyltryptamine and somatostatin on GppNHp binding reached 61, 68, 43, 49 and 81 % of

those in Group C. The corresponding effects of dopamine and DA_2R-agonist bromocriptine changed a little.

IS weakly influenced the regulatory effects of hormones inhibiting AC via Gi proteins in the brain of animals in Group C-S. In Group D-S the IS treatment led to a significant restoration of both AC inhibitory effects of hormones and their stimulation of GTP-binding (Figures 4,5,6). The stimulating effects of norepinephrine, serotonin, 5-nonyloxytryptamine, 5-MeO-DMT and somatostatin on GppNHp binding in Group D-S covered 78, 92, 74, 79 and 83 % of those in Group C-S. These values are higher compared with those of untreated diabetic animals, especialy in the case of 5-HTR agonists. According to the obtained data, IS gives a significant impact to the stimulation of GppNHp binding of G_i proteins by hormones inhibiting AC activity in the diabetic brain, and this effect is most pronounced in serotonin-regulated G_i-coupled AC pathway.

The spatial memory and learning of diabetic and control rats under the influence of IS

The learning process was estimated according to the duration and dynamics of the latent period for finding the hidden platform. The latent period in Group D in the first series was 3.5 times and in the second series 4–4.5 times longer compared with Group C and the dynamics of time reduction in locating the platform was less pronounced (Figure 7). IS did not change the duration and dynamics of the latent period in control animals, but significantly improved the learning process in diabetic rats. On the 4th day of the first series the escape latency reached the plateau and the information about the location of platform was maintained throughout the experiment. In Group D-S the latent period in both series was lower compared with Group D and the difference was significant ($P < 0.05$). The maximal effect of IS was 4 times, at most, the reduction of the latent period on the first day of the second series (35th day of MWM experiment). In both series there was a significant difference in the trajectories of swimming to the remote platform in Groups D and C, especially in the beginning of the second series (Figure 8). IS did not influence the swimming tracking in Group C-S,

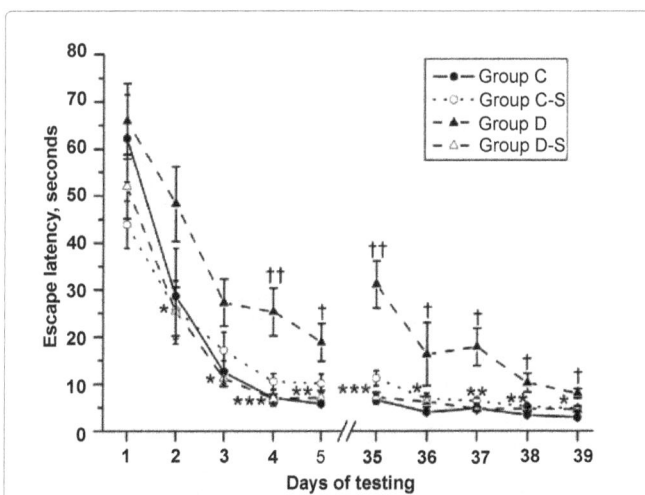

Figure 7: The duration and dynamics of latent period to find the platform by untreated and IS-treated diabetic and control rats in MWM test.
1 – Group C; 2 – Group C-S; 3 – Group D; 4 – Group D-S. Abscissa – the days of testing; ordinate – the escape latency, seconds. The first series covers days 1-5; the second days 35–39.
The data is presented as the mean ± SEM. †, †† - denotes the statistically significant difference between Groups D and C at $P < 0.05$ and $P < 0.01$; *, **, *** - denotes the statistically significant difference between Groups D-S and D at $P < 0.05$, $P < 0.01$ and $P < 0.001$, respectively.

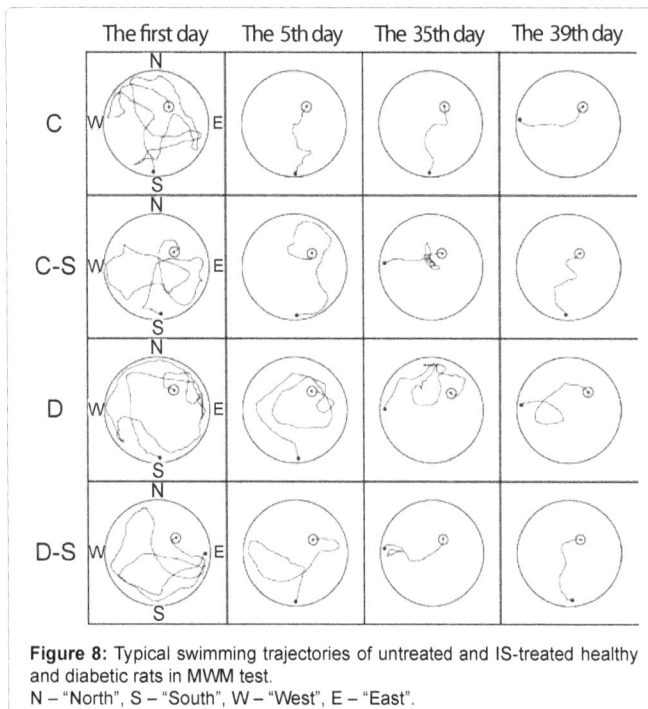

Figure 8: Typical swimming trajectories of untreated and IS-treated healthy and diabetic rats in MWM test.
N – "North", S – "South", W – "West", E – "East".

Rats	The first series, 5th day	The second series, 39th day
Group C (n = 9)	5.8 ± 2.0	7.0 ± 1.0
Group C-S (n = 8)	6.8 ± 1.5	6.6 ± 2.8
Group D (n = 7)	3.1 ± 2.5	4.6 ± 1.8**
Group D-S (n = 7)	5.4 ± 1.6#+	7.9 ± 2.3##

The number of annulus crossings over the platform location was recorded on the fifth day of the first and second series when 40 minutes after the basic testing the animals were placed for 60 seconds in the pool where the hidden platform was removed.
C – control animals, C-S – IS-treated healthy animals, D – diabetic animals; D-S – IS-treated diabetic animals. Values are the mean ± SD of three individual experiments. ** - the statistically significant difference between Groups D and C at $P < 0.01$; #, ## - the statistically significant difference between Groups D-S and D at $P < 0.05$ and $P < 0.01$, respectively; + - the statistically significant difference between Groups D-S and C-S at $P < 0.05$.

Table 2: The number of annulus crossings in the experiments with IS-treated and untreated control and diabetic rats in Morris water-maze test.

but in Group D-S the trajectories were much shorter compared with Group D and similar to those of control rats.

On the last day of testing in the first and the second series there was no difference in the number of annulus crossings between Groups C and C-S (Table 2). However, in diabetic rats there was a 45 % decrease in the first series and a 40 % decrease in the second, compared with Group C and the treatment with IS significantly increased these parameters in both series. In the first and the second series the number of annulus crossings in Group D-S, on average, exceeded 1.7 times that of Group D. Paradoxically, in the second series the number of annulus crossings in Group D-S was larger than in Groups C and C-S (Table 2). This furnishes grounds for us to say that IS improves the long-term spatial memory in rats with neonatal model of T2DM, making it similar to healthy animals. A decrease of time to search the platform and an increase of the number of annulus crossings in Group D-S shows the serotonin-induced improvement of cognitive functions in diabetic rats.

Discussion

Cognitive deficit with impaired abstract reasoning and complex

psychomotor functioning are likely to occur on the late stages of T2DM due to the triggering of neurodegenerative processes in the brain of diabetic patients [29]. However, the molecular mechanisms responsible for these processes in the diabetic brain are poorly understood, which hampers the development of effective approaches for the management and prevention of DM-induced CNS complications. Currently, it is commonly accepted that in DM especially disturbed is the signaling network regulated by insulin, insulin-like growth factor-1 and leptin, the principal hormones to be affected in diabetes; this leads to the disturbances of the growth, differentiation, metabolic and apoptotic processes in neuronal and glial cells. However, in addition to these hormones, there are a large number of other hormones and growth factors, as well as the signaling cascades regulated by them which are also involved in the etiology and pathogenesis of DM and its complications [5].

In this work we showed that in the brain of female rats with neonatal T2DM the brain signaling cascades regulated by biogenic amines and polypeptide hormones do indeed undergo a significant change and the most pronounced alterations are manifested in G_i protein-coupled cascades. The changes were found to occur in the AC system sensitive to AR agonists, serotonin, dopamine, and polypeptide hormones, which agrees very well with the data on the alterations and abnormalities in the adrenergic, serotonergic, dopaminergic and peptidergic neurotransmitter systems in the diabetic brain and on their role in the development of neurodegeneration [5].

We showed that in the diabetic brain the stimulating effects of norepinephrine and isoproterenol on AC activity and GppNHp binding mediated via G_s-coupled β-AR are reduced, so is the AC inhibitory effect of norepinephrine mediated via G_i-coupled α_2-AR. The abnormalities in adrenergic signaling in DM are likely, on the one hand, to have a negative influence on the synaptic transmission provoked by impairment of the mechanism involving increase of intracellular cAMP concentration and protein synthesis *de novo*, which leads to memory impairment and cognitive deficit [30], and on the other, to be responsible for DM-associated disturbances in the cerebral microvessels whose functions are controlled via different signaling systems, the adrenergic in particular [31]. It was shown earlier that in the hypothalamus of 4–16-weeks old *db/db* mice the number of β-ARs was reduced, which demonstrates a marked modification of the adrenergic signaling [32]. In the brainstem of rats with STZ-induced T1DM the affinity of α_2-ARs to agonists was significantly reduced and restored by insulin treatment [33]. The number of β-ARs in cerebral microvessels of fatty (*fa/fa*) and STZ rats is markedly decreased, and isoproterenol-stimulated AC activity in the microvessels of diabetic rats is much lower than that in control, giving evidence for the weakening of β-AR-mediated regulation of cAMP-dependent signaling [31].

In our study pronounced alterations of G_i-coupled serotonin signaling in the brain of diabetic rats are likely to be one of the direct causes of DM-induced behavioral abnormalities, so much so as the brain serotonergic system regulates many physiological functions, and the changes in serotonergic transmission in the diabetic brain provoke disturbances of neuronal processing and the altered plasticity of neurotransmission. We showed that the regulatory effects of 5-HT$_{1B/1D}$R-agonist 5-nonyloxytryptamine and 5-HT$_{1/2}$R-agonist 5-MeO-DMT were markedly reduced, which indicates a weakening of serotonin signaling mediated via 5-HT$_1$R in the brain of rats with neonatal T2DM . The data is available that the flat body posture of STZ diabetic and non-diabetic rats induced by 5-HT$_{1A}$R agonist 8-hydroxy-2-(dipropylamino)tetralin hydrobromide (8-OH-DPAT) changed, but not alike, which means that STZ-induced T1DM profoundly affects the sensitivity to drugs acting via 5-HT$_{1A}$R [34]. One-week insulin treatment restored 8-OH-DPAT-induced behavioral effects. We showed earlier that the sensitivity of G$_i$-coupled AC system to agonists of 5-HT$_1$R was significantly decreased in the brain of STZ rats with T1DM [35], but there was no alteration of AC sensitivity to agonists of G$_s$ protein-coupled 5-HTR. This is consistent with the data obtained in the present study, i.e. that the efficiency of transduction of AC stimulating serotonin signal in the brain of rats with neonatal T2DM is not altered as compared with control. It seems quite possible that the decrease of efficiency of G$_i$-coupled serotonin signaling pathways may well be associated with reduced expression and with decreased functional activity of G$_i$ proteins, which might indeed be the case as in the brain of rats with neonatal DM was also detected a decrease of activity of the G$_i$-coupled cascades which undergo regulation by norepinephrine and somatostatin.

However, studying dopamine signaling in the diabetic brain, we showed that regulatory effects of dopamine and DA$_2$R-agonist bromocriptine on AC system mediated via G$_i$-coupled DA$_2$R did not change significantly, while stimulating effects of dopamine on this system mediated via G$_s$-coupled DA$_1$R increased. In our view, here a decreased expression of G$_i$ proteins was fully compensated by an increased expression of DA$_2$R or by the changes of their binding characteristics. This suggestion finds confirmation in the recent investigations showing that B$_{max}$ of a total DAR binding and the expression of DA$_2$R in the cerebral cortex of STZ rats with T1DM are increased significantly [36]. In the diabetic brain of T1DM rats the expression of DA$_1$R was also increased, which explains the increase of stimulating influence of dopamine on AC, as in the case of rats with neonatal DM in our investigation.

As far as the role of polypeptide hormones somatostatin, PACAP-38 and relaxin in the functioning of CNS is concerned, they are shown to be involved in the regulation of neuronal differentiation, synaptic plasticity, cognitive functions [37-39]. However, the data on functional activity of the brain signaling systems regulated by these hormones in DM are scarce. The information is available now that the intracerebral level of somatostatin and the expression of some types of brain somatostatin receptors are reduced in animal models of T1DM [40]. We showed that in the brain of rats with neonatal T2DM the regulatory action of somatostatin and relaxin on AC activity is decreased. This allowed a suggestion that somatostatin- and relaxin-sensitive AC system is involved in pathogenesis of T2DM and is a candidate to serve as a marker of this disease. At the same time, we found no significant changes in the response of AC in the diabetic brain to PACAP-38. It seems likely that the maintenance of AC stimulating effect of PACAP-38 is due to its important role in the protection of the brain from damage and neurodegenerative changes induced by DM [41].

The well-coordinated regulation of AC system in the normal brain is disrupted in T2DM, and the synergistic effect of alterations in this system leads to neurodegenerative changes in different brain areas. This is confirmed by our data on the impairment of the cognitive functions in rats with neonatal T2DM in MWM test. The diabetic rats demonstrated the problems in intellectual development and learning. The deterioration of the time allocated to search the platform and the increase of swimming trajectory in the second series indicates the impairment of spatial memory in neonatal T2DM. A number of reports are available describing a cognitive deficit associated with abnormalities in the hippocampus activity in obese rats [42]. Female KKAy mice with hyperinsulinemia and impaired glucose tolerance showed a significant impairment of cognitive functions evaluated by the shuttle avoidance and MWM tests [43]. The rats with T2DM induced by high fat diet and low-dose STZ treatment had deterioration of stroke-induced brain

damage and cognitive deficit, as was illustrated by the impairment of the performance of rats in the MWM test [44].

One of the usual approaches used to restore the neuronal network in T2DM is the treatment of diabetic patients with glucose-lowering drugs and, at the late stages of disease, with insulin. Another approach is to treat patients with neurohormones and drugs controlling their synthesis, secretion and uptake, these substances can be used alone or in combination with insulin therapy. The best studied among them are the selective 5-HT reuptake inhibitors having antidepressant activity and DA$_2$R agonist bromocriptine widely used in the treatment of hyperprolactinemia, galactorrhoea and Parkinson disease [16,17]. The 5-HT reuptake inhibitors contribute to lowering the level of hyperglycemia, improve metabolic control through their positive effect on weight loss, thereby improving insulin resistance, and restore cognitive functions impaired in DM. The treatment of 60 patients with depression associated with T1DM and T2DM by fluoxetine, selective 5-HT reuptake inhibitor, reduced depressive symptoms and increased the sensitivity of the brain and the peripheral tissues to insulin [16]. Consequently, the approach leading to an increase of the brain 5-HT level is a successful strategy to treat DM [17]. Proceeding from this data, we applied IS for restoration of activity of the brain AC system and improvement of cognitive deficit of rats with neonatal T2DM. The intranasal route of serotonin administration has been chosen so that the hormone could be delivered to the brain areas, the targets of this action, more effectively. This method is successfully used to treat migraine by 5-HT$_{1B/1D}$R-agonist sumatriptan and its analogues [45]. In the diabetic brain IS restores hormonal sensitivity of AC system, and its positive effect was observed in the case of hormones, especially of serotonin and 5-HT$_1$R agonists, acting via G$_i$ proteins. A considerable restoration of 5-HT$_1$R-mediated signaling in the brain of IS-treated diabetic rats should be ascribed to an increase of the activity of serotonin-sensitive AC system as a result of normalization of the expression of components of this system, and to an increase of the efficiency of interaction between serotonin-regulated and the other signaling systems due to restoration of integrative signaling network in the neuronal and the glial cells impaired in DM. The restoration of the brain AC signaling regulated by neurotransmitters and polypeptide neurohormones leads to the improvement of cognitive functions. The evidence for this is considerable improvement of spatial memory and learning in IS-treated diabetic rats in MWM test. The cognitive functions we evaluated in this test did not differ from those of healthy rats treated as well as untreated with IS.

Summing up, in the brain of diabetic rats with neonatal T2DM the functional activity of hormone-sensitive AC signaling system is subject to changes, the most significant alterations being observed in G$_i$-coupled cascades that mediate the inhibition of AC activity. These alterations were associated with cognitive deficit and manifested as impaired learning and spatial memory. The intranasal delivery of serotonin improves both the brain AC system and cognitive functions of diabetic rats, which opens up a new avenue to correct and prevent the alterations and disturbances in the brain signaling and to improve cognitive functions in T2DM.

Acknowledgment

This work was supported by Grant No. 09-04-00746 from the Russian Foundation of Basic Research and Program "Fundamental Sciences – Medicine" (2009-2011). The authors are grateful to Inga Menina for linguistic assistance.

References

1. Stiles MC, Seaquist ER (2010) Cerebral structural and functional changes in type 1 diabetes. Minerva Med 101: 105-114.

2. Biessels G, Smale S, Duis S, Kamal A, Gispen W (2001) The effect of γ-linolenic

acid-α-lipoic acid on functional deficits in the peripheral and central nervous system of streptozotocin-diabetic rats. J Neurol Sci 182: 99-106.

3. Scheen AJ (2010) Central nervous system: a conductor orchestrating metabolic regulations harmed by both hyperglycaemia and hypoglycaemia. Diabetes Metab 36: S31-S38.

4. Muniyappa R, Montagnani M, Koh KK, Quon MJ (2007) Cardiovascular actions of insulin. Endocr Rev 28: 463-491.

5. Shpakov A, Chistyakova O, Derkach K, Bondareva V (2011) Hormonal signaling systems of the brain in diabetes mellitus: Neurodegenerative Diseases. (R.C. Chang, ed.), Intech Open Access Publisher, Rijeka, Croatia. 349-386.

6. Palmer TM, Taberner PV, Houslay MD (1992) Alterations in G-protein expression, Gi function and stimulatory receptor-mediated regulation of adipocyte adenylyl cyclase in a model of insulin-resistant diabetes with obesity. Cell Signal 4: 365-377.

7. Hashim S, Li Y, Nagakura A, Takeo S, Anand-Srivastava MB (2004) Modulation of G-protein expression and adenylyl cyclase signaling by high glucose in vascular smooth muscle. Cardiovasc Res 63: 709-718.

8. Shpakov AO, Kuznetsova LA, Plesneva SA, Bondareva VM, Guryanov IA, et al. (2006) Decrease in functional activity of G-proteins hormone-sensitive adenylate cyclase signaling system, during experimental type II diabetes mellitus. Bull Exp Biol Med 142: 685-689.

9. Shpakov A, Kuznetsova L, Plesneva S, Kolychev A, Bondareva V, et al. (2006) Functional defects in adenylyl cyclase signaling mechanisms of insulin and relaxin action in skeletal muscles of rat with streptozotocin type 1 diabetes. Cent Eur J Biol 1: 530-544.

10. Shpakov AO, Kuznetsova LA, Plesneva SA, Pertseva MN (2007) The disturbance of the transduction of adenylyl cyclase inhibiting hormonal signal in myocardium and brain of rats with experimental type II diabetes. Tsitologiia 49: 442-450.

11. Shpakov AO, Chistyakova OV, Derkach KV, Moiseyuk IV, Bondareva VM (2012) Intranasal insulin affects adenylyl cyclase system in rat tissues in neonatal diabetes. Central Eur J Biol 7: 33–47.

12. Ovalle F (2010) Clinical approach to the patient with diabetes mellitus and very high insulin requirements. Diabetes Res Clin Pract 90: 231-242.

13. Henkin RI (2010) Intranasal insulin: from nose to brain. Nutrition 26: 624-633.

14. Chistyakova OV, Bondareva VM, Shipilov VN, Sukhov IB, Shpakov AO (2011) Intranasal administration of the insulin eliminates long-term memory deficits in rats with neonatal diabetes mellitus. Dokl Biochem Biophys 440: 216-218.

15. Kerr J, Timpe E, Petkewicz K (2010) Bromocriptine mesylate for glycemic management in type 2 diabetes mellitus. Ann Pharmacother 44: 1777-1785.

16. Lustman P, Freedland K, Griffith L, Clouse R (2000) Fluoxetine for depression in diabetes: a randomized double-blind placebo-controlled trial. Diabetes Care 23: 618–623.

17. Zhou L, Sutton GM, Rochford JJ, Semple RK, Lam DD, et al. (2007) Serotonin 2C receptor agonists improve type 2 diabetes via melanocortin-4 receptor signaling pathways. Cell Metab 6: 398-405.

18. Guidelines for the treatment of animals in behavior research and teaching (2006) Animal Behaviour. 71: 245-253.

19. Hemmings S, Spafford D (2000) Neonatal STZ model of type II diabetes mellitus in the Fischer 344 rat: characteristics and assessment of the status of the hepatic adrenergic receptors. Int J Biochem Cell Biol 32: 905-919.

20. Sharma AK, Srinivasan BP (2009) Triple verses glimepiride plus metformin therapy on cardiovascular risk biomarkers and diabetic cardiomyopathy in insulin resistance type 2 diabetes mellitus rats. Eur J Pharm Sci 38: 433-444.

21. Thyssen S, Arany E, Hill DJ (2006) Ontogeny of regeneration of beta-cells in the neonatal rat after treatment with streptozotocin. Endocrinology 147: 2346-2356.

22. Nicholson JM, Arany EJ, Hill DJ (2010) Changes in islet microvasculature following streptozotocin-induced beta-cell loss and subsequent replacement in the neonatal rat. Exp Biol Med (Maywood) 235: 189-198.

23. Blondel O, Bailbé D, Portha B (1989) Relation of insulin deficiency to impaired insulin action in NIDDM adult rats given streptozocin as neonates. Diabetes 38: 610-617.

24. Suryanarayana P, Patil MA, Reddy GB (2011) Insulin resistance mediated biochemical alterations in eye lens of neonatal streptozotocin-induced diabetic rat. Indian J Exp Biol 49: 749-755.

25. Thorne RG, Pronk GJ, Padmanabhan V, Frey WH (2004) Delivery of insulin-like growth factor-I to the rat brain and spinal cord along olfactory and trigeminal pathways following intranasal administration. Neuroscience 127: 481-496.

26. Shpakov A, Shpakova E, Tarasenko I, Derkach K, Vlasov G (2010) The peptides mimicking the third intracellular loop of 5-hydroxytryptamine receptors of the types 1B and 6 selectively activate G proteins and receptor-specifically inhibit serotonin signaling via the adenylyl cyclase system. Int J Pept Res Ther 16: 95-105.

27. Shpakov A, Shpakova E, Tarasenko I, Derkach K, Chistyakova O, et al. (2011) The influence of peptides corresponding to the third intracellular loop of luteinizing hormone receptor on basal and hormone-stimulated activity of the adenylyl cyclase signaling system. Global J Biochem 2: 59-73.

28. Van Dam D, Lenders G, De Deyn PP (2006) Effect of Morris water maze diameter on visual-spatial learning in different mouse strains. Neurobiol Learn Mem 85: 164-172.

29. Biessels GJ, Deary IJ, Ryan CM (2008) Cognition and diabetes: a lifespan perspective. Lancet Neurol 7: 184-190.

30. Tully K, Bolshakov VY (2010) Emotional enhancement of memory: how norepinephrine enables synaptic plasticity. Mol Brain 3: 15.

31. Mooradian AD, Scarpace PJ (1992) Beta-adrenergic receptor activity of cerebral microvessels in experimental diabetes mellitus. Brain Res 583: 155-160.

32. Garris DR (1990) Age- and diabetes-associated alterations in regional brain norepinephrine concentrations and adrenergic receptor populations in C57BL/KsJ mice. Brain Res Dev Brain Res 51: 161-166.

33. Padayatti PS, Paulose CS (1999) $α_2$-Adrenergic and high affinity serotonergic receptor changes in the brain stem of streptozotocin-induced diabetic rats. Life Sci 65: 403-414.

34. Li JX, France CP (2008) Food restriction and streptozotocin treatment decrease 5-HT1A and 5-HT2A receptor-mediated behavioral effects in rats. Behav Pharmacol 19: 292-297.

35. Shpakov AO, Kuznetsova LA, Plesneva SA, Guryanov IA, Vlasov GP, et al. (2007) Identification of disturbances in hormone-sensitive adenylyl cyclase system in the tissues of rats with types 1 and 2 diabetes using functional probes and synthetic peptides. Tekhnologii zhivykh system 4: 96-108.

36. Robinson R, Krishnakumar A, Paulose CS (2009) Enhanced dopamine D1 and D2 receptor gene expression in the hippocampus of hypoglycaemic and diabetic rats. Cell Mol Neurobiol 29: 365-372.

37. Epelbaum J, Guillou J, Gastambide F, Hoyer D, Duron E, et al. (2009) Somatostatin, Alzheimer's disease and cognition: an old story coming of age? Prog Neurobiol 89: 153-161.

38. McGowan BM, Minnion JS, Murphy KG, White NE, Roy D, et al. (2010) Central and peripheral administration of human relaxin-2 to adult male rats inhibits food intake. Diabetes Obes Metab 12: 1090-1096.

39. Moody TW, Ito T, Osefo N, Jensen RT (2011) VIP and PACAP: recent insights into their functions/roles in physiology and disease from molecular and genetic studies. Curr Opin Endocrinol Diabetes Obes 18: 61-67.

40. Bruno JF, Xu Y, Song J, Berelowitz M (1994) Pituitary and hypothalamic somatostatin receptor subtype messenger ribonucleic acid expression in the food-deprived and diabetic rat. Endocrinology 135: 1787-1792.

41. Reglodi D, Kiss P, Lubics A, Tamas A (2011) Review on the protective effects of PACAP in models of neurodegenerative diseases in vitro and in vivo. Curr Pharm Des 17: 962-972.

42. Greenwood CE, Winocur G (2005) High-fat diets, insulin resistance and declining cognitive function. Neurobiol Aging 26: 42-45.

43. Sakata A, Mogi M, Iwanami J, Tsukuda K, Min LJ, et al. (2010) Female exhibited severe cognitive impairment in type 2 diabetes mellitus mice. Life Sci 86: 638-645.

44. Zhang T, Pan BS, Zhao B, Zhang LM, Huang YL, et al. (2009) Exacerbation of poststroke dementia by type 2 diabetes is associated with synergistic increases of beta-secretase activation and beta-amyloid generation in rat brains. Neuroscience 161: 1045-1056.

45. Cittadini E, May A, Straube A, Evers S, Bussone G, et al. (2006) Effectiveness of intranasal zolmitriptan in acute cluster headache: a randomized, placebo-controlled, double-blind crossover study. Arch Neurol 63: 1537-1542.

Permissions

List of Contributors

Vincenzo De Leo, Maria Concetta Musacchio, Valentina Cappelli, Alessandra Di Sabatino, Claudia Tosti and Paola Piomboni
Molecular Medicine and Development Department, Obstetrics and Gynecology Clinic, University of Siena, Italy

Brian Miller
School of Sport Science & Wellness Education, The University of Akron, Akron, OH; Doctoral Student, Health Education and Promotion, School of Health Sciences, Kent State University, Kent, OH, USA

Mark Fridline
Department of Statistics, The University of Akron, Akron, OH, USA

Jing Liu, Ju-xiang Liu, Jin-xing Quan, Li-min Tian, Jia Liu, Yan-jia Xu, Qi Zhang and Xiao-hui Chen
Department of Endocrinology, Gansu Provincial People's Hospital, 204 West Donggang Road, Lanzhou City 730000, Gansu Province, China

Xiao-feng Huang, Shu-lan Zhang and Rui-lan Niu
The First Clinical College of Lanzhou University, Lanzhou City 730000, Gansu Province, China

Xiao-juan Huang
State Key Laboratory for Oxo Synthesis & Selective Oxidation, Lanzhou Institute of Chemical Physics, Chinese Academy of Sciences, Lanzhou 730000, China

Junki Yoshida, Akiko Tateishi, Yuko Fukui, Mitsuhiro Zeida and Nobuyuki Fukui
Research Division, Suntory Global Innovation Center Limited (Suntory SIC), Seikadai, Seika-cho, Soraku-gun, Kyoto 619-0284, Japan

Ibrahim S Ismail, Ameh D Amodu, Atawodi S Ene-ojoh and Umar I Alhaji
Department of Biochemistry, Ahmadu Bello University Zaria, Nigeria

Aye M and Cabot JSF
Department of Medicine, UniKL Royal College of Medicine, Perak, Malaysia

Razak MSA
State Health Department, Ministry of Health, Perak, Malaysia

María Eugenia Velasco-Contreras Grado
Unit of Primary Attention of Health, Coordination of Comprehensive Health Care for the First Level of Care; Division of Information and Medical Support, Mexican Institute of Social Security, Mexico

R Aller, O Izaola, R Bachiller, E Romero and DA de Luis
Center of Investigation of Endocrinology and Nutrition, Medicine School and Department of Endocrinology and Investigation, Hospital Clinico Universitario, University of Valladolid, Valladolid, Spain

Rocío Aller
Center of Investigation of Endocrinology and Nutrition, Medicine School, Spain

Daniel de Luis, Olatz Izaola, Primo D and Romero E
Center of Investigation of Endocrinology and Nutrition, Medicine School, Spain
Department of Endocrinology and Nutrition, Hospital Clínico Universitario, Spain

Kanishka N Nilaweera
Teagasc Food Research Centre, Moorepark, Fermoy, Cork, Ireland

Liam McAllan
Teagasc Food Research Centre, Moorepark, Fermoy, Cork, Ireland
Department of Pharmacology and Therapeutics, University College Cork, Cork, Ireland

Paul D Cotter
Teagasc Food Research Centre, Moorepark, Fermoy, Cork, Ireland
Alimentary Pharmabiotic Centre, University College Cork, Cork, Ireland

Helen M Roche
UCD Conway Institute of Biomolecular & Biomedical Research, & UCD Institute of Food & Health, University College Dublin, Belfield Dublin 4, Ireland

Riitta Korpela
Institute of Biomedicine, Biomedicum Helsinki, P.O. Box 63, FI-00014 University of Helsinki, Finland

Zhanxiang Wang
Herman B Wells Center for Pediatric Research, Basic Diabetes Group, Department of Pediatrics, Indiana University School of Medicine, USA

Hongji Zhang
Department of Urology, Indiana University School of Medicine, USA

Jhuma KA
Department of Biochemistry, Medical College for Women & Hospital, Plot-4, Road-9, Sector-1, Uttara Model Town, Dhaka-1230, Bangladesh

Giasuddin ASM
Department of Medical Laboratory Science, State College of Health Sciences & Adjunct Professor, State University of Bangladesh, Dhanmondi, Dhaka-1209, Bangladesh

Haq AMM and Huque MM
Department of Medicine, Medical College for Women & Hospital, Plot-4, Road-9, Sector-1, Uttara Model Town, Dhaka-1230, Bangladesh

Mahmood N
Department of Medicine, (Nephrology Unit), Medical College for Women & Hospital, Plot-4, Road-9, Sector-1, Uttara Model Town, Dhaka-1230, Bangladesh

Francisco Avilés-Plaza and Soledad Parra-Pallarés
Clinical Analysis Service, Biochemical Section of University Hospital Virgen de la Arrixaca, Murcia, Spain

Juana Bernabé, Begoña Cerdá, Javier Marhuenda, Pilar Zafrilla and Juana Mulero
Department of Food Technology and Nutrition, Catholic University of San Antonio, Murcia, Spain

Tânia O. Constantino
Faculty of Pharmacy, University of Porto, Porto, Portugal

Cristina García-Viguera and Diego A. Moreno
CSIC, CEBAS, Department of Food Sci & Technol, Res Group Qual Safety & Bioactiv Plant Food, Murcia, Spain

José Abellán
Chair of Cardiovascular Risk, Catholic University of San Antonio, Murcia, Spain

Yohannes Addisu and Akine Eshete
College of Health and Medical Sciences, Dilla University, Ethiopia

Endalew Hailu
Department of Nursing, College of Public Health and Medical Sciences, Jimma University, Ethiopia

DedinskáI, Laca L and Miklušica J
Surgery Clinic and Transplant Center, University Hospital Martin and Jessenius Faculty of Medicine, Comenius University, Slovak Republic

Stančík M, Kantárová, Galajda P and Mokáň M
Clinic of Internal Medicine I, University Hospital Martin and Jessenius Faculty of Medicine, Comenius University, Slovak Republic

Ulinako J
Department of Plastic Surgery, F.D.Roosevelt's Faculty Hospital in Banská Bystrica, Slovak Republic

Janek J
Department of Vascular Surgery, F.D.Roosevelt's Faculty Hospital in Banská Bystrica, Slovak Republic

Jingyan Chen, Tingting Li, Helin Ding and Jin Zhang
Department of Endocrinology, Sun Yat-Sen Memorial Hospital of Sun Yat-Sen University, Guangzhou, PR China

Hua Zeng, Zhixian Zhang and Lei Bi
Department of Clinical Laboratory, Sun Yat-Sen Memorial Hospital of Sun Yat-Sen University, Guangzhou, PR China

Duarte-Vázquez Miguel Ángel and Jorge Luis Rosado
CINDETEC A.C. Avenida Jurica, Industrial Park Querétaro, Querétaro, México
Nucitec, S. A. de C. V. Avenida Jurica, Industrial Park Querétaro, Querétaro, México

Gómez-Solís María Antonieta, Gómez-Cansino Rocio, Reyes-Esparza Jorge and Rodríguez-Fragoso Lourdes
Faculty of Pharmacy, Autonomous University of the State of Morelos, Cuernavaca, Morelos, México

Sermin Kesebir, Merih Altıntaş, Elif Tatlıdil Yaylacı, Boray Erdinç and Nevzat Tarhan
Uskudar University, Turkey

Shinichi Iwai, Masayuki Arai, Kanji Furuya, Shinichi Kobayashi and Katsuji Oguchi
Department of Pharmacology, Showa University School of Medicine, 1-5-8 Hatanodai, Shinagawa-ku, Tokyo 142-8555, Japan

Keiichiro Ohba and Go Koizumi
Department of Pharmacology, Showa University School of Medicine, 1-5-8 Hatanodai, Shinagawa-ku, Tokyo 142-8555, Japan

Department of Pharmacogenomics, St. Marianna University Graduate School of Medicine, 2-16-1 Sugao, Miyamae-ku, Kawasaki, Kanagawa 216-8511, Japan

Naoki Matsumoto
Department of Pharmacology, St. Marianna University School of Medicine, 2-16-1 Sugao, Miyamae-ku, Kawasaki, Kanagawa 216-8511, Japan

Toshio Kumai and Go Oda
Department of Pharmacogenomics, St. Marianna University Graduate School of Medicine, 2-16-1 Sugao, Miyamae-ku, Kawasaki, Kanagawa 216-8511, Japan

Minoru Watanabe
Institute for Animal Experimentation, St. Marianna University Graduate School of Medicine, 2-16-1 Sugao, Miyamae-ku, Kawasaki, Kanagawa 216-8511, Japan

Biswabandhu Bankura, Madhusudan Das, Arup Kumar Pattanayak and Bidisha Adhikary
Department of Zoology, University of Calcutta, 35 Ballygunge Circular Road, Kolkata-700 019, West Bengal, India

Rana Bhattacharjee, Soumik Goswami, Subhankar Chowdhury and Ajitesh Roy
Department of Endocrinolgy, Institute of Post Graduate Medical Education & Research, 244 A J C Bose Road, Kolkata-700 020, West Bengal, India

Surabhi Nanda and Ranjit Akolekar
Harris Birthright Research Centre for Fetal Medicine, King's College Hospital, London, UK
Department of Fetal Medicine, Medway Maritime Hospital, Gillingham (Kent), UK

Kypros H Nicolaides
Harris Birthright Research Centre for Fetal Medicine, King's College Hospital, London, UK
Department of Fetal Medicine, Medway Maritime Hospital, Gillingham (Kent), UK
Department of Fetal Medicine, University College Hospital, London, UK

Isabela C Acosta and Dorota Wierzbicka
Harris Birthright Research Centre for Fetal Medicine, King's College Hospital, London, UK
Department of Fetal Medicine, University College Hospital, London, UK

de Luis DA, Aller R, Primo D, Izaola O, Fuente B and Romero E
Center of Investigation of Endocrinology and Nutrition, Medicine School and Dpt of Endocrinology and Investigation, Hospital Clinico Universitario, University of Valladolid, Valladolid, Spain

Nanlan Luo and Yuchang Fu
Department of Nutrition Sciences, University of Alabama at Birmingham, Birmingham, AL 35294-3360, USA

Timothy W. Garvey
Department of Nutrition Sciences, University of Alabama at Birmingham, Birmingham, AL 35294-3360, USA
Birmingham VA Medical Center, Birmingham, AL 35233, USA

Da-Zhi Wang
Department of Cardiology, Boston Children's Hospital, Harvard Medical School, Boston, MA 02115, USA

Federica Giampetruzzi and Gabriella Garruti
Section of Internal Medicine, Endocrinology, Andrology and Metabolic Diseases, Department of Emergency and Organ Transplantation (DETO), University of Bari "Aldo Moro", School of Medicine, Bari, Italy

Shivaram Prasad Singh, Preetam Nath, Ayaskanta Singh, Jimmy Narayan, Prasant Parida, Pradeep Kumar Padhi and Girish Kumar Pati
Department of Gastroenterology, S.C.B. Medical College, 753007 Cuttack, India

Chudamani Meher and Omprakash Agrawal
Department of Radiology, Beam Diagnostics Centre, Bajrakabati Road, 753001 Cuttack, India

Nalin Siriwardhana, Arnold M Saxton, Naima Moustaid-Moussa and Jay Wimalasena
Department of Animal Science and Obesity Research Center, University of Tennessee, Knoxville, Tennessee 37996

Rett Layman, Ayub Karwandyar, Shiwani Patel, Blair Tage, Matthew Clark, Jessica Lampley, Courtney Rhody and Erica Smith
Department of Obstetrics and Gynecology, Graduate School of Medicine, University of Tennessee Medical Center, Knoxville, Tennessee 37920

Nfor O Nlinwe
Department of Medical Laboratory Science, University of Bamenda, Cameroon

Manopriya T
MAPIMS, Chennai, India

Khalid G
Chettinad Dental College, Chennai, India

Alshaari AA and Sheriff DS
Faculty of Medicine, Benghazi University, Benghazi, Libya

Priscilla O Okunji
Howard University College of Nursing and Allied Health Sciences, Washington, DC, USA

Johnnie Daniel
Department of Sociology and Anthropology, Washington, DC, USA

Anthony Wutoh
College of Pharmacy, Washington, DC, USA

Gomes DC, Pinto-Neto AM and Costa-Paiva L
State University of Campinas (UNICAMP), Campinas, SP, Brazil

Akl LD
State University of Campinas (UNICAMP), Campinas, SP, Brazil
Eduardo de Menezes Hospital (HEM), Belo Horizonte, MG, Brazil

Valadares ALR
State University of Campinas (UNICAMP), Campinas, SP, Brazil
José do Rosário Vellano University (UNIFENAS), Belo Horizonte, MG, Brazil

Thirumagal Kanagasabai, Jason X. Nie and Chris I. Ardern
School of Kinesiology and Health Science, York University, Toronto, Ontario, Canada

Caitlin Mason
University of Washington Health Promotion Research Center, Seattle, Washington, USA

Thomas H Braunstein, Niels-Henrik Holstein-Rathlou
The National Research Foundation Center for Cardiac Arrhythmia, Denmark
Department of Biomedical Sciences, Faculty of Health Sciences, University of Copenhagen, Denmark

Helena Domínguez
The National Research Foundation Center for Cardiac Arrhythmia, Denmark
Department of Biomedical Sciences, Faculty of Health Sciences, University of Copenhagen, Denmark
Department of Cardiology Y, Bispebjerg Hospital, Frederiksberg Section, Frederiksberg, Denmark

Anna Fossum
Biotech Research and Innovation Center, FACS Facility, University of Copenhagen, Copenhagen, Denmark

Christian Torp-Pedersen
Department of Health Science and Technology, Aalborg University, Aalborg, Denmark

Beray Selver and Yildiz Dallar
Department of Pediatrics, Ankara Research and Training Hospital, Ankara, Turkey

Enver Simsek
Department of Pediatrics, Division of Endocrinology, Eskisehir Osmangazi University, School of Medicine, Eskisehir, Turkey

Ugur Kocabas
Department of Cardiology, Ankara Research and Training Hospital, Ankara, Turkey

Jian-hua Jiang, Jing Cheng, Bao Zhang, Shi-xia Guan and Li-li Hou
Department of Clinical Nutriology, the First Affiliated Hospital of Anhui Medical University, Hefei, China

Cecilia Ramírez-Murillo, Elizabeth Guillot-Sánchez, Elizabeth Artalejo-Ochoa Q B, Alma E. Robles-Sardin, José A. Ponce-Martínez, María I Grijalva-Haro, Graciela Caire-Juvera, María I. Ortega-Vélez and Martha N. Ballesteros-Vásquez
Centro de Investigación en Alimentación y Desarrollo, A.C. Carretera a la Victoria km 0.6, Hermosillo, Sonora México

Radina Eshtiaghi
Department of Internal Medicine, Faculty of Medicine, AJA University of Medical Sciences, Tehran, Iran

Ali Reza Khoshdel
Department of Epidemiology, Faculty of Medicine, AJA University of Medical Sciences, Tehran, Iran
Department of Nephrology, John Hunter Hospital, The University of Newcastle, NSW, Australia

Alexander O Shpakov, Kira V Derkach, Oksana V Chistyakova, Ivan B Sukhov, Valery N Shipilov and Vera M Bondareva
Sechenov Institute of Evolutionary Physiology and Biochemistry, Russian Academy of Sciences, Thorez av. 44, 194223 St. Petersburg, Russia

Index

www.ingramcontent.com/pod-product-compliance
Lightning Source LLC
Chambersburg PA
CBHW080508200326
41458CB00012B/4131